SARCOIDOSIS
AND OTHER
GRANULOMATOUS DISORDERS

SARCOIDOSIS
AND OTHER
GRANULOMATOUS DISORDERS

Proceedings of the XI World Congress on Sarcoidosis
and other Granulomatous Disorders, Milan,
6–11 September 1987

Editors:

CARLO GRASSI

Director, Institute for Respiratory Disease
Pavia University, Pavia, Italy

GIANFRANCO RIZZATO

Director, Sarcoidosis Clinic
Niguarda Hospital, Milan, Italy

ERNESTO POZZI

Director, Chair of Pulmonary Physiopathology
Turin University, Turin, Italy

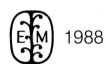 1988

EXCERPTA MEDICA, Amsterdam – New York – Oxford

International Congress Series No. 756
ISBN 0 444 80983 x

Published by:
Elsevier Science Publishers B.V.
(Biomedical Division)
P.O. Box 211
1000 AE Amsterdam
The Netherlands

Sole distributors for the USA and Canada:
Elsevier Science Publishing Company Inc.
52 Vanderbilt Avenue
New York, NY 10017
USA

Library of Congress Cataloging in Publication Data:

```
World Congress on Sarcoidosis and Other Granulomatous Disorders (11th
    : 1987 : Milan, Italy)
    Sarcoidosis and other granulomatous disorders : proceedings of the
XI World Congress on Sarcoidosis and Other Granulomatous Disorders,
Milan, 6-11 September 1987 / editors, Carlo Grassi, Gianfranco
Rizzato, Ernesto Pozzi.
       p.   cm. -- (International congress series ; no. 756)
    Includes indexes.
    ISBN 0-444-80983-X (U.S.)
    1. Sarcoidosis--Congresses.  2. Granuloma--Congresses.
I. Grassi, Carlo.  II. Rizzato, Gianfranco.  III. Pozzi, Ernesto.
IV. Title.  V. Series.
    [DNLM: 1. Granuloma--congresses.  2. Sarcoidosis--congresses.  W3
EX89 no. 756 / QZ 140 W927 1987s]
RC182.S14W67 1987
616--dc19
DNLM/DLC
for Library of Congress                                    88-7135
                                                               CIP
```

Printed in The Netherlands

INTRODUCTION

The traditional, triennial World Congress on Sarcoidosis gathers together scientists and clinicians involved in research on this 'fascinating' disease; fascinating, of course, for the problems it poses and for solutions which, from the point of view of etiopathogenesis and therapy, always seem to be within reach and yet are not. These Congresses, as is evident from the Proceedings, have delineated the steps of the evolution of research both in experimental and clinical fields. From a prevalence of histological studies, from rudimentary immunology and clinics we have progress to more sophisticated knowledge on the immunological, molecular, genetic mechanisms underlying the production of sarcoid granuloma. New technologies of course have had a great impact on the new achievements. The same can be said for the functional and clinical studies.

The etiopathogenetic, epidemiological and clinical aspects of this proteiform disease have been the object of lectures, papers and posters which have been grouped into eight sessions of the scientific program;
1. The sarcoid granuloma formation - immunology
2. Pathology (from granuloma to fibrosis)
3. Epidemiology
4. Clinical aspects of pulmonary and extrapulmonary sarcoidosis
5. Assessment of sarcoid activity
6. Functional impairment
7. Treatment
8. Other granulomatous disorders

There is no doubt that the most important development has been registered in immunology, where progress in the methods and in the recognition of function and significance of different sections of the immune system has led to the comprehension of some pathogenetic mechanisms regulating the granuloma formation. Moreover, these researches may open new possibilities for the definition of the stages of the diseases and, hopefully, for the therapeutic approach in the future.

The modern and sophisticated techniques of molecular biology, of which we have seen the first steps in some presentations, will offer a new dimension to the comprehension of the most subtle mechanisms at the basis of the cellular growth leading to the formation of granuloma and its perpetuation. From the possibility that the new technologies offer the possibility to combine information of immunologic and genetic origin at the molecular level, we expect a definitive answer to the intriguing problem of the etiology of sarcoidosis. However, the final goal has not been reached and this Congress once again proves that we do not surrender, but that we believe that our common efforts will succeed in achieving this goal. I should like to underline the necessity of combining the efforts of the experts in different fields in order to obtain fruitful and rewarding results in a faster way. Immunologists, molecular biologists, pharmacologists, radiologists, and clinicians should coordinate their efforts in order to avoid dispersing them.

This Congress always presents a good opportunity to exchange ideas in a friendly atmosphere. Infact the 'sarcoidologists' have become a sort of exclusive club; they vi

know each other. I must however add that just like members of many other clubs, they sometimes display oddness and adhere to their own ideas. The club nevertheless has greatly expanded during the years. By chance I found the photograph of the participants of the IV International Conference held in Paris in 1966 and I am pleased to see many of them here, a little older, but always faithful to sarcoidosis as witnesed by their presence.

To organize a World Congress is a heavy task and it would not have been possible for me to do so without the invaluable help of Professors Rizzato and Pozzi, who had to work very hard during the two years spent in organizing it. I am also very grateful to all the members of the scientific and organizing secretariat, who did their utmost for the success of the Congress.

Another point to be taken into account when a congress is being organized is its location: a beautiful town from the artistic or natural point of view presents the possibility to offer some diversions or recreations to the participants. It seems that Milan cannot compete with other famous Italian towns such as Rome, Florence, Venice; it is a busy town, foggy and cold in winter, hot and humid in summer with few artistic monuments. However, the Duomo, the Sforza Castle, the Last Supper in the Cloister of Santa Maria delle Grazie, some beautiful palazzi, represent some of the interesting landmarks. Its past is also full of important events for the history of Italy and Europe. I would like to recall the four periods of its maximum historical splendour: when it was one of the capitals of the Western Roman Empire (from the 4th to the 5th century); then from the 11th to the 13th century when the town formed itself as a free Common. In the 14th and 15th the town was the capital of the Duchy of Milan first under the Viscontis, and then under the Sforzas. At the beginning of the 19th century Milan became the capital of the Regno Italico (Italic Kingdom) under Napoleon and from that period it started its modern development. It was under the Viscontis and Sforzas that the town was enriched with its most famous monuments, the Duomo, the Castello Sforzesco, S. Maria delle Grazie, the Ospedale Maggiore, etc., and in that period Bramante and Leonardo da Vinci were active in the town.

Our Congress takes place in the buildings that were the Hospital (the Ospedale Maggiore) planned by Filarete at the order of Francesco Sforza in the 14th century and enlarged in the following centuries. It was commonly called the 'Ca' Granda' in the Milanese dialect to signify it was conceived as a house to be open to everybody, above all to the poor people. And now it is open to the free exchange of ideas and experiences as University and center of congresses and seminars in any field of science and culture.

Since olden times Milan has shown its business-minded talent. But besides business, Milan has also an artistic soul that has been made concrete in the great musical tradition, constantly handed on, from generation to generation in the Scala Theatre. There is more of course, but I limit myself to the ones already mentioned in my remarks at the opening ceremony hoping that these few facts about the historical and cultural background of this town will highlight the fame and the atmosphere in which the XI World Congress on Sarcoidosis has taken place.

Carlo Grassi
President of the
XI World Congress on Sarcoidosis

LIST OF PARTICIPANTS

ARGENTINA

Lebron, R.E.F. Les Americas Professional Center, Ave. Domenech 400 Suite 607, Hato Rey PR00918

AUSTRALIA

Alpers, J. Flinders Medical Centre, Adelaide, SA 5042
Basil, W.W. 141 Doncaster Avenue, Kensington, Sydney, NSW 2033
Lawson, J. 231 Macquarie Street, Sydney, NSW 2000

AUSTRIA

Braun, O.M. Paussauerplatz 4, 3424 Zeiselmauer
Klech, H. 2 Med. Department, Wilhelminenspital, Montlearstraße 37, 1171 Vienna
Vetter, N. Pulmologische Zentrum der Stadt Wien, Sanatoriumstraße 2, 1145 Vienna

BELGIUM

Macklem, P. Inst de Recherche Interdisc. sur la Biologie, Humana et Nucleare, Hopital Afrasma, Rue Laennec, 1070 Bruxelles
Pannier, R. Augustijnerei 7, 8000 Brugge
Sibille, Y. Cliniques Universitaires de Mont-Godinne, 5180 Yvoir

CANADA

Dales, R. Ottawa General Hospital Soi Smyth Ro, Ottawa, Ontario K1H 8L6
Grossman, R.F. Suite 427, Mount Sinai Hospital, 500 University Avenue, Toronto, Ontario M5G 1X5
Mannix, S. 3615 University Apt 5, Montreal H3A 2B3
Morse, J.L.C. Dept of Medicine, St. Joseph's Hospital, McMaster University, 50 Charlton Avenue East, Hamilton, Ontario L8N 4A6
Renzi, G. Notre-Dame Hospital, 1560 Sherbrooke Street, Est, Montreal, P.Q. H2L 4K8

CHINA

Zheng Yuanrang Guangzheu

CZECHOSLOVAKIA

Kolek, V. Kischova 3, Olomouc
Vitkova, E. Statni Ustav pro Kontrolu Leciv, Srobarova 48, post. prihr 87, 10041 Prague
Votava, V. 1st University Lung Clinic, Katerinska 19, 12800 Prague 2

DDR

Eckert, H. Hartriegelstrasse 45, 1197 Berlin
Eule, H. Wilhelm-Kulz Strasse 7a, 1406 Hohen Nevendorf, Birkenwerder 3779
Scharkoff, T. Pestalozzistrasse 07, 7500 Cottbus

DENMARK

Romer, F.K. Department of Medicine, Silkeborg Central Hospital, 8600 Silkeborg
Frederiksen, J. Bovang 42, 2660 Broendby Strand
Sorensen, P.G. Klovervenget 20 B 101, 5000 Odense

FINLAND

Elo, J.J. Huhtamaki oy Pharmaceuticals, P.O. Box 415, 20101 Turku
Gronhagen-Riska, C. IVth Department of Medicine, University of Helsinki, Unioninkatu 38, 00170 Helsinki
Karma, A. Suvantokatu 1B, 33100 Tampere
Koivunen, E. Hallituskatu 29 A 22, 33200 Tampere
Oksanen, V. Parkkimaentie 16/1, 13600 Hameenlinna
Sallinen V. Pl 3, 20501 Turku
Tiitinen, H. Kuikkarinne 20, 00200 Helsinki

FRANCE

Basset, F. 11 rue Alphonse de Neuville, 75017 Paris
Chinet, T. INSERM U 214, Hôpital Laennec, 42 rue de Sevres, 75007 Paris
Chretien, J. Hôpital Laennec, 42 rue de Sevres, 75007 Paris
Delaval, P. 34 Clos Sevigne, 35510 Cesson
Dugas, M. Dept de Pneumologie, Hôpital Calmette, Bld du Pr. J. Laclerc, 59037 Lille
Fortin, F. Dept de Pneumologie, Hôpital Calmette, Bld du Pr. J. Laclerc, 59037 Lille
Harf, R. Centre Hospitalier Lyon Sud, Service du Pr Perrin Fayolle, 69310 Pierre Benite
Kerbourc'h, J.F. Service Courcous C.H.R.U., B.P. 824, 29285 Brest Cedex
Leguern, G. Hôpital Laennec, 42 rue de Sevres, 75007 Paris
Maffre, J. Service de Pneumologie, C.H.R. Angers, 49033 Angers Cedex
Mordelet, M. Hôpital Laennec, 42 rue de Sevres, 75007 Paris
Pacheco, Y. Centre Hospitalier Lyon Sud, 69310 Pierre Benite
Perrin-Fayolle, M. 21 Cours F. Roosevelt, 69006 Lyon
Takiya, C. Institut Pasteur, 77 rue Pasteur, 69365 Lyon
Vergnon, J.M. Hôpital Nord, Dept de Pneumologie, Av. Albert Raimond, 42277 St Priest en Jarez Cedex
Voisin, C. Cl Pneumo Ptisiologique Hôpital Calmette, Bld du Pr. J. Laclerc, 59037 Lille

GREECE

Angomachalelis, N. University of Thessaloniki, 19,25th Martiou Avenue, 546 45 Thessaloniki
Giotaki, E. Akadhnias 4, 453 32 Joannina
Hourzamanis, A. Nicplastira 73 Kalamaria, 551 32 Thessaloniki
Papadopoulus S. 40 Parashon Street, 114 74 Athens
Scotti F. Trelessinas 25, 154 52 Athens
Veslemes M. 19 Riga Ferraiou Street, Chalandri, 152 32 Athens

INDIA

Bambery, P. Department of Internal Medicine, P.G.I.M.E.R., 160012 Calcutta
Dutta, S.K. No 2 Ram Chandra Das Row, 700013 Calcutta
Gupta, S.K. Flat No 15, 105, Park Street, 16 70016 Calcutta

IRAN

Amoli, K. 1 Safrang Lane Enghelanb Ave, nr Ferdowsi Square, Tehran 11318

IRELAND

Fitzgerald, M. St Vincent's Hospital, Dublin 4
O'Connor, C.M. Department of Medicine, University College Dublin, "Woodview" Belfield, Dublin 4
Pratt, I. Department of Pharmacology, University College, Dublin 4
Ward, K. St Vincent's Hospital, Elm Park, Dublin 4

ISRAEL

Bruderman, I. Chest Department, Meir Hospital, 44281 Kfar Saba
Fireman, E. Institute of Pulmonary and Allergic Disease, Tel Aviv Medical Center,
6 Weizman Street, 67239 Tel Aviv
Toplisky M. 40 Tagor Street, Tel Aviv

ITALY

Agati, G. Via Torrione 32/C, 89100 Reggio Calabria
Agostini, C. Via Fusinato 55/1, 35100 Padova
Aiolfi, S. Divisione Pneumologica Ospedale Civile, 26013 Crema -CR
Albano, A. Largo Montebello 35, 10100 Torino
Albera, C. Osp. S. Luigi Gonzaga, Regione Gonzole, 10, 10043 Orbassano -TO
Alessandrini, A. Ospedale G Cantu' 20081 Abbiategrasso -MI
Allegra, L. Via Gian Galeazzo 3, 20100 Milano
Amaducci, S. Ospedale San Carlo, Via Pio II 3, 20153 Milano
Azzolini, L. Via Lago di Bolsena 8, 41012 Carpi
Babolini, G. Via Regina Elena 165, 98100 Messina
Baldi, F. Via Ventimiglia 108, 10100 Torino
Barbolini, G. Ist Anatomia Universita', Via Berengario 4, 41100 Modena
Bariffi, F. Univ degli studi Fac Medicina e Chirurgia, Cl Tisiologica, Via
Bianchi, 80131 Napoli
Baritussio, A. Ist Med Int Patologia Medica 1a Univ Padova, Via Giustiniani 2,
35100 Padova
Baroni, M. Via del Tago, 12, 20161 Milano
Belli, F. Via Luigi Biolchini, 21, 00145 Roma
Bernasconi, A. Via Molino di Sotto 2, 21050 Clivio -VA
Bertini, L. Via Togliatti, 5, 58022 Follonica -GR
Bertoletti, R. Istituto Forlanini, Via Taramelli, 5, 27100 Pavia
Berton, G. Istituto di Patologia Generale, Strada le Grazie, 37134 Verona
Beulche, G. Ospedale San Carlo, Via Pio II 3, 20156 Milano
Beverelli, B. Istituto Forlanini, Via Taramelli 5, 27100 Pavia
Bianco, S. Via dei Tufi 1, 53100 Siena
Biondi, A. Via Imbriani 60, 50019 Sesto Fiorentino -FI
Bisetti, A. 1° Cl. Tisiopneumologica Univ. di Roma, Osp. Carlo Forlanini
(Monteverde Nuovo), 00151 Roma
Blasi, A. Corso Europa, 9, 80127 Napoli
Boari. L. c/o Sig. Ferrari Giancarlo, Via Mantovana 89, 37137 Verona
Bocceri, M.G. Via S Margherita del Gruagno, 45, 33100 Udine
Bracco, I. Via Po 14, 10034 Chivasso -TO
Brenna, M. Via Plinio 25, 22036 Erba -CO
Capecchi, V. Via Cavazzoni 25, 40139 Bologna
Carratu', L. Via Salita Scudillo,20, 80136 Napoli
Carriero, G. Ist Tisiologia e Malattie App Respiratorio, Via Tufi 1, 53100 Siena
Castrignano, L. Via Famagosta 28, 20142 Milano
Catena, E. Istituto di Cl Tisiologica e Malattie App Respiratorio, Ospedale
Monaldi, 80100 Napoli
Cattivelli, M. Via Monti di Pietralata 268, 00157 Roma
Cavone, E. Via Pagano 28, 70123 Bari
Cazzola, M. P.le Tecchio 49, 80125 Napoli
Ceresatto, P. Via Monache 14, 34170 Gorizia
Chilosi, M. Anatomia Patologica Universita' Verona, 37100 Verona
Cipriani, A. Divisione Pneumologica - Ospedale Civile, 35100 Padova
Cocco, G. XXXI Div di Pneumologia e Allergologia Resp, Osp Cardarelli, Via
Cardarelli 9, 80131 Napoli
Codecasa, A. Via Arzaga 30, 20100 Milano
Collodoro, A. c/o Massobrio, Via Vecchie Fornaci 10, 17028 Spotorno -SV-
Comi, F. Via Varaita 4, 10100 Torino
Consigli, G. Via Abba 12, 43100 Parma
Conti, A. Via Chiantigiana 65, 50012 Bagno A Ripoli -FI-
Cremoncini, M. V. Le Famagosta 28, 20142 Milano

Crimi, N. CL Tisiologica Malattie Resp Univ, Osp Tomaselli, Via Passo Gravina 187, 95125 Catania
Curti, P. Ospedale e. Morelli, Via Zubiani 33, 23039 Sondalo
Daddi, G. Via Barberini 36, 00187 Roma
Dadduzio, F. C. So Vittorio Emanuele 224, 70051 Barletta
Dantes, M. Reparto Medicina Ospedale San Carlo, Via Pio II 3, 20153 Milano
De Felice, C. c/o Ist de Angeli Spa, Via Serio 15, 20139 Milano
Delli Veneri, F. Via Monte Donzelli 48/B, 80128 Napoli
Di Filippo, A. Via Giotto 43, 81100 Caserta
Di Pisa, G. Ospedale Generale Climatico Regionale, 23035 Sondalo -SO-
Di Stefano, A. Via Leopardi 10, 23035 Sondalo -SO-
Dondi, A. Ospedale G Cantu', 20081 Abbiategrasso -MI-
Donghi, M. c/o Sig. Bianchi Massimo, Viale M. Masia 37, 22100 Como
Fabbri, L. Ist Med dl Lavoro Universita' degli Studi, Via Jacopo Facciolati 71, 35127 Padova
Fabbri, M. c/o Dir Marketing Recordati SpA, Via Civitali 1, 20148 Milano
Fanti, O. c/o Ist de Angeli SpA, Via Serio 15, 20139 Milano
Fantini F. P.zza Arnoldo Mondadori 2, 20122 Milano
Fazzi P. Istituto di Fisiologia Cl CNR, Via Savi 8, 56100 Pisa
Ferrara, G. Via dei Tufi 1, 53100 Siena
Ferretti G. c/o Emiliano Locatelli, Via Aldo Moro7, 27058 Voghera
Festi, G. Via Bomporti 3, 35100 Padova
Finotto, S. Via Poerio 14/4, 35137 Padova
Fiora, G. Via Trento, 13051 Biella -VC-
Foresti, V. Via Kennedy 32, 20097 S Donato Milanese -MI-
Frigerio, L. c/o Pagliari Gabriella, Via della Brianza 8, 00161 Roma
Genghini, M. Ospedale Generale Regionale, Via Zubiani 33, 23039 Sondalo
Giagnoni, E. Servizio Cardiologia C.P.A., Viale Zara 81, 20159 Milano
Ginesu, F. Via Principessa Jolanda 16, 07100 Sassari
Giobbi, A. C.P.A., Via Le Zara 81, 20159 Milano
Gioia, V. Via Principe Villafranca 32, 90141 Palermo
Girbino, G. Via Chiesa dei Marinari 12, 98100 Messina
Giuliano, V. Ospedale Maggiore, 28100 Novara
Giura, R. Ospedale Sant'Anna, Via Napoleone 60, 22100 Camerlata -CO-
Gramiccioni, R. Via Casaletto 671, Villino G, 00151 Roma
Grassi, C. Via Frua 19, 20146 Milano
Grechi, A. Ospedale Legnano, Fisiopatologia Resiratoria (Med. 1^), 20025 Legnano -MI-
Iacono, G. Ospedale Sacco Pao 3, Via GB Grassi 74, 20157 Milano
Ignazi, P. Via Molino Vecchio 31, 40026 Imola
La Monica, G. Via Redipuglia 8, 90144 Palermo
Leonarduzzi, B. Casella Postale 356, 20100 Milano
Leproux G.B. c/o Ist de Angeli SpA, Via Serio 15, 20139 Milano
Libertucci, D. Corso Tessoni 79/3, 10100 Torino
Lizzi, G. c/o Ist de Angeli SpA, Via Serio 15, 20139 Milano
Lo Cicero, G. Ospedale Niguarda, Piazza Ospedale Maggiore 3, 20165 Milano
Lombardo, G. Via V.E. Orlando 55, 98028 S.Teresa Riva -ME-
Longhini, E. Ospedale di Sesto S. Giovanni, Corso Matteotti, 20099 Sesto San Giovanni -MI-
Lucchesi, M. Via Tor Fiorenza 38, 00199 Roma
Luisetti, M. Istituto Forlanini, Via Taramelli 5, 27100 Pavia
Luppis, B. Istituto di Fisiologia Clinica, 56100 Pisa
Lusuardi, M. Centro Medico di Riabilitazione, 28010 Veruno -NO-
Maggi, L. Via Carducci 368, 24100 Bergamo
Mantero, O. Via Lamarmora 6, 20100 Milano
Marangio, E. Osp Prov Spec G Rasori Pneumologico, Vle G Rasori 10, 43100 Parma
Marazzini, L. Ospedale di Sesto San Giovanni, Corso Matteotti, 20099 Sesto San Giovanni -MI-
Marcatili, S. Ist; di Clinical Tisiologica e Malattie App Respiratorio, Ospedale Monaldi, 80100 Napoli
Marsico, S. Via Schiavi 18, 88100 Catanzaro
Massaglia, G.M. Via Bianze' 8, 10148 Torino

Massei, V. Via Zara 1, 60123 Ancona
Mastaglio, C. Via Stelvio 97, Delebio- Sondrio
Mastrangeli, A. 1°Cl Tisipneumologia Universita di Roma, Osp Carlo Forlanini (Monteverde Nuovo), 00151 Roma
Matteucci, S. Via Paolo Sabi 151, 55049 Viareggio -LU-
Melillo, G. XXXI Div di Pneumologia e Allergologia Resp, Ospedale Cardarelli, Via Cardarelli 9, 80131 Napoli
Messi, G. Via Manzoni 2, 22100 Como
Migliaccio, A. c/o Locatelli Emiliano, Via Aldo Moro 7, 27058 Voghera
Minore G. Ospedale M. Malpighi, Via Palagi, 9, 40138 Bologna
Mistretta, A. Cl Tisiologica Malattie Resp Universita', Osp Tomaselli, Via Passo Gravina 187, 95125 Catania
Montemurro, L. Via Mac Mahon 73, 20155 Milano
Nava, A.M. C.P.A., Via Marconi 22, 25124 Brescia
Nunziati, F. Ospedale Forlanini, Via Portuense 332, 00100 Roma
Olivieri, D. Clinica Pneumologica, Ospedale Rasori, 43100 Parma
Ossi, E. Via S Mattia 18, 25100 Padova
Palla, A. Ist di Fisiologia Clinica CNR, 56100 Pisa
Paruccio, P. Via Bolognese 247, 50139 Firenze
Pazardjiklian, M. Policlinico Div Litta, Via F Sforza 35, 20123 Milano
Pellati, R. c/o Ist de Angeli SpA, Via Serio 15, 20139 Milano
Pescetti, G. Via R Gessi 18, 10100 Torino
Pezza, A. Corso Vittorio Emanuele 697, 80122 Napoli
Pozzi, E. Via Volta 25, 27100 Pavia
Prandi, E. Via A Veneri 20, 42100 Reggio Emilia
Prediletto, R. Ist Fisiologia Cl CNR, Via Savi 8, 56100 Pisa
Puccini, G. Via Gramsci 731, Firenze
Rantzer, G. Ospedale Maggiore, Piazza Ospedale Maggiore 3, 20100 Milano
Rimoldi, G. Ospedale di Circolo, Via Luigi Borri 57, 21100 Varese
Rizzato, G. Via Juvara 9, 20100 Milano
Rossi, A. Via Mincio 20, 27100 Pavia
Rossi, G.A. Via Costa Scioa' 3, 16100 Genova
Rottoli, P. Ist di Tiosologia dell'Universita', Via dei Tufi 1, 53100 Siena
Sabbioni, E. Div Radiochimica Centro Comune di Richerch, 21027 Ispra -VA-
Sada, E. Via Cadorna, 22100 Como
Salvaterra, A. Via Zara 17, 38066 Riva Del Garda -TN-
Sanduzzi, A. Via Aniello Falcone 56, 80127 Napoli
Sanguinetti, C. Divisione di Pneumologia, Ospedale Regionale di Torrette, 60020 Ancona
Savoia, G. Via Marchese di Villabianca 70, 90143 Palermo
Sbressa, S. Ospedale Niguarda, Piazza Ospedale Maggiore 3, 20162 Milano
Scaglione, R. Via Lombardia 9, 90144 Palermo
Scagliotti, G. Via Madama Cristina 15, 10100 Torino
Scevola, M. Via Tommaseo 25, 30035 Mirano -VE-
Sciaraffa, A. Via IV Novembre 15, 28038 Domodossola -MO-
Scolari, N. Via Oslavia 15, 20099 Sesto S Giovanni MI
Semenzato, G. Via Nazareth 2, 35128 Padova
Sergi, M. Ospedale L Sacco, Via G.B. Grassi 74, 20100 Milano
Sivieri, G. Via Paolo Sabi 151, 55049 Viareggio -LU-
Siviero, F. Via Cereria 32, Bassano del Grappa -VC-
Sofia, M. Istituto Clinica Tisiologica, Ospedale Monaldi, Via L Bianchi, 80131 Napoli
Spatafora, M. Ist Fisiopatologia Resp Consiglio Nazionle Richerche, Via Trabucco 180, 90146 Palermo
Spina, G. Viale Buozzi 99, 00197 Roma
Spinelli, F. Ospedale Niguarda, Pizza Osp Maggiore 3, 20100 Milano
Stanziola, A. c/o Camillo Corvi SpA, Marchesini, Viale dei Mille 3, 29100 Piacenza
Tassi, G. Ospedale Civile, Reparto Pneumologia, 25047 Darfo -BS-
Tommasini, A. Via Ongarello 10, 35100 Padova
Tosi, G. c/o Camillo Corvi SpA, Viale dei Mille, 3, 29100 Piacenza
Trentin, L. Clinica Medica 1, Via Giustiniani, 2, 35100 Padova
Vagliasindi, M. Via Martino Cilestri 41, 95129 Catania

Valenti, S. Clinica Tisiologica Osp Marigliano, Via SS Mosso 8, 16132 Genova
Velluti, G. Istituto Tisiologia - Policlinico, Via del Pozzo 71, 41100 Modena
Vignali, F. Via Masotto 23, 20100 Milano
Villa, R. Via IV Novembre 55, 24100 Bergamo
Zambello, R. Ist di Medicina Clinica Universita', Via Giustiniani 2, 35100 Padova
Zaurino, M. Via Primaticcio 32, 20100 Milano

JAPAN

Arai, I. Dept. Pathology, Faculty of Medicine, Kyoto Univiversiy, Konoe-cyo Yoshida
Sakyo-Ku, 606 Kyoto.
Chikazawa, C. Saishunso Hospital National Sanatorium, Suya 2639 Nishgoshi-machi
Kikuchi-Gun, Kumamoto 86111
Eishi, Y. Dept. of Pathology, Tokyo Medical & Dental University, 1-chome, Yushima,
Bunkyo-ku, Tokyo 113
Fujii, K. 3262, Sekigahara-cho, Fuwa-Gun, Gifu-Pref. 503-15 Fuwa-Gun, Gifu-Pref.
Fujimura, N. Red Cross Hospital, 1-1-1 Abuno Takatsuki 569, Osaka
Gemma, H. The Second Dept. of Internal Medicine, Hamamatsu University School of
Medicine, 3600 Handa-cho, Hamamatsu 431-31
Hongo, O. Dermatology Dept. Tokyo Metropolitan, Komagome Hospital -3-18-22
Hngomagome Bunkyo-ku, Tokyo 113
Hosoda, Y. Radiation Effects Research Foundation, 5-2 Hijiyama Park Minami-Ward,
Hiroshima 732
Ikeda, S. Misumi Hospital National Sanatorium, Hata 1 775 Misumi Machi Uto Gun,
Kumamoto 86932
Ina, Y. Second Dept. of Internal Medicine, Nagoya City University Medical School,
Kawasumi, Mizuho, Nagoya 467
Izumi, T. Chest Disease Research Institute, Kyoto University, Sakyo, Kyoto 606
Kitaichi, M. Chest Disease Research Inst., Kyoto University, Sakyo, 606 Kyoto
Kiyoshi, S. 1-1-60, Koto, 862 Kumamoto
Kusama, S. Internal Med. School of Medicine Shinshu Univ, Asahi 3-1-1, 390
Matsumoto
Masayoshi, S. 51-2 Sturugamatz, Nara
Masayuki, A. 1st Dept. Internal Medicine Kumamoto University Medical School, 1-1-1
Honjo, 860 Kumamoto
Matsui, Y. 4-1-22, Hiroo, Shibuya-ku, Japanase Red Cross Medical Center, 150 Tokyo
Mikami, R. National Sagamihara Hospital 18-1 Sakuradai, 228 Sagamihara
Mochizuki, I. Shinshu University School of Allied Med. Science, Asahi 3-1-1,
Matsumoto 390
Morishita, M. 3-41, Ohno-machi, Tokoname-shi, Aichi-ken 479
Nagai, S. Chest Disease Research Institute, Kyoto University, Sakyo, Kyoto 606
Nakashima, H. First Department of Medicine, Kumamoto University Medical School,
1-1-1 Honjo Kumamoto 860
Nishimura, K. Chest Disease Research Institute, Kyoto University, Sakyo, Kyoto 606
Nishimura, M. Dept. of Dermatology, Medical Institute of Bioregulation, Kyushu
University, Tsurumibaru 4546, 874 Beppu
Noda, M. Second Dept. of Internal Medicine, Nagoya City University Medical School,
Kawasumi, Mizuho-ku, 467 Nagoya
Osamu, A. 1-3-6 Higashicho Kichijoji Musashinoshi, 180 Tokyo
Oshima, S. Chest Disease Research Institute, Kyoto University, Sakyo, 606 Kyoto
Sato, A. 3600, Handa-cho, 431-31 Hamamatsu
Shigematsu, N. 3-1-1 Maidashi Higashiku, 812 Fukuoka
Shinnosuke, F. Komagome 1-7-6, Toshima-ku, 170 Tokyo
Sugimoto, M. First Department of Internal Medicine, Kumamoto University Medical
School, 1-1-1 Honjo, Kumamoto 860
Takahara, T. 3-51-6 Wakamiya Nakano-ku, 165 Tokyo
Takemura, T. 1-7-14, Koenjikita, Suginami-ku, Tokyo 166
Tamura, S. Kanto Teishin Hospital, 22 9 5 Higashigotanda Shinagawa-ku, 141 Tokyo
Tanimoto, H. Nakano-ku Saginomya 6-31-21, Tokyo
Tawaraya, K. 1-7-1-608 Aoyama Niigata-shi Niigata-ken, 950-21 Niigata
Yagawa, K. Kyushu University Medical School Dept of Resp Disease, 812 Fukuoka
Yamaguchi, M. 1 044 Domiiru Gobanchou 12-7 Gobanchou, Chiyoda Ku, 102 Tokyo

Yamamoto, M. 2nd Dpt. Internal Medicine, Nagoya City University Medical School, 1-Kawasumi, Mizuho-cho, Mizuho-ku, Nagoya 467

JORDAN

Abandhe, I. P.O. Box 777, Irbid
Haj, H.A.R. Amman 2030
Samara, N. Jordan University Hospital, 922613 Amman

NETHERLANDS

Alberts, C. De Bosporus 34, 1183 GJ Amstelveen
Beumer, H.M. Longarts, Militair Hospitaal Dr. A. Mathijsen, Postbus 90.000, 3509 AA Utrecht
Durkstra, S. Jekerstraat 114, 1078 MJ Amsterdam
Hoogsteden, H. Breitnerstraat 61B, 3015 XB Rotterdam
Rothova, A. Academic Medical Centre Dept. Ophthalmology, Meibergdreef 9, 1005 AZ Amsterdam
Van Maarseeveen, T. Pathology, Academic Hospital Free University, De Boelelaan 1117, 1081 HV Amsterdam
Van Weeldem, B. Groenhovenweg 411, 2803 DK Gouda
Withaar, A. Jekerstraat 114, 1078 MJ Amsterdam

NORWAY

Bjornstad Pettersen, H. Arne Garborgs Veg 45E, 7000 Trondheim

PORTUGAL

De Avila, R. Dept. de Pneumologia Hopital Pulido Valente, A La Meda Dal Linas de Torres 117, 1700 Lisboa
Freitas E Costa, M. Clinica de Doencas Pulmonares - Fac. De Med. de Lisboa -1699 Lisboa Codex
Monteiro, J.T. Clinica de Doencas Pulmonares Faculdade Med., Av Prof. Egas Moniz, 1699 Lisboa
Teles De Araujo, A. Clinica de Doencas Pulmonares F.M.L., Av. Prof. Egas Moniz, 1699 Lisboa

SOUTH AFRICA

Rossouw, D.J., Dept. of Pathology Univ Stellenbosch, Med. School PO Box 63N, Tygerberg 7505
Suzman Moses, M. 101 Tower Hill Kotze Street Hillbrow, 2001 Johannesburg

SPAIN

Badrinas Vancells, F. Hospital de Bellvitge Princeps de Espanya, L'Hospitalet, 08907 Barcelona
Morera Prat, J. Aussias March 113 4° 1a, 08013 Barcelona
Rose, Laboratorios Castejon S.A., Appartado de Correos 14 602, 28080 Madrid

SWEDEN

Andersson, B. Goteborgs Univ Avdelningen For Klinisk, Immunology, Guldhedsgatan 10, 413 46 Goteborg
Andersson, L. Salviagatan 63 4TR, 424 40 Angered
Blanking, S. Torevagen 6, 352 51 Vaxio
Blaschke, E. Dept. of Clinical Chemistry, Karolinska Hosp., 104 01 Stockholm
Bradvik, I. Sofiaparken 5 C, 222 41 Lund
Eklund, A. Dept. of Thoracic Medicine, Karolinska Hosp., 104 01 Stockholm
Engstrom, C.P. Islandsvagen 19, 161 54 Bvomma Stockholm

Harngren, A. Dept. of Thoracic Medicine, Karolinska Sjukhuset, 104 01 Stockholm
Hernbrand, R. Dept. of Clinical Chemistry, Karolinska Hosp. 104 01 Stockholm
Ripe, E. Dept. of Pulmonary Medicine, Huddinge University Hospital, 141 86 Huddinge
Schmekel, B. AB Draco, Box 34, 221 00 Lund
Selroos, O. AB Draco, Box 34, 221 00 Lund
Sternby, E. AB Draco, Box 34, 221 00 Lund

SWITZERLAND

Herzog, H. Bethesda Spital, Gellerstrasse 144, 4052 Basel
Noelpp, B. Boehringer Ingelheim GmbH, Peter-Marian Strasse 19/21, CH 4002 Basel

THAILAND

Bovornkitti, S. Dept. of Medicine, Siriraj Hospital, Bangkok 10700

UNITED KINGDOM

Davies, B., Asthma Research Unit, Sully Hospital, CF6 2YA South Glamorgan
Fleming, H.A. Cardiac Unit, Papworth Hospital, Papworth Everard, Cambridge CB3 8RE
Foley, N. Medical Unit - The Middlesex Hospital, Mortimer Street, London W1N 8AA
James, D.G. Royal Northern Hospital, Holloway Road, London N7 6LD
Jones, K. Asthma Research Unit, Sully Hospital, Sully South Glamorgan
Jones-Williams, W. Pathology Dept. Llandough Hospital, Penarth South Glamorgan CF6
  1XX, Cardiff
Mier, A. 42, Heathfield Road, London W3
Reynolds, S. Asthma Research Unit, Sully Hospital, South Glamorgan
Sherlock, S. Royal Free Hospital, Pond Street - Hampstead, London NW3 2QG
Siltzbach Hansi-Bohm, S. 39 Ordnance Hill, 6PS London NW8
Solias, R. Royal Northern Hospital, Holloway Road, N7 6LD London
Studdy, P. 76 Grosvenor Road, N10 2DS London
Turner-Warwick, M. Cardiothoracic Institute, Brompton Hospital, Fulham Road,
  London SW3

U.S.A.

Albrecht, G. 7311 S.W. 62nd Avenue Suite 202, South Miami FL 33143
Alvarez, J. 260 Lakeland, Grosse Pointe, MI 48230
Andrews, J.L. 17 Dorset Road, Newton-Waban MA 02168
Auerbach, R. Lab of Developmental Biology University of Wisconsin, Madison WI 53705
Baughman, R.P. Pulmonary Disease Division Mail Location 564, 231 Bethesda Avenue,
  Cincinnati, OH 45267
Castriotta, R.J. Pulmonary Diseases Mount Sinai Hospital, 500 Blue Hills Avenue,
  Hartford, CT 06112
Chang Jui, C. Bronx VA Medical Center-Pul., 130 West Kingsbridge Road, Bronx, NY
  10468
Colp, C. 301 East 79 St., New York, NY 10021
Crystal, G.R. National Institute of Health, Bethesda, MD 20205
De Remee, R. 200 1st St. S.W., Rochester, MM 55905
Della Rocca, A. 4002 E. Montebello, Phoenix, AZ 85018
Douglas, W.W. 200 First Street SW, Rochester MN 55905
Du Bois, R. Building 10 Room 6D 12 N.I.H., Bethesda, MD 20892
Du Brow, E. 13000 N. 103 Avenue 99, Sun City, AZ 85351
Epstein, W. Dermatology University of California, San Francisco CA 94143-0536
Foster, S. 243 Charles Street, Boston MA 02114
Fukuyama, K. Dermatology University of California, San Francisco CA 94143-0536
Graham, D.Y. V.A. Medical Center, 2002 Holcombe Blvd, Houston, Texas 77211
Hackney Jr R.L. Howard University Hospital Pulmonary Division, 2041 Georgia Avenue,
  N.W., Washington, DC 20060
Hewlett, R. 320 Superior, Suite 310, Newport Beach, CA

Holter, J.F. Dept. of Medicine- Pulmonary, E.C.U. School of Medicine, Greenville, NC 27858

Israel, H.L. Thomas Jefferson University, 1025 Walnut Street, Room 804, Philadelphia, PA 19107

Johns-Johnson, C. Johns Hopkins University, 720 Rutland Avenue, Baltimore MD 21205

Karetzky, M. 201 Lyons Ave, Newark, NJ 07112

Kataria, S. East Carolina University School of Medicine Dept. of Pediatrics - Greenville, NC 27858-4354

Kataria, Y.P. East Carolina Univ. School of Med. Pulm. Div., Greenville, NC 27858-4354

Katz, S. Georgetown University Hospital, Washington DC 20007

Kleinhenz, M.E. Dept. of Medicine University Hospital of Cleveland, 2074 Abington Road, Cleveland, OH

Langer, B. 777 N Michigan, Chicago IL 60611

Latimer, R. 24 Portland Pl, Montclair NJ 07042

Lawrence, E.C. 6535 Eannin F 907, Houston, TX 77030

Lieberman, J. Veterans Administration Medical Center, 16111 Plummer St., Sepulveda, CA 91343

Lopez-Majano, V. Cook County Hospital, 1825 W. Harrison Street, Chicago IL 60612

Lower, E. Univ. of Cincinnati Medical Center Hematology, Oncology Div. 231 Bethesda Avenue, Cincinnati, OH 45267-4233

Lundborg, R. 66 Makakai Place, Hilo, HI 96720

Markeisch, D. VA Medical Center (111D), 2002 Holcombe Blvd. Room 612, Houston, TX 77030

Markham, T. Brush Wellman Inc., 1200 Hanna Building, Cleveland, OH 44115

McLean, R. 2736 Waldorf Circle, Winston Salem, NC 27106

Millard, M. 7400 SW 62 Ave South Miami Hospital, 331 South Miami, FL

Miller, A. Mount Sinai Hospital, Box 1232, New York NY 10029

Mishra, B.B. 4427 Wickford Road, Baltimore MD 21210

Mootz, A. 9519 Robin Meaclow Dr, Dallas, TX 75243

Newman, L. National Jewish Center for Immunology and Resp. Med., 1400 Jackson St., Denver CO 80206

Patrick, H. Jefferson Medical College, 1025 Walnut Street, Philadelphia PA 19107

Pavesi, M. 88 McGregor Street, Suite 202, Manchester NH 03102

Phan Sem H. Dept. of Pathology-Box 0602 Univ. Michigan Medical School 1500 E. Medical Center Drive, Ann Arbor, MI 48109-0602

Pincelli, C. Department of Dermatology, University of California, San Francisco CA 94143-0536

Reynolds, H. Pulmonary Section Dept. of Internal Medicine, Yale University School of Medicine 105 LCI, PO Box 333, New Haven, CT

Robbins, R. Pulmonary Med Univ of Nebraska Medical Center, 42nd and Dewey Avenue, Omaha, NE 68105

Rockoff, S.D. G. Washington University Medical Center, 901 23rd St Nw, Washington DC 20037

Rohrbach, M. Thoracic Disease Research Unit, Rochester MN 55905

Saltini, C. NIH Bldg 10 Rm 6D18, Bethesda MD 20025

Sharma O.P. 717 Domingo Drive, San Gabriel CA 91775

Sider, L. Northwestern Memorial Hospital, 710 N. Fairbanks Ct., Chicago IL 60611

Staton, G.W.J. The Crawford W. Long Memorial Hospital, 35 Linden Avenue, N.E., Atlanta GA 30365

Stewart, G.L. Internal Medicine Associates, 2841 Debarr Road 50, Anchorage, AK 99508

Stone, D. 41 Abington Ave, Ardsley, NY 10502

Sulavik, S. P.O. Box 191, 4 West Mountain Road, Canton Center CT 06020

Teirstein, A.S. Pulmonary Division The Mount Sinai Medical Center - One Gustave Levy Place, New York, NY 10029

Weissler, J. 5323 Harry Hines, Blvd - Pulmonary Division, Dallas, TX 75235-9034

Wilder, N. 2841 Debarr Road 50, Anchorage, AK 99508

WEST-GERMANY

Barth, J. I Medizinsche Universitatsklinik, Schittenhelmstr. 12, D-2300 Kiel

Buhl, R. Lerchesbergring 86, D 6000 Frankfurt 70
Costabel, U. Abt. Pneumologie, Med. Univ. Klinik, D-7800 Freiburg
Jasch, K.D. Holostein Str. 18 E, Wiesbaden D 6200
Jungbluth, H. Klinik Seltersberg Gaffkys Tr. 9, Giessen D 6300
Kreipe, H. Hopitalstr. 42, Institute Fur Pathologie, 2300 Kiel
Meier-Sydow, J. Z. Der Innere Medizin der Johan Goethe Univ., Abt. fur Pneumologie
    Theodor Stern Kaj 7, 6000 Frankfurt Am Meim
Nolle, B. 1 Med. Department University of Kiel, Schittenstrasse 12, D 2300 Kiel
Petermann, W. I Medizinische Universitatsklinik, Schittenhelmstr, 12, D-2300 Kiel
Rennch, H. C/o Karl Thomre GmbH, Abteilung Medizin, Biberbach An der Riss
Rust, M. Abt. Pneumologie Zim Klinikum JW Goethe Univ., D 6000 Frankfurt
Sprenger, H. Boehringer Ingelheim Zentrale GmbH, Medical Department, 6507 Ingelheim
    An Rhein
Wegener, F. Nibelungenstrasse 141, D 2400 Luebeck 1

YUGOSLAVIA

Djuric, O. Institute For Pulmonary Diseases and TBC, Ul Visegradska 26 - 11000
    Belgrade
Djuric', B. Institut ZA Plucne Bolesti, 21204 Sremska Kamenica, Novi Sad
Stern, S. 1st. Za Pljucne Bolzei, Golnik

CONTENTS

INVITED LECTURES

The many faces of sarcoidosis
  D.G. James   1
The Kveim Siltzbach test in 1987
  A.S. Teirstein and L.K. Brown   7
Death from sarcoid heart disease. United Kingdom series 1971–1986.
300 cases with 138 deaths
  H.A. Fleming   19
Biological characteristics and significance of subclinical inflammatory
alveolitis in extrathoracic granulomatous disorders
  C. Voisin, B. Wallaert, M. Dugas, P. Bonniere, A. Cortot, J.B. Martinot
  and Y. Sibille   35
Wegener's granulomatosis, new concepts of classification and treatment
  R.A. DeRemee   51
The liver–lung interface
  S. Sherlock   59

THE SARCOID GRANULOMA FORMATION — IMMUNOLOGY

The sarcoid granuloma formation — Immunology. State of the art
  G. Semenzato   73
Detection of IL-1B in bronchoalveolar lavage fluids from sarcoid patients
by RIA
  C. O'Connor, A. VanBreda, K. Ward, C. Odlum and M.X. Fitzgerald   89
Interleukin-2 dysregulation in circulating mononuclear cells of patients
with active sarcoidosis
  J.L. Johnson and M.E. Kleinhenz   97
Prednisolone treatment and alveolar lymphocyte–macrophage
cooperation in sarcoidosis
  T. van Maarsseveen, H. Mullink, M. de Haan, J. Stam and J. de Groot   101
The relationship between BAL immunocytology and clinical indices in
sarcoidosis
  G.M. Ainslie, R.M. Dubois and L.W. Poulter   105
Alveolar macrophages recovered from the lung of patients with active
sarcoidosis display a monocyte–like phenotype and the property to
release Type IV collagenase
  C. Agostini, S. Garbisa, R. Zambello, A. Cipriani, A. Negro,
  M. Masciarelli, M. Luca and G. Semenzato   109
Phenotyping of alveolar macrophage subpopulations in pulmonary
sarcoidosis. Relation to intracellular interleukin-1 production
  H. Klech, C. Neuchrist, W. Pohl, E. Schenk, C. Sorg, W. Knapp,
  Th. Luger, O. Scheiner and D. Kraft   115
Regulation of neutrophil mobility by alveolar macrophages from patients
with sarcoidosis
  Y. Sibille, W.W. Merrill, S.B. Care, G.P. Naegel, J.A.D. Cooper Jr and
  H.Y. Reynolds   123

The effect of angiotensin II (A-II) on the accessory function of BALF
macrophages – A possible autostimulatory mechanism of T lymphocyte
alveolitis in sarcoidosis
    S. Nagai, T. Izumi, M. Takeuchi, K. Watanabe and S. Oshima   129
Mast cells in sarcoidosis
    P. Rottoli, L. Rottoli, M.G. Perari, C. Vindigni, A. Collodoro,
    M. Cintorino and S. Bianco   135
Cutaneous granulomata in response to injection with autologous
bronchoalveolar lavage cell preparations in sarcoidosis patients
    J.F. Holter, Y.P. Kataria and H.K. Park   139
Pathogenesis of granuloma formation in lymph nodes with sarcoidosis
    Y. Eishi, T. Takemura, Y. Matsui and S. Hatakeyama   143
Antigen presenting capacity in sarcoidosis
    Y. Ina, S. Sado, M. Yamamoto, K. Takada, M. Morishita, M. Asai,
    K. Arakawa and M. Noda   147
In-vitro sarcoid granulomas – Differences between active and inactive
disease
    B.B. Mishra, S.M. Phillips, H. Patrick and H. Israel   151
Monocytes derived multinucleated giant cells: Immunophenotype and
functional analysis
    H. Kreipe, H.J. Radzun, P. Rudolph, J. Barth, K. Heidorn,
    W. Petermann and M.R. Parwaresch   155
Decreased phosphatidylethanolamine methyltransferase (PMT) activity in
T lymphocytes in sarcoidosis: An indicator of T cell immaturity
    Y. Pacheco, F. Gormand, P. Fonlupt, M. Dubois, M. Perrin-Fayolle
    and H. Pacheco   157
Isolation of cell wall–defective acid–fast bacteria from skin lesions of
patients with sarcoidosis
    D.Y. Graham, D.C. Markesich, D.C. Kalter and H.H. Yoshimura   161
Immune–response of peripheral T lymphocytes to SCW antigen and
circulating immune complexes levels as prognostic factors in patients
with active sarcoidosis
    K. Yagawa, S. Hayashi, N. Kamikawaji, K. Ogata, K. Matsuba and
    N. Shigematsu   165
Anergy: A correlate of granulomatous inflammation in sarcoidosis
    M.E. Kleinhenz   169
Autologous mixed lymphocyte reactions probe macrophage function in
sarcoidosis
    M. Spiteri and L.W. Poulter   173
Ocular manifestations of sarcoidosis preceeding systemic manifestation
    C.S. Foster   177
Characterization of alveolar macrophages from sarcoidosis patients
using different monoclonal antibodies of the Ki-series
    J. Barth, W. Petermann, P. Entzian, H. Kreipe, H.J. Radzun and
    M.R. Parwaresch   183
Correlation between PGE_2 production and suppressor cell activity of
alveolar macrophages in interstitial lung diseases
    E. Fireman, S.B. Efraim, J. Greif, A. Alguetti, D. Ayalon and
    M. Topilsky   185

A genotypic and phenotypic analysis of T cells proliferating in the lung of patients with active sarcoidosis
  R. Zambello, L. Trentin, G. Casorati, F. Siviero, M. Masciarelli, A. Tommasini and C. Agostini   187

Suppression of local immunoglobulin production in active pulmonary sarcoidosis by oral prednisone therapy
  M. Spatafora, A. Mirabella, A. Bonanno, L. Riccobono, A. Merendino, V. Bellia and G. Bonsignore   191

Outlook
  T. Izumi   193

PANEL DISCUSSION
THE CELLULAR ORIGIN OF SACE AND THE VARIOUS FACTORS IN REGULATING ITS PRODUCTION

The cellular origin of angiotensin converting enzyme (ACE) and the various factors regulating its production (Introduction to a panel discussion)
  R.A. DeRemee   201

ACE in physiologic and pathologic conditions
  C. Grönhagen-Riska, V. Koivisto, H. Riska, E. von Willebrand and F. Fyhrquist   203

Angiotensin converting enzyme inducing factor (AIF): A potential mediator of the increased angiotensin converting enzyme levels in sarcoidosis
  M.S. Rohrbach, U. Specks, Z. Vuk-Pavlovic and A.K. Conrad   213

Comparison of an intrinsic serum–ACE inhibitor to captorpril and enalapril in man
  J. Lieberman, A. Sastre and F. Zakria   221

SACE related to other markers, as clinical perspective
  Ph. Delaval, B. Desrues, P. Bourguet, C. Pencole and J.P. L'Huillier   227

PATHOLOGY FROM GRANULOMA TO FIBROSIS

Sarcoidosis – From granuloma formation to fibrosis. State of the art
  F. Basset, P. Soler and A.J. Hance   235

Isolation and preparation of acellular granuloma (sarcoid matrical complex, SMC)
  C. Takiya, A. Calle, L.E. Cardoso, S. Peyrol, J.-F. Cordier and J.-A. Grimaud   247

Immunohistochemical analysis of sarcoid granulomas: Evidence of proliferating lymphocytes and presence of cells with cytoplasmic interleukin-1 (IL-1)
  M. Chilosi, P. Capelli, M. Lestani, L. Montagna, G. Pizzolo, A. Cipriani, C. Agostini, L. Trentin, R. Zambello and G. Semenzato   255

Fibronectin (FN) in sarcoidosis: Evaluation of plasma levels and distribution in lung tissue
  C. Albera, L. Viberti, B. Bartone, P. Ghio, F. Bardessono, G. Scagliotti, F. Gozzelino, L. Pescetti and G. Pescetti   259

Generation of superoxide anion by alveolar macrophages in sarcoidosis
  M.A. Cassatella, G. Berton, C. Agostini, R. Zambello, L. Trentin,
  A. Cipriani and G. Semenzato   263
Effects of muramyldipeptide and indomethacin on schistosome
egg–induced granulomatous inflammation in the lung
  S.H. Phan and S.L. Kunkel   267
Relationship between markers of macrophage and fibroblast activity in
bronchoalveolar lavage fluid in sarcoidosis
  E. Blaschke, A. Eklund, R. Hällgren, R. Hernbrand and Å Hanngren   271
Pathology from granuloma to fibrosis. Outlook
  A. Blasi   273

EPIDEMIOLOGY

Epidemiology of sarcoidosis. State of the art
  Y. Hosoda   279
Familial sarcoidosis: Clinical, immunologic, and genetic features of an
unusual variant
  J.L. Andrews Jr, T.C. Campbell, R.E. Rocklin and M.R. Garovoy   291
Antibodies to TWAR – a novel type of chlamydia – in sarcoidosis
  C. Grönhagen-Riska, P. Saikku, H. Riska, B. Fröseth and
  J.T. Grayston   297
Retrospection of an unique mode to obtain complete epidemiological
data in sarcoidosis
  T. Scharkoff   303
Results of the 1984 nationwide prevalence survey in Japan
  Y. Hosoda, M. Odaka, M. Yamaguchi, Y. Hiraga, T. Izumi,
  T. Tachibana and K. Aoki   307
Statistics of sarcoidosis autopsies during these 26 years in Japan
  K. Iwai, T. Tachibana, Y. Hosoda and Y. Matsui   309
Sarcoidosis in North India: An emerging clinical spectrum
  P. Bambery, D. Behera, A. Gupta, U. Kaur, S.K. Jindal, S. Sehgal,
  S.K. Malik and S.D. Deodhar   311
Sarcoidosis deaths – The Howard University Hospital experience
1975–1987
  R.L. Hackney Jr, R.C. Young Jr, O.D. Polk Jr and E.M. Armstrong   313
Smoking does not affect prevalence or short term functional outcome of
sarcoidosis in Ireland
  K. Ward and M.X. Fitzgerald   315
Sarcoidosis in Barcelona: Spring cluster of Löfgren syndrome
  F. Badrinas, J. Morera, J. Mañá, E. Fité, J. Valverde, R. Vidal and
  J. Ruiz-Manzano   317
Sarcoidosis and tuberculosis of lymph nodes: An epidemiological study
of 25 years
  K. Gourgoulianis, A. Stefis, S. Gougoulakis, F. Scotti and
  V. Tsakraklides   319
Ocular sarcoidosis in the Netherlands
  A. Rothova, C. Alberts, A. Kijlstra, E. Glasius and A.C. Breebaart   321
Final results of 15-years follow-up study of 168 sarcoid patients
  B. Djurić, N. Žafran and D.J. Považan   323

A continuation of the worldwide study on sarcoidosis
 *B. Djurić, A.G. Khomenko, M. Mayer, G. Rizzato, O. Schweiger,
 R. Christ and N. Sečen*   325
Sarcoidosis and cancer: A prospective study
 F.K. Rømer   327
Epidemiology of sarcoidosis. Outlook
 M. Freitas e Costa   329

FUNCTIONAL IMPAIRMENT

Functional impairment in sarcoidosis. State of the art
 O.P. Sharma   341
The spectrum of airways obstruction in sarcoidosis
 A. Miller, A.S. Teirstein, M. Pilipski and L.K. Brown   351
Bronchial hyperreactivity in sarcoidosis
 K. Shima, S. Takenaka, K. Fukuda and K. Teramoto   355
The effect of corticosteroid therapy on the breathing pattern in interstitial
lung disease (ILD)
 P.M. Renzi and G.D. Renzi   361
Respiratory clearance of 99Tc-DTPA and granuloma surface area in rat
lung granulomatosis induced by complete Freund adjuvant
 *M. Mordelet-Dambrine, G. Stanislas-Leguern, D. Henzel, L. Barritault,
 J. Chretien and G. Huchon*   367
Sarcoidosis, bronchial reactivity and BAL
 *A. Collodoro, A. Ferrara, P. Rottoli, L. Rottoli, A. Sturman,
 M.G. Pieroni, M. Refini, N. Chilaris, A. Perrella and S. Bianco*   369
Impaired airway function in sarcoidosis Stage II
 W. Petermann, J. Barth, P. Entzian and S. Hoppe-Seyler   371
Ventilation–perfusion relationships in pulmonary sarcoidosis
 *Z. Zwijnenburg, C. Alberts, C.M. Roos, H.M. Jansen and
 H.R. Marcuse*   373
Multiple inert gas elimination technique in interstitial lung disease:
Analysis of ventilation–perfusion relationships
 *R. Prediletto, B. Formichi, G. Viegi, E. Fornai, E. Begiomini,
 A. Santolicandro and C. Giuntini*   375
Radiological pulmonary changes in sarcoidosis: A modification of
international staging system
 S.K. Gupta and S.K. Sharma   377
Comparison of new CSF, neurophysiological and neuroradiological
studies in neurosarcoidosis
 V. Oksanen   381
Retroperitoneal involvement in sarcoidosis
 L. Castrignano, G. Fasolini, M. Nozza and A. Schieppati   383
Conclusive summarizing remarks and outlook
 H. Herzog   385

CLINICAL ASPECTS OF PULMONARY SARCOIDOSIS

Sarcoidosis: Clinical aspects. State of the art
  S.K. Gupta   397
Elevated serum levels of soluble interleukin-2 receptor is characteristic
of but not specific for active pulmonary sarcoidosis
  E.C. Lawrence, V.A. Holland, M.B. Berger, K.P. Brousseau,
  R.J. Wallace Jr, L.E. Mallette, C.E. Kurman and D.L. Nelson   407
Sarcoidosis and trace metals as investigated by neutron activation
analysis
  R. Pietra, J. Edel, E. Sabbioni and G. Rizzato   411
The course and management of 53 patients with hemoptysis in sar-
coidosis
  C.J. Johns, S.A. Schonfeld and P.P. Scott   417
Factors which adversely affect the course of sarcoidosis: An analysis of
111 autopsied cases of sarcoidosis
  O.P. Sharma and E. Klatt   421
Smoking causes an alteration of BALF cell findings in patients with BHL
sarcoidosis but no evidence could be found that smoking affects the
natural course of BHL sarcoidosis
  T. Izumi, S. Nagai, M. Kitaichi and S. Oshima   423
Value of bronchoalveolar lavage lymphocyte subpopulations for the
diagnosis of sarcoidosis
  U. Costabel, A. Zaiss, D.J. Wagner, R. Baur, K.H. Rühle and
  H. Matthys   429
Early neutrophil alveolitis in Lofgren syndrome
  J.Ph. Maffre, E. Tuchais, M.F. Chretien and M. Oury   433
Analysis of unusual thoracic manifestations of sarcoidosis: A review of
radiographic features
  S.D. Rockoff and P. Rohatgi   437
Pulmonary sarcoidosis in the elderly: Incidence and roentgenographic,
physiologic, bronchoalveolar lavage, and scintigraphic characteristics
  C.M. Sanguinetti, B. Balbi, F. Vassallo, C. Albera, S. Gasparini,
  P. Ghio and G.A. Rossi   441
CT versus radiography in sarcoidosis
  L. Sider and E.S. Horton Jr   445
Adverse effect of chronic tonsillitis on regression of bilateral hilar
lymphadenopathy in sarcoidosis
  T. Ikeda, H. Kotoh, K. Watanabe and N. Shigematsu   447
High resolution computed tomography in sarcoidosis
  G. Stanislas-Leguern, J. Frija, P. Morel, A. Hirsch, M. Laval-Jeantet
  and J. Chretien   449
Transbronchial lung biopsy in the diagnosis of sarcoidosis
  A. Cipriani, G. di Vittorio, G. Festi and A. Tommasini   451
Clinical findings and bronchoscopic abnormalities in sarcoidosis
  C. Melissinos, M. Veslemes, D. Bouros, D. Zarifis, M. Zahariadis and
  J. Jordanoglou   453
Recent pulmonary sarcoidosis mimicking idiopathic pulmonary fibrosis
  F. Bart, C. Delerive and V. Massart   455

Lymphocyte karyotypes in pulmonary sarcoidosis
    Y. Pacheco, C. Charrin, G. Cozon, F. Gormand, M. Perrin-Fayolle and
    D. Germain   457
Clinical risk assessment in sarcoidosis. Outlook
    H. Klech   461

CLINICAL ASPECTS OF EXTRAPULMONARY SARCOIDOSIS

Synovial sarcoidosis in children. Report of six cases
    F. Fantini, V. Gerloni, M. Murelli, M. Gattinara, A. Negro and
    T. Sciascia   485
On the existence of microangiopathy in sarcoidosis
    R. Mikami, M. Sekiguchi, Y. Ryujin, F. Kobayashi, Y. Hiraga,
    Y. Shimada, I. Mochizuki and S. Tamura   489
Ophthalmic changes in sarcoidosis: A prospective study of 308 patients
    M.R. Angi, F. Forattini, A. Cipriani, P. Capelli and G. Semenzato   493
Phosphocalcic metabolism, bone quantitative histomorphometry and
clinical activity in 10 cases of sarcoidosis
    J.M. Vergnon, D. Chappard, D. Mounier, A. Emonot and
    C. Alexandre   499
Diagnostic significance of two-dimensional echocardiography in sarcoid
infiltrative cardiomyopathy
    N. Angomachalelis and A. Hourzamanis   503
Vectorcardiography versus echocardiography in the diagnosis of silent
myocardial involvement in sarcoidosis
    E. Giagnoni, L. Beretta and A. Sachero   505
Evaluation of lung T-cell subsets in uveitis patients with normal chest
roentgenograms
    M. Sugimoto, M. Ando, H. Nakashima, H. Kohrogi and S. Araki   509
Longitudinal study of ocular sarcoidosis
    A. Karma   511
Angiotensin–converting enzyme levels in tears and sera: Potential
predictor of ocular sequela in North Carolina Afro-Americans
    P.S. Ellison Jr and J.C. Merritt   513
Fine needle aspiration biopsy in granulomatous diseases
    J.J. Elo, H. Joensuu and P.J. Klemi   515
A combinatorial analysis of ^{67}Ga scanning of the head and thorax in the
diagnosis of sarcoidosis – The Panda sign
    S.B. Sulavik, D. Weed, R. Spencer, H. Shapiro and R. Castriotta   517
Gallium 67 scintigraphy in the localization of sarcoidosis
    V. Lopez-Majano, P. Muthuswamy and G. Renzi   519
Methodology for Gallium 67 scintigraphy in sarcoidosis
    P. Sansi, V. Lopez-Majano and P. Muthuswamy   521

ASSESSMENT OF SARCOID ACTIVITY

Assessment of sarcoid activity. State of the art
    J. Chretien   525

Magnetic resonance imaging in sarcoidosis
B.G. Langer, V. Lopez-Majano, R. Rhee and D.G. Spigos 541
Long-term follow up of Ga^{67} scans and BAL lymphocytes in untreated
sarcoid patients. A worldwide study from 9 centres in 7 different
countries
G. Rizzato, C. Alberts, F. Badrinas, A. Cipriani, P. Delaval,
M. Granata, T. Izumi, M. Perrin-Fayolle, P. Rohatgi and T. Sharkoff 545
Mast cell-derived mediators in pulmonary sarcoidosis
A. Miadonna, A. Pesci, A. Tedeschi, E. Leggieri, G. Bertorelli,
M. Froldi, D. Olivieri and C. Zanussi 557
Elevation of serum Type III procollagen N-terminal peptide levels in
thoracic sarcoidosis: A possible index for fibroblast activity
M. Luisetti, C. Aprile, L. Bacchella, V. de Rose, V. Peona and E. Pozzi 563
The clinical application of bronchoalveolar T-cell subsets in the follow-up
of pulmonary sarcoidosis
M.G. Perari, G. Carriero, P. Rottoli, L. Rottoli, A. Collodoro, G. Coviello
and S. Bianco 567
Gallium-67 lung scan in the evaluation of pulmonary sarcoidosis
R. Scaglione, G. Parrinello, G. Capuana and G. Licata 571
Urinary neopterin for assessing the follow-up of pulmonary sarcoidosis
J. Lacronique, B.M. Traore, A. Auzeby, P. Soler, Y. Touitou and
J. Marsac 575
Prognostic assessment of BAL and Gallium 67 scan in sarcoidosis less
than 2 years after the onset
M. Yamamoto, M. Noda, Y. Hosoda, Y. Hiraga, T. Izumi,
T. Tachibana, K. Shima and A. Sato 579
Increased procoagulant activity of bronchoalveolar lavage cells in
patients with sarcoidosis: Relationship steroid treatment, forced vital
capacity, gallium uptake, and bronchoalveolar lavage percent
lymphocytes
R. Perez, G. Staton, M. Kidd and I. Check 581
Bronchoalveolar lavage in patients with erythema nodosum
K. Ward, C. Odlum, C. O'Connor, A. van Breda and M.X. Fitzgerald 585
The role of broncho–alveolar lavage in predicting the outcome of
pulmonary sarcoidosis
N.M. Foley, K. Tung, A.P. Coral, D.G. James and N.Mcl. Johnson 587
Circulating monocytes from patients with sarcoidosis express cell
surface laminin
M. Nishimura, T. Koga, K. Matsuba and N. Shigematsu 589
Assessment of disease activity in pulmonary sarcoidosis: A
clinico–pathological correlation
D.J. Rossouw, J.R. Joubert and C.C. Chase 591
Spontaneous secretion of hydrogen peroxide by alveolar macrophages
of patients with sarcoidosis
R.P. Baughman, S. Strohofer and E.E. Lower 593
Prognostic value of ACE, lysozyme and pulmonary lymphocytosis in
sarcoidosis: Results of multicentric prospective study
R. Harf, N. Biot, M.P. Fayolle and the EMMEANS Cooperative Study
Group 595

Marked elevation of serum angiotensin converting enzyme activity –
Clinical correlates
    H.L. Israel, H. Patrick, J.E. Gottlieb and R.M. Steiner   599
Angiotensin converting enzyme (ACE) inhibitors in sarcoidosis sera with
markedly elevated ACE activity
    H. Patrick, J.W. Gray, K.J. Shepley and H.L. Israel   601
Serum angiotensin–converting enzyme (SACE) activity as an indicator of
total body granuloma load and prognosis in sarcoidosis
    P.P. Muthuswamy, V. Lopez-Majano, M. Ranginwala and
    W.D. Trainor   603
Activity assessment and treatment decisions. Outlook
    H.L. Israel, J.E. Gottlieb, H. Patrick and R.M. Steiner   605

TREATMENT

Treatment of pulmonary sarcoidosis. State of the art
    M. Turner-Warwick   621
Reducing osteoporosis in chronic long-term steroid therapy: Usefulness
of calcitonin
    G. Rizzato, G. Tosi, C. Mella, L. Montemurro, D. Zanni and S. Sisti   631
Further experiences with inhaled budesonide in the treatment of
pulmonary sarcoidosis
    O. Selroos   637
Corticosteroid therapy of pulmonary sarcoidosis (PS): Efficacy and
tolerability of deflazacort (DFZ) vs prednisone (PR)
    G. Velluti, O. Capelli, L. Azzolini, E. Prandi, A. Fontana,
    M.O. Guaglianone and C. Dragonetti   641
Steroid aerosols in systemic sarcoidosis in India
    S.K. Gupta   643
Sparing hospitalizations and steroids: The role of a sarcoidosis clinic in
Italy
    L. Montemurro, F. Durante, L. Castrignano and T. Loglisci   645
Therapeutic trial of pulmonary sarcoidosis with sulfathiazole: A possible
etiotropic treatment
    A. Giobbi, G. Martignoni and E. Miradoli   649
Effect of treatment of sarcoidosis in India
    S.K. Gupta, S.K. Dutta, K. Mitra and M. Roy   651
The orally active angiotensin–converting enzyme inhibitors in sarcoidosis
    S. Panayeas, A. Michalopoulos, C. Tsiroyiannis, A. Papapaschali,
    N. Siafakas and S. Papadopoulos   653
The treatment of sarcoidosis. Outlook
    R. Ávila   657

OTHER GRANULOMATOUS DISORDERS

Granulomas in the diagnosis of sarcoidosis. State of the art
    W. Jones Williams   661

A study into the effects of direct and indirect antigenic challenge on
bronchoalveolar lavage fluid findings in pigeon breeders disease
  S.P. Reynolds, E.D. Jones, K.P. Jones, J.H. Edwards and B.H. Davies   675
Environmental and immunologic studies on the causative agent of
summer-type hypersensitivity pneumonitis
  *M. Ando, K. Yoshida, T. Sakata, K. Soda, M. Sugimoto, M. Suga,
  H. Nakashima and S. Araki*   681
Abnormalities of lipid composition of bronchoalveolar lavage (BAL) in
respiratory diseases induced by dust inhalation (RDID)
  *A. Teles-de-Araújo, J.M. Reis-Ferreira, M. Freitas-e-Costa and
  J. Benveniste*   685
Beryllium skin disease
  W. Jones Williams, W.R. Williams, D. Kelland and P.J.A. Holt   689
Light and electron microscopy of experimental cutaneous granulomas in
mice treated with cyclosporine
  C. Pincelli, A. Fujioka, H. Suya, K. Fukuyama and W.L. Epstein   691
Association of pulmonary tuberculosis and Crohn's disease
  *G.M. Massaglia, A. Ardizzi, S. Barberis, F. Galietti, G.E. Giorgis,
  C. Miravalle and P.C. Giamesio*   695
The influence of anabolic steroids during the course of treatment for
tuberculosis
  *G.D. Renzi, P.M. Renzi, S. Sekely, V. Lopez Majano, P.J. Feustel and
  R.E. Dutton*   697
Studies on antigens and cellular components in bronchoalveolar lavage
fluid with hypersensitivity pneumonitis
  H. Gemma, A. Sato, K. Chida, M. Iwata and I. Shichi   703
Cytotoxic mechanisms in the lung of patients with hypersensitivity
pneumonitis
  L. Trentin, R. Zambello, G. Festi, R. Bizzotto, M. Luca and C. Agostini   705
Respiratory distress from mulitple stenosis of the tracheal and of the
bronchial tree during system vasculitis
  F. Fortin, F. Bart, J.M. Degreef, B. Gosselin and J.J. Lafitte   707
Pneumoconiosis caused by hard metals. A case series
  *G.M. Massaglia, G. Avolio, S. Barberis, M. Cacciabue, F. Galietti,
  G.E. Giorgis and C. Miravalle*   709
Characteristics of the lymphocytary alveolitis of sarcoidosis and mineral
dust inhalation induced pulmonary granulomatosis
  *A. Teles de Araújo, A.C. Mendes, J.T. Monteiro and
  M. Freitas e Costa*   711
Pulmonary injury from silica dust evaluated with broncho–alveolar
lavage (BAL)
  *M. Lusuardi, E.L. Spada, A. Capelli, A. Braghiroli, S. Zaccaria and
  C.F. Donner*   713
Antigen–specific T cells in a mouse model of beryllium disease
  L. Newman   715
Histology of granulomatous inflammation in nude rats lungs induced by
complete Freund's adjuvant (CFA)
  J. Chang, J. Jagirdar, T. Faraggiana and F. Paronetto   717
Other granulomatous diseases – How can they help understanding
sarcoidosis? Outlook
  H.Y. Reynolds   719

ROUND TABLE
DIFFUSE PANBRONCHIOLITIS

Introduction
  G. Rizzato   739
Pathology of diffuse panbronchiolitis from the view point of differential
diagnosis
  M. Kitaichi   741
Radiologic findings of patients with diffuse panbronchiolitis (DPB)
  K. Nishimura and H. Itoh   747
A nation-wide survey of diffuse panbronchiolitis in Japan and the high
incidence of diffuse panbronchiolitis seen in Japanese respiratory clinics
  T. Izumi   753
Diffuse pan bronchiolitis
  M. Turner-Warwick   759
Diffuse panbronchiolitis – How to place it into the framework of chronic
bronchiolitis in adults?
  J. Meier-Sydow   761

INDEX OF AUTHORS   765

SUBJECT INDEX   771

INVITED LECTURES

© 1988 Elsevier Science Publishers B.V. (Biomedical Division)
Sarcoidosis and other granulomatous disorders
C. Grassi, G. Rizzato, E. Pozzi, editors

THE MANY FACES OF SARCOIDOSIS

D GERAINT JAMES MA MD FRCP

ROYAL NORTHERN HOSPITAL

LONDON N7 6LD

INTRODUCTION

During the course of this World Congress, we shall be discussing nine
aspects of sarcoidosis in different symposia, and also probably many more
aspects during informal discussion. What questions and answers do we
anticipate from each of these sessions? I shall ask the question now
and I hope to receive the answers by the end of the Congress. These
answers will be the 1987 update, embodied in a prestigious Transactions of
the Xl World Congress on Sarcoidosis, which you are now reading.

1. IMMUNOLOGY

At about this time last year in Vienna, Ron Crystal brought us up-to
-date by reminding us that leu 3+ helper/inducer cells expressing DR
(HLA Class II) antigens are central to the pathogenesis of sarcoidosis.[1]
The sarcoid granuloma is a battlefield between invading antigen and the
cellular and humoral defences of the body. Such new techniques as
immunofluorescence, histochemistry, monoclonal antibodies and ELISA have
provided new insights in this immunologic battlefield for it is now
possible to identify the uniforms of the participating warriors. The
activated T helper lymphocyte releases interleukin-2 (IL2) in abundance.
The initiating signal for this exaggerated response has not yet been
recognised but it seems that local stimuli in the battlefield maintain
this exaggerated state of alert. The activation of the IL-2 gene is
compartmentalised, for lung T cells express IL2 m RNA transcripts but
peripheral blood T cells do not have this property. Soluble interleukin-
2 receptors have elevated levels in serum and bronchoalveolar lavage
fluid in active sarcoidosis.[2] But if IL2 is present in abundance, why is
there no dramatic response to treatment with cyclosporin?

2. PATHOLOGY

In about 10% of sarcoidosis patients the granulomas persist with the
development of extensive patchy fibrosis, mainly affecting the upper and
middle lobes. What are the steps from granuloma to fibrosis? The
alveolar macrophage hastens fibrogenesis via fibronectin and a
progression growth factor, both of which influence fibroblasts to cause

recruitment-attachment and to produce collagen type 1 fibrosis. Chemical
mediators maintain a continuous cascade to fan on this process. The
monocyte-macrophage lineage possess calcitriol receptors, promoting the
metamorphosis of cells and to granuloma formation.[3]

What are the best markers of this ongoing fibrosis? Is it electron
microscopy, histochemistry, humoral mediators, monoclonal antibodies, or
magnetic resonance, or a combination of all of them.

Another question is why the predominance of fibrosis in the lungs?
It is inconspicuous and infrequent in the liver and other organs. Is it
possible that a foreign-body giant cell reaction is the inciting nidus.
Under certain circumstances this initial foreign body reaction progresses
inexorably to granuloma formation and fibrosis. In the absence of
co-factors this accelerated response fizzles out harmlessly. This theory
is dictated by the like behaviour of the Kveim-Siltzbach test.

3. THE KVEIM-SILTZBACH TEST

The Kveim-Siltzbach skin test is no longer used as frequently for
three reasons. It is not commercially available so it is difficult to
obtain the antigen. Secondly, it takes a month for a result, and a month
in which systemic steroids must be avoided for this would suppress the
test. But the most important is that fibreoptic bronchoscopy provides
histological confirmation within a day or so. Nonetheless, it remains
most helpful in delineating sarcoidosis as a cause of uveitis, erythema
nodosum, hepatic granulomas, hilar adenopathy and hypercalciuria.

What remains of considerable academic interest is the way in which
it expresses granuloma formation so vividly. Serial biopsies of the
developing Kveim papule at two weeks displays a dense perivascular
infiltration of T4 and T8 lymphocytes and HLADR + dendritic cells. The
latter are RFD+ indicating their macrophage lineage. There is progressive
serial development to acid-phosphatase-positive epithelioid cells and to
true granuloma formation.[4,5]

The question surrounding this test is its longterm future. Many of us
are dedicated to its value in diagnosis and monitoring progress of the
disease. But for many it has an even greater academic future, for it
expresses the natural history of an evolving granuloma and of sarcoidosis
itself. What new techniques are there to study this phenomenon? Is it
just a favourable foreign-body reaction in a favourable terrain of
co-factors?

4. EPIDEMIOLOGY

Every World Congress on sarcoidosis gathers increasing snowball support because the disorder is now universally recognised.[4] There are, of course, areas of high and of low prevalence, or should we say that there are sophisticated communities where it is well-recognised and developing countries where it is still ill-recognised. When comparative studies are made in different parts of the world, the pattern of sarcoidosis is surprisingly similar.

It is hoped that the Milan Congress will expand the composite of figures of the prevalence already gathered from various previous conferences. (Table 1). Please help to update this information.

Table 1 PREVALENCE OF PULMONARY SARCOIDOSIS PER 100,000 OF POPULATION EXAMINED.

AREA	PREVALENCE
NEW YORK BLACKS	80
PUERTO RICANS	30
SWEDEN	55-64
URUGUAY	60
DENMARK	53
GERMANY	41
HUNGARY	40
EIRE	40
WEST BERLIN	30
UNITED KINGDOM	27
CAPE TOWN BLACKS	27
COLOUREDS	17
CAUCASIANS	6
NORWAY	26
NEW ZEALAND	6-24
CZECHOSLOVAKIA	23
HOLLAND	21
LONDON	19
SWITZERLAND	16
LEIPZIG	13
JAPAN	12
ITALY	11
YUGOSLOVIA	11
POLAND	10
NORTHERN IRELAND	10
FRANCE	10
CANADA	10
FINLAND	9.2
AUSTRALIA	9
SCOTLAND	8
ARGENTINA	1-5
SPAIN	3
ISRAEL	1.6
KOREA	1
BRAZIL	0.2
PORTUGAL	0.2
RUMANIA	120 (total)
TAIWAN	6 (total)

Ten years ago sarcoidosis was rare in India, but it is now increasingly recognised because it is being distinguished more easily from tuberculosis. It is hoped that other areas of the world can contribute in comparative studies in the way that India has already done. (Table 2).

Table 2

PERCENTAGE COMPARISON OF SARCOIDOSIS IN INDIA COMPARED WITH WORLDWIDE SERIES AND EASTERN EUROPE

FEATURE	INDIA	WORLDWIDE	EASTERN EUROPE
FEMALE	41	57	57
INTRATHORACIC INVOLVEMENT	98	87	96
SKIN LESIONS	20	26	16
OCULAR INVOLVEMENT	10	15	4
PAROTID INVOLVEMENT	7	4	1.5
NERVOUS SYSTEM	10	4	1
POSITIVE KVEIM TEST	89	78	73
NEGATIVE TUBERCULIN SKIN TEST	71	64	58
HYPERCALCAEMIA	47	11	12
HYPERGLOBULINAEMIA	44	44	44

Is sarcoidosis becoming more evident in the Chinese and Greeks in whom it is infrequently reported at present?

And finally the vexed problem of sarcoidosis in the West Indies. Is it recognised as often in their home countries as it is in those who came from the Caribbean to London, Paris and New York.[4]

5. CRITERIA OF ACTIVITY

We are inundated with numerous markers of activity - clinical bedside techniques including lung function and fluorescein angiography; biochemical markers; immunological changes; radioactive scanning; and magnetic resonance. Each of these has its advocates, but let us not spend the week arguing which is the better. We know that each and every one of these tests is nonspecific. Rather should we interpret the peculiar value of each test and what does it reflect from the functional standpoint. For instance, fluorescein angiography reveals leakage of dye due to retinal vasculitis in posterior uveitis. This is already well known. What of further progress by the Japanese on the use of this technique to define the bronchial circulation?

And what of new markers of activity, such as serum neopterin which bears a close relationship with lymphocytic alveolitis in active sarcoidosis? It seems that activated T lymphocytes produce gamma interferon which stimulates alveolar macrophages to release neopterin. Thus, it reflects activated cellular immunity. Is this also destined to be a nonspecific feature of pulmonary granulomatoses?

6. FUNCTIONAL IMPAIRMENT

In every World Congress on Sarcoidosis many papers are presented showing functional impairment of the respiratory tract. What about functional impairment of other organs? Corticosteroid therapy has changed the natural history of sarcoid uveitis. Patients no longer become blind due to ocular fibrosis and secondary cataract and glaucoma if recognised and treated early. Magnetic resonance may do the same for the brain and heart. Are we able to recognise renal involvement at an early reversible stage?

7. CLINICAL ASPECTS

When a new technique is introduced to medicine a new dimension is added to the picture of sarcoidosis. Fluorescein angiography provided a new view of posterior uveitis and magnetic resonance has unfolded otherwise latent myocardial sarcoidosis, spinal involvement and sarcoid basal meningitis. Immunofluorescence, histochemistry and monoclonal antibody techniques have clarified the sarcoid granuloma, and ELISA provides a novel method of assessing soluble interleukin-2 receptors and yet another marker of activity.

Hidden ill-defined clinical aspects carrying the highest mortality are the heart and brain. New torchlights are still needed to shed light on cardiac and neurosarcoidosis.

8. TREATMENT

Corticosteroid therapy is the mainstay of treatment around the world. It has radically changed the course of sarcoid uveitis and of abnormal calcium metabolism and has given symptomatic relief to most sufferers. Second-best alternatives include indomethacin, methotrexate, chloroquine and azathioprine.

What we wish to learn this week is the therapeutic role of cyclosporin in view of its immunological significance. We have found it to be disappointing for sarcoidosis although it is of considerable value in posterior uveitis due to Behcet's disease, in the field of transplantation, and of emerging value in many autoimmune disorders.

9. OTHER GRANULOMATOUS DISORDERS

All that glitters is not sarcoidosis for it has numerous mimics, due to infections and other causes of vasculitis. Even more important are the many overlap syndromes, which may lead us towards the cause of sarcoidosis.

How near is sarcoidosis to Crohn's disease and primary biliary cirrhosis now that it has been shown that lymphocytic alveolitis is very similar in all three granulomatous disorders?

How near is sarcoidosis to extrinsic allergic alveolitis (EAA or hypersensitivity pneumonitis). Their pathology is similar but at the site of invasion, the battlefield, there is a T helper excess in Sarcoidosis and a T suppressor excess in EAA. What is the explanation for this differing response?

REFERENCES

1. Crystal, R.G, Saltini, C, Moller, D, Supurzen, J, Muller-Querheim, J, Wewers, M.
    The lymphocyte and sarcoidosis
    Sarcoidosis 1986; 3: 112

2. Lawrence E.C, Burger M.B, Broussea K.P, et al.
    Elevated serum levels of soluble interleukin-2 receptors in active pulmonary sarcoidosis.
    Sarcoidosis 1987; 4: 25-27

3. Ohta M, Okabe T, Ozawa K et al
    In vitro formation of macrophage-epithelioid cells and multinucleated giant cells by 1 , 25-dihydroxyvitamin D3 from human circulating monocytes.
    Ann N.Y Acad. Sci. 1986; 465: 211-220

4. James D.G, Jones Williams, W
    Sarcoidosis and Other Granulomatous Disorders.
    Philadelphia: W B Saunders. 1985

5. Mishra, B.B, Poulter L.W, Janossy G, Sherlock S, James D.G.
    The Kveim-Siltzbach Granuloma: a model for sarcoid granuloma formation.
    Ann. N.Y Acad. Sci. 1986: 465: 164-175

THE KVEIM SILTZBACH TEST IN 1987

ALVIN S. TEIRSTEIN MD, LEE K. BROWN MD

Pulmonary Division, Mount Sinai Medical Center, Box 1232, New York, NY
10029 USA

Supported in part by The Catherine and Henry J. Gaisman Foundation

INTRODUCTION

As in the book of Genesis, it is customary to introduce a state of the
art review with a historical recapitulation starting with "In the beginning".
While devoutly proclaiming my debt and devotion to our forebearers, I intend
to omit the usual obeisance to the works of Kveim[1], Nickerson[2], Nelson[3],
Putkonen[4], James[5], Chase[6], and even Siltzbach[7] and concentrate
primarily on the Kveim-Siltzbach (K-S) test, as I view it in the last
quarter of 1987 - more than one-half century after Kveim's first report.

Unfortunately, at the outset, I must take a detour on the road to the
present in the hope that once, and for all time, the controversy concerning
the diagnostic specificity of the K-S test can be put to rest. Naively
assuming that all but a few well-known, respected, authorities agree that
the K-S test is a valid procedure for the diagnosis of sarcoidosis, I would
have preferred to omit discussion of the controversy which erupted more than
30 years ago. However, repeated questioning by colleagues, several recent
publications and unfortunate erroneous comments at national meetings, impel
me, once again, to review the controversy.

The K-S debate began in 1955 with the report of Israel and Sones of 14
positive tests in 33 patients with active tuberculosis[8]. In 1962 Daniel
and Schneider found false-positive reactions in 8 of 13 patients with
granulomatous diseases other than sarcoidosis; histoplasmosis, coccidiomyco-
sis and tuberculosis[9]. The controversy reached a crescendo from 1969
through 1972 with false-positive tests recorded in significant numbers of
patients with Crohn's disease by Karlish et al[10] and Mitchell et al[11],
false-positive reactions in diseases other than sarcoidosis in which hilar
adenopathy was prominent, such as infectious mononucleosis, tuberculosis,
and lymphoma by Israel and Goldstein[12] and in collagen vascular diseases
by Bringle[13]. Izumi obtained the most disturbing array of false-positive
K-S reactions in more than one-half of 135 patients who had a variety of
cancers, silicosis and in 13 of 29 normal subjects[14]. Thus, by 1972 the
K-S test was all but thoroughly discredited. It is probable that the task
of defense is much more difficult than that of prosecution. However, unlike
politicians and our colleagues in the legal profession, scientists have the

advantage of objective data and the results of years of investigation which can be marshalled at times of attack. Thus, Siltzbach with the staunch support of James, noted that a subsequent report by Israel revealed no positive K-S tests in patients with tuberculosis[15]. Similarly, the same pathologists who found false-positive K-S reactions in the study of patients with granulomatous diseases other than sarcoidosis, by Daniel and Schneider, found no false-positive tests in patients with non-sarcoidal diseases using a different validated K-S suspension[16]. In addition, using the same validated test material, no false-positive reactions were obtained in patients with collagen vascular diseases. Finally, we must all bow to Izumi[14], whose meticulous records yielded the clue that uncovered the production and world-wide distribution of faulty Commonwealth Serum Laboratories' (CSL) K-S suspensions. His data clearly demonstrated the epidemic of false-positive tests was due to lack of validation of the subsequent batches of test suspensions produced by the CSL Laboratories, after they had successfully produced and validated initial batches of test material. Only Mitchell's finding of false-positive K-S tests in a substantial number of patients with granulomatous bowel disease and adult celiac disease remains unexplained[11]. Multiple studies before, and since, and a new ongoing study at the Mount Sinai Medical Center, New York, the home of Crohn, have failed to yield significant numbers of false-positive K-S tests in patients with granulomatous bowel disease[17].

It is easy to produce K-S suspensions. A competent technician strictly adhering to the simple methodolgy outlined by Chase[6] will have no difficulty. However, the essence of acceptable K-S suspensions is validation and not production and rests in Israel's statement that "were the Kveim reaction truly a reliable test for demonstrating the presence or absence of sarcoidosis, its use would still be desirable"[18]. Reliability demands the ability to validate test suspensions. This can only be accomplished by testing the newly manufactured product, in tandem with previously validated material in patients with and without sarcoidosis[19]. For example, Table I shows that with a new team of investigators since Siltzbach's death, we have produced 10 batches of K-S test material and implanted test doses in 1,133 patients.

TABLE I

RESULTS OF KVEIM-SILTZBACH (K-S) TESTS IN 1133 PATIENTS SINCE 1981

	Total number	Positive K-S	(%)	Negative K-S	(%)
Sarcoidosis	849	671	79%	178	221%
Non-Sarcoid	284	1	0.004%	283	99%

849 had sarcoidosis and 284 had non-sarcoidal diseases or were normal.
In patients with sarcoidosis 671 (79%) were positive and only 1 of the 284
patients without sarcoidosis gave a false-positive reaction; results comparable to Siltzbach's. After the report of the international study conducted
by the International Committee on Sarcoidosis, the Third International
Congress suggested that validated K-S test material should yield no more
than 3% false-positive results[20]. Our experience strongly suggests that
this value is too high and that a false-positive rate of less than 3% is
readily attainable. Simply put, K-S suspensions which give a false-positive
result in a significant percentage of patients with diseases other than
sarcoidosis or in normals are not K-S suspensions. Instead of reporting a
plethora of false-positive tests, this faulty material should be discarded.

The following criteria for acceptable K-S material have been modified
from the report given at the Third International Congress of Sarcoidosis:

1. The K-S test should give a positive histologic result in at least
    60% of patients with sarcoidosis.

2. There should be no more than 1% false-positive results in patients
    without sarcoidosis or normals.

3. Clearly discernible noncaseating epitheliod granulomas with or
    without giant cells should be microscopically visible with hematoxy-
    lin and eosin staining.

4. All K-S test material must be validated by simultaneous comparison
    with a previously validated suspension in patients with and without
    sarcoidosis.

Strict adherence to these criteria will yield a valuable, risk-free, relatively
inexpensive diagnostic test - the only test available which is diagnostic of
sarcoidosis.

The issue of diagnostic specificity of the K-S test should be firmly
placed behind us. In 1987 we should be concentrating on possible roles for
the K-S test other than in diagnosis. I will concentrate on the following
two: 1) Is the K-S test an in-vivo model of the immunopathology and biochemical events that occur in sarcoidosis? 2) Can the K-S test tell us anything
about the etiology of sarcoidosis?

Kataria has shown an orderly progression from a subcutaneous lymphocytic
inflammatory infiltrate in 48 hours to a mature lymphoid graunuloma within
21 to 34 days of intracutaneous injections of K-S suspensions[21]. The infil-
trating lymphocytes are predominantly Leu-3A helper T-lymphocytes. Mishra,
et al have confirmed the presence of helper T4 positive lymphocytes throughout
the granulomatous reaction, surrounded by T8 positive suppressor lymphocytes[22].
Pierard, et al have suggested that the K-S reaction parallels the evolution

of the pulmonary lesions in sarcoidosis. In 80 patients with sarcoidosis
they found that the more exuberant K-S reactions occurred during the stage
of overt pulmonary granulomatous infiltration, while a more bland response
to the skin test was noted when the lungs exhibited chronic fibrotic disease[23].

Studies of leukocyte, lymphocyte and monocyte migration and monocyte
inhibition factor with validated K-S suspensions have yielded varying
results. Hardt and Wanstrup[24], Becker et al[25], and Goldstein et al[26]
have reported decreased migration of leukocytes in the presence of K-S
suspensions. Mandell et al noted diminished monocyte migration when incubated with K-S test material but noted no direct chemotactic activity and no
lymphocyte production[27]. On the other hand, Topilsky et al found no
enhancement of migration inhibition factor by lymphocytes from normals or
sarcoidal lymphocytes when exposed to K-S suspensions[28]. Izumi et al,
noted no increased incorporation of labelled thymidine by lymphocytes of
patients with active sarcoidosis when the cells were stimulated by K-S
fractions[29]. Horshmanheimo et al, found no K-S induced inhibition of
leukocyte migration or lymphocyte transformation in-vitro in 23 patients
with sarcoidosis[30]. However, Jones Williams, et al demonstrated the
presence of a guinea pig macrophage migration inhibition factor in 21 of 30
patients with sarcoidosis when the lymphocytes were stimulated in-vitro with
K-S material[31]. Favez and Leuenberger reported circulating antibodies to
K-S suspensions in more than 95% of patients with sarcoidosis and in only
8.6% of controls[32]. Studies of the effect of K-S suspensions on lymphocytes and macrophages obtained by bronchoalveolar lavage have been equally
inconclusive.

Not discouraged by these conflicting reports and utlizing validated
suspensions, several groups are proceeding with further studies of the
effect of K-S suspensions on the immunologic events occurring in sarcoidosis. Carpel and Bloom[33], at the Albert Einstein Medical Center in New
York, are studying the effect of K-S suspensions on immune effector cells
obtained at bronchoalveolar lavage and peripheral blood cells from patients
with sarcoidosis. In addition, they are performing T-cell cloning in an
attempt to establish T-cell lines that are specific for sarcoidosis.
They have already cloned T-cells from patients with tuberculosis and are
working arduously to compare the differences and similarities of these cells
with those obtained from patients with sarcoidosis.

At the Mount Sinai Medical Center in New York, Marom and Kalb are
proceeding with studies of the immunogenetics of sarcoidosis[34]. It is
known that immune reactivity is controlled by genes termed immunoresponse
(Ir) genes. These genes are located within the major histocompatibility

complex which codes for transplantation antigens. The product of Ir genes, immunoresponse associated or Ia molecules, are potent transplantation antigens. Ia molecules are not present on every nucleated cell in the body. Their expression is limited to B-lymphocytes, antigen presenting cells such as macrophages, and activated T-cells. It is clear that the expression of Ia molecules by antigen presenting cells determines whether or not antigens are appropriately seen by T-cell receptors. In other words, Ia molecules may exert their effect by influencing the way in which antigens are presented to T-cells.

Through the use of recombinant DNA technology, it has been possible to identify 3 Ir gene families in humans: the HLA-DR, the HLA-DQ and the HLA-DP gene families. Several groups of investigators have attempted to demonstrate a significant association between a specific Ir gene and clinical disorders. An association between a single HLA-DR serotype in a given disease has already been achieved. Given that there is a significant association between Ir genes and disease, the relevance of this finding remains to be explored. Marom and Kalb are studying the site specific immune responsiveness demonstrated in the lungs of patients with active sarcoidosis by examining the role of class II histocompatibility molecules: DR, DQ and DP and the immune regulatory cells on whose surface these molecules are expressed. They have extended previous observations by demonstrating an enhanced expression of DP antigen on the surface of macrophages obtained by bronchoalveolar lavage of patients with sarcoidosis. Utilizing K-S suspensions, the functional capacity of DP, DR and DQ in T-cell proliferate assays is under study. They plan to employ K-S suspensions in autologous T-cell response assays obtained from patients with positive K-S reactions. Their aim is to demonstrate disease specific responsiveness to this "antigen". In a similar in-vitro system, the role of so-called mucosal immunity in the lung of patients with sarcoidosis is being investigated. They are hypothesizing a role for respiratory epithelium as an alternate immune competent antigen presenting cell in an analagous fashion to epithelium immune responsiveness demonstrated in the gut of patients with Crohn's disease and the thyroid in patients with Graves' disease. Preliminary results demonstrate the presence of DR antigen on the surface of respiratory epithelial cells. Further studies are underway to examine the regulation of epithelial histocompatibility antigen expression as well as in-vitro T-cell proliferation responsiveness to epithelial cells in allogenic and K-S pulsed autologous systems. Through these studies they hope to obtain a model in which site specificity in sarcoidosis is determined by the central role of tissue elements in the lung as initiators of immune responsiveness. Finally, the same investigators have been studying the

effect of K-S suspensions on the production of Il-2 from leukocytes and granulomas obtained at bronchoscopic lavage and biopsy. Initial studies have
yielded a T-cell growth factor that could not be identified as Il-1 or Il-2.
This growth factor was elaborated only after treatment with K-S suspensions.

In addition to the cellular immunoresponse to K-S suspensions, new data
suggest that the K-S reaction also mimics the enzymatic and biochemical events
seen in the naturally occurring sarcoid granuloma. Silverstein et al have
shown that sarcoid tissue produces angiotensin converting enzyme (ACE)[35].
This is further supported by the demonstration of ACE in bronchoalveolar
lavage fluid obtained from patients with active sarcoidosis[36,37]. Selroos
has reported a battery of serum enzymes and other biochemical substances
including beta-2 microglobulin, ACE and Lysozyme which parallel the course
of sarcoidosis[38]. He has noted that serum beta-2 microglobulin is elevated
in patients with acute sarcoidosis and when relapses occur during the course
of the disease. On the other hand, serum ACE levels may be normal during
the most acute stages of the disease, for example, erythema nodosum, and
becomes elevated with increased mass of granulomas. Almenoff et al have
described another thermolysin metalloendopeptidase (TME) which complements
serum ACE in sarcoidosis[39]. While ACE was elevated in patients with active
disease and tended to become normal in the most chronic stages of sarcoidosis
and when patients were receiving adrenocorticosteroid medication, TME identified patients with chronic active sarcoidosis and did not appear to be affected
by the exhibition of adrenocorticosteroid therapy. We are currently engaged
in studies of the enzymes produced by the cells partaking in the positive
K-S granuloma[40]. We have performed preliminary studies on the skin of
normal patients, unaffected skin from sarcoidosis patients, naturally
occurring sarcoid skin lesions and positive K-S biopsy tissue (Table II).
TABLE II

PRELIMINARY RESULTS OF TISSUE ENZYMES IN SKIN OF NORMALS, NORMAL &
GRANULOMATOUS SKIN IN SARCOIDOSIS AND K-S GRANULOMAS PRINT 1.1/2 Lines AT 1

	ACE*	TME	CATHEPSIN-D	PROLINE ENDO-PEPTIDASE
NORMAL	18	22	201	34
SARCOID-NORMAL	72.8	108.5	382	111
SARCOID-GRANULOMA	473	452	1042	149
K-S GRANULOMA	334	550	1261	228

* All determinations in nm/mg/hr

Preliminary results show that there is an increase in TME, ACE, cathep-
sin-D and prolene endopeptidase when comparing normal skin from patients
with sarcoidosis with normal skin from subjects without disease. A much
more marked elevation was noted comparing the enzymes extracted from sarcoid
skin lesions and positive K-S granulomas with normal skin taken from sarcoidosis
patients and from normal volunteers. There was a four to five-fold increase
in all four enzymes in the granulomatous lesions when compared with non-granulomatous skin and normal skin. The enzyme levels of both granulomatous
tissues, naturally occurring and K-S reaction, were similar.

This overwhelming emphasis on the host response to the sarcoidosis
inciting agent or agents, would suggest that the reaction to the K-S
suspension, similar to the disease, lies with the host and not the elusive,
mysterious, active principal. Perhaps the K-S suspension is only a soup of
fragments from a sarcoid granuloma which are, in themselves, nonspecific
evoking the typical epitheliod granuloma only in patients whose disease
presents the ideal substrate, acquired and/or genetically endowed, necessary
to mount an immunologic response. In this hypothesis the role of the host
is paramount. In an attempt to address this question, a clinical study of
the approximately 20% of patients with sarcoidosis who failed to react to
K-S suspensions with a granulomatous response is of interest (Table III).
TABLE III

CLINICAL STATUS OF 63 PATIENTS WITH SARCOIDOSIS
AND NEGATIVE K-S TESTS

Disease ❭2 YRS	39	62%
Disease Waning	11	17%
Disease ❬2 YRS	8	13%
Indeterminate	5	8%

We reviewed the status of the last 63 patients with probable sarcoidosis
and a negative K-S test[41]. Of these 63, 39 had clinical evidence of
sarcoidosis, usually radiographic abnormalites, uveitis and/or cutaneous
lesions, for more than two years prior to the performance of the test.
Bronchoscopic biopsy, skin biopsy and/or scalene lymph node biopsy proved
the diagnosis of sarcoidosis in all of these patients. Of the remaining 24,
11 patients exhibited clearing of the radiographic abnormalities during the
four weeks that the K-S test was maturing and subsequently cleared their
disease completely without further diagnostic procedures. While it is
possible that these 11 had another disease, for our purposes we assume them
to have had sarcoidosis with negative K-S tests. Of the remaining 13

patients, 8 had evidence of disease of less than 2 years' duration by virtue
of conversion of a recent normal radiograph to a radiographic stage typical
of sarcoidosis, or recent onset of dyspnea, uveitis or sarcoid skin lesions.
In the final 5 patients with negative K-S tests and sarcoidosis, the onset
of the illness could not be accurately dated. Thus, 62% of the patients
with negative K-S tests had disease of more than 2 years' duration, a
finding in keeping with earlier studies which noted that repeated K-S tests
in the same patient yielded decreasing frequency of positive reactions with
time, the rate of positivity approaching only 50% in the same patients five
years after the initial positive K-S test[20,42]. 17% of the negative K-S
tests occurred in subjects who were recovering from their disease. In the
first instance, the data suggest that a positive K-S test occurs with
greatest frequency during the first two years of the disease in patients
whose illness is relatively fresh and florid. Indeed, the majority of these
39 patients with disease of greater than two years' duration at the time of
the K-S implantation had no clinical or laboratory evidence of active
sarcoidosis at the time that the K-S test was performed. Nevertheless,
tissue biopsies continued to reveal diagnostic granulomas. While it is true
that many of these specimens revealed hyalinization of the granulomas
suggesting an aging lesion, still others presented reactions indistinguishable
from those seen in fresh sarcoidosis. At the other end of the spectrum, the
11 patients with negative K-S tests whose sarcoidosis was already on the
wane at the time of implantation, gave additional support to the concept
that the process must be active in order for the host to mount a positive
reaction to K-S suspensions. There remains, however, 8 subjects with
negative tests, apparently in the acute stages of their disease, who confound
all theories of the role of the host by failing to produce a positive
reaction to validated K-S suspensions. After viewing these data, one is
forced to nod in agreement with Munro and Mitchell who entitled their
elegant paper "The Kveim response: still useful, still a puzzle"[43].

However, confusing, Kataria and Mishra's studies of immunopathology and
on-going studies of enzyme elevations strongly support the hypothesis
that the K-S reaction is an _in-vivo_ model of the immunologic and biochemical
events which occur during the naturally occurring disease. It follows that
this unique reaction should lend itself to further investigations elaborating
these, and other alterations which undoubtedly will be identified in the
near future. Furthermore, the K-S reaction would appear to be a good
model in which to study, and perhaps predict, the efficacy of future therapeutic agents on the host's response.

We come to the final question: Can the K-S test reveal anything about

the etiology of sardoidosis? Siltzbach, and others, spent a good part of
their lives peering into the murky suspension and wondering what was the
active principle that provoked patients with active sarcoidosis to form a
nodule which recapitulates the disease at the site of the injection.
Siltzbach considered his inability to identify this causative agent to be
his greatest failure. Is the etiologic agent, or some part of it, trapped
within that small vial? Simplistically, the answer would appear to be "no".
All microscopic and sublight microscopic examinations of the injected
material have failed to demonstrate bacteria, mycobacteria, fungus, virus,
inorganic or organic chemical, or fragments of these, which might be
identified as the causative agent. No patient has ever contracted sarcoidosis after being injected with K-S suspension. No patient with sarcoidosis
has suffered an exacerbation of his disease following an intracutaneous
injection of the test material.

In a search for the active principle in K-S suspensions, Chase and
Siltzbach attempted to refine their material[44]. Using differential
centrifugation they were able to reduce by one-half the alcohol precipitable
dry weight of the test material and still maintain specificity and sensitivity comparable to the original crude suspension. Activity remained in small
particles minute enough to pass through bacteria retaining Pyrex glass
filters. Major activity was in particles that sedimented in 15 minutes at
5500 g and 45 minutes at 10,000 g. Cohn, et al, examined a homogenate
extracted from sarcoidal lymph nodes[45]. Cell fractions of the homogenate
obtained by differential or gradient centrifugation were examined by high
resolution phase contrast microscopy and in a few instances were studied by
electron microscopy. The majority of the active material was found to
sediment below 10,000 g. Using sucrose gradients, K-S activity was associated with cytoplasmic particles that equilibrated between 50 and 70 p.
100 sucrose. Electron microscopy and acid phosphatase assays suggested that
K-S activity resided in membrane bound dense bodies. They theorized that
these dense bodies were derived from histiocytic and epithelioid cells. In
our laboratory, complete solubilization of K-S suspensions eliminated all
activity. It can be concluded that the active principle is membrane
bound and is present in particulate matter which is lost in solubilized
fractions. This observation is supported by the work of Boros and Warren
who noted that in the animal model, soluble degradable antigens are incapable
of inducing granulomatous reactions[46]. Insoluble particles of bentonite,
latex and/or synthetic beads acting as a nidus for adsorbed antigens were
required for experimental granuloma formation. The resulting granulomas
appeared to be a combined foreign body, macrophage and T-cell mediated

reaction. In a like fashion it can be hypothesized that in sarcoidosis the K-S suspensions contain the foreign body component which may be a complex of peptidoglycan and group C polysaccaride similar to that found in experimental granulomas[47]. Perhaps, in sarcoidosis the K-S suspensions supply the granulomagenic foreign body and the sarcoid host supplies the macrophages and lymphocytes.

K-S suspensions are remarkably stable. Shelf supplies have been reported to remain active for more than five years[48]. Siltzbach and Ruttenberg subjected their suspensions to a multitude of physical and chemical challenges[49]. Activity was not lost when exposed to 0.1 N HCL or 50% trichlorocetic acid at 0° centigrade and 90° centigrade. The suspensions were not inactivated by formalin, extraction with 2 M NaCl, ethanol, butanol, ether or chloroform. The suspended particles withstood digestion with pepsin, trypsin, papain, subtilisin, hyaluronidase, neuraminidase, hydroxylamine, carbohydrases, neucleases and denaturing with 8M urea and 5M guanidine hydrochloride. Boiling for one-half hour and 0.05 N NaOH diminished activity and autoclaving, alkali at pH 11.9 and 8M urea plus mercaptoethanol completely abolished activity. Thus, the elusive active principle must be extremely stable.

The primary role of physicians is to prevent or alleviate disease. The most effective prevention and treatment is derived from a knowledge of etiology. We are deeply indebted to the work of Reynolds, Crystal, Hunninghake, Semenzato, Rossi and many others in giving us insight into the cellular and biochemical products elaborated by the lungs of patients with sarcoidosis. While these monumental studies have yielded profound knowledge of host immunology, we must not lose sight of pathogenesis. For our existing knowledge of the pathogenesis of granulomatous diseases we owe a major debt to the work of basic scientists such as Epstein[50], Spector[51], Adams[52] and, in particular, Boros[53]. Their labors should point the way for renewed interest in the study of the etiology of sarcoidosis. Utilizing many different experimental models, it has been demonstrated that the granulomatous response is induced by non-degradable particulate tissue toxins. These irritants cause a continuous stimulus for macrophage and lymphocyte activity. Nematodes, fungi, bacilli, paracyte ova and some protein fractions have been shown to be granulomagenic. All of these agents persist in the host tissues evoking a cell mediated immune response. Boros has asked, "What is the causative agent of sarcoidosis?" He concludes that this question is not currently answerable. To date, all efforts invested in the isolation, identification and propagation of putative transmissable or infectious agents of sarcoidosis remain unsuccessful. However, according to the

lessons of the experimental models, the inciting agent of sarcoidosis should
be of a persisting non-degradable nature. Recalling that the only intracutaneous tests similar to the K-S test, the Lepromin, zirconium and beryllium
skin tests, contain the active disease causing substance or a fraction thereof,
it is time that we turn again to the K-S suspension and its demonstrated
persisting granulomagenic fractions in a search for the answer to Munro and
Mitchell's puzzle and to complete Siltzbach's work.

REFERENCES

1.   Kveim A (1941) Nord Med 9:169-172

2.   Nickerson DA (1941) Arch Dermat Syph 43:172-173

3.   Nelson CT (1949) Arch Dermat Syph 60:337-389

4.   Putkonen T (1943) Acta Dermat-Venereol 23 (Supp. 10):1-194

5.   James DG, Thomson AD (1955) Quart J Med 24:49-59

6.   Chase MW (1961) Am Rev Respir Dis 84:86-88

7.   Siltzbach LE, Ehrlich JC (1954) Am J Med 16:790-803

8.   Israel HL, Sones M (1955) Ann Intern Med 43:1269-1282

9.   Daniel TM, Schneider GW (1962) Am Rev Respir Dis 86:98-99

10. Karlish AJ, Cox EV, Hampson F, et al (1970) Lancet 2:977

11. Mitchell DN, Cannon P, Dyer NH, et al (1969) Lancet 2:571

12. Israel HL, Goldstein RA (1971) N Engl J Med 284:345-349

13. Bringle C (1972) La Sarcoidoise. Reports of the European Symposium on
     Sarcoidosis, Geneva pp 34-35

14. Izumi T, Kobara Y, Morioka S, et al (1974) In: Iwai K, Hosoda Y (eds):
     Proceedings of the VI International Conference on Sarcoidosis. Tokyo,
     University of Tokyo Press pp 77-78

15. Israel HL (1958) N Engl J Med 259:365-369

16. Siltzbach LE (1964) Am Rev Respir Dis 90:308

17. Siltzbach LE, Vieira LOBD, Topilsky M, et al (1971) Lancet 2:634-636

18. Israel HL)1983) In: Fanburg BL (ed): Sarcoidosis and Other Granuloma-
     tous Diseases of the Lung. New York, Marcel Dekker pp 273-286

19. Siltzbach LE (1974) In: Ingelfinger FJ (ed): Controversy in Internal
     Medicine. Philadelphia, WB Saunders pp 339-348

20. Siltzbach LE (1964) Acta Med Scand 176 (Suppl 425):73-78

21. Kataria YP, Park HK (1986) In: Johns CJ (ed) Ann of the NY Acad
     of Sci. New York, 465:221-232

22. Mishra BB, Poulter LW, Janossy G, et al (1983) Clin Exp Immunol 54:705-715

23. Pierard GE, Damseaux M, Franchimont C, et al (1982) Am J Dermatopathology
     4(1):17-23

24. Hardt F, Wanstrup J (1969) Acta Path Microbiol Scand 76:493-494

25. Becker FW, Krull P, Deicher H, et al (1972) Lancet 1:120-123

18

26. Goldstein RA, Janicki BW, Schultz KE (1974) In: Iwai K, Hosado Y (eds): Proceedings of the VI International Conference on Sarcoidosis. Tokyo, University of Tokyo Press pp 42-43

27. Mandell GL, Sullivan GW, Siltzbach LE, et al (1979) Journal of the Reticuloendothelial Society 26(5):525-530

28. Topilsky M, Siltzbach LE, Williams M, et al (1972) Lancet 1:117-120

29. Izumi T, Nilsson BS, Ripe E (1973) Scand J Resp Dis 54:123-127

30. Horsmanheimo M, Horsmanheimo A, McKee KT, et al (1978) Br J Dermatol 79:263-270

31. Jones Williams W, Pioli E, Jones DJ, et al (1972) J Clin Path 25:951-954

32. Favez G, Leuenberger P (1982) J Clin Lab Immunol) 9:87-91

33. Bloom BR, Karpel JP (1987) personal communication

34. Marom Z, Kalb TH (1987) personal communication

35. Silverstein E, Pertschuk LP, Friedland J (1979) Proc Natl Acad Sci 76:6646-6648

36. Lanzillo JJ, Fanburg B (1979) Lancet I, 1200

37. Perrin-Fayolle M, Pacheco Y, Harf R, Montagnon B, Biot N (1981) Thorax 34, 790

38. Selroos OB (1986) Clin Lab Sci 24:185-216

39. Almenoff J, Teirstein AS (1987) Amer J of Med 82:33-38

40. Teirstein AS, Wilk E, Brown LK unpublished data

41. Teirstein AS, Brown LK unpublished data

42. Mikhail JR, Mitchell DN (1971) Postgrad Med J 47:698-704

43. Munro CS, Mitchell DN (1987) Thorax 42:321-331

44. Chase MW, Siltzbach LE (1967) In: Turiaf J, Chabot J (eds) La Sarcoi-ose. Rapports de la IV Conference Internationale. Paris, Masson & Cie pp 150-153

45. Cohn ZA, Fedorko Me, Hirsch JG et al (1967) In: Turiaf J, Chabot J (eds) La Saroidose. Rapports de la IV Conference Internationale. Paris, Masson & Cie pp 141-149

46. Boros DL, Warren KS (1973) Immunology 24:519-529

47. Abdulla EM, Schwab JH (1966) J. Bacteriol 91:374-383

48. Kataria YP, Sharma OM, Israel H, et al (1980) In: Williams WJ, Davies BH (eds) Proceedings of the VIII International Conference on Sarcoidosis and Other Granulomatous Diseases Cardiff, Wales, Alpha Omega Press pp 660-667

49. Siltzbach LE, Ruttenberg MA (1971) In: Levinsky L, Macholda F (eds) Vth International Conference on Sarcoidosis. Praha, University Karlova pp 371-374

50. Epstein WL (1977) Pathobiol 7: pp 1-30

51. Spector WG (1969) Int Rev Exp Pathol 8:1-55

52. Adams DO (1976) Am J Pathol 84:164-192

53. Boros DL (1983) In: Fanburg BL (ed) Sarcoidosis and Other Granulomatous Diseases of the Lung. Marcel Dekker, NY pp 403-449

DEATH FROM SARCOID HEART DISEASE. UNITED KINGDOM SERIES 1971-1986.
300 CASES WITH 138 DEATHS.

HUGH A FLEMING

Cardiac Unit, Papworth Hospital, Cambridge, England.

This paper presents an analysis of the deaths in the first 300 cases of
sarcoid heart disease in the United Kingdom series personally collected by the
author. Since the first major report in 1974 (1) the study has continued and
progress reports have been made (2,3). In 1984 a report to the last meeting of
this Society in Baltimore (4) discussed the prognosis of sarcoid heart disease
and suggested that it was not necessarily as bad as had been previously thought.

A total of 350 cases has now been collected and the basic details of the
initial 300 of these will be presented first, to set the scene for the death
report.

The series consisted of 161 men and 139 women. Two hundred and seventy-nine
were white and only 15 black and 6 Asian. This is in contrast to the heavy
preponderance of black cases in the North American literature (5).

The age at cardiac presentation is shown in Fig 1.

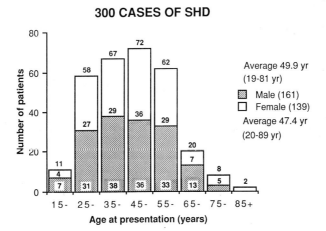

300 CASES OF SHD

Average 49.9 yr (19-81 yr)
Male (161)
Female (139)
Average 47.4 yr (20-89 yr)

The age range is wide - from 19-81 years with the main incidence between 25 and 65 years - so this is a disease important in the prime years of life. Most of the cases presented as cardiac problems (2) and clinical features of sarcoid elsewhere were frequently inconspicuous. The presenting cardiac features are shown in Table 1.

TABLE 1

300 CASES OF SARCOID HEART DISEASE:
PREDOMINANT CARDIAC FEATURES AT PRESENTATION.

	Number	% of Total
Ventricular arrhythmia	134	45
Supraventricular arrhythmia	85	28
Complete heart block	77	26
"Cardiomyopathy"	71	24
RBBB	69	23
Partial HB	68	23
Mitral valve involvement	67	22
Sudden death	49	16
LBBB	45	15
Simulating myocardial infarction	15	5
Pericarditis	9	3
Transplantation	3	1

These features are frequently multiple and the diagnosis should indeed be suspected in any difficult form of heart disease, particularly with varied and intractable rhythm problems. Arrhythmia, heart block, heart failure, mitral systolic murmur and sudden death are the most frequent methods of presentation.

GEOGRAPHICAL DISTRIBUTION

It is emphasized that this collection of cases is not the entire United Kingdom series. However, the strikingly high reported incidence in East Anglia continues to be remarkable (Fig 2).

In the East Anglian Health Region there is an incidence of over 63/million of population. The nearest approach to this is 10/million in the Oxford Region and the lowest 0.64/million in the South West Region. The only reasonable explanation for these figures would appear to be awareness of the diagnosis - though even this theory does not entirely fit the facts.

FIG 2

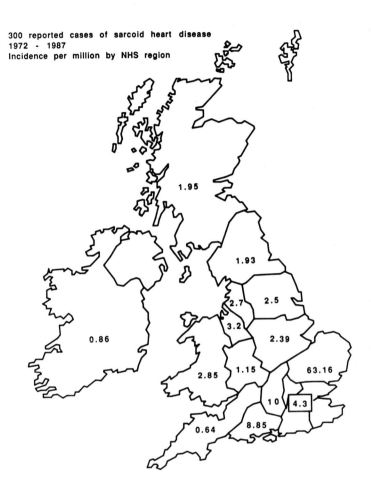

300 reported cases of sarcoid heart disease
1972 - 1987
Incidence per million by NHS region

These deaths will now be discussed in detail.

One hundred and sixty-two cases have survived and are being followed. One hundred and thirty-eight have died and there have been 103 necropsies.

Seventy-seven died suddenly, 35 in congestive cardiac failure and 26 from other causes.

22

TABLE 2

MODE OF DEATH ACCORDING TO PRESENTATION

PRESENTATION (often multiple)	NUMBER OF CASES	% death		
		CHF	SUDDEN	OTHER
"Cardiomyopathy"	40	62	22	16
Complete Heart Block	33	30	37	33
Ventricular arrhythmia	59	38	49	13
Supraventricular arrhythmia	34	29	47	24
Sudden	49		1·00	

   TABLE 2 shows that congestive heart failure and sudden death occurred in all types of sarcoid heart disease - I always felt that this table should mean more but the multiple modes of presentation rather obscure things.

   Of the 77 sudden deaths, 49 were first diagnosed at coroner's post-mortem. The age and sex distribution of these is shown in Fig 3.

FIG 3

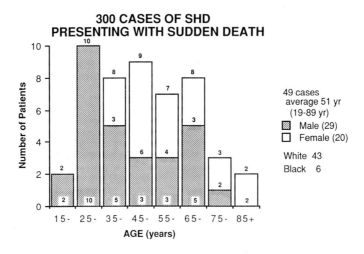

   The high incidence in young men is noteworthy. There were 17 men below the age of 45 years and 12 below the age of 35 years. None of these cases was suspected of having heart disease in life, but retrospective analysis of their records shows that in fact 14 of them were known to have sarcoidosis of other organs before death.

The distribution of these clinical features is shown in Table 3.

TABLE 3

PRESENTATION - SUDDEN DEATH   -
49 PATIENTS

Retrospective symptoms or signs	
Lungs	12
Nodes	10
Eyes	7
Skin	2
Liver	1
Spleen	1

These features are widely distributed but, as with general sarcoidosis, the emphasis is on intrathoracic organs and the eyes.

In the Sudden Death Series as a whole, modes of presentation are shown in Table 4.

TABLE 4

SUDDEN DEATH IN 77 CASES

Modes of Presentation - Often Multiple	
Undiagnosed	49
Ventricular arrhythmia	28
R or LBBB	22
Supraventricular tachycardia	17
Partial heart block	13
Complete heart block	12
"Cardiomyopathy"	8
Simulating myocardial infarction	3
Pericarditis	0

Arrhythmias and degrees of heart block are common and it is therefore not surprising that sudden death is also common.

Little could be done to avoid death in those patients presenting at necropsy, as the problem had not been suspected. However, sarcoidosis was known to be present in 14 cases and this should have led to an awareness that the heart might be involved and that, therefore, sudden death was a possibility.

The 28 cases of known sarcoid heart disease who subsequently died suddenly were analysed in detail in an unsuccessful attempt to determine whether their fate could have been predicted.

Table 5 lists the sarcoid occurring in other organs.

24

TABLE 5

SUDDEN DEATH IN 28 KNOWN CASES

Clinical Evidence in Other Organs	
Lungs	28
Nodes	21
Eye	13
Skin	4
Liver	2
Spleen	2
Other	6

These appeared to be typical cases of sarcoidosis in the involvement of other organs. Cardiac and sarcoid presentation are shown in Tables 6 and 7.

SUDDEN DEATH IN 28 KNOWN SHD

TABLE 6

Type of Cardiac Presentation	
Ventricular arrhythmia	12
"Cardiomyopathy"	11
Supraventricular arrhythmia	11
Complete heart block	10
BBB	8
Simulating myocardial infarction	3
Chest pain	2
Pericarditis	0

TABLE 7

Sarcoid Presentation	
Heart	16
Lung	11
Nodes	8
Skin	4
Eye	4
Bone	1

Cardiac presentation was not notably different from the series as a whole, nor was mode of sarcoid presentation.

SURVIVAL

In known cases of sarcoid heart disease that have died suddenly, survival ranged from 0-13 years with an average of 3.6 years.

Age at diagnosis 26-76 years (average 47 years).

Age at death 31-76 years (average 51.5 years).

In patients still alive in the total series we have many who have survived for longer than 13 years. Thirty-six have, in fact, survived for more than 10 years, and 7 for more than 20 years from the time of cardiac diagnosis (4).

DIAGNOSIS

Biopsy confirmation of sarcoid is considered very desirable and the results
here are shown in Table 8.

TABLE 8

SUDDEN DEATH IN 28 KNOWN SHD.

Biopsy Results

	+VE	-VE
Kveim	8	3
Node	3	1
Bronchial	2	2
Skin	2	1
Liver	1	1
Heart	1*	1*

* Both in same patient

Obviously, negative results make thorough review of the diagnosis essential,
but they do not exclude the diagnosis. We have negative results from all areas
in cases subsequently proved at necropsy. Positive endomyocardial biopsy is
diagnostic but a negative is of no value (6).

Of the known cases dying suddenly, 18 were male and 10 female, 27 white and
only one black.

There were 26 necropsies but in 9 of these, the quality of examination was
poor. Fourteen of the cases had been known to the author in life and often
only this fact and the resultant persistent enquiries led to the correct
necropsy diagnosis being made.

Some pathologists are reluctant to attribute sudden death to anything other
than coronary artery disease, even when no such disease is demonstrable.
Macroscopic diagnoses made in these cases were "ischaemic heart disease with
normal coronary arteries" (which appeared several times) "Hodgkins disease ",
"lymphoma", "carcinomatosis", "tuberculosis", "miliary tuberculosis" and "normal
heart".

Usually, the heart was considerably enlarged with obvious involvement, often
with masses of sarcoid tissue. The heart was not always weighed but the
recorded figures are as follows:-

26

TABLE 9

HEART WEIGHTS

	NUMBER	WEIGHT	AVERAGE
Known Cases	20	350-750gms	474gms
Presenting Cases	30	275-830gms	462gms

In other cases the heart was described as "massively enlarged"

Occasionally, the heart was macroscopically normal and only meticulous histological examination led to the correct diagnosis. The interventricular septum was particularly rewarding in producing positive histology.

Sudden death is by definition unexpected. The gross involvement of the heart in patients with sarcoid heart disease leading a normal or even an athletic life, until the time of death, is a recurrent source of surprise. Sudden death has been noted in this series in the course of the following activities:- walking, washing dishes, eating, driving a car, in bed, boxing, rugby, cricket, karate, flying a plane and playing skittles.

We have already published brief case histories illustrating these various points and I would refer you to the following examples:-

1. A 27 year old Police Sergeant who died suddenly. He had massive cardiac involvement. (3) (Case 1) 2. A 25 year old man who died suddenly at home. He had an apical LV aneurysm and the conducting system was entirely replaced by sarcoid granuloma. (3) (Case 3)

3. A 32 year old man who died suddenly after a good recovery from an illness resembling myocardial infarction. He had an enormous amount of sarcoid granulomatous tissue comprising much of the total heart weight of 830gms. (1) (Case 4)

4. Sudden death with a heart that macroscopically looked normal and only on microscopy showed sarcoid granulomata. (1) (Case 7)

Sudden death is, therefore, not rarely due to sarcoid heart disease. It is astonishing that various epidemiological studies of sudden death (7,8,9,10,11) do not even consider it as a possibility, limiting their interest to coronary artery disease.

PATHOLOGY

Detailed studies of the conducting system in fatal cases demonstrate how frequently this is extensively involved; indeed, often completely replaced by sarcoid granulomatous material. I have already reported (12) a histological study by my colleague, Dr P G I Stovin, demonstrating this frequency. Again, this is in keeping with the high incidence of sudden death, arrhythmias and heart block.

This fact needs wider recognition and recent detailed studies fail to note this point adequately if at all (13,14).

DEATH IN CONGESTIVE CARDIAC FAILURE

There were 39 patients in this category, 26 male and 13 female. The age of cardiac presentation is shown in Fig 4.

FIG 4.

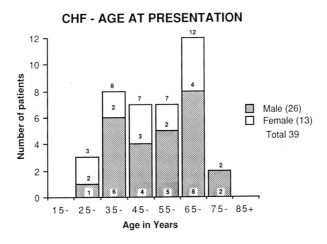

The ages are older than the sudden death series, and indeed older than the series as a whole.

The modes of cardiac presentation are shown in Table 10.

TABLE 10

C.H.F. PRESENTATION - 39 CASES (often multiple)

	No	%
CHF	25	62.5
VE & VT	22	55
MSM	14	35
CHB	12	30
Supra vent arrhythmia	11	27.5
RBBB	10	25
Partial HB	9	22.5
LBBB	7	17.5

The clinical evidence of sarcoid in other organs is shown in Table 11 with similar figures for the total series of 300 (there is no striking difference).

TABLE 11

CLINICAL EVIDENCE IN OTHER ORGANS
(total 300 in brackets)

	%	
Nodes	50	(49)
Lungs	47.5	(46)
Eyes	25	(21)
Liver	12.5	(5.6)
Skin	12.5	(18.3)
Spleen	7.5	(6)
Nerve	5	(4.3)
Bone	2.5	(4.3)
Other	5	(8)

This group of patients with rather insidious onset of symptoms and necropsies often of a poor standard was difficult to analyse, so 10 cases with necropsies of high standard were selected for study in detail. There were 9 men (aged 34-69 years - average 50 years) and one female aged 51 years. The duration of the illness was 1-5 years. Correct diagnosis in life was made in 6 and at necropsy the heart weights ranged from 590-880gms (average 650gms), often with active vasculitis.

Other organs were involved in all cases and steroids had been given in 5 cases, but in none effectively. There had been clinical evidence of sarcoidosis elsewhere, particularly the lungs or the nodes, in 6 cases sometimes many years before (5-12 years).

All cases had severe arrhythmias in addition to congestive heart failure - namely ventricular ectopics, ventricular tachycardia or heart block. However, in many of them, the diagnosis of sarcoidosis had not been made. In a number the possibility of considering sarcoid was mentioned in the case notes, but never followed up and never appropriately treated. Therefore, there is still the need to emphasize a high index of suspicion for the diagnosis.

COMPLETE HEART BLOCK

Complete heart block is common in sarcoid heart disease and in the series of 300 there have been 77 cases. We have demonstrated (15) that the age of development of complete heart block is much younger in the sarcoid patient than in the general population. Indeed, sarcoid heart disease should be suspected in any younger patient developing complete heart block.

Ten paced patients with complete heart block died in congestive cardiac failure. Steroids had not been used and in at least 2 men, aged 49 years, it is possible they could have been beneficial. However, sarcoid heart disease was not diagnosed in life.

An example was Dr A, a physician who was aged 49 at the time of his death (3) (Case 2). He presented 3 years previously with complete heart block and had been paced with a return to full activity. One year before his death he slipped into severe congestive heart failure which was treated medically. Sarcoidosis was suggested by the house physician's notes but no action was taken and the diagnosis was only made by the pathologist after his death in intractable heart failure.

Sarcoid granulomata were found in the lungs, nodes, and the spleen. The heart weighed 620gms and the myocardium was extensively infiltrated (Fig 5) - as was the conducting system which was almost entirely replaced. The major coronary arteries were normal but the small vessels showed a very active sarcoid vasculitis (Fig 6).

Figs 5 and 6 over:- Fig 5: Dr A. Section of the upper part of the ventricular septum and the AV ring showing extensive replacement of the myocardium by granulomatous tissue. Fig 6: Small coronary artery involved in an active granulomatous process with giant cells.

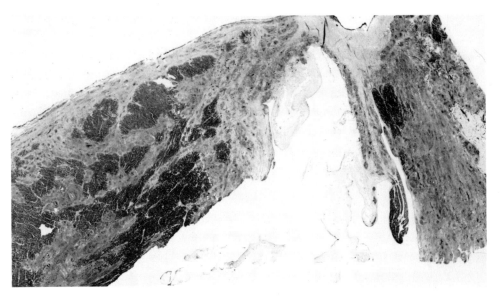

FIG 5

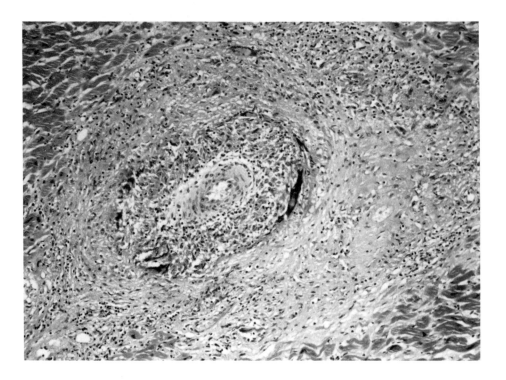

FIG 6

Seven paced patients died relatively suddenly. Four of these were cases of true sudden death, none had been diagnosed as having sarcoidosis in life. It is possible that the correct diagnosis, a more strict search for arrhythmia, and appropriate treatment might have prolonged life.

Once again the necessity for suspicion and pursuit of the correct aetiological diagnosis is emphasized. Sarcoidosis is still very frequently not considered.

The assessment of patients with possible sarcoid heart disease will not be dealt with here; it has been discussed elsewhere (3).

Treatment of sarcoid heart disease to avoid death will involve pacing and all cardiac drugs as necessary. It is increasingly evident that steroids should be used more aggressively and for a more prolonged period of time. The presence of acute vasculitis in some cases is quite striking and as has been suggested (16,17) this could be a fundamental part of the pathological process and could be very responsive to steroids. Limiting or improving myocardial damage has been reported (18,19,20,5) as has improvement in heart block or serious arrhythmia (21,22,23,24).

There is now a considerable body of evidence on clinical grounds, electrocardiographic grounds, thallium scanning and echocardiography that steroids can be of benefit in the individual case. Variable pathology and clinical course make assessment difficult and controlled trial impossible.

SUMMARY

Three-hundred and fifty cases of sarcoid heart disease in the United Kingdom have been collected over a 15 year period, and 300 of these are analysed in detail. The majority presented with cardiac manifestations. One hundred and thirty-eight patients have died, 77 of them suddenly, and 49 presented as sudden death. There were 103 necropsies. Sarcoidosis was often overlooked even by the pathologist.

Normal life was frequently possible in spite of the grossest of cardiac pathology.

Thirty-nine patients died in congestive cardiac failure, again, often without the diagnosis of sarcoid heart disease.

A high index of suspicion, a diagnosis of sarcoid heart disease, and careful monitoring with adequate treatment using steroids energetically where indicated should improve the prognosis.

ACKNOWLEDGEMENTS

  Thanks are due to the many colleagues who have contributed cases, to
Mrs Sheila Bailey, Mrs Jean Pulley and Mr Doug Shaw for help in collection and
handling of data, and to my wife Julia for much assistance. The Departments of
Medical Illustration at Addenbrooke's Hospital, Cambridge and Hinchingbrooke
Hospital, Huntingdon are responsible for the figures.

REFERENCES

1.   Fleming HA (1974) Sarcoid Heart Disease. Br Heart J 36:54-68

2.   Fleming HA, Bailey SM, (1981) Sarcoid Heart Disease. Report of 197 UK
     cases with necropsy confirmation in 62. J R Coll Phys Lond 15:245-53

3.   Fleming HA (1986) Cardiac Sarcoidosis. Cl in Derm 4:143-9

4.   Fleming HA, Bailey SM (1986) The prognosis of sarcoid heart disease in the
     United Kingdom. Ann NY Acad Sci 465:543-50

5.   Lorell B, Alderman EL, Mason JW (1978) Cardiac sarcoidosis: diagnosis with
     endomyocardial biopsy and treatment with corticosteroids. Am J Cardiol
     42:143-6

6.   Sekiguchi M, Numao Y, Imai M, Furuie T, Mikami R (1980) Clinical and
     histopathological profile of sarcoidosis of the heart and acute idiopathic
     myocarditis. Concepts through a study employing endomyocardial biopsy. I.
     Sarcoidosis. Jpn Circ J 44:249-63

7.   W.H.O Technical Report Series No 726 (1985) Sudden Cardiac Death. W.H.O.
     Geneva.

8.   Kannel WB, Schatzkim A (1985) Sudden death: Lessons from subsets in
     population studies. Am Coll Cardiol 5:141B-149B

9.   McCabe WC, Morganroth J (1985) Sudden death revisited. Cardiovasc. med
     10:10-14

10. Campbell RWF (1987) Sudden Death. Current Opinion in Card 2:13-18

11. Buxton AE (1986) Sudden Cardiac Death. Ann intern Med. 104:716-7

12. Fleming HA (1985) Sarcoid Heart Disease. Sarcoidosis 2:20-4

13. Davies MJ, Anderson RH, Becker AE. (1983) In: Conduction Systems of the
     Heart. Butterworth. London p 315

14. Warnes CA (1986) The pathology of sudden death. Current Opinion in Card
     1:837-41

15. Fleming HA (1986) Sarcoid heart disease and complete heart block. Sarcoidosis 3:78

16. James TN (1977) Clinicopathologic correlations. De subitaneis mortibus XXV, Sarcoid Heart Disease. Circulation 56:320-6

17. Mikami R, Sekiguchi M, Ryuzin F et al (1986) Changes in the peripheral vasculature of various organs in patients with sarcoidosis - possible involvement of microangiopathy. Heart and Vessels 2:129-139

18. Stein E, Stimmel E, Siltzbach LE (1976) Clinical course of cardiac sarcoidosis. Ann NY Acad Sci 278:470-4

19. Forman MB, Sandler MP, Sacks GA, Kronenberg MW, Powers TA (1983) Radionuclide imaging in myocardial sarcoidosis; demonstration of myocardial uptake of technetium pyrophosphate 99m and gallium. Chest 83:578-80

20. Ishikawa T, Kondoh H, Nakagawa S, Koiwaya Y, Tanaka K (1984) Steroid therapy in cardiac sarcoidosis. Increased left ventricular contractility concomitant with electrocardiographic improvement after prednisolone. Chest 85:445-7

21. Gozo EG, Cosnow I, Cohen HC, Okun L (1971) The heart in sarcoidosis. Chest 60:379-88

22. Friedman HS, Parikh NK, Chander N, Calderon J (1976) Sarcoidosis with incomplete bilateral bundle branch block pattern disappearing following steroid therapy: an electrophysiological study. Eur J Cardiol 4:141-50

23. Yamamoto M, Muramatsu M, Suzuki T (1980) Successful corticosteroid treatment of seven cases of probable myocardial sarcoidosis. Proceedings of 8th International Conference on Sarcoidosis. In: Sarcoidosis and Other Granulomatous Disorders 1979. Jones WJ, Davies BH (Eds) Alpha Omega Publishing Ltd, Cardiff p 615-23

24. Sekiguchi M et al. (1983) Long-term prognosis of cardiac sarcoidosis patients with permanent pacemaker implantation. A Japanese Study. Proceedings of 9th International Conference on Sarcoidosis - Paris 1981. In: Sarcoidosis. Chretien J, Marsac J, Saltiel JC (Eds) Published by Pergamon Press. p 658

© 1988 Elsevier Science Publishers B.V. (Biomedical Division)
Sarcoidosis and other granulomatous disorders
C. Grassi, G. Rizzato, E. Pozzi, editors

BIOLOGICAL CHARACTERISTICS AND SIGNIFICANCE OF SUBCLINICAL INFLAMMATORY ALVEOLITIS IN EXTRATHORACIC GRANULOMATOUS DISORDERS.

CYR VOISIN*, BENOIT WALLAERT*, MARIO DUGAS*, PHILIPPE BONNIERE**, ANTOINE CORTOT**, JEAN BENOIT MARTINOT***, YVES SIBILLE***

  * Département de Pneumologie, Hôpital Calmette et Institut Pasteur, Lille, FRANCE.
 ** Service de Gastro-entérologie, Hôpital Régional, Lille. FRANCE.
*** Pulmonary section and Experimental Medicine Unit, International Institute of cellular and molecular Pathology, Catholic University of Louvain, BELGIUM.

INTRODUCTION

In the past decade it has become clear that alveolitis, i.e, the accumulation of immune and inflammatory cells in the lower respiratory tract, was the earliest manifestation of interstitial lung disorders that preceded and was responsible for the development of fibrosis (1, 2). However recent reports demonstrated that a subclinical inflammatory alveolitis may be present in the lung of asymptomatic patients with systemic disorders (3 - 8). Recent studies from our department demonstrated that a subclinical alveolitis was present in a high proportion of patients with extrathoracic sarcoidosis (9). In addition, the distribution and the state of activation of bronchoalveolar cells was similar to the one described in patients with pulmonary granulomatous disease (10). Subsequently, lymphocyte alveolitis was observed in Crohn's disease (11-13) and in patients with primary biliary cirrhosis (PBC) (14).These data raised the intringuing question of the significance of subclinical alveolitis in extrathoracic granulomatous disorders. The aim of this study was to determine the biological characteristics and the prognostic value of subclinical alveolitis in extrathoracic sarcoidosis, Crohn's disease and PBC and to compare our results with those observed in pulmonary sarcoidosis.

PATIENTS AND METHODS

Patients

Eighty-two untreated patients with extrathoracic granulomatosis were included in the study. None had symptoms or signs of respiratory involvement and all had normal chest radiograph as judged by two radiologists who were unaware of the clinical data. None had history of occupational or drug exposure known to be associated with interstitial lung disease. The distribution of the patients is shown on table I : there were 41 patients with Crohn's disease (20 were smokers), 15 non smoking patients with PBC, 26 non smoking patients with extrathoracic sarcoidosis.

Control groups consisted of 30 healthy controls (13 non smokers) and 30 non smoking patients with pulmonary sarcoidosis.

Bronchoalveolar lavage

Informed consent was obtained from all subjects. BAL was performed after premedication with atropine under local anesthesia with lignocaine using a wedged fiberoptic bronchoscope (Olympus model BF-B$_3$; Olympus Corps of America, New Hyde Park, N.Y.) and 250 ml of sterile saline solution was applied in five 50-ml aliquots with immediate gentle vacuum aspiration after each aliquot. The aspirated fluid was collected into sterile siliconized jugs and immediatly transported on ice of the laboratory. BAL was filtered through several layers of sterile surgical gauze and the cells were separated from the fluid by low speed centrifugation at 800 g (10 min). After three washings, the cells were resuspended in 10 ml of Hank's balanced salt solution (HBSS) and evaluated for their total number and for a differential cell count. The cellular viability of alveolar macrophages (AM's) was assessed by trypan blue exclusion.

Lymphocyte subpopulations

Lymphocytes were separated from AM's by centrifugation at 400 g (20 min, 4° C) on a continuous gradient of Percoll. The resulting pellet was washed twice, and RPMI-SVF medium was added so that a lymphocyte-enriched suspension 5 x 10^6 cells/ml) could be obtained. Each of three 200-µl aliquots of the suspension was preincubated on ice for 30 min with a different murine monoclonal antibody, that is, with 5µl of OKT$_3$, OKT$_4$, or OKT$_8$ (Ortho Pharmaceutical, Raritan, NJ). Another aliquot was preincubated with 5µl of medium alone. Fluorescein-conjugated goat antimouse immunoglobulin reagent was added to each aliquot in ice for 30 min, and medium was added until the reagent was diluted 1 : 40. The final volume of the suspension was 200µl. After two washings, the cells were examined on slide by epifluorescence microscopy ; 200 lymphocytes were counted on each slide. Only 2 % of the lymphocytes on the control slide (which were preincubated with medium aione) were fluorescent.

Alveolar macrophage chemiluminescence

To assess the respiratory burst activity of AM's, chemiluminescence (CL) assay was performed using a lucigenin-dependent CL method adapted from Williams and Cole (15, 16) in which lucigenin (bis-N-methylacridinium nitrate ; Sigma chemical co, St. Louis, Mo) served as a chemilumigenic probe. Lucigenin $10^{-4}M$ was dissolved in HBSS buffered with 18 mM HEPES (N-2-hydroxyethyl-piperazine-N-2-ethane sulfonic acid). PMA (Sigma Chemical co) was dissolved in dimethylsulfoxide and the resulting concentration was 0.5 mg/ml. Alveolar cells were washed with HBSS, centrifuged at 800 g (10 min, 4° C) and resuspended in HBSS-HEPES to a concentration of 1×10^{6} viable AM's/ml. The suspension was kept on ice in a siliconized glass container until use. Chemiluminescence was measured at 37° C using a Luminometer (Lumac System AG, BASEL). A 500μl aliquot of the AM suspension was added to each to four vials ; each vial contained a 900-μl aliquot of the lucigenin solution and a 50-μl aliquot of a 3 % gelatin solution. A 100-μl aliquot from a 2μl/ml PMA solution was added to one of the vials ; a 100-μl aliquot from a 120μg/ml superoxide dismutase (SOD) solution was added to another ; and one vial contained 100-μl aliquots of both PMA and SOD. The total volume in each vial was brought to 1.650 ml by adding the appropriate amount of HBSS-HEPES. All the vials were incubated in parallel. Intensity of luminescence was integrated for 60 sec after a 12-min incubation (37° C). The CL responses were determined by substracting background CL values from the mean recorded CL responses. The results were expressed in relative luminescent units (RLU) per 0.5×10^{6} viable AM's.

Protein assays

An immunoradiometric assay (IRMA) was used for measurement of the proteins in BAL. This assay previously described in detail (17), provides as sensitivity in the range of the nanogram per milliliter and was performed on a non concentrated BAL fluid. BAL samples were diluted in 20 % goat serum in phosphate buffered saline, pH 7.4. Serum levels of the different proteins were determined by immunophelometry. Results are expressed in coefficient of excretion relative to albumin (RCE) :

$$RCE = \frac{(protein)\ BAL}{(protein)\ serum} \bigg/ \frac{(albumin)\ BAL}{(albumin)\ serum}$$

Pulmonary function tests

Pulmonary function tests (PFT) were performed at rest and included Forced Vital Capacity (FVC) and Forced Expiratory Volume in one second (FEV_1). Residual Volume (RV) was determined with the helium dilution method. Total Lung Capacity (TLC) was calculated from RV + IVC (Inspiratory Vital Capacity). The diffusing capacity (DLCO) was obtained by single breath method and corrected for alveolar volume and hemoglobin. The predicted values for each subject, based on sex, age, and height were obtained from standard table (18). All data were expressed as percentage of the predicted values.

Follow-up studies

All 82 patients with extrathoracic granulomatosis were examined at hospital consultation and has chest roentgenograms at 6 and/or 12 month intervals after initial evaluation. Twenty-six of them were studied 18 to 24 months after initial evaluation with pulmonary function tests (PFT). The four functional parameters (TLC, FVC, FEV_1, and DLCO) were measured to regroup each patient as "no change", "improvement",or "deterioration." This characterization of PFT was establihed using criteria based on the percent change in lung function. For each parameter, the percent change in that parameter was determined using the formula : percent change = (absolute value of the parameter at the second evaluation – absolute value of the parameter at the initial evaluation) x 100/(absolute value of the parameter at the initial evaluation). A significant change in each functional parameter was defined as a percent change greater than 10 %. In addition a second BAL was performed on 20 patients at 12 months.

RESULTS

I.Bronchoalveolar lavage

I.1 Cellular characteristics

Results of BAL studies are summarized in table I.

Total BAL volume of fluid recovery, total cell yields, percentage and total number of alveolar macrophages were not significantly different between patients with extrathoracic granulomatosis and control subjects with regard to smoking habits. However, patients with pulmonary sarcoidosis showed an increased but non significant number of cells. The main finding of our study was the presence of a lymphocyte alveolitis which was characterized by an increased number of lymphocytes (> mean control value + 3 standard deviation : > 2.6×10^4 cells/ml) in a high proportion of patients. Lymphocyte alveolitis was observed in 40/82 (49 %) patients with extrathoracic granulomatosis (respectively 51 % in

Crohn's disease, 33 % in PBC and 54 % in extrathoracic sarcoidosis) and in 24/30 (80 %) patients with pulmonary sarcoisosis. In contrast, distribution of other BAL inflammatory cells, that is neutrophils and eosinophils, was normal in all groups.

TABLE I. TOTAL AND DIFFERENTIAL BRONCHOALVEOLAR LAVAGE CELL COUNTS

Patients	n	Cells 10^4/ml	AM %	Lymphocytes %	10^4/ml	Neutro %	Eosino %
Healthy non smokers	13	9.7 ± 4.4	88.2 ± 7.1	9.6 ± 5.3	0.91 ± 0.69	1.38 ± 2.7	.15 ± 0.37
smokers	17	24.5 ± 16.9	93.5 ± 5.5	4.8 ± 5.2	0.8 ± 0.45	0.88 ± 1.2	0.35 ± 0.7
Crohn's non smokers	21	14.2 ± 12.4	72.3 ± 21.8	24.6* ± 21.1	3.7* ± 3.6	1.8 ± 1.8	0.17 ± 0.45
smokers	20	30.3 ± 31.7	24.8 ± 13.0	13.6* ± 12.8	3.6* ± 4.0	1.5 ± 1.4	0.05 ± 0.2
PBC	15	12.7 ± 6.1	74.2 ± 24.1	23.5* ± 22.3	3.7* ± 5.0	2.0 ± 2.1	0.13 ± .35
Extrathoracic sarcoidosis	26	12.3 ± 8.7	65.8 ± 18.4	30.1* ± 17.4	4.0* ± 5.0	2.7 ± 3.4	0.1 ± 0.35
Sarcoidosis	30	24.6 ± 41.9	58.7* ± 14.4	39.5* ± 14.3	9.8* ± 14.2	1.5 ± 1.1	0.24 ± 0.8

* the difference is statistically significant ($p < 0.05$) when compared to healthy controls with regard to smoking habits.
Results are expressed as mean ± SD

The percentage of BAL lymphocytes that stained positively with monoclonal antibodies CD4+ and CD8+ are shown in table II. The relative proportion of the helper/inducer and suppressor/cytotoxic subsets are expressed as CD4 : CD8 ratio. The percentage of T lymphocytes was normal in patients with extrathoracic granulomatosis but significantly

TABLE II. T LYMPHOCYTE SUBPOPULATIONS IN BRONCHOALVEOLAR LAVAGE AND
CHEMILUMINESCENCE OF ALVEOLAR MACROPHAGES.

Patients	CD4+ (%)	CD8+ (%)	CD4:CD8	Spontaneous CL	PMA induced CL
Healthy non smokers	46 ± 6.1	28 ± 5.6	1.7 ± 0.35	800 ± 329	16670 ± 3900
smokers	51 ± 9.1	27 ± 5.5	1.9 ± 0.56	1134 ± 468	15600 ± 5210
Crohn's non smokers without alveolitis	47.9 ± 3.3	28.6 ± 9.3	1.82 ± 0.6	6804* ± 3228	30291* ± 14920
non smokers with alveolitis	55.6 ± 18.2	22.1 ± 10.4	3.3* ± 1.9	5487* ± 4980	25129* ± 13209
smokers without alveolitis	32.8 ± 19.8	40.3 ± 13.4	1.08 ± 0.6	4993* ± 6315	19325* ± 5921
smokers with alveolitis	49.0 ± 10.2	27.8 ± 8.6	1.98 ± 10.7	2688* ± 1694	18040* ± 6582
PBC without alveolitis	51.8 ± 11.3	30.6 ± 5.6	1.8 ± 0.66	3450* ± 3021	23222* ± 12211
with alveolitis	64.0 ± 8.7	16.3 ± 7.6	4.5* ± 1.8	7619* ± 3130	31688* ± 10993
Extrathoracic sarcoidosis without alveolitis	51.3 ± 5.9	27.2 ± 4.5	1.92 ± 0.34	3947* ± 3232	29868* ± 12532
with alveolitis	41 ± 5.4	26.7 ± 2.5	1.54 ± 0.14	2067* ± 410	19474* ± 5624
Pulmonary sarcoidosis without alveolitis	73.2* ± 10.7	19.7 ± 8.2	4.7* ± 2.5	1702* ± 522	27955* ± 2606
with alveolitis	77.2* ± 6.5	14.7 ± 8.2	6.4* ± 2.4	4543* ± 4119	29129* ± 12945

* the difference is statistically significant ($p < 0.05$) when compared
to healthy controls with regard to smoking habits.
Results are expressed as mean ± SD

increased in the patients with active pulmonary sarcoidosis. CD4 : CD8
ratio was increased in the groups of non smoking patients with Crohn's
disease and of patients with PBC which exhibited a lymphocyte
alveolitis, and in patients with pulmonary sarcoidosis.

Both spontaneous and PMA-induced CL of BAL cells were markedly increased in patients with extrathoracic granulomatosis and in patients with pulmonary sarcoidosis regardless the magnitude of alveolar lymphocytosis. However in PBC and in pulmonary sarcoidosis, increased CL response of AMs was associated with an expansion of the lung T-lymphocyte population.

1.2 Biochemical characteristics

The results of BAL alpha-2-macroglobulin content, expressed as RCE are shown in fig 1. Patients with Crohn's disease which exhibited a

ALPHA 2 MACROGLOBULIN

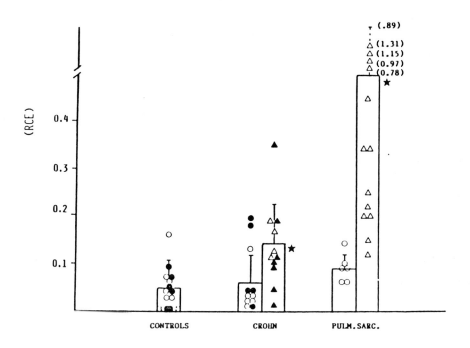

Fig 1. Alpha-2-macroglobulin levels (RCE) in Bronchoalveolar lavage fluid from patients with Crohn's disease and with pulmonary sarcoidosis according to the presence of a lymphocyte alveolitis.
* p < 0.05 when compared to controls and to patients without lymphocyte alveolitis.

lymphocyte alveolitis, had a significant increase of alpha-2 macroglobulin compared to normals and patients with Crohn's disease without lymphocyte alveolitis. As previously reported (17), patients with pulmonary sarcoidosis and lymphocyte alveolitis, showed a dramatic increased RCE alpha-2-macroglobulin whereas the level was normal in patients with pulmonary sarcoidosis with normal BAL. Levels of IgG, IgM and alpha-1-antitrypsin were not significantly different between patients with Crohn's disease with normal BAL and controls whereas they were increased in patients with Crohn's disease with lymphocyte alveolitis and in patients with pulmonary sarcoidosis (Table III).

TABLE III. BIOCHEMICAL CHARACTERISTICS OF BRONCHOALVEOLAR LAVAGE FLUID

	CCNTROLS	CROHN		SARCOIDOSIS	
		without alveolitis	with alveolitis	without alveolitis	with alveolitis
IgG	0.75 ± 0.28	0.72 ± 0.4	1.57* ± 0.75	1.22 ± 0.41	1.93* ± 0.88
IgM	0.095 ± 0.04	0.03 ± 0.02	0.19* ± 0.24	0.17 ± 0.7	0.49* ± 0.41
SeC	0.20 ± 0.12	0.12 ± 0.08	0.35 ± 0.25	0.21 ± 0.12	0.12 ± 0.06
α^2M	0.05 ± 0.06	0.062 ± 0.05	0.14* ± 0.08	0.09 ± 0.03	0.49* ± 0.39
α^1AT	1.27 ± 0.48	0.72 ± 0.4	1.35 ± 0.9	1.11 ± 0.48	1.98 ± 0.77

* $p < 0.05$ when compared to healthy controls and to patients without alveolitis

SeC = Secretory Component ; α^2 M = α^2 macroglobulin

α^1AT = α^1antitrypsin

II.Correlation between BAL characteristics and clinical data

II.1. Pulmonary function Tests

Pulmonary function tests were carried out in the 82 patients at entry
to the study. The mean values of TLC, FVC, FEV$_1$ and DLCO were normal in
all group except for DLCO in smoking patients with Crohn's disease and
with lymphocyte alveolitis which was significantly lower than in smoking
patients with Crohn's disease without lymphocyte alveolitis and than in
non smoking patients (fig 2).

DLCO

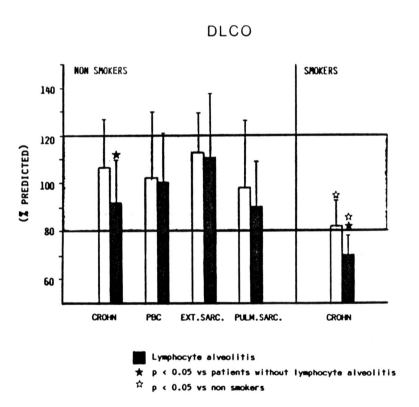

Fig 2. Diffusing capacity in patients with extrathoracic granulomatosis
and with pulmonary sarcoidosis according to the presence of a lymphocyte
alveolitis
* p < 0.05 when compared to controls and to patients without lymphocyte
alveolitis.

II.2. <u>Follow-up</u> <u>studies</u>

Fourteen patients with Crohn's disease (10 of them showed a lymphocyte alveolitis at initial evaluation) and 9 patients with extrathoracic sarcoidosis (4 with lymphocyte alveolitis) were evaluated by pulmonary function tests 18 to 24 months later. The mean value of TLC, FVC, FEV_1 and DLCO was not significant different at the second evaluation when compared to initial value. In addition, three patients with PBC did not show significant changes in pulmonary function tests over a 12-month period.

II.3. <u>Sequential</u> <u>evaluation</u> <u>of</u> <u>alveolitis</u>

Among the 82 patients, 20 were evaluated by BAL 13 to 30 (mean 24) months after initial evaluation. As shown in fig 3, lymphocyte

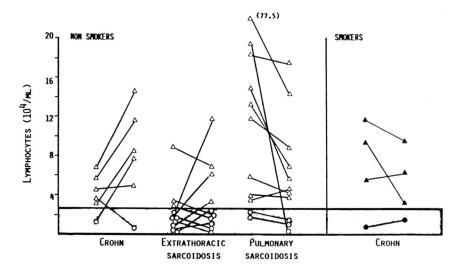

Fig 3. Sequential evaluation of alveolitis

alveolitis appeared to be a persitent finding in the lower respiratory tract of patients with extrathoracic granulomatosis. Seven patients with Crohn's disease showed persistent lymphocyte alveolitis whereas one returned to normal BAL, one with normal BAL exhibited a lymphocyte alveolitis and one showed persistent normal BAL. In extrathoracic sarcoidosis, three of studied patients showed initial lymphocyte alveolitis whereas four demonstrated lymphocyte alveolitis at the second evaluation. As previously reported (10), this was largely related to the persistance and evolution of the extrathoracic lesions.

DISCUSSION

Our study clearly demonstrated the existence of a high proportion of subclinical lymphocyte alveolitis assessed by bronchoalveolar lavage in patients with extrathoracic granulomatosis free of clinical pulmonary symptoms and with normal chest roentgenograms (fig 4). Although alveolitis is a diagnosis based in histologic finding through lung

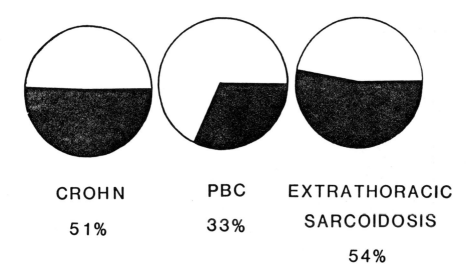

CROHN   PBC   EXTRATHORACIC

51%   33%   SARCOIDOSIS

54%

Fig 4. Frequency of subclinical lymphocyte alveolitis in extrathoracic granulomatous disorders.

biopsy, there is now evidence that an increased number of lymphocytes (>
2.6 x 10^4/ml) in BAL does characterize an inflammatory process of the
lower respiratory tract. Our data lead us to define the new concept of
subclinical inflammatory alveolitis in extrathoracic granulomatous
disorders.

Subclinical alveolitis has been also reported in patients exposed to
organic or inorganic particles without evidence of occupational lung
disorders. For example, previous studies demonstrated that a high
proportion of asymptomatic dairy farmers or of asymptomatic pigeon
breeders exhibited a lymphocyte alveolitis in the same extent than did
symptomatic patients (19, 20). In addition, none of these asymptomatic
patients have developed clinical or radiological features of the
disease (hypersensitivity pneumonitis) over a 4-yr period (21). Taken
together these data support the view that inflammatory alveolitis does
not necessarily lead to a clinically significant interstitial pulmonary
process per se.

Strikingly, the biological characteristics of subclinical alveolitis
in extrathoracic granulomatosis are similar to those described in
pulmonary granulomatosis like sarcoidosis but none of the patients had
evidence of pulmonary involvement. Although the lymphocyte component of
alveolitis had not an increased proportion of T lymphocytes, the CD4/CD8
ratio was increased in BAL from patients with extrathoracic
granulomatosis and with lymphocyte alveolitis. Alveolar macrophages were
activated as indicated by increased chemiluminescence. In addition,
antiproteases and immunoglobulins, which are potentially reflecting the
processus regulating the alveolitis, were also increased in BAL fluid
from patients with Crohn's disease with lymphocyte alveolitis. Thus, all
these data demonstrate that an active alveolar inflammation mimicking
the alveolitis of pulmonary sarcoidosis is associated with extrathoracic
granulomatosis, especially with Crohn's disease.

The significance of subclinical alveolitis remains unclear and may be
different according to the disease. Pulmonary function tests results
were normal in PBC and in extrathoracic granulomatosis. In marked
contrast, in patients with Crohn's disease, the presence of a
subclinical lymphocyte alveolitis is associated with more severe
impairment of diffusing capacity and of pulmonary perfusion scanning
(22) supporting the hypothesis that the role of alveolitis may be quite
different between Crohn's disease, PBC, and extrathoracic sarcoidosis.

The mechanisms responsible for lymphocyte accumulation in the lung and for alveolar macrophage activation are unknown. The subclinical alveolitis may be the first step of pulmonary involvement. However, obvious pulmonary disorder have been rarely described in Crohn's disease (23-25) or in PBC (26-28). In addition, in our series, only one patient (with extrathoracic sarcoidosis) developped interstitial lung disease. Lastly the presence of lymphocyte alveolitis is not associate with a deterioration of pulmonary function. Thus, another hypothesis is that subclinical alveolitis reflect a local expression of a systemic immunological disorder.

REFERENCES

1. Keogh BA, Crystal RG (1982) Alveolitis : the key to the interstitial lung disorders. Thorax 37 : 1 - 10

2. Crystal RG, Bitterman PB, Rennard SI, Hance AJ, Keogh BA (1984) Interstitial lung diseases of unknown cause. Disorders characterized by chronic inflammation of the lower respiratory tract. N Engl J Med 310 : 154 - 166 and 235 - 244

3. Voisin C., Wallaert B., Devulder B., Hatron PY (1985) Alvéolites chroniques latentes au cours de connectivites. Détection par le lavage broncho-alvéolaire et signification. Bull Acad Natle Med 169 : 1453 - 1459

4. Garcia JGN, Parhami N, Killam D, Garcia PL, Keogh BA (1986). Bronchoalveolar fluid evaluation in rheumatoid arthritis. Am Rev Respir Dis 133 : 450 - 454

5. Wallaert B, Hatron PY, Grosbois JM, Tonnel AB, Devulder B, Voisin C (1986). Subclinical pulmonary involvement in collagen-vascular disease assessed by bronchoalveolar lavage. Relationship between alveolitis and subsequent changes in lung function. Am Rev Respir Dis 133 : 574 - 580

6. Bitterman PB, Rennard SI, Keogh BA, Wewers MD, Adelberg S, Crystal RG (1986). Familial idiopathic pulmonary fibrosis. Evidence of lung inflammation in unaffected family members. N Engl J Med 314 : 1343-1347

7. Hatron PY, Wallaert B, Gosset D, Tonnel AB, Gosselin B, Voisin C, Devulder B (1987). Subclinical lung inflammation in primary Sjögren's syndrome. Arthritis Rheum (in press)

8. Wallaert B, Prin L, Hatron PY, Ramon Ph, Tonnel AB, Voisin C (1987). Lymphocyte subpopulations in bronchoalveolar lavage in Sjögren's syndrome. Evidence for an expansion of cytotoxic/suppressor subset in patients with alveolar neutrophilia. Chest (in press)

9. Wallaert B, Ramon Ph, Fournier E, Tonnel AB, Voisin C (1982) Bronchoalveolar lavage, serum angiotensin-converting enzyme and Gallium-67 scanning in extrathoracic sarcoidosis. Chest 82 : 553 - 555

48

10. Wallaert B, Ramon Ph, Fournier E, Prin L, Tonnel AB, Voisin C (1986) Activated alveolar macrophage and lymphocyte alveolitis in extrathoracic sarcoidosis without radiological mediastinopulmonary involvement. Ann NY Acad Sci 465 : 201 - 210

11. Wallaert B, Colombel JF, Tonnel AB, Bonniere Ph, Cortot A, Paris JC, Voisin C (1985) Evidence of lymphocyte alveolitis in Crohn's disease. Chest 87 : 363 - 367

12. Wallaert B, Aerts C, Bonniere Ph, Cortot A, Tonnel AB, Paris JC, Voisin C (1985) Superoxide anion generation by alveolar macrophage in Crohn's disease. N Engl J Med 312 : 444 - 445

13. Smiejan JM, Cosnes J, Chollet-Martin S, Soler P, Basset F, Le Quintrec Y, Hance AJ (1986) Sarcoid-like lymphocytosis of the lower respiratory tract in patients with active Crohn's disease. Ann Intern Med 104 : 17 - 21

14. Wallaert B, Bonniere Ph, Prin L, Cortot A, Tonnel AB, Voisin C (1986). Primary biliary cirrhosis : Subclinical Inflammatory Alveolitis in Patients with Normal Chest Roentgenograms. Chest 90 : 842 - 848

15. Williams AJ, Cole PJ (1981). Investigation of alveolar macrophage function using lucigenin dependent chemiluminescence. Thorax 36 : 866 - 869

16. Aerts C, Wallaert B, Grosbois JM, Voisin C (1986). Superoxide anion release by alveolar macrophages in pulmonary sarcoidosis. Ann NY Acad Sci 465 : 193 - 200

17. Delacroix DL, Marchandise FX, Francis C, Sibille Y (1985). Alpha-2-macroglobulin, monometric and polymeric immunoglobulin A, and immunoglobulin M in bronchoalveolar lavage. Am Rev Respir Dis 132 : 829 - 835

18. Quanger PH (1981). Standardized lung function testing Report working party "Standardization of lung function tests". Luxembourg: European Community for Coal and Steel

19. Solal-Celigny P, Laviolette M, Hebert J, Cormier Y (1982). Immune reactions in the lung of asymptomatic dairy farmers. Am Rev Respir Dis 126 : 964 - 967

20 Keller RH, Fink JN, Lyman S, Pedersen G (1982). Immunoregulation in hypersensitivity pneumonitis : I. Difference in T-cells and macrophage suppressor activity in symptomatic and asymptomatic pigeon breeders. J Clin Immunol 2 : 46 - 54

21. Cormier Y, Belanger J, Laviolette M (1986). Persistent bronchoalveolar lymphocytosis in asymptomatic farmers. Am Rev Respir Dis 133 : 843 - 847

22. Bonniere P, Wallaert B, Cortot A, Marchandise X, Riou Y, Tonnel AB, Colombel JF, Voisin C, Paris JC (1986). Latent pulmonary involvement in Crohn's disease : biological, functional, bronchoalveolar lavage and scintigraphic studies. Gut 27 : 38 - 44

23. Eade OE, Smith CL, Alexander JR, Whorwell PJ (1980). Pulmonary function in patients with inflammatory bowel disease. Am J Gastroenterol 73 : 145 - 156

24. Pasquis P, Colin R, Denis PH, Baptiste P, Galmiche JP, Hecketsweiller PH (1981). Transient pulmonary impairment during attacks of Crohn's disease. Respiration 41 : 56 - 59

25. Heatley RV, Thomas P, Prokipchuk EJ, Gauldie J, Sieniewcz DJ, Bienenstock J. (1982). Pulmonary function abnormalities in patients with inflammatory bowel disease. Quart J Med 203 : 241 - 250

26. Ahrens EH Jr, Payne MA, Kunkel HG(1950). Primary biliary cirrhosis. Medicine 29 : 299 - 364

27. Sherlock S, Scheuer PJ (1973). The presentation and diagnosis of 100 patients with primary biliary cirrhosis.N Engl J Med 289 : 674-678

28. Schaffner (1975). Primary biliary cirrhosis. Clin Gastroenterol 4 : 351 - 366

SUMMARY

Cellular and biochemical characteristics of bronchoalveolar lavage were studied in 82 patients with extrathoracic granulomatosis (Crohn's disease : 41 ; Primary biliary cirrhosis : 15; extrathoracic sarcoidosis : 26), 30 patients with pulmonary sarcoidosis and 30 healthy controls. A subclinical inflammatory alveolitis similar to the one associated with pulmonary sarcoidosis (comprising activated alveolar macrophages and CD4+ T-lymphocytes) was demonstrated in 51% patients with Crohn's disease, 33 % patients with PBC and 54 % patients with extrathoracic sarcoidosis. In addition, IgG, IgM and alpha-2-macroglobulin levels were increased in BAL fluid from patients with Crohn's disease with lymphocyte alveolitis and from patients with active pulmonary sarcoidosis. Pulmonary function tests results were normal in patients with extrathoracic granulomatosis but DLCO was significantly decreased in patients with Crohn's disease and with lymphocyte alveolitis. Follow-up studies suggest that subclinical alveolitis may persist over a 36-month period and is not associated with a significant deterioration of pulmonary function. Whether subclinical alveolitis in extrathoracic granulomatosis is the first step of pulmonary involvement or represents the local expression of a systemic disorder remains to be elucidated.

This work was supported in part by INSERM (Réseau de Recherche Clinique, Participation des Cellules Inflammatoires en Pathologie Respiratoire) and by Université de Lille II.

WEGENER'S GRANULOMATOSIS, NEWER CONCEPTS OF CLASSIFICATION AND TREATMENT

RICHARD A. DeREMEE, M.D.
Professor of Medicine, Mayo Medical School, Consultant in Thoracic Diseases
and Internal Medicine, Mayo Clinic, Rochester, Minnesota 55905, USA

INTRODUCTION

On May 7-9, 1986, an "International Colloquy on Wegener's Granulomatosis"
took place at Mayo Clinic, Rochester, Minnesota. With my colleagues, Drs.
T. J. McDonald and L. H. Weiland, I had the pleasure of organizing the affair
and acting as host to over 100 physicians from six countries. I am happy to
report that Dr. Friedrich Wegener, who turned 80 this April, is living and
well in Lübeck, Germany. Doctor Wegener was our special guest in Rochester
with his wife and it was his lively presence that made the meeting a great
success. Let us briefly review the historical background to this disease we
now call Wegener's granulomatosis.

In 1931, Klinger[1] described two patients having what he called
Grenzformen der Periarteritis Nodosa (borderline forms of periarteritis
nodosa). His patients differed from those having classic periarteritis nodosa
(PAN) in that the pathology involved unusual sites such as the lung and upper
respiratory tract. Moreover, in addition to vasculitis there were
granulomatous changes not typical of PAN. Nevertheless, the disease
manifested by these patients was considered in the spectrum of PAN.
Subsequently, in 1936 and 1939, Friedrich Wegener[2,3] published his classic
works that convincingly demonstrated the uniqueness of the disease that now
bears his name. He described three cases embracing a characteristic clinical
course of four to seven months beginning with nasal congestion, evolving with
necrotizing lesions of the nose and sinuses and ending in renal failure and
death. Pathologically, there was generalized vasculitis reminiscent of
periarteritis nodosa plus necrotizing granulomas of the upper respiratory
tract and other organs. He called this disease "Rhinogenic Granulomatosis,"
undoubtedly because of the prominence of the pathology in the nose and
paranasal sinuses. Subsequently, Godman and Churg,[4] in 1954, set down formal
criteria for the diagnosis as follows: 1) necrotizing granulomas of the upper
or lower respiratory tract or both, 2) generalized focal necrotizing
vasculitis involving both arteries and veins, almost always in the lung and
more or less widely disseminated in other sites, and 3) glomerulitis
characterized by necrosis and thrombosis of loops or lobes of the capillary
tuft, capsular adhesion and evolution as a granulomatous lesion. Godman and

Churg proposed the term "necrotizing respiratory granuloma, angiitis, and nephritis."

Fienberg,[5] in 1955, recognized the incomplete expression of pathologic changes similar to those described by Wegener. He proposed the term "pathergic granulomatosis" subdivided into "disseminated" for the complete syndrome of Wegener, and "focal" for the incomplete forms. Carrington and Liebow,[6] in 1966, proposed the classification of limited Wegener's granulomatosis to encompass those cases having involvement of the lung without evidence of glomerulitis. Those patients seem to have a more favorable prognosis compared to classic Wegener's granulomatosis. Fienberg[7] has also commented on the protracted lesions of skin and respiratory mucosa that may antedate the complete syndrome by as many as 18 years. Thus, there has been a developing awareness of the possibility of a spectrum of involvement and developmental tempo in patients with identical pathology who respond to similar forms of treatment. This realization led our group to propose the ELK classification.[8] In this scheme, a number of combinations of major site involvement can be recognized at first encounter. E stands for the ENT system or upper respiratory tract, L for the lung, and K for the kidneys. Any of these major sites may be involved alone or in combination, except that isolated kidney involvement is not accepted by modern criteria, since the lesion of focal necrotizing glomerulitis is not specific for Wegener's granulomatosis. The presence of renal involvement must be confirmed by typical lesions of the upper and/or lower respiratory tracts. According to this classification, the complete syndrome would be designated ELK.

A newly emerging test for Wegener's granulomatosis, namely the anti-neutrophile cytoplasmic antibody (ANCA) or anticytoplasmic antibody (ACPA)[9] theoretically may allow us to include isolated kidney involvement if the test were to be positive. Developmental work on this test is proceeding in Denmark, Germany, Great Britain, Holland, and the United States. In the very near future the medical community should have a clearer conception of the role this test will play in our diagnosis and management of Wegener's granulomatosis. Early data suggests the test to be highly specific for the disease.

In spite of the various names proposed for this disease that may have more precise scientific meaning, the eponym Wegener's granulomatosis has held fast in the literature, appropriately recognizing the seminal contribution of Friedrich Wegener. It was his perceptive analysis of the clinical and pathologic data that has led the international medical community to recognize the uniqueness of his observations.

PRESENTATION AND CLINICAL COURSE

The presentation and clinical course is extremely variable. There may be a long history of nasal congestion and crusting with occasional epistaxis prior to the development of other signs of involvement in the lungs, kidneys, the skin, central nervous system, or other organs. Or, the presentation may be explosive, occurring over a few days, with extensive necrotizing lesions of the upper and lower respiratory tracts, infarctive lesions of the skin, mononeuritis multiplex, and evidence of glomerulonephritis. Colby[10] has recently written about pulmonary hemorrhage as an early manifestation of Wegener's granulomatosis. He has described generalized capillaritis in the lung that may exist without the classic granulomatous changes. From 1965 through 1985, our group studied 151 patients at the Mayo Clinic. One hundred twenty eight (85%) had lesions of the upper respiratory tract or E. Of particular interest is the so-called saddle nose deformity, which can also be seen in relapsing polychondritis. The lung was involved in 57% of patients with multiple nodular lesions with or without cavitation. The kidneys were involved in 62 patients or 41%, an incidence somewhat lower than other series, such as reported by Fauci[11] and associates. Although the upper and lower respiratory tracts and kidneys are the major sites of involvement, other tissues and organs are occasionally affected, as already mentioned, such as the skin and peripheral nervous system. In addition, the eye and orbit may be affected, producing proptosis, or there may be episcleritis, keratitis, and conjunctivitis. Visual loss may be a consequence of lesions of the optic nerve, retina, or uveal tract. A late sequel of cicatricial healing of a nasal lesion may be obstruction of the nasolacrimal duct with chronic epiphora. The skin may be involved in 15-50% of patients with a variety of lesions, including necrotic papullonodules, urticaria, vessicles, or pyoderma gangrenosum. Mononeuritis multiplex is the foremost expression of nervous system involvement. Other signs may include multiple cranial nerve palsies, symmetric peripheral neuropathy, amaurosis fugax, cerebral infarction, seizures, and transverse myelitis. The overall incidence of neurologic signs was 29% in our series. Arthralgias and frank polyartheritis are frequently observed and tend to reflect the intensity of disease activity. Joint deformity, as occurs in rheumatoid arthritis, is not seen. Virtually any organ system can be involved with vasculitis, and we have observed perforations of the bowel due to vasculitis and granulomatous vasculitis involving the prostate.

TREATMENT

Before 1951, no effective treatment was available for Wegener's granulomatosis. In 1951, Henry Williams[12] of the Mayo Clinic reported with his associates the first patient to be successfully treated with cortisone, that had been recently discovered at Mayo Clinic. The effect was dramatic and encouraging. Over the next 20 years, in addition to glucocorticoids, a number of cytotoxic drugs were reported to be effective, and these included nitrogen mustard, methotrexate, chlorambucil, azathioprine, and cyclophosphamide. However, it was noted that patients thusly treated frequently died of infections. By 1970, the standard regimen became cyclophosphamide with or without prednisone. With the emergence of such regimens, prognosis of patients with Wegener's granulomatosis has dramatically improved. In a review by Walton[13] in the 1950's, he reported 80% of the patients to be dead by the first year after diagnosis, and 93% dead by two years. In contrast, our data derived from 151 patients shows the overall mortality rate to be 28%, with our longest survival being 19½ years. Survivorship was 90% at one year, 87% at two years, and 76% at five years. It has been thought that kidney involvement is most decisive in outcome. In earlier reports, the leading causes of death were renal failure and sepsis. In our series, kidney involvement was of significant importance only in the first year, after which the survival curve parallels that of the entire group. This came as a great surprise to me, as did the apparent importance of lung involvement. Lung involvement proved to be the most significant factor in overall survivorship, not only during the first year, but throughout the period of observation. Another factor which was of significance in survivorship was age, as one might expect.

In analyzing causes of death, we found 11 patients dead of renal failure, 7 within the first year. I would emphasize that 12 patients died of infections of an apparent opportunistic nature. In addition, malignant neoplasms were associated with death in 5 patients. Two patients died of cytotoxic lung. Other causes of death included pulmonary hemorrhage (4), stroke (4), pancreatitis (2), bone marrow failure (1), and pulmonary embolism (1). It is reasonable to assume that our treatment, namely glucocorticoids with or without cytotoxics, was responsible for the opportunistic infections in 12 patients, and that cyclophosphamide was the cause of the cytotoxic lung disease in 2 patients. It is even possible that the five neoplasms may have in some way been related to immunosuppressant therapy by way of impaired immune surveillance. Conceivably, then, 19 of the 43 deaths could be attributable directly or indirectly to treatment. Such statistics cause one to reflect on the possibility we may be overtreating some patients and we should be more cautious in our use of these powerful immunosuppressant agents. It is also important to note that we have detected 3 carcinomas of the urinary bladder in patients treated with cyclophosphamide.

In the context of an ominous disease such as Wegener's granulomatosis, it is understandable why physicians feel compelled to use strong treatment. Our experience would suggest, however, that there may be room for more judicious use of glucocorticoids and cyclophosphamide. In this regard, experience has led me to a few generalizations. In the acutely ill patient who may have necrotic lesions of the skin as well as the respiratory tract serving as large portals for infection, the simultaneous use of glucocorticoids and cyclophosphamide appears to invite serious systemic infection. Therefore, I would recommend doses of prednisone of 60-80 mg daily (parenteral if necessary) alone until the acute inflammation is brought under control and healing has begun. This may take seven to ten days. When control is perceived, cyclophosphamide can be introduced at 2 mg/kg/day. The effect of cyclophosphamide on the primary disease process appears to be delayed for two to three weeks. When the effect of cyclphosphamide has been established, prednisone can be withdrawn over a period compatible with the patient's improving or stable status. The use of bolus, high dose, intravenous glucocorticoids, such as Solu-Medrol is, in my mind, of questionable value and I know of no good data to support its use in Wegener's granulomatosis. I have customarily continued cyclophosphamide one year beyond last evidence of disease activity. This is an entirely arbitrary duration, although shorter periods of administration seem to be associated with higher rates of relapse. I customarily monitor leukocyte counts at three weeks intervals, interrupting cyclophosphamide when leukocyte counts drop below 3000 per mm^3.

If the patient presents with an indolent, slow moving course, it may be appropriate to begin with cyclophosphamide alone. Activity may be assessed from a number of parameters which must be individualized. These may include direct observation of lesions of the respiratory mucosa or skin, the chest roentgenogram, hemoglobin, erythrocyte sedimentation rate, urine sediment, and tests of renal function.

Chlorambucil and azathioprine are agents of second choice, to be tried in patients who are unable to tolerate cyclophosphamide.

Appreciating the causes of death that may be attributable to immunosuppressant treatment, an effective treatment of low toxicity and high tolerance seems highly desirable in the late 1980's. In 1985, we[14] published our initial experience with 12 patients having Wegener's granulomatosis who were treated either primarily or secondarily with trimethoprim/sulfamethoxazole combination (T/S). This experience was grown to 28 patients. When last analyzed, two patients experienced no response and were shifted to conventional regimens. Three patients died after failing both conventional regimens with prednisone and cyclophosphamide as well as T/S. However, it is encouraging to note that 23 of our patients have experienced significant improvement on T/S. In 11 patients, T/S was the sole agent used. Our first patient began treatment in 1975 and is living without evidence of active Wegener's granulomatosis at the time of this writing. She continues to take trimethoprim/sulfa daily and has experienced no measurable side-effects. I reported these interesting observations ten years after the original was made, as I wanted to be absolutely certain of their validity.

The addition of T/S to our armamentarium provides us with an exciting and safe alternative to glucocorticoids and cytotoxics. I would hasten to emphasize that all patients to not respond to T/S, but neither do many to conventional regimens including prednisone and cyclophosphamide. What is the current place for T/S in our considerations for treatment? Since we are early in our experience, I would continue to advise cautious application to those patients having indolent courses. For those having explosive presentations with renal disease and other evidence of widespread systemic vasculitis, I would continue to initiate treatment with glucocorticoids with a subsequent addition of cyclophosphamide. However, a trial of glucocorticoids plus T/S would not be unreasonable even in the acute patient. For those with indolent courses, particularly for lesions confined to the upper respiratory tract, I feel T/S should be initial treatment given a six to eight week trial before considering addition of other more toxic agents.

Recently, Dr. Harold Israel[15] of Jefferson Medical School in Philadelphia has communicated to me his experience with T/S, having now accumulated eight patients who have responded to such treatment. Furthermore, in patients treated previously with standard regimens he feels the relapse rate has been significantly reduced by the addition of T/S for long-term treatment.

How does T/S work? This I cannot tell you. Two main hypotheses are raised. T/S could act as an anti-inflammatory immunosuppressant agent such as glucocorticoids and cytotoxic agents. Alternatively, Wegener's granulomatosis may be caused by a microbe sensitive to T/S. I know of no firm evidence to support either hypothesis. Experience with T/S implicating a possible microbial infection supports the theory propounded by Wegener 50 years ago.

The current mystery surrounding the effect of T/S should serve as a provocative stimulus for future research into the cause of this fascinating disease.

REFERENCES
1. Klinger H (1931) Frankfurter Ztschr Path 42:455-480
2. Wegener F (1936) Verh Dtsch Path Ges 29:202-210
3. Wegener F (1939) Beitr Zur Path Anat 102:36-68
4. Godman GC, Churg J (1954) AMA Arch Path 58:533-553
5. Fienberg R (1955) Am J Med 19:829-831
6. Carrington CB, Liebow AA (1966) Am J Med 41:497-527
7. Fienberg R (1981) Human Path 12:458-467
8. DeRemee RA, McDonald TJ, Harrison EG Jr, Coles DT (1976) Mayo Clin Proc 51:777-781
9. Van der Woude FJ, Rasmussen N, Lobatto S, Wiik A, Permin H, Van Es LA, Van der Giessen M, Van der Hem GK, The TH (1985) Lancet 23:425-429
10. Colby TV (In Press) Sem Resp Med
11. Fauci AS, Haynes BF, Katz P, Wolff SM (1983) Ann Int Med 98:76-85
12. Moore PM, Beard EE, Thoburn TW, Williams HL (1951) Laryngoscope 61:320-331
13. Walton EW (1958) Brit Med J 2:265-270
14. DeRemee RA, McDonald, TJ, Weiland LH (1985) Mayo Clin Proc 60:27-32
15. Israel H Personal communication

© 1988 Elsevier Science Publishers B.V (Biomedical Division)
Sarcoidosis and other granulomatous disorders
C. Grassi, G. Rizzato, E. Pozzi, editors

THE LIVER-LUNG INTERFACE

SHEILA SHERLOCK

Royal Free Hospital School of Medicine, Pond Street, London NW3 2QG, England

INTRODUCTION

The interests of the Pneumonologist and the Hepatologist overlap in many ways (1). Pulmonary changes, particularly in the circulation, are a feature of hepato-cellular failure. The lungs and liver may be involved simultaneously in a pathological process, for instance, sarcoidosis, an infection such as Q fever, or a metabolic abnormality, for instance, alpha-1-antitrypsin deficiency. Diseases which are considered autoimmune can affect both organs. A disease may commence in the lung, but be diagnosed because of hepatic involvement, for instance, lung cancer. Finally, the selection of patients for liver transplantation and the pulmonary complications developing after the operation must be considered.

Pulmonary Changes Complicating Chronic Hepatocellular Disease (Table 1)

Hypoxia

Intrapulmonary shunting

Ventilation-perfusion mismatch

Reduced transfer factor

Pleural effusion

Raised diaphragms

Basal atelectasis

Primary portal hypertension

Porto-pulmonary shunting

Chest X-ray mottling

Reduced arterial oxygen saturation and cyanosis are found in about a third of patients with hepatic cirrhosis. These are due largely to intra-pulmonary shunting through microscopic arterio-venous fistulae. The peripheral branches of the pulmonary artery are markedly dilated. Rarely actual pulmonary arterio-venous shunts can be demonstrated by pulmonary angiography including angioscintography (2). Such shunts may be confirmed by infusions of micropaque gelatin into the pulmonary vascular tree at autopsy (3). The picture at angiography is of a spongy appearance of the basal pulmonary vessels corresponding to the infiltrates seen on chest roentgenograms in patients with chronic liver disease (4).

PULMONARY CHANGES IN LIVER FAILURE

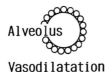 Arteriovenous shunting

Alveolus   Ventilation – perfusion
                        mismatch

Vasodilatation

Capillary   Transfer factor ↓

Wall thickened

Reduction of diffusing capacity is present without a restrictive
ventilatory defect (5).   This is likely to be due to dilatation of small
pulmonary blood vessels, a complication of advanced cirrhosis (6).
Reduction in transfer factor is a consistent finding, perhaps related to
thickening of the walls of the small veins and capillaries by a layer of
collagen (6).   Lung perfusion studies show dilated pulmonary capillaries
and/or arterio-venous communications (7).   The pulmonary vaso-dilation is
associated with a low pulmonary vascular resistence which fails to respond
to hypoxia (8).   This leads to failure of the lung to match perfusion with
ventilation (9).   Even in those who retain hypoxic pulmonary vaso-constriction,
the pulmonary artery pressure is low in the face of hypoxia and a raised
carbon dioxide.

   Porto-pulmonary anastomoses have been demonstrated but are unlikely to
contribute to arterial oxygen desaturation as the portal vein has a high
oxygen content.   Moreover, the flow through them is probably small.

   The pulmonary changes of hepato-cellular failure may thus be summed up
as pulmonary vaso-dilation with pulmonary arterio-venous shunting combined
with ventilation-perfusion inequality (10).   The mechanisms remain uncertain.
A pulmonary vaso-dilator is probably responsible, but whether this is due to

failure of production by the diseased liver or failure of metabolism is uncertain. False sympathetic neuro-transmitters, such as octopamine or hydroxyphenylethanolamines coming from the gut and bypassing the diseased liver have been incriminated. However, although there is substantial sympathetic innervation in the pulmonary vasculature, endogenous norepinephrine has little effect on resting pulmonary vascular tone. Circulating false neuro-transmitters would thus be unlikely to lower pulmonary artery pressures or to interfere with hypoxic pulmonary vaso-constriction (11). Endotoxin inhibits pulmonary hypoxic vaso-constriction in the experimental animal (12). Ferritin is another candidate (13). Plasma vaso-active intestinal peptide is increased, but its role in the circulatory changes is uncertain (14). An immuno-reactive substance, "P", is markedly increased in the plasma of patients with hepatic coma. This is associated with decreased systemic vascular assistance and increased cardiac index (15). Finally, the endogenous prostaglandins recontribute to the increased cardiac output and general diminished vascular resistence observed in cirrhosis of the liver (16). There have been very few studies of actual levels of possible vaso-dilator substances in patients with cirrhosis and pulmonary changes. However, in two patients with cirrhosis and hypoxia due to pulmonary arterio-venous shunting, hormone levels (sex hormones, serotonin, prostaglandins and intestinal hormones) were normal, and treatment with oestrogens, CPD choline and indomethacin was ineffective (16).

Primary pulmonary hypertension is a rare complication of cirrhosis (17). It has been associated with severe hepato-cellular disease, with or without a portal systemic shunt. It can also accompany extra-hepatic portal hypertension and a large portal-systemic collateral circulation (18). Histometric investigation of the muscular-type arteries of the pulmonary vasculature may show dilatation and thickening of the wall and rarely thrombi (19). Plexogenic pulmonary arteriopathy - that is, focal dilatation of pulmonary arteries of 10 to 200 m in diameter, endothelial cell proliferation surrounding vascular channels and within the vessel lumen, and concentric fibrosis of the interma, once thought to be pathognomonic for pulmonary hypertension have been found at autopsy in patients with cirrhosis (19). The patients with clinical pulmonary hypertension have dilated main pulmonary arteries in chest X-rays (17). The cause of the pulmonary hyper-tension is not known. It may be part of the general hyperdynamic circulatory state of cirrhosis with its high cardiac output. Diversion of splenic blood into the pulmonary circulation may be important (17).

Pulmonary hypertension can follow multiple tumour emboli to the pulmonary microvasculature in patients with hepatocellular carcinoma (20).

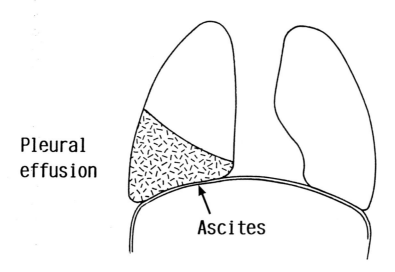

A pleural effusion is found in about 6% of cirrhotic patients and in 67% of these it is right-sided (21).   It is due to defects in the diaphragm allowing ascites to pass into the pleural cavity.   Pleural effusions may even develop in the absence of ascites.   Here ascitic fluid is believed to be drawn through defects in the diaphragm directly into the pleural space by intrathoracic-peritoneal pressure gradients (22).

Finally, pulmonary function in cirrhotics may be reduced by the high diaphragm secondary to hepatomegaly or massive ascites.

Liver Involvement in Granulomatous Pulmonary Diseases

Granulomas are found in 4 to 10% of needle liver biopsies and in 10% of these no cause is found even after noting specific histological characteristics, staining for causative organisms and culture of the specimen (23).   The granulomas vary between 50 and 200 m .   This compares with an aspiration liver biopsy specimen having a width of 1000 m .   Serial sections must therefore be cut and stained if granulomas are to be identified. Hepatic tranulomas are always part of a generalised disease process. Their presence in the liver as part of a predominantly pulmonary disease may allow diagnosis of the chest condition and assist in prognosis.

The Liver in Sarcoidosis

Granulomas are found in liver biopsies from about 67% of patients with pulmonary sarcoidosis (1).   Liver biopsy may offer a diagnosis where less invasive techniques have failed.   The hepatic granulomas are not usually associated with symptoms.   Occasionally, they may result in a rise in serum alkaline phosphtase.   However, massive hepatic involvement leads to healing with fibrosis and the histological picture resembles hepatic cirrhosis. In some patients, portal zone granulomas and fibrosis result in pre-sinusoidal portal hypertension, oesophageal varices and haematemesis (24). Sinusoidal fibrosis may contribute (25).   Sometimes severe intrahepatic cholestasis can complicate sarcoidosis (26, 27).   The patients are usually young blacks.   The clinical picture mimics primary biliary cirrhosis very closely (28) (table 2).   The overlap is stressed by four patients who showed positive serum mitochondrial antibodies (diagnostic of primary biliary cirrhosis) with hepatic granulomas and three of whom had lung granulomas. All had predominant pulmonary symptoms with pleuritic pain, dyspnoea and dry cough.   Hepatic histology suggested primary biliary cirrhosis (29).

HEPATIC GRANULOMAS ASSOCIATED WITH CHOLESTASIS

	Sarcoidosis	Primary biliary cirrhosis
Hepatic histology	?	?
SACE	↑	↑
Sex F:M	Equal	8:1
Respiratory	Yes	No
Kveim	+ve	-ve
S.Mitochondrial Ab	-ve	+ve (99%)

The similarities between sarcoidosis and primary biliary cirrhosis is also stressed by the finding of T-lymphocytes (predominantly T-4 positive cells) and activated alveolar macrophages by broncho-alveolar lavage in patients with primary biliary cirrhosis, similar findings to those of sarcoidosis (30).

Sarcoidosis has also been reported in association with the Budd-Chiari syndrome. The hepatic veins were narrowed by sarcoid granulomas forming the mechanical basis for venous stasis and extensive thrombotic occlusions (31).

Pulmonary Changes in Autoimmune Liver Diseases

Autoimmune "lupoid" chronic active hepatitis: over the years various pulmonary complications have been described in association with autoimmune "lupoid" chronic active hepatitis, a recognised multisystem disease (1). Unfortunately, few are documented by pulmonary histology or function studies. Earlier series, published before the identification of hepatitis B markers, undoubtedly included examples of chronic viral active hepatitis. Nevertheless, there does seem to be an association between autoimmune chronic active hepatitis, pleurisy and transitory pulmonary infiltrations when the disease is active (32).

Primary Biliary Cirrhosis: the overlap between cholestatic sarcoidosis and primary biliary cirrhosis has already been discussed.

Abnormal pulmonary gas transfer studies have been reported often associated with an abnormal chest roentgenogram showing nodules and interstitial fibrosis. Lung biopsies show interstitial lung disease (33, 34). Pulmonary interstitial giant cell granulomas have also been described (26).

The CREST syndrome can complicate primary biliary cirrhosis and is accompanied by interstitial pneumonitis and pulmonary vascular abnormalities (34).

THE LIVER IN THE ACQUIRED IMMUNODEFICIENCY SYNDROME (AIDS)

Pulmonary infections, particularly opportunistic, are features of the AIDS syndrome. The liver is similarly involved in these infections, often with granuloma formation. Liver biopsy may be an appropriate method for diagnosis and for confirmation of the causative organism. Patients with AIDS show modest increases in serum transaminase levels. Serum alkaline phosphatase is usually increased if hepatic granulomas are present.

Liver biopsy shows fatty change, focal necrosis (often due to cytomegala infection) and Kupffer cell iron (35). Granulomas are frequent, about a third of AIDS sufferers showing these lesions in the liver (36, 37).

Similarly, pulmonary granulomas are frequently found. These granulomas are usually ill-defined and formed largely of foamy histocytes. They have a lack of peripheral lymphocyte cuffing and a paucity of T-4 cells. It is perhaps surprising that hepatic granulomas are so frequent in these immuno-compromised patients as factors known to suppress the activity of T-lymphocytes have been shown to have a suppressive effect on the expression of granulomatous hypersensitivity. However, such inefficient ill-formed histocyte granulomas have been associated with a decreased ratio of helper to suppressor T-cells (38).

PULMONARY COMPLICATIONS OF OESOPHAGEAL SCLEROTHERAPY

Oesophageal varices may be obliterated by the injection of a sclerosant introduced via the endoscope (1). This may be done followed by a later course of sclerotherapy so that all the varices are obliterated. The sclerosants used include sodium morrhuate, ethanolamine oleate, polydocanol and sodium tetradecyl sulphate. Fever, chest pain, usually retrosternal and non-pleuritic, and dysphagia are frequent complications (39). The pain is probably due to tissue extravasation and sometimes to oesophageal ulceration. Pleural effusions, right, left or bilateral have been identified after 31 of 65 (48%) sclerotherapy sessions (40). They are most frequent in those who suffer chest pain and have a large volume of sclerosant injected. At thoracentesis the pleural fluid has the characteristics of an exudate. It is probably due to inflammation of the mediastinal parietal pleura. Others have found a much lower prevalence of pleural effusion after sclerotherapy and have found no significant differences in lung function, gas exchange or ventilation/perfusion scans before and after the procedure (41). The reduced incidence has been related to the use of sodium tetradecyl sulphate rather than sodium morrhuate.

Aspiration pneumonia is another complication (42). Multiple invasions of large venous channels through a needle contaminated with salivary microflora might be expected to be associated with a high frequency of bacteremia, especially in cirrhotic patients with a compromised immune system. This would contribute to the aspiration pneumonia.

Acute respiratory distress syndrome may complicate oesophageal sclerotherapy with sodium morrhuate. It is suggested that the sclerosant causes pulmonary hypertension and pulmonary oedema due to increased efflux of fluid with a relatively low protein concentration from the pulmonary vasculature. This suggestion is based on studies in a sheep model and has not been confirmed by measurement of oedema fluid protein concentration in patients who undergo oesophageal sclerotherapy.

Broncho-esophageal fistula formation has been described after endoscopic sclerotherapy (43). Severe hypoxaemka due to right to left shunting with a PaO2 of less than 50 mm/Hg is anabsolute contra-indication to transplantation (44). In the presence of any infection, including pulmonary, the one year survival drops from 60 to 70% to 30 to 40%.

Involvement of the lungs and liver in a metabolic process such as alpha-1-antitrypsin deficiency may contra-indicate the operation. However, patients with severe cirrhosis due to this cause have undergone successful transplantation and the lung lesions are said to regress. In other patients, intrahepatic shunts have not closed even though the liver transplant was successful (45).

In the early days after hepatic transplantation, mechanical factors contribute to pulmonary complications. Air emboli in the venous system passing through an abnormal pulmonary vasculature can cause cerebral air emboli (45). This has been prevented by improved surgical techniques. The right diaphragm is paralysed and right lower lobe atelactasis is common. This results in significant respiratory embarrassment (45,46). This is treated by physiotherapy, and if necessary, therapeutic bronchoscopy. In one series 20% underwent bronchoscopy, and this is now often being carried out repetitively at the bedside in the intensive care until until there is complete resolution of the atelectasis (45).

Pleural effusion occurs in almost all patients. However, in only about 18% is aspiration necessary (46).

After transplant, the pulmonary consultant plays an important part in identifying and treating pulmonary infections in patients who have undergone a six to eight hour abdominal operation and who are being given immuno-suppressive drugs including cyclosporin, corticosteroids and often azathioprine. Intense prophylactic treatment with antibiotics contributes (47). About 18.7% have pulmonary infections including pneumonia, empyema and lung abscesses (46). Intense prophylactic treatment with antibiotics contributes. Causes include a variety of bacterial, viral and fungal agents, as well as Legionella and pneumocysts carinii. Many of these infections occur after discharge from the hospital in patients with well-functioning liver grafts. Fungal infections (candida, aspergillosis and cryptococcus) are particularly common. Candidiasis may be disseminated with grave pulmonary manifestations and a very poor prognosis (48).

Cytomegaly infection is common and usually asymptomatic. Epstein-Barr, herpes simplex and varicella-zoster can also be associated with pulmonary infection.

During the operation and post-operatively, intravenous administration of

blood products may lead to circulatory overload and pulmomary oedema (49).
Azathioprine has been related to interstitial pneumonitis (50), and
pulmonary oedema (51, 52).

Intravenous cyclosporin given soon after liver transplantation has been
related to two patients dying from fatal adult respiratory distress
syndrome (53).   This is presumably related to the high concentrations of
cyclosporin in the pulmonary veins.   It does not seem to follow peripheral
intravenous use of the drug.   Aspiration pneumonia is another possible
cause.

SUMMARY

Chronic liver failure (cirrhosis) is marked by pulmonary circulatory
changes summed up as pulmonary vaso-dilatation with pulmonary arterio-
venous shunting combined with ventilation-perfusion inequality.
Fulminant hepatic failure is associated with pulmonary oedema.

Pleural effusion in cirrhotic patients is largely due to defects in
the diaphragh allowing the passage of ascitic fluid from the abdomen.

Hepatic granulomas have numerous causes but in 10% the aetiology
remains unknown even after the fullest possible investigation.

Cholestasis in a small proportion of patients with chronic sarcoidosis
mimics primary biliary cirrhosis very closely.   Hepatic granulomas are
surprisingly frequent in patients with the AIDS syndrome.   They may
give the diagnosis of the associated opportunist infection.

Patients having sclerotherapy for oesophageal varices have frequent
pulmonary complications including chest pain, pleural effusion and
aspiration pneumonias.   The patient having a hepatic transplant has
many pulmonary complications.   They may simply be those expected from a
long serious operation.   Intensive antibiotic and immunosuppressive
therapy contributes.   Pulmonary fungal infections may b e persistent
and fatal.

REFERENCES

1.   Sherlock S (1983) In: Diseaeses of the Liver and Biliary System.
      7th ed. Blackwell Scientific Publications Oxford

2.   Vergnon J M, de Bonadona J F, Riffat J et al (1986)   Rev
      mal Resp 3: 145-151

3.   Berthelot P, Walker J G, Sherlock S, Reid L (1986)   N Engl
      J Med 274: 292-298

4.   Sang O H K, Bender T M, Bowen A, Ledesma-Medina J (1983)
      Paediat Radiol 13: 111-115

5.   Stanley N M, Woodgate D J (1972)   Thorax 27: 315-323

6.   Stanley N N, Williams A J, Dewar G A, Blendis L M, Reid L
      (1977) Thorax 32: 457-471

7.   Wolfe J D, Tashkin D P, Holly F E et al (1977) Am J Med 63:
      746-753

8.   Dauod F S, Reeves J H, Schaefer J W (1972)   J Clin Invest 51:
      1076-1080

9.   Furukawa T, Hara N, Yasumoto K, Inokuchi K (1984)   Am J Med
      Sci 287: 10-13

10.   Yao E H, Kong B, Hsue G et al (1987) Am J Gastro 81: 352-354

11.   Naeije R, Melot C, Hallemans R, Mans P, Lejeune P (1985)   Sem
      Resp Med 7: 164-170

12.   McDonnell P J, Toye P A, Hutchins G M (1983)   Am Rev Respir Dis
      127: 437-441

13.   Keren G, Boichis H, Zwas T S, Frand M.   Pulmonary arterio-
      venous fistulae in hepatic cirrhosis   Arch Dis Child 58: 302-304

14.   Henriksen J H, Staun-Olsen P, Fahrenkrug P, Ring-Larsen H (1980)
      Scand J Gastroent 15: 787-792

15.   Hortnagel H, Singer E A, Lenz K, Kleinberger G, Lochs H (1984)
      Lancet 1: 480-483

16.   Bruix J, Bosch J, Kravetz D, Mastai R, Rhodes J (1985)
      Gastroenterology 88: 430-435

17.   Lebrec D, Capron J P, Dhubaux D, Benhamou J P (1979)   Am Rev
      Resp Dis 120: 849-855

18.   Cohen M D, Rubin L J, Taylor W E, Cuthbert J A (1983)
      Hepatology 3: 588-592

19.   Matsubara O, Nakamura T, Uehart T, Kasuga T (1984)   J Path 143:
      31-37

20.   Willett I R, Sutherland R C, O'Rourke M F, Dudley F J (1984)
      Gastroenterology 87: 1180-1184

21.   Lieberman F L, Hidemura R, Peters R L, Reynolds T B (1966)
      Ann intern Med 64: 341-351

22.   Vargas-Tank L, Escobar C, Fernandez G et al (1984)   Scand J
      Gastroenterol 19: 294-298

23.   Scheuer P J (1980)   In: Liver Biopsy Interpretations 3rd ed.
      Bailliere-Tindall, London

24.   Tekeste H, Latour F, Levitt R E. (1984)   Am J Gastroenterol
      79: 389-396

25. Valla D, Pessegueiro-Miranda H, Degott C et al (1980)   Quart
     J Med 63 NS: 531-544

26. Stanley N N, Fox R A, Whimster W F, Sherlock S, James D G (1972)
     New Engl J Med 287: 1282-1284

27. Rudzki C, Ishak K G, Zimmerman H J (1975)   Am J Med 59: 373-387

28. Bass N M, Burroughs A K, Scheuer P J, James D G, Sherlock S (1982)
     Gut 23: 417-421

29. Fagan E A, Moore-Gillon J C, Turner-Warwick M (1983) New Engl
     J Med 30': 572-575

30. Wallaert B, Bonniere P, Prin L et al (1986)   Chest 90: 842-848

31. Russi E W, Bansky G, Pfaltz M, Spinas G, Hammer B, Senning A
     (1986) Am J Gastro 81: 71-75

32. Golding P L, Smith M, Williams R (1973)   Am J Med 55: 772-782

33. Weissman E, Becker N H (1983)   Am J Med Sci 285: 21-27

34. Davidson A G, Epstein O (1983)   Thorax 38: 316-317

35. Lebovics E, Thung S N, Schaffner F, Radensky P W (1985) Hepatology
     3: 293-298

36. Gordon S C, Reddy K R, Gould E E et al (1986)   J Hepatol (Amsterdam)
     2: 475-484

37. Jagad H A, Andavolu R H, Huang C T (1985)   Am J Clin Path 84:
     298-602

38. Modlin R I, Hofman F M, Meyer P R, Sharma O P, Taylor C R, Rea T H
     (1983)   Clin Exp Immunol 51: 430-438

39. Ayres S J, Goff J S, Warren G H (1983)   Ann intern Med 98:
     900-903

40. Bacon B R, Bailey-Newton R S, Connors A F Jr (1985) Gastroenterology
     88: 1910-1914

41. Korula J, Baydur A, Sassoon C, Sakimura I (1984) Gastrointest
     Endosc 30: 134-135 (abstract)

42. Larson A W, Cohen H, Zweiban B et al (1986)   JAMA 255: 497-500

43. Carr-Locke D L, Sidky K (1982)   Gut 23: 1005-1007

44. Iwatsuki S, Shaw B W Jr, Starzl T E (1983)   Sem Liv Dis 3: 173-180

45. Krowka M J, Cortese D A (1985) Mayo Clin Proc 60: 407-418

46. Wood R P, Shaw B W Jr, Starzl T E (1985) Sem Liv Dis 5: 377-384

47. Dummer J S, Hardy J, Poorsattar A, Ho M (1983)   Transplantation
     36: 259-267

48. Wajsczuk C P, Dummer J S, Ho M et al (1983)   Transplantation 36:
     347-353

49. Van Thiel D H, Schade R R, Gavaler J S, Shaw B W Jr, IwatsukiS,
     Starzl T E (1983)   Hepatology 4 suppl: 79-83

50. Bendrossian C W M, Sussman J, Conklin R H, Kahan B (1984) Am J
     Clin Path 82: 148-154

51. Sloane J P, Depledge M H, Powles R L, Morgenstern G R, Trickey B S,
     Dady P J (1983)   J Clin Pathol 36: 546-554

70

52. Barrett A J, Kendra J R, Lucas C F, Joss D V, Joshi R, Pendharkar
     P, Hugh-Jones K (1982)   Br Med J 285: 162-166

53. Powell-Jackson P R, Carmichael F J L, Calne R Y, Williams R (1984)
     Transplantation 18: 341-343

THE SARCOID GRANULOMA FORMATION — IMMUNOLOGY

© 1988 Elsevier Science Publishers B.V. (Biomedical Division)
Sarcoidosis and other granulomatous disorders
C. Grassi, G. Rizzato, E. Pozzi, editors

THE SARCOID GRANULOMA FORMATION - IMMUNOLOGY

STATE OF THE ART

Gianpietro Semenzato

Padua University School of Medicine, Department of Clinical Medicine,

1st Medical Clinic and Clinical Immunology Branch, 35128 Padua, Italy

Recent immunological studies have greatly improved our understanding of

several pathogenetic mechanisms in sarcoidosis (1-3). First of all, full credit

for advances in this field must be given to the bronchoalveolar lavage (BAL) and

to the immunohistological techniques. Although the role of BAL as a routine

diagnostic procedure is still controversial, it has been invaluable in providing

access to cell populations derived from the sites of active inflammation and

granuloma formation, in particular allowing to recover the cells accounting for

the alveolitis in sarcoid lung (4-6). In this regard, consistent evidence has

been provided for a concordance between the types of cells present in the lung

parenchyma and those present in the lavage fluid (7-9). On the other hand,

immunohistological analysis allows the study of tissue sections from both the

lung and different sites of disease involvement (10-15). In fact, sarcoidosis is

a multisystem disorder in which multiple organs need to be studied

simultaneously. The availability of these techniques, coupled with the technology

of monoclonal antibodies, cell culture facilities, and the possibility to assay

many of mediators of immune responses, have led to the fundamental concept that the alveolitis, as well as the cellular infiltration in involved organs, is characterized by activated helper Í cells and macrophages (1-15).

To make a traditional state of the art review, at this point I should analyze in depth and describe the different steps that lead to the T helper cell compartmentalization and their aggregation with macrophages to form discrete granulomas. Since these concepts have been extensively reviewed (2,3,16,17), it seems rather appropriate for me to make a brief historical overview herein of the key events in the conceptual development of sarcoid immunology over the last decades up to this point and to discuss those areas that I believe will offer comparable intellectual challenges and upon which the progress of this field may be built.

In the seventies, immunological studies were focused on the analysis of phenotypical and functional evaluations of mononuclear cells in the blood of sarcoid patients using the traditional markers, notably E rosetting, surface immunoglobulins and phytohemoagglutinin in vitro response. However, we did not have very much in terms of comprehension of the pathogenesis of this disease from blood studies. Major clues to the understanding of pathogenetic events have come from the evaluation of cells at sites of disease activity, mainly from the study of cells recovered from the bronchoalveolar lavage. These studies were performed in the late seventies and early eighties and presented at the Cardiff, Paris, and Baltimore Conferences. In Cardiff, in 1978, for the first time the concept of cellular compartmentalization was introduced. Since then, studies at the different sites of disease activity have been focused upon and have drawn the interests of sarcoidosis immunologists. At the time of the Paris conference, in 1981, monoclonal antibodies had become available and the evaluation of cells recovered from the lavage with these reagents greatly improved our knowledge. At the Baltimore Conference immunological studies focused on the analysis of different lymphokines accounting for cell accumulation and growth at different sites of disease activity.

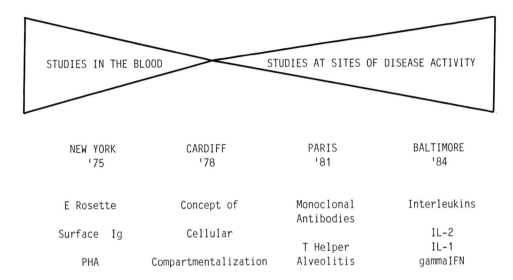

NEW YORK '75	CARDIFF '78	PARIS '81	BALTIMORE '84
E Rosette	Concept of	Monoclonal Antibodies	Interleukins
Surface Ig	Cellular	T Helper	IL-2 IL-1
PHA	Compartmentalization	Alveolitis	gammaIFN

Figure 1.   Life history of immunological studies in sarcoidosis

What about studies performed in the years between Baltimore and Milan? Many of the results of different research programs conducted during this period are reported in papers included in the present book. It is anticipated herein that the evaluation of the lymphocytic component of alveolitis has been further investigated. The idea that Interleukin(IL)-2 is the major substance accounting for an exaggerated, relatively uninhibited, proliferation of lung T cells has been further substantiated and the cell subset releasing this substance precisely characterized (18). In addition, the release of an inhibitor of macrophage migration has been demonstrated, which may contribute to the macrophagic accumulation (19). More importantly, studies during these last three years have been directed towards the phenotype and function of alveolar macrophages in sarcoidosis. With regard to the phenotype, it has been shown that alveolar

76

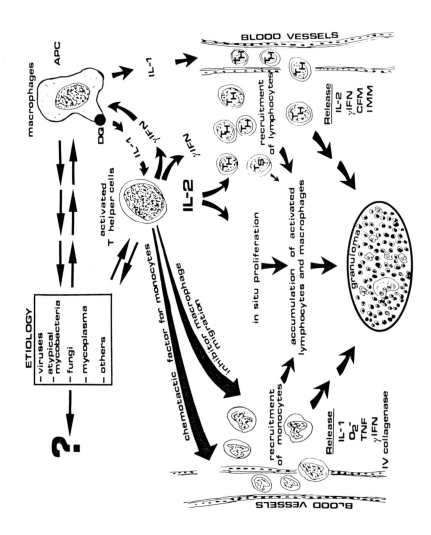

Figure 2. Mechanisms leading to the granuloma formation

macrophages express IL-2 receptors (20,21) and determinants usually present on peripheral monocytes (20,22). In terms of functional properties, besides IL-1, a number of new substances released by activated macrophages have been evidenced, including cytotoxic factors (23), superoxide anion (24), type IV collagenase (25), gamma interferon (26,27), and tumor necrosis factor (28). The latter has been demonstrated to display a chemotactic function on monocyte (29).

Another topic that has been investigated is the relationship between lymphocytes and macrophages and other antigen-presenting cells. An ehanced surface density of Class II molecules of the major histocompatibility complex has been demonstrated on alveolar macrophages from sarcoid patients (30,31). In this regard, the density of antigenic molecules involved in the antigen presentation is crucial to understanding the mechanisms leading to the intercellular communications. In fact, cell interactions are regulated by these antigenic molecules, in particular the DQ molecules. Also, the magnitude of the proliferative response is a function of the product of antigen concentration and the number of Ia molecules expressed on antigen presenting cells, in particular on macrophages. All these studies allowed the delineation of the pathogenetic events leading to granuloma formation as illustrated in Figure 2. Under the influence of an unknown inciting stimulus and following cooperation with macrophages, activated helper T lymphocytes proliferate in an exaggerated way and release a series of mediators. All together, these lymphokines contribute in maintaining the granuloma formation by amplifying the immune responses through the induction of cellular growth at sites of ongoing inflammation and by the accumulation of newly recruited lymphocytes and macrophages from the bloodstream.

In this model however, several doubts still persist. One concerns IL-2. If IL-2 does in fact mediate the in situ activities during granuloma formation, then the ineffectiveness of cyclosporin on sarcoid patients remains a mystery (32). We could tentatively presume that the cyclosporin does not reach the lung. Alternatively, we could suppose that IL-2 does not behave as the central activator, with other substances perhaps playing the crucial role in initiating all these mechanisms, for instance those released by activated macrophages (23-28). Since cyclosporin is not effective on cells belonging to the monocyte/macrophage lineage, this could be the reason why this drug is not helpful in sarcoidosis. Of course other possibilities exist; keep in mind that we are at the very beginning of understanding the physiological rules governing immunity in sarcoidosis. For instance, we still do not know the role of substances such as IL-3 and IL-4 in sarcoid patients. IL-3 is a colony stimulating factor which can recruit new cells from the bone marrow (33) while IL-4 is able to activate both macrophages and B lymphocytes and represents an autocrine growth factor for some helper T cells (34-36). These lymphokines have been recently discovered and have been demonstrated to play an essential role in immunoregulation. Their role in the mechanism of granuloma formations still remains elusive however. Always in terms of biological response modifiers, I would like to quote a paper recently published by a Canadian group which describes a case of pulmonary sarcoidosis following interferon therapy (37). Which came first the chicken or the egg ? A mechanism not yet totally proven in the model represented in the Figure 2 is the release of Interleukin-1 by alveolar macrophages. Some authors suggest that a spontaneous production does exist, while other investigators claim that the T cell activation in sarcoidosis is an IL-1 independent mechanism (38-41). Alternatively, the IL-1 could be released by other cell types at sites of disease activity. Despite the advances that have been made in our understanding of the regulation of immune responses in this disorder, the etiology of sarcoidosis remains an enigma. Unfortunately, we still do not know the inciting stimulus that drives the cellular activation and granuloma formation. I'll discuss the matter of etiology in more detail in a moment.

Up until now, much attention has been payed to lymphocytes and macrophages. However, other populations need further investigation: for instance endothelial and epithelial cells which may be relevant to the regulation of immunological phenomena taking place in sarcoid lung. In fact, endothelial cells express surface Ia antigens and studies at the molecular level have documented the ability of vascular endothelial cells to express the gene for the major form of Interleukin-1 found on human monocytes and are capable of producing significant IL-1 activity in response to appropiate stimuli (42). Thus, this cellular population could represent an alternative source for the IL-1. The solution to this matter could eventually explain the discrepancies I mentioned before in terms of spontaneous production of IL-1 (38-41). In turn, gamma interferon, which is produced by activated cells in sarcoid lung (26,27), could play a crucial role in triggering endothelial cells. Even more, why is IL-1 present in epithelioid cells but not in multinucleated giant cells (43) ? Beside offering an explanation for an alternative source of IL-1, this finding suggests a model for the fate of the sarcoid granuloma. Another cell population that has been studied in the last years is the mast cells and their soluble products, such as histamine (44). In other words, endothelial cells, epithelial cells and perhaps mast cells are pressing to come into the picture illustrated in figure 2 and find their proper place in the scheme of things.

Basic and clinical immunology have progressed rapidly in these days; certainly one of the fields in which major advances have been made is the area of molecular biology. This science, coupled to the recombinant DNA technology, has provided the solution to one of the most vexing of questions, that is the chemical nature of the T cell receptor for antigen. The cloning of genes for the alfa- and beta-chains of the T cell receptor and the determination of the structure of molecules bearing T cell clonotypic determinants has opened the door to rapid progress in the understanding of the structural and genetic basis of the exquisite T cell specificity for antigen. With the methodologies available today we can precisely study the first steps of the cascade of events leading to the granuloma formation, that is the process of interaction between the inciting antigen and cells mediating the immune responses in sarcoidosis. Using the molecular biology technology, we can precisely determine the genes that encode for surface proteins, define the genes turned on and the clonality of the cells we are dealing with. Furthermore, different oncogenes and their products, viral sequences and the viral DNA integration must be determined. Perhaps in this way we can approach the intriguing, but still unsolved problem, of the etiology of sarcoidosis.

The editor of The Lancet in a recent issue of his Journal through an editorial stated ".....what is the etiology of sarcoidosis? This fundamental question remains unanswered. Between 1980 and 1985 there were over seven hundred English-language publications on sarcoidosis; of these only one was an experimental study relating to aetiology. Perhaps it is time for a change of emphasis" (45). In other words, he is claiming that immunological studies were inconclusive. I, personally do not think that it is time to change emphasis. The time has come to utilize the methodologies available today to study the etiology of this disease. As a matter of fact, only now the has molecular biology offered the right techniques to solve this problem. In fact, reviewing the literature on sarcoidosis published between 1960 and 1970 we realize that it is overflowing with papers on the etiology of this disease. Atypical mycobacteria, fungi, mycoplasma, viruses, transmissible agents, allergy, ect. have been explored as potential causes of this disorder. Unfortunately, all these papers were inconclusive. That of course, is not because of the inability of the authors, but because at that time the methodologies to approach the problem were not yet available. How could, for instance, viruses be studied twenty years ago without facilities provided by techniques available today ?

At this conference , a paper will be presented describing the posivitity of a consistent number of sarcoidosis sera for HBLV (46). This is a newly discovered herpes virus which infects B cells (47,48). Is there any relationship with the hypergammaglobulinemia in sarcoidosis? What is the etiological role, if any, of this virus? Does it have a direct role or act only as a co-factor like in some lymphomas? The virus therefore could not represent the final causative event. This could be induced by genetic rearrangements involving the activation of transforming oncogenes in proximity to the cell relevant genes. In this regard, chromosomal abnormalities in sarcoidosis should be investigated and the genes should be mapped especially in those rare cases of familiar sarcoidosis. Of course we can not pretend to find the etiological agent immediately. Perhaps we must suffer for years, step by step. However, do not worry about the Editor of The Lancet. In the next years many papers will be published on the topic of the etiology of sarcoidosis, not in spite of immunology but because of it.

Unfortunately every day these immunological methods seem to become more difficult and sophisticated and often they are not available in every lab. In this regard, I want you to keep in mind that the goal of immunological studies is twofold:

1) the search of the pathobiology and of course the etiology of the disease

2) the search of tests useful for the diagnosis and management of patients

The message I would like to give to all the investigators in the field of immunology of sarcoidosis is that they persue the first route, always keeping in mind the acquisition of the second objective also. The experience of these years has tought us that sarcoidosis is too complex a disorder to be staged using one parameter alone. We can improve the accuracy of our staging by adding new parameters. The clinician needs a test which can indicate the activity of the disease; this test should be: repetitive, suitable, not too disturbing to the patient and, last but not least, easy and quick. For instance, the quantitation of the IL-2 spontaneously released by helper lung T cells or their evaluation in terms of IL-2 mRNA transcripts could be extremely useful (49,50) but, how many centers have the facilities to perform this test ? Can a physician from a small hospital include these parameters in his protocol ? I do not think so. The best test which is not annoying to the patient is the serum sample. In fact, from an instrumental point of view, it is easier to gain access to the blood than to the lung and certainly more repetitive.

Recently two lines of evidence have revealed that markers of disease activity may also be found in the peripheral blood; 1) circulating T cells expressing the interleukin-2 receptor gene (51), and 2) high levels of soluble IL-2 receptors (IL-2R) in the serum of sarcoidosis patients (52,53). Both issues involve the activation pathway related to the IL-2 system. The first point is covered in another part of this book. I would like to comment on the second point. Current concepts on T cell activation (Figure 3) point out that the specific interaction between antigen and major histocompatibility complex restricted T3-Ti receptor structure leads to the transcription and translation of IL-2 and IL-2R genes followed by IL-2 interaction. In turn, this growth hormone

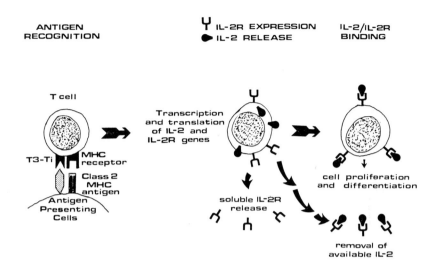

Fig. 3 Model for the IL-2 mediated T cell activation.

system triggers the cascade of events leading to cellular proliferation and then

represents an autocrine apparatus for modulating the immune response. It has been

recently demonstrated that, under specific in vivo and in vitro conditions, the

IL-2R may be released from the cell surface in a soluble form (54,55). It may be

measured using a simple enzyme-linked immunosorbent assay based on the use of two

antibodies developed against two different epitopes of the IL-2R molecules.

Two papers recently published have independently reported an increase of the

soluble IL-2R in the serum of sarcoid patients (52,53). It is reasonable to

suppose that alterations of serum levels of sIL-2R may affect the fine balance

between IL-2 and IL-2R molecules. As a consequence, a down modulation of the

immune response would occur, leading to a defective immunoregulation which could

contribute to the cell abnormalities observed in sarcoid patients. In particular,

since the sIL-2R, like its cellular counterpart, is capable of binding IL-2, it could exert a blocking activity responsible for the removal of the IL-2 necessary for an optimal immune response. This starvation of IL-2 could explain the finding of reduced in vitro proliferative response to mitogens and the impaired helper activity, all these functions being basically mediated by IL-2. Thus, the blocking activity of sIL-2R could represent the major source of the still not defined inhibitory serum factors extensively reported in the peripheral blood of sarcoid patients (56-58). In terms of clinical correlations, Dr. Lawrence and co-workers (53) have demonstrated that a relationship exists between the levels of sIL-2R and the activity of the disease. In a few patients, we measured the soluble IL-2R during the follow-up and we found decreased levels when the clinical course of the disease improved. Further longitudinal studies are needed to assess the suitability of this parameter as a biological marker of disease activity. The evaluation of serum soluble IL-2R may be an effective, non invasive method for estimating different phases of sarcoidosis.

I will close emphasizing the role of immunology, not only in the comprehension of the etiopathogenesis of sarcoidosis, but also in finding new tests useful for the clinical management of these patients, including therapeutical decisions. The major problem nowdays is to ensure that advances of basic research are being creatively and effectively translated into clinical applications. To this end, my final message is to gain a strict collaboration between clinicians and basic reseachers.

REFERENCES

1.   Semenzato G, James DG (1984) Sarcoidosis 1:24

2.   Crystal RG, Bitterman PB, Rennard SI, Hance AJ, Keogh BA (1984) N Engl J Med 310:235

3.   Thomas PD, Hunninghake GW (1987) Am Rev Respir Dis 135:747

4. Reynolds HY (1987) Am Rev Respir Dis 135:250

5. Crystal RG, Reynolds HY, Kalica AR (1986) Chest 90:122

6. Davis GS (1986) Am Rev Respir Dis 133:181

7. Semenzato G, Chilosi M, Ossi E, Trentin L, Pizzolo G, Cipriani A, Agostini C, Zambello R, Marcer G, Gasparotto G (1985) Am Rev Respir Dis 132:400

8. Campbell DA, du Bois RM, Poulter LW (1985) Am Rev Respir Dis 132:1300

9. Paradis IL, Dauber JH, Rabin BS (1986) Am Rev Respir Dis 133:855

10. Semenzato G, Pezzutto A, Chilosi M, Pizzolo G (1982) N Engl J Med 306:48

11. Mishra BB, Poulter LW, Janossy G, James DG (1983) Clin Exp Immunol 54:705

12. Modlin RL, Hofman FM, Meyer PR, Sharma OP, Taylor RR, Rea TH (1983) Clin Exp Immunol 51:430

13. Semenzato G, Pezzutto A, Pizzolo G, Chilosi M, Ossi E, Angi MR, Cipriani (1984) Clin Immunol Immunopathol 30:29

14. van Maarsseveev ACMTH, Mullink H, Alons CL, Stam J (1986) Human Pathol 17:493

15. Semenzato G, Agostini C, Zambello R, Trentin L, Chilosi M, Angi MR, Ossi E, Cipriani A, Pizzolo G (1986) Ann N Y Acad Sci 465:56

16. Daniele RP, Rossman MD, Kern JA, Elias JA (1986) Chest 89:174S

17. Semenzato G (1986) Sem Respir Med 8:17

18. Saltini C, Spurzem JR, Lee JJ, Pinkston P, Crystal RG (1986) J Clin Invest 77:1962

19. Campbell PB, Tolson TA (1986) Am Rev Respir Dis 134:1029

20. Agostini C, Trentin L, Zambello R, Luca M, Masciarelli M, Cipriani A, Marcer A, Semenzato G (1987) J Clin Immunol 7:64

21. Hancock WW, Muller WA, Cotran RS (1987) J Immunol 138:185

22. Hance AJ, Douches S, Winchester RJ, Ferrans V, Crystal RG (1985) J Immunol 134:284

23. Kan-Mitchell J, Hengst JCD, Kempf RA, Rothbart RK, Simons SM, Brooker AS, Kortes VL, Mitchell MS (1985) Cancer Res 45:453

24. Cassatella MA, Agostini C, Luca M, Masciarelli M, Tommasini A, Chilosi

M, Berton G, Semenzato (1986) Sarcoidosis 3:154

25. Garbisa S, Ballin M, Daga-Gordini D, Gastelli G, Mazzoli D, Naturale M, Negro A, Semenzato G, Liotta KA (1986) J Biol Chem 261:2369

26. Robinson BWS, McLemore TL, Crystal RG (1985) J Clin Invest 75:1488

27. Nugent KM, Glazier J, Monick MM, Hunninghake GW (1985) Am Rev Respir Dis 131:714

28. Bachwich PR, Lynch III JP, Larrick J, Spengler M, Kunkel SL (1986) Am J Pathol 125:421

29. Ming WJI, Bersani L, Mantovani A (1987) J Immunol 138:1469

30. Lem VM, Lipscomb MF, Weissler JC, Nunez G, Ball EJ, Stastny P, Toews GB (1985) J Immunol 135:1766

31. Poulter LW, Campbell DA, Butcher RG, du Bois RM (1986) Sarcoidosis 3:155

32. James DG (1988) This Volume

33. Metcalf D (1986) Blood 67:257

34. Grabstein K, Eisenman J, Mochizuki D, Shanebeck K, Conlon P, Hopp T, March C, Gillis S (1986) J Exp Med 163:1405

35. Crawford RM, Finbloom DS, Ohara J, Pawl WE, Meltzer MS (1987) J Immunol 139:135

36. Lichtman AH, Kurrt-Jones EA, Abbas AK (1987) Proc Natl Acad Sci USA 84:824

37. Abdi EA, Nguyen GK, Ludwig RN, Dickout WJ (1987) Cancer 59:896

38. Hunninghake GW (1984) Am Rev Respir Dis 129:569

39. Kleinhenz ME, Fujiwara H, Rich EA (1986) Ann N Y Acad Sci 465:91

40. Eden E, Turino GM (1986) J Clin Immunol 6:326

41. Hudspith BN, Flint KC, James DG, Brostoff J, Johnson NMcI (1987) Thorax 42:250

42. Bank I, Stern DM, Nawroth PP, Cassimeris J, Chess L (1985) Clin Res 33:556A

43. Chilosi M, Bonetti F, Menestrina F, Lestani M, Montagna L, Pizzolo G, Trentin L, Zambello R, Cipriani A, Semenzato G (1988) This Volume

44. Rankin JA, Kaliner M, Reynolds HY (1987) J Allergy Clin Immunol 79:371

45. Editorial (1987) Lancet ii:195

46. Ablashi D, Salahuddin SZ, Imam P, Biberfeld P, Dalghliesh A, Eklund A, Hanngren A, Gallo R. XI Congress on Sarcoidosis, Milan 6-11 September 1987, Abs. p68

47. Salahuddin SZ, Ablashi DV, Markham PD, Josephs SF, Kaplan M, Halligan G, Biberfield P, Wong-Staal F, Kramarsky B, Gallo RC (1986) Science 234:596

48. Josephs SF, Salahuddin SZ, Ablashi DV, Schachter F, Wong-Staal F, Gallo RC (1986) Science 234:601

49. Pinkston P, Bitterman PB, Crystal RG (1983) N Engl J Med 308:793

50. Muller-Quernheim J, Saltini C, Sondermeyr P, Crystal RG (1986) J Immunol 137:3475

51. Konishi K, Saltini C, Moller D, Spurzem J, Crystal RG (1987) Am Rev Respir Dis 135:A28

52. Semenzato G, Cipriani A, Trentin L, Zambello R, Masciarelli M, Vinante F, Chilosi M, Pizzolo G (1987) Sarcoidosis 4:25

53. Lawrence EC, Berger MB, Brousseau KP, Rodriguez TM, Siegel SJ, Kurman CC, Nelson DL (1987) Sarcoidosis 4:87

54. Rubin LA, Kurman CC, Fritz ME, Biddison WE, Boutin B, Yarchoan R, Nelson DL (1985) J Immunol 135:3172

55. Osawa H, Josimovic-Alasevic O, Diamantstein T (1986) Eur J Immunol 16:467

56. Belcher RW, Carney JF, Nankervis GA (1974) Int Arch Allergy 46:183

57. Mangi RJ, Dwyer JM, Kantor FS (1974) Clin Exp Immunol. 18:519

58. Semenzato G, Amadori G, Cipriani A, Tosato F, Gasparotto G (1976) Schweiz Med Wscher 107:1744

DETECTION OF IL-1B IN BRONCHOALVEOLAR LAVAGE FLUIDS FROM SARCOID PATIENTS BY RIA.

C. O'CONNOR[1], A. VanBREDA[1], K. WARD[2], C.ODLUM[2], M.X. FITZGERALD[2].
[1]Dept. of Medicine, University College Dublin. [2] St. Vincent's Hospital, Dublin, Ireland.

INTRODUCTION

Interleukin 1 (IL-1) is one of a group of potent mediators produced by activated monocytes/macrophages which modulate inflammation and tissue regeneration. "In vitro" studies indicate that IL-1 stimulates the production of lymphokines by T-lymphocytes, the proliferation and differentiation of B lymphocytes and the proliferation and activation of fibroblasts (1,2). In addition, IL-1 acts as a chemotactic factor for T-lymphocytes, particularly T-helper cells (3) and as an up-regulator of T-helper phenotype expression (1). As the sarcoid alveolitis is characterised by an increasing number of T-lymphocytes, particularly T-helper cells (4), an examination of the role of IL-1 in sarcoidosis may serve to elucidate disease mechanisms.

The most commonly employed system for detection of IL-1 activity is the thymocyte proliferation or LAF assay. However, in this assay system the presence of IL-1 can be masked by the presence of inhibitors and other effectors. In the present study, a recently introduced radioimmunoassay (RIA) was employed to assess levels of IL-1B directly in bronchoalveolar lavage fluids from patients with sarcoidosis. IL-1B is the major form of IL-1 produced by monocytes/macrophages(5). The sensitivity of the RIA is similar to that of the LAF assay but, unlike the latter, the RIA can detect IL-1B despite the presence of inhibitors or other mediators (such as IL-2, Tumor Necrosis Factor, Interferons or Transforming Growth Factor).

To assess the relationship between IL-1B and the disease process in sarcoidosis, we measured levels of
(i) T-lymphocyte subsets, which reflect alveolitis intensity (4);
(ii) angiotensin converting enzyme (ACE), which reflects granuloma burden(6);
(iii)fibronectin, which acts as a chemoattractant and progression factor for
     fibroblasts (7) and
(iv) Type III procollagen peptide (PCP), which is produced by activated
     fibroblasts (8).

MATERIALS AND METHODS

Study Population

Twenty four newly presenting sarcoid patients (13M, 11F) of mean age 33.4±9.7 yr (range 20-62 yr) underwent bronchoalveolar lavage (BAL). Diagnosis was confirmed by biopsy of various sites (11 node biopsies, 3 lung biopsies and 10 Kveim biopsies). Nine were current smokers. Five healthy volunteers were included in the study as a control group. Pulmonary function tests, performed prior to BAL, indicated normal lung function in control subjects. All subjects gave their informed consent for BAL.

Bronchoalveolar lavage

Before bronchoscopy, patients were given atropine (0.6mg) and pethidine (50mg) i.m. and the upper respiratory tract was anaesthetized with lignocaine spray and lignocaine 2% solution. A fibreoptic bronchoscope (Olympus Model B3R) was securely wedged in a subsegmental bronchus in the right middle lobe, 180 ml of sterile 0.9% saline at 37°C was infused in three 60ml aliquots and gentle suction applied after each infusion. The volume of aspirated fluid was recorded and the fluid strained through sterile surgical gauze to remove mucus. The fluid was then centrifuged at 400g for 15min and the supernatant stored at -20°C for subsequent analysis.

Analysis of BAL cells

The cells recovered from lavage fluid were washed twice in Hank's balanced salt solution (HBSS) without Ca^{++} and Mg^{++} (Gibco Ltd. Scotland), resuspended in HBSS containing 0.5% bovine serum albumin and counted. Cell density was adjusted to 2×10^6 cells/ml and analysed for the presence of Leu-1 +ve (pan T-cells), Leu-2a +ve (cytotoxic/suppressor), Leu-3a +ve (helper/inducer) cells using murine monoclonal antibodies (Becton-Dickinson, Mechelen, Belgium). In brief, cells were incubated with the respective monoclonal antibody at 4°C for 45 min. They were then washed twice in Dulbeccos phosphate buffered saline (PBS, Oxoid, UK) containing 20mM sodium azide. FITC-conjugated goat anti-mouse IgG (Tago Inc. California, USA) was added and samples incubated at 4°C for a further 30 min. Following washing (x3), the cells were re-suspended in a small amount of 90% glycerol and placed on a microscope slide. Fluorescent labelled cells were then counted using a Leitz Dialux 22AB epifluorescent microscope. A mimimum of 200 cells were counted per slide.

BAL Fluid Analysis

IL-1B was measured directly in BAL fluid by radio-immunoassay (Cistron Biotechnology, New Jersey, USA). The detection limit of the assay was 0.25 ng/ml. Fibronectin was measured by an ELISA system as described by Gomez-Lechon and Castell (11). In brief, samples and standards of purified fibronectin (Boehringer Mannheim, GmbH, D-6800 Mannheim 31, FRG) were incubated in 96 well plates (0.1ml/well) at 37°C, pH9.6 for 30min. Following washing (x10) with PBS containing 0.1% Tween-20, rabbit antibody to human fibronectin (Boehringer) was added and plates incubated for 1hr @ 37°C. Unbound antibody was removed by washing (x5) prior to the addition of goat anti-rabbit antiserum

(Hoechst-Behring, Behringwerke AG, Marburg, FRG.). Following a further
incubation (30min, 37°C) wells were again washed (x5) and peroxidase-labelled
rabbit anti-goat serum added (Sigma Chemicals Ltd., Poole, Dorset, UK). After
incubation and thorough washing (x10) o-phenylenediamine and H_2O_2 (pH 5.0) were
added and colour development monitored at 405nm after 30 mins using a Biotech
ELISA plate reader. Sample controls, without the addition of fibronectin
antibody, were included for each sample. The detection limit of the assay was
5ng/ml.

Radiology

Chest roentgenograms were scored according to the Siltzbach classification
system i.e. 0 = no lung involvement; I = hilar adenopathy alone; II = hilar
adenopathy with lung infiltrates and III = lung infiltrates alone.

Statistical Methods

Between group comparisons on BAL data was performed using the Rank Sum test.
Pulmonary function data are expressed as means ± standard error of the mean.

RESULTS

IL-1B was not detected in BAL fluid from any of the control subjects.
However, varying levels of IL-1B were detected in 7(29%) sarcoid patients (mean
level = 0.68ng/ml; range 0.32-1.15ng/ml) (Fig. 1). There was no apparent
association between smoking status and IL-1B. 43% of patients with detectable
IL-1B levels were smokers compared to 35% of those with undetectable IL-1B
levels.

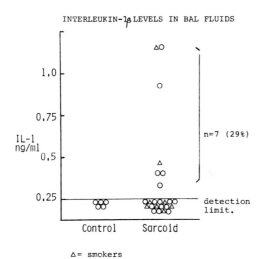

Fig. 1. Interleukin-1Blevels in BAL fluids from control and sarcoid patients

T-lymphocyte subsets

The number of T-lymphocytes (Leu 1+ve) recovered on BAL was significantly elevated in sarcoid subjects (mean = 4.15×10^6, range $0.72-19.4 \times 10^6$) compared to controls (mean = 1.07×10^6, range $0.42-3.3 \times 10^6$; $p < 0.01$). This increase in T-lymphocytes was largely attributable to an increase in helper T-cells, as the number of Leu 3+ve cells was similarly increased in sarcoid patients (mean = 3.46×10^6; range $0.46-15.7 \times 10^6$) compared to controls (mean = 0.4×10^6; range $0.32-2.62 \times 10^6$; $p < 0.01$) whereas the number of suppressor T-cells (Leu 2a+ve) was not significantly elevated (sarcoid group: mean = 0.88×10^6, range $0.17-2.56 \times 10^6$; control group; mean = 0.38×10^6, range $0.17-0.74 \times 10^6$). However, no difference was observed between sarcoid patients with detectable BAL IL-1B levels (IL-1B +ve) and those without detectable BAL IL-1B levels (IL-1B -ve) in relation to T-lymphocyte subsets. The number of helper and suppressor T-cells were similar in both sarcoid groups.(Fig. 2) In all groups, the same pattern was observed whether T-lymphocytes and subsets were expressed as total numbers of cells or as a proportion of the cells recovered on BAL.

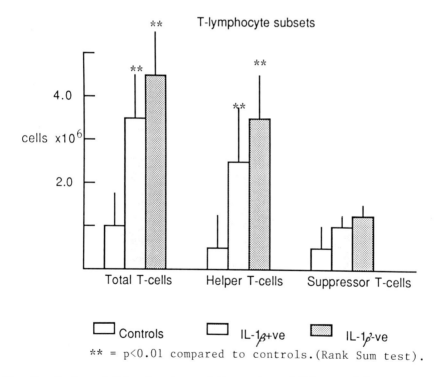

Fig. 2. Number of T-lymphocytes and the number of Helper and Suppressor T-cells in BAL fluids from controls, IL-1B +ve and IL-1B -ve sarcoid patients.

BAL fluid proteins

BAL levels of ACE, fibronectin and PCP in sarcoid patients were
significantly elevated compared to controls (Table 1). Interestingly, levels
of all 3 proteins were markedly increased in the IL-1B +ve group compared to
the IL-1B -ve group (Fig. 3) and the observed increase in these proteins in the
entire sarcoid group was largely accounted for by this marked increase in the
IL-1B +ve group.

TABLE 1:   BAL FLUID PROTEINS IN CONTROL AND SARCOID PATIENTS

	Control	Sarcoid
Fibronectin ug/ml	0.345; 0.075-0.525	0.744; 0.3-3.2**
ACE units/ml	0.034; 0.0-0.20	0.146; 0.0-1.07*
PCP ng/ml	0.008; 0.0-0.18	0.574; 0.0-6.8*

Values are expressed as means; ranges. * $p < 0.05$; ** $p < 0.01$ compared to
controls.

Pulmonary Function and Radiographic Classification

At the time of BAL the majority of sarcoid patients displayed normal
pulmonary function. Mean value of FEV% (84.2±5.0); FVC%(89.7±7.7) and DLCO%
(85.6±21.7) were within normal range. Only 4 patients displayed FVC% values of
< 80% predicted and 7 patients DLCO% values of < 80%. There was no significant
difference in pulmonary function between patients with or without BAL IL-1B ,
nor was any difference noted between the two groups with respect to
radiographic disease staging (TABLE 2).

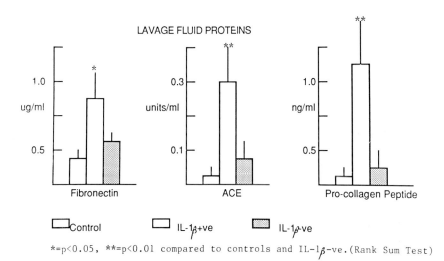

*=$p < 0.05$, **=$p < 0.01$ compared to controls and IL-1β-ve.(Rank Sum Test)

Fig. 3. Levels of Fibronectin, ACE and PCP in BAL fluids from controls,
IL-1B +ve and IL-1B -ve sarcoid patients.

TABLE 2:   PHYSIOLOGICAL PROFILE OF SARCOID PATIENTS

	IL-1+ve	IL-1 -ve
N	7	17
FEV1%	81.5 ±12.0	85.3 ±5.4
FVC%	86.3 ± 8.5	91.0 ±4.2
DLCO%	73.3 ± 8.9	90.5 ±5.3
Radiographic Stage 0	0	2(EN)*
Stage I	2	8
Stage II	4	6
Stage III	1	1

Values are means SE. *2 patients without lung involvement on chest
roentgenograms had active erythema nodosum.

Disease "Outcome"

   Five of the original 24 patients were placed on corticosteroid treatment at
various times after initial diagnosis and BAL. The decision to treat was taken
purely on clinical grounds, without knowledge of BAL IL-1B levels. Only 2 of
these 5 patients had raised IL-1B levels at BAL. Functional and radiographic
assessment of untreated patients over time (mean follow-up time = 10.3 months,
range 6-20 months) indicated spontaneous improvement in a further five
patients. Criteria for assessing improvement were (i) an increase in DLCO% of
>10% and/or (ii) a change in radiographic stage (from II to I, or I to 0).
Again, 2 of these patients were IL-1B +ve. The remaining 14 patients (3 IL-1B
+ve; 11 IL-1B -ve) remained stable without treatment.

DISCUSSION

   BAL IL-1B levels were found to be elevated in 29% of the sarcoid patients
studied. However, these patients did not display a more active alveolitis, as
determined by number or proportion of T-lymphocytes, than patients without BAL
IL-1B. In "in vitro" studies, Hunninghake (12) demonstrated the spontaneous
production of IL-1 by alveolar macrophages (AMs) from patients with active
sarcoidosis. Kleinhenz et al (13) failed to replicate this finding and
indicated that an inhibitor of IL-1 activity is also produced by AMs from
sarcoid patients. Thus, the overall "in vivo" response of T-cells would be
expected to reflect a balance between the production of IL-1 and inhibitor,
which may explain why some patients with elevated BAL IL-1B levels did not
display a T-cell alveolitis. The presence of increased numbers of
T-lymphocytes in the lungs of patients with undetectable levels of IL-1B is
more difficult to interpret. However, Hunninghake et al (3) have demonstrated
that IL-1 can act as a chemo-attractant for T-lymphocytes at concentrations
several orders of magnitude lower than that detected by the LAF assay. Thus it

may be that the RIA employed in this study, which has a similar sensitivity to the LAF assay, is not sensitive enough to detect the low levels of IL-1B which are sufficient to induce a T-cell response. Alternatively, other factors, such as IL-2, may be responsible for the induction of T-lymphocytes into the lung and enhancing their proliferation.

As a group, patients with elevated IL-1B levels also displayed elevated ACE, fibronectin and PCP levels. Like IL-1B, fibronectin is also produced by activated macrophages. Fibronectin acts both as a chemoattractant and a progression factor for fibroblasts, priming fibroblasts for the action of IL-1B and other competence-type growth factors (7). Thus, the presence of elevated levels of both fibronectin and IL-1B would reflect a situation ideal for the proliferation and activation of fibroblasts. The high levels of PCP observed in this group of patients would indicate that fibroblasts are indeed activated and producing increased quantities of Type III collagen. However, despite the presence of "ideal" conditions for fibroblast growth and collagen production, only two of the seven patients in this group deteriorated on follow-up and a further two improved significantly. Thus it may be that elevated BAL levels of IL-1B, fibronectin and PCP reflect the normal healing process following acute lung inflammation in early sarcoidosis and it is only in cases where feed-back regulators of these mediators fail that chronic inflammation and fibrosis ensues.

ACKNOWLEDGEMENTS

This work was supported by the Medical Research Council of Ireland.

REFERENCES

1. Durum SK, Schmidt JA, Oppenheim JJ. Interleukin-1: an immunological perspective: Ann Rev Immunol 1985; 3: 263-87.

2. Dinarello CA. Interleukin-1. Rev Infect Dis 1984; 6: 57-95.

3. Hunninghake, GW, Grazier, AJ, Monick, MM, Dinarello CA. Interleukin-1 is a chemotactic factor for human T-lymphocytes. An Rev Respir Dis. 1987; 35: 66-71.

4. Hunninghake GW, Crystal RG. Pulmonary sarcoidosis: a disorder predicted by T-lymphocyte activity at sites of disease activity. N Engl J Med 1981, 305: 425-34.

5. March CJ, Mosley B. et al. Cloning, sequence and expression of two distinct human interleukin-1 complementary DNAs. Nature 1985; 315: 641-647.

6. Silverstein E, Pertschuk LP, Friedland J. Immunoflourescent localisation of antiotensin converting enzyme in epithelioid and giant cells of sarcoidosis granulomas. Proc Natl Acad Sci USA 1979; 76: 6648-8.

7. Rennard SI, Hunninghake GW, Bitterman PB, Crystal RG. Production of fibronectin by the human alveolar macrophage: a mechanism for the recruitment of fibroblasts to sites of tissue injury in the interstitial lung diseases. Proc Natl Acad Sci USA 1981; 78:7147-51.

8. Fessler JH & Fessler LI. Biosynthesis of procollagen. Ann Rev Biochem 1978; 47:129-62.

9. Gomez-Leclow MJ, Castell JV. Enzyme-linked immunoassay to quantify fibronectin. Anal Biochem 1985; 145: 1-8.

10. Lieberman J. Elevation of serum angiotensin converting enzyme levels in sarcoidosis. Am.J.Med 1975; 59:365-72.

11. Cotes JE. Lung Function throughout life: determinants and reference.

12. Hunninghake GW. Release of interleukin-1 by alveolar macrophages of patients with active pulmonary sarcoidosis. Am Rev Respir Dis 1984; 129: 569-572.

13. Kleinhenz ME, Fujuwaria H, Rich EA. Interleukin-1 production by blood monocytes and bronchoalveolar cells in sarcoidosis. Annals N Y Acad Sci. 1986; 465: 91-97.

INTERLEUKIN-2 DYSREGULATION IN CIRCULATING MONONUCLEAR CELLS
OF PATIENTS WITH ACTIVE SARCOIDOSIS

J.L. JOHNSON, M.D. and M.E. KLEINHENZ, M.D.
Department of Medicine, Case Western Reserve University, University
Hospitals of Cleveland, Cleveland, Ohio

INTRODUCTION

Current concepts of sarcoidosis suggest that dysregulation of
interleukin-2 (IL-2) metabolism at tissue sites of granuloma formation is
central to pathogenesis of this disorder (1,2). Systemic cellular immune
responses require elaboration of this immunopotentating lymphokine as well
as cellular expression of surface receptors (IL-2R) which permit specific
uptake of IL-2. Decreased IL-2 production has been correlated with
depressed _in vivo_ and _in vitro_ antigen reactivity in a variety of disease
states including tuberculosis (3) and lepromatous leprosy (4) while soluble
IL-2R have been recovered in increased amounts from serum of patients with
active sarcoidosis (5). To assess whether a constitutive defect in IL-2
metabolism contributes to the depressed antigen responsiveness observed in
sarcoidosis, we examined antigen-induced IL-2 production and IL-2R
expression by blood mononuclear cells from patients with active and
corticosteroid treated sarcoidosis.

METHODS

Human Subjects. Samples of venous blood were obtained from 26 patients
with biopsy-proven sarcoidosis; 15 patients had active sarcoidosis and 11
patients were studied during treatment with corticosteroids. The mean age
(± 1 SD) of the active and treated patient groups was 38.9 ± 11 and 38.7 ±
8.6 years respectively. A blood sample was obtained from healthy, age and
sex matched individuals on the same day as each patient study.

Mononuclear Cells. Blood mononuclear cells (PBMC) were separated from
whole blood by Ficoll-Hypaque density gradient centrifugation. A T cell
enriched fraction was prepared by sequential depletion of cells adherent to
plastic petri dishes and nylon wool columns (3). The adherent cell
monolayer was recovered from the plastic petri dishes and was 85% monocytes
by peroxidase cytochemistry.

Antigen Induced Responses. Mononuclear cell responsiveness to the recall
antigen streptolysin O (SLO) was assayed as _in vitro_ blastogenesis, IL-2

production, and surface IL-2R expression. PBMC and T cell blastogenesis in
response to SLO was assayed as tritiated thymidine incorporation (3HTdR) in
a standard microculture assay (3). IL-2 activity in culture supernatants of
SLO-stimulated T cells was determined as mitogenicity for the mouse
cytotoxic T cell line CTLL-20. IL-2 activity was calculated by modified
probit analysis and expressed as units/ml (3). Cellular expression of
surface IL-2R by SLO-stimulated T cells was assayed by indirect
immunofluorescence microscopy using murine anti-TAC antibody (the kind gift
of Dr. T.A. Waldmann).

Interleukin-1 (IL-1) Production. IL-1 activity in culture supernatants of
lipopolysaccharide-stimulated blood monocytes was determined in a direct
mitogenic assay using thymocytes of C3H/HeJ mice (Jackson Labs, Bar Harbor,
ME.) IL-1 activity was calculated by modified probit analysis and expressed
in units/ml. (6).

RESULTS

SLO-induced 3HTdR and IL-2 production by PBMC and T cells from patients
with sarcoidosis was not normally distributed. The distribution of
SLO-induced 3HTdR by PBMC and T cells of patients with active sarcoidosis
differed significantly from the responses observed in studies of controls
[p=0.001 and p=0.01, respectively, Mann-Whitney U test (M-W-U)] with
SLO-induced 3HTdR in patients skewed toward lower activity than controls.
IL-2 activity observed in supernatants of patient T cells incubated for 48
hours with SLO was different from that detected in control supernantants
(Fig 1, p=0.01, M-W-U). No IL-2 activity was detected in the supernatants of
T cells from 5 patients with active sarcoidosis. IL-2R expression assayed
as surface staining for TAC antigen by resting and SLO-stimulated cells from
patients with active sarcoidosis and controls was comparable at 0, 48, 96
hours (Table 1). Mean IL-1 activity in supernatants of monocytes from
untreated patients 9.9± 7.3 units/ml (± 1SD) however was not different from
controls (12.4 ± 12.3).

In eleven sarcoidosis patients studied while receiving corticosteroid
therapy, SLO-induced 3HTdR of PBMC was significantly different from that of
patients with active sarcoidosis (p<0.01, M-W-U) but within the range
observed in controls. Similarly, SLO-induced IL-2 activity from
corticosteroid treated patients was increased compared to the active
sarcoidosis patients (p=0.01, M-W-U) and not different from values detected
in controls.

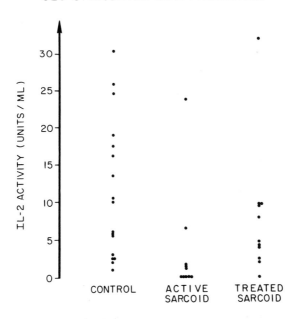

Fig.1 SLO-induced IL-2 activity in culture supernatants of T cells from
controls and patients with sarcoidosis.

DISCUSSION

   These data demonstrate that depressed systemic antigen reactivity
coincides with low levels of IL-2 activity in supernatants of
antigen-stimulated blood T cells from patients with active sarcoidosis.
Measurements of surface IL-2R and production of the monokine IL-1 revealed
no differences between controls and sarcoidosis patients. Thus availability
of IL-2 appears to limit T cell antigen responsiveness in patients with
active sarcoidosis. Due to the experimental technology available for
determining IL-2 activity, it is not clear whether deficient numbers or
output of IL-2 producing cells underlies the impaired systemic cellular
immune responses. Exaggerated T cell consumption or absorption of IL-2
during the interval of lymphokine generation also could reduce IL-2 activity
detected in the mitogenic assay. This possibility is unlikely since
comparable IL-2R expression was observed in the freshly isolated T cells of
controls and patients with active sarcoidosis. Binding of IL-2 with
soluble IL-2R would inactivate this lymphokine and decrease IL-2 activity
detected in the mitogenic assay.

Normalization of the cellular turnover of IL-2R would be anticipated effect of corticosteroid treatment of sarcoidosis which would explain at least in part, the recovery of systemic IL-2 activity observed during treatment of sarcoidosis as well as the paradoxical effect of corticosteriods on systemic antigen responsiveness in sarcoidosis.

TABLE I

T CELL REACTIVITY WITH ANTI-TAC ANTIBODY

	0°	48°	96°
CONTROLS (n=25)	$1.2 \pm 1.1*$	9.2 ± 6.4	19.7 ± 9.9
ACTIVE SARCOID (n=15)	1.1 ± 1.0	10.8 ± 4.5	20.2 ± 6.9
TREATED SARCOID (n=11)	0.6 ± 9.0	9.0 ± 7.3	18.5 ± 10.1

*(mean % $\pm$ 1 S.D.)

REFERENCES

1. Muller-Quernheim J, Saltini C, Sondermayer, Crystal RG (1986) J. Immunol. 137:3475-3483

2. Kataria YP, Padgett RC, English LS (1986) Ann N.Y. Acad. Sci 465:157-163

3. Toossi Z, Kleinhenz ME, Ellner JJ (1986) J. Exp. Med. 163:1162-1172

4. Kaplan G, Weinstein GE, Steinman RM, Levis WR, Elvers V, Patarroyo ME, Cohn ZA (1985) J. Exp. Med. 162:917-929

5. Semenzato G, Cipriani A, Trentin L, Zambello R, Masciarelli M, Vinante F, Chilosi M., Pizzolo G (1987) Sarcoidosis 4:25-27

6. Fujiwara H, Kleinhenz ME, Wallis RS, Ellner JE (1986) Am. Rev. Resp. Dis. 133:73-77

PREDNISOLONE TREATMENT AND ALVEOLAR LYMPHOCYTE-MACROPHAGE COOPERATION IN SARCOIDOSIS

TON VAN MAARSSEVEEN, HENDRIK MULLINK, MEENY DE HAAN, JAAP STAM, JAN DE GROOT.

Departments of Pathology and Pulmonology, Academical Hospital, Free University, De Boelelaan 1117, 1081 HV Amsterdam, The Netherlands.

INTRODUCTION

The activity of pulmonary Sarcoidosis can be assessed by characterization of the mononuclear cell infiltrate obtained by bronchoalveolar lavage (BAL) (1). This activity correlates with the alveolar lymphocytosis in sarcoidosis (2). The disease may resolve or may lead to pulmonary fibrosis and respiratory impairment. Steroid therapy is effective in relieving these symptoms (3, 4, 5). It is described (5-8) that macrophages and lymphocytes in the BAL's of sarcoidosis patients form rosettes. We studied the kind of lymphocytes involved in these "tight macrophage-lymphocyte aggregates" (MLA) and it's dependence on steroid treatment of the disease.

MATERIALS AND METHODS

The BAL was done with 2 aliquots of 50 ml of 37°C Hanks solution. The lavage fluid was filtered by gauze immediately and the cells were recovered after washing 3 times. Cytospin slides were prepared, air-dried and stored at -20°C until staining. T4+ and T8+ cells were simultaneously stained using a double immunoenzyme staining technique as described earlier (9) and combined with an acid phosphatase staining for macrophages (10). From the triple stained slides, at least 1,000 leucocytes were characterized as macrophages, T4+, T8+ or TO lymphocytes. As MLA's were considered only those macrophages, with closely attached lymphocytes (fig. 1). Because of the low percentage of B-lymphocytes (±2%) as seen in cell suspensions by means of immunofluorescense (11), we decided to accept the not-stained lymphocytes present in the triple stained preparations as TO lymphocytes. In this way in one preparation the blue T4+, brown T8+ and unstained TO lymphocytes could be seen simultaneously, lying free or in close association (MLA's) with the red-stained macrophages. BAL's were evaluated without knowledge of the clinical status

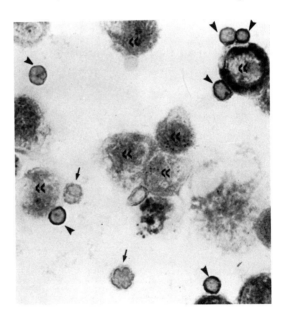

Fig. 1. Cytospin slide stained by a double immunoenzyme staining combined with acid phosphatase staining. Yellow T8+ lymphocytes (▶) strongly adhered to a red macrophage (≪) can be distinghuised from blue T4+ lymphocytes (✓) 250 x.

and the results were grouped accordingly to disease, clinical activity and treatment.

RESULTS

The BAL's from Sarcoidosis patients mostly consist of lymphocytes and macrophages. Steroid treatment did not influence the number of T4+ cells, but the number of T8+ cells was augmented significantly (p=0.025) resulting in a lower T4/T8 ratio (p<0.005) (table 1). By counting the MLA's per 1,000 leucocytes (table 2), significant higher values of macrophages with T8 lymphocytes (MLA-T8) could be found in the BAL of steroid-treated patients as compared with the non-treated patients (p<0.01). As there was a great variation in the number of lymphocytes among the patients, the possibility exists that in BAL's with a low number of lymphocytes, hardly MLA's could be seen. Therefore these values were corrected and expressed as MLA/1,000 lymphocytes. Within the T8+ lymphocyte subset it was found that steroid therapy influences the number of MLA. The promillage of MLA-T8 varied between 20-96 in untreated patients and was increased in the treated patients to 158-272 (p=0.005) (table 2). No such variations were observed in the MLA-T4 or MLA-T0 subset of lymphocytes (table 2). Besides these described MLA's, also macrophages were present which have 2 or sometimes 3 different lymphocyte types like T4, T8 or T0 to one and the same macrophage. It could be shown that all kinds

Table I

Lymphocyte phenotypes present in the BAL.

	NO TREATMENT		STEROID TREATMENT	
	%	$\times 10^6$	%	$\times 10^6$
Lymphocytes	41 ±14	4,9 ±5,0	25 ±14	2,8 ±1,1
T lymphocytes	62 ±7	3,3 ±4,3	65 ±5	1,8 ±0,3
T_4 "	47 ±12	1,8 ±1,3	53 ±6	1,4 ±0,4
T_8 "	6,2±2,8	0,3 ±0,3	21 ±3	0,6 ±0,2
$\frac{T_4}{T_8}$ Ratio	6,6 ±2,7		1,3 + 0,8	
Anti-Ig tot.cells	2,2 ±1,7	0,06 ±0,06	1,0 ±1	0,03 ±0,03

The mean ± sd for six patients are presented.

Table 2

Quantitation of macrophage-lymphocyte aggregates.

Patient	P	Lympho %	T4/T8	MLA-Tx/10^3leuco's			MLA-Tx/10^3lympho's		
				T8	T4	T0	T8	T4	T0
1	−	22	4,9	19	77	25	86	350	114
2	−	25	5,9	24	74	17	96	296	68
3	−	39	9,8	11	125	23	28	320	159
4	−	40	3,6	21	59	19	52	147	47
5	−	45	10	11	48	17	24	107	38
6	−	61	5,3	12	96	5	20	157	8
7	+	12	2,2	19	68	5	158	567	42
8	+	13	1,9	35	61	10	269	469	77
9	+	29	0,5	79	31	6	272	107	21
10	+	31	2,3	67	60	21	216	193	68
11	+	35	1,9	61	47	5	174	134	14
12	+	48	1,8	74	93	11	159	194	23

Quantitation of macrophages with adherent lymphocytic subtypes (MLA-T8, MLA-T4, MLA-T0) related to the total number of leucocytes or lymphocytes.
P=Patients treated (+) or not (−) with prednisolone.
T4/T8=T-helper/suppressor cell ratio.
Lympho %=Percentage of lymphocytes obtained by BAL.

of MLA were present over a wide range in both groups of patients. MLA-T4-T8's were the predominant type in both groups.

DISCUSSION

Current concepts of the pathogenesis of sarcoidosis suggest that macrophages locally play a central role in this disorder. Variations in distribution of the lymphocyte subsets provide evidence for different kinds of inflammatory reactions (12). Cooperation between these lymphocytes and macrophages exists (13) and can be observed in the alveolitis (14). The different functional properties between T4+ and T8+ lymphocytes are well known (15). The T4+ lymphocytes mostly are responsible for the cellular immune inflammatory response, also known as high intensity alveolitis (1, 12) whereas T8+ cells tend to dampen this reaction (16, 17). From our study it can be seen that prednisolon induces a significant accumulation of T8+ lymphocytes in the lung. Therefore the decreased T4/T8 ratio can be explained by the augmented number of alveolar T8 cells in patients under prednisolon treatment. In our BAL's lymphocyte-macrophage clusters (MLA) were noticed, which were also reported before (5-8). To evaluate this intercellular phenomenon we quantitated and characterized the adhered lymphocyte population in the MLA's. Only significant more MLA-T8 were found in the treated patients (table 2). This could mean that the direct influence of the T8+

Table 3

Thelper/suppressor lymphocyte ratio's.

	$\dfrac{T_4}{T_8}$	$\dfrac{MLA\text{-}T_4}{MLA\text{-}T_8}$
Steroid treatment	$1,3 \pm 0,8$	$1,4 \pm 0,6$
No treatment	$6,6 \pm 2,7$	$6,8 \pm 2,9$
	$p < 0,005$	

Ratio's obtained from sarcoidosis patients with or without prednisolon treatment. Comparison between the overall ratio, estimated by means of immunofluorescence on cell suspensions and the T4+ and T8+ lymphocytes which are adhered to macrophages and estimated by means of a triple staining.

lymphocyte on the alveolar macrophage is necessary and results in suppression of some inflammatory reactions. Macrophages adhered by two or three subtypes of lymphocytes together were also seen; from this MLA-T4-T8 were present in all sarcoidosis patients independent of treatment. A good correlation between this MLA-T4-T8 number and the alveolar lymphocytosis was found.
It could be proven (table 3) that the overall balance between T4+ and T8+ lymphocytes, expressed by the T4/T8 ratio fits well ($p < 0.005$) with the balance of macrophages with adhered T4+ or T8+ cells. And this could mean that the exchange of immunological information between macrophages and lymphocytes as demonstrated by our cell adhesions (MLA) are reflected by the overall T4/T8 ratio.

In conclusion:
The vigorous high intensity alveolitis, observed in many sarcoidosis patients is cut off by means of steroid treatment. Application of prednisolon is followed by an increase of T8+ lymphocytes. Direct interference of these T8+ lymphocytes with alveolar macrophages might result in suppression of the inflammatory reaction.

REFERENCES

1. Crystal RG, Roberts WC, Hunninghake GW et al (1981) Ann Intern Med 94: 73-94.
2. Hunninghake GW and Crystal RG (1981) New Engl J Med 305: 429-434.
3. Johns CJ, McGregor MI, Zachary JB et al (1976) Ann N Y Acad Sci 278: 722-731.
4. DeRemee RA (1977) Chest 71: 388-392.
5. Herscowitz HB (1985) Ann All 55: 634-648.
6. Hunninghake GW, Gadek JE, Young RC et al (1984) New Engl J Med 302: 594-598.

7. Reynolds HY (1978) Lung 155: 225-242.
8. Yeager H, Williams HC, Beekman JF et al (1977) Am Rev Respir Dis 116: 951-955.
9. Mullink H, Henzen-Logmans SC, Alons- v Kordelaar JJM et al (1986) Virch Arch B 52: 55-65.
10. Maarsseveen v TC, Mullink H, Haan de M et al (1987) submitted.
11. Hunninghake GW, Kawanami O, Ferrans v J et al (1981) Am Rev Respir Dis 123: 407-412.
12. Ceuppens JC, Laquet LM, Marien J et al (1984) Am Rev Respir Dis 129: 563-568.
13. Unanue ER (1980) New Engl J Med 303: 977-985.
14. Lem VM, Lipscomb MF, Weissler JC et al (1985) J Immunol 135: 1766-1771.
15. Janossy G (1982) In: Janossy G (Ed) Clinics in Haematol vol 11, Saunders Comp. London, pp 631-660.
16. Chensue SW, Wellhausen SR, Boros DL (1981) J Immunol 127: 363-367.
17. Chudwin DS, Cowan MJ, Wara DW et al (1983) Clin Immunol Immunopathol 26: 126-136.

THE RELATIONSHIP BETWEEN BAL IMMUNOCYTOLOGY AND CLINICAL INDICES IN SARCOIDOSIS

GILLIAN M. AINSLIE, R.M. DUBOIS, L.W. POULTER.
Depts. of Thoracic Medicine and Immunology, Royal Free Hospital and School
of Medicine, London, England.

INTRODUCTION

There has been a continuing search to find a parameter in sarcoidosis
which will identify those patients with active disease and predict future
disease course. Bronchoalveolar lavage (BAL), differential counts, T cell
subsets, gallium 67 scanning and serum angiotensin converting enzyme have
all been investigated but the data is as yet inconclusive,(1-3).

Alveolar macrophages and lymphocytes are thought to be important in the
underlying immune mechanisms of sarcoidosis,(4). It is thought that an
as yet undefined antigen is processed by alveolar macrophages and presented
to lymphocytes that become activated, secrete lymphokines attract further
macrophages and lymphocytes,resulting in alveolitis and granuloma formation.

Previous studies have shown alveolar macrophages to be very heterogeneous,
with no clear difference demonstrated between normals and various types
of interstitial lung disease (5,6). The aim of our studies was to use a
panel of monoclonal antibodies against both alveolar macrophages and lymphocytes from patients with sarcoidosis, in order to correlate cell membrane
markers with clinical criteria of disease activity.

METHODS
Study population.

This consisted of 10 normal controls and 22 patients with histologically
proven sarcoidosis. In an attempt to produce an index of clinical activity
an arbitary scoring system was applied to each patient,(Table 1).

TABLE 1. CLINICAL ACTIVITY SCORE.

	Score. 0	1	2	3
Symptoms	Absent	Present		
Signs	Absent	Present		
CXR	Clear	BHL	ILS1	ILS2,3
FVC	80%	70-80%	70%	
DLCO	80%	70-80%	70%	
SACE	Normal	Raised		

This gives a maximum score of 10 and those patients with a score of 5 or more were adjudged clinically active.

BAL.

This was performed in the standard way with routine total cell count and differentials done. Standard cytocentrifuge slides were made and stored for subsequent immunocytology.

Immunocytology.

The following panel of McAbs. were used. Their specificity in normal tissues is given in brackets. RFD1,(dendritic cells); RFD7,(mature macrophages); RFD9,(epithelioid cells); RFDR1,(HLA.DR); UCHM1,(monocytes); RFT2,(CD7, T blasts) RFT8,(CD8,suppressor/cytotoxic cells); Leu3a,(CD4,helper/inducer cells); RFTmix, (CD2,7,8. all T cells), Tac,(CD25,IL2 receptors). were employed and the percentage of alveolar macrophages and lymphocytes positive for each marker was then identified by the immunoperoxidase method,(7). Double expression of two surface markers was shown by double immuno-fluorescence,(8).

RESULTS

Total Cell and Differential Counts.

The sarcoidosis patients had the expected significant increases in total cell numbers, macrophage numbers and especially lymphocyte numbers and percentages.

Immunocytology.

Normals vs Sarcoidosis Patients

(a) Macrophages:

Compared to normals there were significantly increased RFDI+ cells in sarcoid lavage,(69 + 5% vs 39 + 5%, p- 0.001). There was also an increase in RFD7+ cells (45 + 4% vs 33 + 48), but this not significant. Double immunofluorescence showed that the proportion of D1+/D7+ cells was very significantly increased (36 + 3% in sarcoids vs 10 + 2% in normals, p- 0.0001). Almost all macrophages both in normals and sarcoidosis express HLA-DR (86% v 92%). In normals, very small numbers of cells express RFD9 (epithelioid cell marker) or UCHMI (circulating monocyte marker), and this was significantly increased for both in sarcoidosis (RFD9: 29 + 4%, UCHM1: 28 + 5% vs 7 + 3%, p- 0.01).

(b) Lymphocytes:

The CD4:8 ratio was significantly increased in sarcoidosis (4.8 vs 1.9, p- 0.01). There was also a significant increase in the proportion of lymphocytes expressing the activation markers: RFT2 (CD7 antigen strongly expressed on lymphoblasts), Tac (CD25 antigen marking interleukin-2 receptors) and RFDR (21 + 4% vs 7 + 2%, 9 + 2% vs 2 + 0.4%. 21 + 4% vs 7 + 1%, all p- 0.05).

Correlation with Clinical Indices.

There was no correlation between the expression of any of these markers and disease duration PFTs or SACE. However, when we looked at chest radiographic type, those patients with evidence of extensive pulmonary parenchymal involvement (ie Types II and III vs I) had significant increases in RFD1+ and RFD7 cells (p- 0.05), and especially joint D1+/D7+ cells (p- 0.005). Figure I.

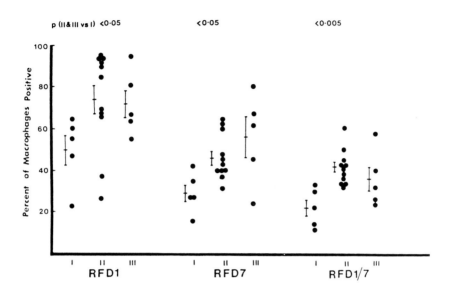

Fig I   The proportions of BAL non-lymphoid mononuclear cells expressing reactivity with McABs RFD1, RFD7 and both (RFD1/7), in sarcoid patients grouped on x-ray stage (I, II, III). Bars represent mean and standard error in each group.

There were also significant increases in the numbers of macrophages positive for RFD9 and UCHM1 but not RDR1. There were also significant increases in RFT2+ and Tac+ lymphocytes (p- 0.45 and - 0.01 respectively), and more HLA - DR+ T-lymphocytes.

Correlation with Activity Score.

We then looked at how these markers correlated with the overall index of clinical activity, comparing the 15 patients judged as active with the 7 inactive.

In the active patients there were significant increases in RFD7+, RFD9+ (p- 0.05), and especially D1+/D7 and UCHM1+ macrophages (p- 0.005). Clinically active patients also had significant increases in the proportions of alveolar lymphocytes expressing RFT2 and Tac. The number of CD4+ and DR+ lymphocytes were also raised, but did not reach significance because of the wide range of the results.

DISCUSSION

We have shown significant variations in the proportions of phenotypically distinct subsets of alveolar macrophages and lymphocytes in sarcoidosis as compared to normals. More importantly, we have shown that the increases in the proportions of certain phenotypes correlate with increased disease activity as determined by clinical criteria.

Most markers however, were increased in patients with Types II and III chest radiographs ie those with evidence of widespread lung involvement. Of especial interest is the increased co-expression of RFD1 and RFD7. RFD1 recognises a cell membrane antigen related to the Class II major histocompatibility complex,(9). Not all DR+ cells however, express RFD1 eg Langerhans cells. This suggests that RFD1 recognises an epitope with restricted expression. It is thought to be functionally related to antigen presentation and this has been confirmed by the fact that RFD1 inhibits the mixed lymphocyte reaction (10).

RFD7 recognises an antigen of mature tissue macrophages which are acid phosphatase positive and very phagocytic (9). RFD1 and D7 expression is mutually exclusive in normal secondary lymphoid tissue (9). Co-expression of D1 and D7 occurs at low levels in normal BAL macrophages and this is raised in sarcoidosis, especially in clinically active patients withextensive radiographic lung involvement. This data suggests that surface antigen expression may be the product of the local immune environment. This hypothesis is supported by the concurrent increase in nymbers of activated T-ılymphocytes. UCHM1+ cells suggests recruitment of increased monocytes to the lungs and increased RFD9+ cells implies that epithelioid cells, are differentiating. This data shows the value of lavage immunocytology in assessing disease activity and providing clues to underlying immuno-pathogenic mechanisma.

REFERENCES

1 Lawrence EC, Teague RB, Gottlieb MS et al Am J Med 1983; 74: 747-56

2 Baughman RP, Fernandez M, Bosken CH et al Am Rev Respir Dis 1984; 129:676-681

3 Cueppens JL, Lacquet LM, Marien G, et al Am Rev Respir Dis 1984; 129: 563-8

4 Venet A Hance AJ, Saltini C et al J Clin Invest 1985; 75: 293-301

5 Campbell DA, Poulter LW, du Bois RM Thorax 1986; 41: 429-34

6 Biondi A Rossing TH, Bennett J et al J Immunol 1984; 132: 1237-43

7 Munro CS, Campbell DA, Collings LA et al Scand J Immunol 1986; 24: 351-57

8 Janossy G, Bofill M, Poulter LW etal J Immunol 1986; 136: 4354-61

9 Poulter LW, Campbell DA, Munro C et al Scand J Immunol 1986; 24: 351-57

10 Poulter LW, Duke O Proc Quatrieme Cours d'Immmunorheumatologie Montpellier 1983; 189-99

ALVEOLAR MACROPHAGES RECOVERED FROM THE LUNG OF PATIENTS WITH ACTIVE SARCOIDOSIS
DISPLAY A MONOCYTE-LIKE PHENOTYPE AND THE PROPERTY TO RELEASE TYPE IV COLLAGENASE

AGOSTINI C. , GARBISA S., ZAMBELLO R., CIPRIANI A., NEGRO A., MASCIARELLI M.,
LUCA M., SEMENZATO G.

Departments of Clinical Medicine, 1st Medical Clinic and Clinical Immunology;
Pneumology and Histology Institutes; University of Padua, Italy.

INTRODUCTION

The alveolitis in the lung of sarcoid patients is characterized by the
accumulation of lymphocytes and macrophages within the alveolar structures.
At least two mechanisms account for this accumulation: a local proliferation
and a cell redistribution from the peripheral blood to the lung (1,2). With
regard to the macrophagic component of the alveolitis, previous studies have
demonstrated that in situ replication partially accounts for the expansion of
mononuclear phagocytic population (3,4). On the contrary, the recruitment of
fresh monocytes from peripheral blood, even if supposed, has not yet been proven.

The present study was carried out to verify the hypothesis that recently
recruited monocytes are present in the lung of patients with sarcoidosis. For
this purpose, alveolar macrophages (PAM) recovered from bronchoalveolar lavage
(BAL) of 30 patients with sarcoidosis (19 patients with active sarcoidosis,
11 patients with inactive disease) have been characterized by a panel of monoclonal antibodies (MoAbs) recognizing determinants expressed by most peripheral
monocytes, but only by a certain degree of tissue macrophages. The phenotypic
analysis has been coupled to the in vitro evaluation of type IV-collagenase
production by PAM. This neutral proteinase is released from circulating
monocytes but not from resident macrophages and plays a relevant role in the
traversal of the endothelium membrane when monocytes migrate from peripheral
blood to tissues (5).

MATERIALS AND METHODS

Study population Thirty patients with biopsy-proven sarcoidosis (16 women and
14 men, mean age 35 ± 5 yrs) were studied. The diagnosis was based on consistent
clinical features and was confirmed by laboratory findings. Disease activity
was evaluated according to (a) clinical features, (b) the percentage and
absolute number of T cells recovered from the BAL, (c) the frequency of T cell
subsets, and (d) the positivity of the ^{67}Ga scan, as previously described (6).
Using these criteria, 19 patients had active sarcoidosis while 11 patients

showed inactive disease. All patients were non-smokers and were studied at the time of diagnosis. Eight normal non-smoking volunteers (5 men and 3 women; average 36 ± 6 yrs) were evaluated as controls.

Purification of PAM from BAL Following morphologic evaluation and differential count, BAL cells were separated by centrifugation on a density gradient, washed and resuspended in RPMI 1460 (Grand Island Biological Co.). PAM were isolated from the entire BAL mononuclear cell population by removing T lymphocytes using rosetting with neuroaminidase-treated sheep red cells (SRBC). The resulting PAM population was more than 95% pure as judged by non-specific esterase staining.

Evaluation with Monoclonal Antibodies PAM were characterized by a panel of MoAbs usually expressed by peripheral monocytes, including those belonging to CD11 (OKM1, Ortho), CD13 (My7, Coulter), CD14 (MoP9 Becton Dickinson; My4, Coulter), and OKM5 (Ortho). In addition, T cell subpopulations were identified by their reactivity with CD4 (OKT4, Ortho) and CD8 (OKT8 Ortho) MoAbs which include helper-and suppressor/cytotoxic-related cells, respectively.

Type IV Collagenolytic activity Type IV-collagen was biosynthetically labeled with ^{14}C proline, as already reported (7). The quantitation of type IV-collagen degradation by PAM in vitro was performed according to the method previously described (7). Briefly, 3×10^5 PAM were plated with 1.0 ml of HB 101 medium in 16-mm wells coated with 2×10^3 or 2×10^4 cpm of ^{14}C-labeled type IV collagen. Control wells contained 1.0 ml HB 101 medium with or without bacterial collagenase (10 μg/ml). Following 3 and 24 hrs of incubation supernatants were harvested and counted. The mean value of triplicate assays was used to calculate the percentage of type IV-collagenolytic activity. The results were expressed as percent of bacterial collagenase control.

Statistical analysis All data were presented by mean ± SD and comparisons between values were made using the Cockran-Cox test.

RESULTS

Differential counts of cells recovered from BAL of patients with sarcoidosis revealed: a) an increase of the total yielded from BAL in patients with active sarcoidosis when compared to the corresponding values obtained from patients with inactive sarcoidosis and controls ($p < 0.01$, and p 0.001, respectively); b) an increase in the percentage and absolute number of lymphocytes recovered from BAL of patients with active disease ($p < 0.001$ both vs inactive sarcoidosis and controls); c) an increase of the absolute number of PAM both in active and inactive sarcoidosis with respect to normal individuals ($p < 0.02$ in both groups).

Evaluation with MoAbs demonstrated that in active sarcoidosis a higher percentage of PAM expresses determinants usually present on the membrane of peripheral blood monocytes . As shown in Tab. 1, the frequency of PAM positivity for OKM1, OKM5, and My7 MoAbs was significantly increased with respect to controls ($p < 0.05$, 0.05, 0.001, respectively). A statistically significant difference has also been observed in the frequency of OKM5+ cells between patients with inactive sarcoidosis and controls. Pulmonary T4/T8 ratio was increased in active sarcoidosis with respect to both inactive sarcoidosis and controls ($p < 0.001$).

TABLE 1

REACTIVITY OF PULMONARY ALVEOLAR MACROPHAGES WITH MONOCLONAL ANTIBODIES

Patients	OKM1 %	OKM5 %	MoP9 %	My4 %	My7 %
a) Active sarcoidosis	67.4 ±5.2	40.3 ±5.6	70.1 ±5.1	35.2 ±6.8	57.1 ±6.0
b) Inactive sarcoidosis	60.1 ±5.6	45.2 ±7.0	69.0 ±8.7	34.3 ±7.0	40.3 ±5.1
c) Controls	49.5 ±4.4	18.7 ±9.6	78.0 ±3.8	30.1 ±4.5	35.2 ±6.6

Significance as follows:

a	vs	b	ns	ns	ns	ns	ns
a	vs	c	<0.05	<0.05	ns	ns	<0.001
b	vs	c	ns	<0.05	ns	ns	ns

Data concerning type IV-collagenolytic activity are shown in Fig. 1. PAM recovered from normal individuals failed to degrade type IV-collagen. Conversely, in PAM recovered from patients with active sarcoidosis very high levels of type IV-collagenolytic activity was observed. The difference was found to be statistically significant with respect to the values obtained both in controls and in patients with inactive disease ($p < 0.001$, and 0.001, respectively). PAM derived from patients displayed intermediate levels of type IV-collagenolytic activity.

Type IV-collagenolytic activity was also tested during a 24-hr collection period. Sarcoid PAM degraded significant amounts of type IV-collagen during the first 24 hrs, with maximum activity being found after 3 hrs. When culture periods were prolonged, the type IV-collagenolytic activity gradually decreased and became undetectable after 5 days (data not shown).

DISCUSSION

Both phenotypic and functional data described in this paper, including the demonstration that PAM show a higher percentage of determinants usually expressed by peripheral blood monocytes and an increased production of type IV-collagenase, support the hypothesis that newly recruited monocytes are

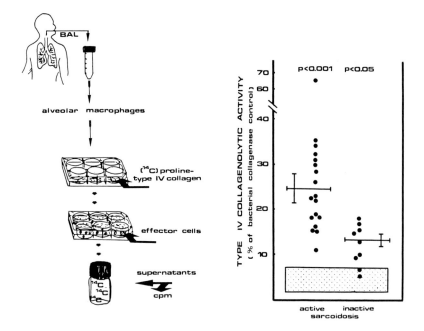

Fig. 1: Evaluation of type IV-collagenolytic activity by PAM recovered from sarcoid patients. The left panel of the figure shows the type IV-collagenolytic assay. The right panel of the figure shows the results. Shaded area represents the normal range.

present in patients with active sarcoidosis.

Recent evidence has been provided that in active sarcoidosis PAM are in a state of hightened activity. These studies include the findings that a higher number of PAM expresses determinants related to the activated monocytes-macrophages (8,9) and the demonstration of an enhanced production of biologic mediators, that is interleukin 1, γ-interferon, tumor necrosis factor, and superoxide anion (10-13). Since in this study we have shown that sarcoid PAM are a heterogeneous population composed of cells with a spectrum age ranging from young, freshly recruited phagocytes to mature macrophages, further studies are needed to establish whether the cells accounting for the increased secretion of biologic mediators are the newly recruited monocytes and/or activated macrophages.

When leaving the blood stream, peripheral monocytes transiently produce a metalloproteinase, called type IV-collagenase, which cleaves type IV-collagen, a structural component of the endothelium basement membrane (14). Data have been recently accumulated demonstrating that the type IV-collagenase production is restricted to a population of young phagocytes. In fact, when monocytes in different tissues differentiate into mature macrophages, they lose the property to release this enzyme (5). According to this interpretation, peripheral monocytes induced by appropriate in vitro culture to differentiate into macrophages fail to degrade type IV-collagen (5). During an inflammatory state (for instance an acute peritonitis) monocytes are quickly recruited to sites of ongoing inflammation and release great amounts of type IV-collagenase (5). The findings herein described that PAM recovered from BAL of patients with active sarcoidosis produce this enzyme suggests that freshly recruited monocytes are present in the lungs of these patients. Further confirmation of this suggestion comes from the evidence that after in vitro culture (3 to 5 days), sarcoid PAM do not release type IV-collagenase, owing to the differentiation of recruited monocytes into macrophages. Since lymphocytes are able to influence the secretory capacity of mononuclear phagocytes through the release of lymphokines (15), additional studies are needed to clarify whether CD4 lymphocytes, which massively infiltrate sarcoid lungs, may regulate the PAM type IV-collagenolytic activity.

REFERENCES

1. Semenzato G (1986) Sem Respir Dis 8: 17
2. Crystal RG, Bitterman PB, Rennard SI et al (1984) N Engl J Med 310: 224
3. Bitterman PB, Saltzman LE, Adelber S et al (1984) J Clin Invest 74: 460
4. Chilosi M, Lestani M, Montagna M (1986) Sarcoidosis 3: 189
5. Garbisa S, Ballin M, Daga-Gordini D et al (1986) J Biol Chem 261: 2369
6. Agostini C, Trentin L, Zambello R et al (1985) Clin Immunol Immunopath 37: 262
7. Garbisa S, Kniska K, Tryggvason K et al (1980) Cancer Lett 9: 359
8. Agostini C, Trentin L, Zambello R et al (1987) J Clin Immunol 7: 64
9. Hance AJ, Douches S, Whinchester RJ et al (1985) J Immunol 134: 284
10. Hunninghake GW (1984) Am Rev Respir Dis 129: 569
11. Robinson BWS, McLenore TC, Crystal RG (1985) J Clin Invest 75: 1488
12. Bachwich PR, Lynch JP, Larraick J et al (1986) Am J Pathol 125: 421
13. Cassatella M, Agostini C, Luca M et al (1986) Sarcoidosis 3: 154
14. Garbisa S, Negro A (1984) Appl Pathol 2: 217
15. Nathan CF (1987) J Clin Invest 79: 319

© 1988 Elsevier Science Publishers B.V. (Biomedical Division)
Sarcoidosis and other granulomatous disorders
C. Grassi, G. Rizzato, E. Pozzi, editors

PHENOTYPING OF ALVEOLAR MACROPHAGE SUBPOPULATIONS IN PULMONARY SARCOIDOSIS, RELATION TO INTRACELLULAR INTERLEUKIN-1 PRODUCTION.

H.KLECH[1],C.NEUCHRIST[2],W.POHL[1],E.SCHENK[1],C.SORG[3],W.KNAPP[4],TH.LUGER[5],O.SCHEINER[2], D.KRAFT[2].

1) Second Med.Dept.Wilhelminenspital, 2)Institute General & Experimental Pathology, Vienna, Austria, 3) Department Experimental Dermatology,Univ.Münster,FRG, 4) Institute for Immunology, 5) 2nd Department Dermatology,Univ.Vienna,Austria.

SUMMARY

Alveolar macrophages (AM) obtained by Bronchoalveolar lavage (BAL) of patients with sarcoidosis had been examined by a panel of monoclonal antibodies in order to further define their phenotypic activity. 14 patients with biopsy proven pulmonary sarcoidosis were included. 12 patients served as control, consisting of patients with extrinsic allergic alveolitis (EAA), tuberculosis, lung cancer and viral pneumonia. As monoclonal antibodies had been used: 1) 27E10 detects a surface antigen which is expressed in peripheral blood monocytes and in acute inflammatory tissues but absent from normal resident mononuclear phagocytes (J.Immunol.13:512-18,1986), 2) 25F9 detects an antigen preferentially expressed on mature tissue fixed macrophages but not in freshly isolated blood monocytes (J.Immunol.134:1487-92,1985), 3) Anti IL-1 is directed against Interleukin-1 (IL-1) of human origin (J.Exp.Med.163:463-68,1986), 4) VID-1 detects cytoplasmatic (human Ia) HLA-DR (Clin.exp.Immunol.59:613-21,1985).
27E10 (immature AM) was significantly expressed only on AM of patients with acute pneumonia. In contrast only patients with sarcoidosis and EAA showed high expression of 25F9 (mature AM) compared to the other group of patients (p<0,01). Lowest percentages for 25F9 were found in patients with tuberculosis and lung cancer. 25F9 positive AM correlated significantly (r_s=0,52) to increased cytoplasmatic distribution of IL-1. In sarcoid patients % of positive 25F9 AM correlated to % of BAL-helper lymphocytes (r_s=0,55). Except from patients with tuberculosis all AMs in all groups showed a consistent high expression of the HLA-DR antigen.Our study emphasizes the important and active role of AM subpopulations, in particular mature 25F9 positive AM, in diseases with enhanced cellular hyperactivity like sarcoidosis and EAA. At first instance we could demonstrate increased cytoplasmatic distribution of IL-1in alveolar macrophages that are suggested to be majorily responsible for the enhanced production of Interleukin-1 in sarcoidosis leading to attraction and proliferation of T-lymphocytes and fibroblasts in the lung resulting in granuloma formation and lung fibrosis.

INTRODUCTION

Although alveolar macrophages (AM) generally function poorly as accessory cells for T-cell activation, relative to their immediate precursors in the blood or macrophage population from sources such as the peritoneal cavity (1,2),there is compelling evidence that in diseases associated with immunological hyperactivity in lung tissue, in particular in pulmonary sarcoidosis, alterations in AM subpopulations are one of the key determinants responsible for the enhanced cellular reactivity in the lung of those patients (3,4,5,6).

AM obtained by bronchoalveolar lavage (BAL) in patients with sarcoidosis spontaneously secrete Interleukin-1 (IL-1) (3) which is thought to activate T-lymphocytes to synthesise Interleukin-2 (7), this in turn may activate other T-lymphocytes to produce lymphokines, including monocyte chemotactic factor. It is suggested that this results in recruitment of monocytes to the inflammatory response and this amplification produces the building block on which the granuloma are formed (8). AM from patients with sarcoidosis, like those from patients with fibrosing alveolitis, secrete increased amounts of fibronectins (9) and alveolar macrophage derived growth factor (10) which activates lung fibroblasts.

The purpose of our study was to further define phenotypes resp. subpopulations of BAL AM's from sarcoid patients compared to a control group by use of a panel of monoclonal antibodies.

MATERIAL AND METHODS

Patients: 26 patients were included in the study. 14 patients with biopsy proven pulmonary sarcoidosis (8 males, 6 females). 10 of those patients showed activity of the disease suggested by recent deterioration of chest radiography, elevated S-ACE levels, positive ^{67}Ga scans, and clinical symptoms.
The control group consisted of 12 patients: 3 patients with extrinsic allergic alveolitis, 3 patients with pulmonary tuberculosis, 3 patients with lung cancer and 3 patients with an acute pneumonia due to viral or mycoplasma infection.

Bronchoalveolar Lavage: BAL was accomplished through a fiberoptic bronchoscope (Olympus) wedged in a subsegmental bronchus of the right middle lobe. 250ml of sterile, warmed 0.9% saline solution was instilled in 5 aliquots to 50ml each recovered by gentle aspiration, trapped in a plast vessel, and filtered through sterile gauze to remove respiratory mucus prior to in vitro analysis and transferred into a sterile bottle containing 50ml medium RPMI 1640 supplemented with 10% fetal calf serum.

Preparation of mononuclear cell population: The cells were centrifuged, the pellet was resuspended in medium RPMI 1640 containing 5% fetal calf serum, washed twice, counted and ajusted to 5 x 10 cells/ml for cytocentrifuge preparations. After air drying for two hours the slides were frozen in present of a desiccans and stored at -20C.

Monoclonal antibodies (MoAbs):
The monoclonal antibody 27E10 belongs to the IgG1 subclass and detects a surface antigen that is expressed by a subset of periperipheral blood monocytes and of monocytes/macrophages being maximally expressed between days 2 and 3 of culture. In situ the antigen is found only in inflammatory tissues and is absent from normal resident mononuclear phagocytes (11).
The monoclonal antibody 25F9 belongs to the IgG1 subclass and detects a differentiation antigen preferentially expressed on mature, tissue fixed macrophages in - cluding AM. It does not react with freshly isolated blood monocytes (12).
The monoclonal antibody Anti IL-1 belongs to the IgG2a subclass. It is directed against Interleukin-1 of human origin. It blocks IL-1 mediated lymphocyte and fibroblast proliferation but does not interfere with the biological effect of other lymphokines, such as Interleukin-2 or Interleukin-3 (13).
The monoclonal antibody VID-1 defines a nonpolymorphic determinant (IgG1 subclass) of human Ia (HLA-DR) (14). As negative controls PBS/10% FCS and ascites from a non producing plasmocytoma cell line were used.

Immunoperoxidase staining: To stain the respective antigens the avidin-biotin
system was used. The monoclonal antibodies were tested for their final dilution,
the secondary antibody (biotinylated sheep anti-mouse immunoglobulin, 5ng Ig/ml
was followed by incubation in avidin peroxidase complex (15 ng/ml). All incuba-
tions were performed in a humid atmosphere at room temperature for 1 h. Peroxidase staining was achieved with diaminobenzidine (Fluka, Basel, Switzerland)
according to Reese and Karnovsky (15). Cells were counterstained with Mayer's
hämalaun (Merck, F.R.G. art. 9249) and mounted in DePex (Serva Nr.18243).

Inhibition of endogenous peroxidase: A mixture of glucose and glucoseoxidase
was added. Slides were immersed in Methanol/H202 for 30 min. between step two
and three. To block unspecific binding to Fc-receptors of cells, 10% human AB-
serum was added to the second step.
To quantify the proportion of positive cells, a minimum of 400 cells was counted.

Differential cell counts were carried out on smears after centrifugation and
May-Grünwald-Giemsa staining.
Lymphocyte subsets were identified by the monoclonal antibodies; OKT 4 for T-helper cells and OKT 8 for T-suppressor cells (Ortho Pharmaceuticals) by the lymphocyte suspension method (4×10^6 cells/ml). After incubation, washing, fluorescin
labelling with goat antimouse immunglobulin and resuspension the cells were examined by fluorescence microscopy.

Statistical Methods
Values were expressed as % of stained cells showing the monoclonal antibody
(mean $\pm$ SD). Since the data are unevenly distributed non parametric tests had
been used (U-Test, Mann Whitney). Correlations tested by the Spearman rank analysis (16).

RESULTS

MAb 27E10 (Fig.1, Table1)
MAb 27E10 was only significantly expressed (64 $\pm$ 2,08%) on AM of patients with
pneumonia. All other patients showed significant lower percentages. Lowest expression was found in patients with tuberculosis and lung cancer. The most intense staining was found on small AM.

Table 1: Expression of various MAb (% positivity) on AM of various patient
groups.

patients	n	27E10	25F9	Anti IL-1
sarcoidosis	14	20,33$\pm$ 5,18	23,28$\pm$4,27	68,42$\pm$11,03
EAA	3	17$\pm$ 6,8	90$\pm$5	68,66$\pm$14,45
Tbc, cancer	6	10,33$\pm$ 4	30$\pm$5,77	0,33$\pm$ 0,33
pneumonia	3	64$\pm$ 2,08	61$\pm$10,69	74,66$\pm$ 5,33

Fig. 1 : 27E10

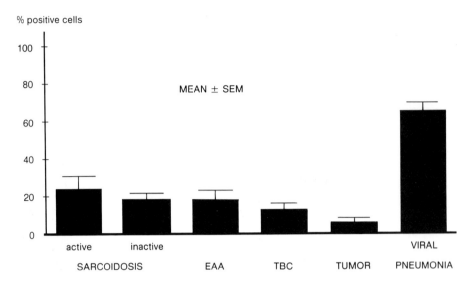

MAb 25F9 (Fig.2, Table1)
Patients with sarcoidosis and EAA showed high expression $(83,28 \pm 4,17\%$, resp. $90 \pm 5\%)$ of 25F9 and were significantly higher than patients in the other groups $(p < 0,01)$, Fig.2. Lowest percentage $(30 \pm 5,77)$ was found in patients with tuberculosis and lung cancer.

Fig. 2 : 25F9

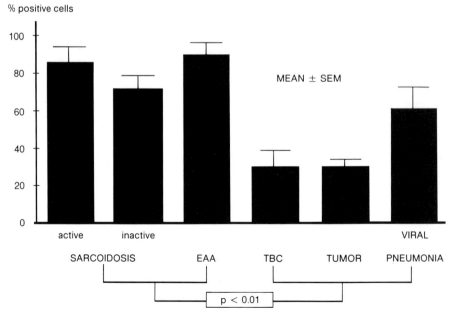

MAb VI D- 1
Except from patients with tuberculosis all AM in the other groups of patients
showed a consistenthigh expression (>90%) of VI D-1.

Fig. 3 :   Anti IL-1

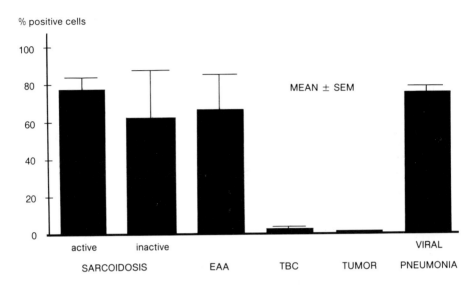

% positive cells

MEAN ± SEM

active   inactive

SARCOIDOSIS   EAA   TBC   TUMOR   VIRAL PNEUMONIA

MAb Anti IL-1   (Fig. 3, Table1)
High percentages of Anti IL-1 positive AM could be observed in patients suffering
from sarcoidosis, EAA and pneumonia, whereas less than 5% of AM from patients
with tuberculosis and neoplasia expressed Anti IL-1 in their cytoplasma. Comparing the results of 25F9 and Anti IL-1, a significant positive correlation
$(r_S=0,52, n=26)$ between those two markers could be established. Patients with
Sarcoid, EAA and pneumonia showing high percentages of 25F9 + AM simultaneously
had incrased numbers of Anti IL-1 positive cells. In accordance, AM of patients
with tuberculosis and neoplasia showing low percentages of 25F9 cells corresponded to low numbers of Anti IL-1 positive cells.

Relation to other BAL-effector cells   (Table 2)
As expected the highest percentages of BAL lymphocytes were observed in patients
with sarcoidosis and EAA. In sarcoidosis % of 25F9 positive cells correlated significantly $(p<0,05)$ to BAL T-helper lymphocytes (T_4). In the total group of patients % of 25F9 positive AM correlated significantly $(p<0,05)$ to % of BAL
lymphocytes (Table 2).

Table 2: Correlation (r_s) %(MAb ÷)AM to % BAL cells or T_4/T_8 ratio.

	n	Sarcoidosis	p-value	n	all patients	p-value
25F9 vs. Lympho	14	0,36		26	0,41	< 0,05
25F9 vs. T-helper	14	0,55	< 0,05	24	0,19	
25F9 vs. T_4/T_8	14	0,49		24	0,17	
Anti IL-1 vs.Lympho	14	0,24		24	0,26	
Anti IL-1 vs.T-helper	14	0,30		24	0,26	
Anti IL-1 vs.T_4/T_8	14	0,28		24	0,26	

DISCUSSION

There is increaseing evidence that AM function of patients with sarcoidosis is distinctively different from the usual behaviour of AM in normal individuals. Functional studies of resident AM from normals exhibited a rather restricted activity of these cells: 1) Under normal conditions they have a decreased capacity to present antigens to various populations of lymphocytes in contrast to blood monocytes (2,4) and 2) release of Interleukin-1 for further T-cell activation may be sufficiently suppressed by AM derived inhibitors, like prostaglandin E_2 (17) Some studies however, emphasize that even the normal AM can exert considerable functional activity if there is a low ratio of AM to T-lymphocytes. Increasing ratios of AM to lymphocytes however, result in suppression by the AM (18).

AM in patients with sarcoidosis obviously behave different. Enhanced cellular immune reactivity in the lower respiratory tract of suffereres (19) is accompanied by increased IL-1 secretion by their AM (3,20), concomitant with increased antigen presenting capacity by these cells (21).

Our study strongly supports those current concepts of activated AM in sarcoidosis. We could demonstrate at least 2 different AM subpopulations which obviously exert different functional activities. 25F9 + AM are predominantly found in the alveoli of our patients with sarcoidosis and EAA. Their phenotype is markedly different from blood monocytes. In strong contrast to the dormant behavior of the normal resident AM, the 25F9 + AM in sarcoidosis appears to be in a high state of activity. The characteristics of those macrophages are their marked intracellular distribution of IL-1 and their significant correlation to % of BAL T-helper cells which are known to be the hallmarks of the alveolitis in sarcoidosis.

However, a couple of questions still need further clarification.
1) Since we have not tested the spontaneous release of IL-1 of the 25F9 +AM from

mononuclear cell culture, we dont know whether the enhanced IL-1 storage is due to enhanced production and subsequent release or due to diminished release resulting in intracellular accumulation. However, as soon IL-1 is released from the AM apparently there is a variety of inhibitors present, which may explain some of the discrepant results reported so far (22).

2) No data are available whether our observed proportion of mature (25F9+) and recently recruited AM (27E10+) will be maintained during the course of the disease. Studies by Hance et al. (23)suggest that in some instances AM phenotypes resembling those of freshly recruited monocytes from the peripheral blood are characteristic as well. More longitudinal data are necessary to shed more light in these questions.

3) It is evident that changes in the AM population may exacerbate T-cell mediated lung damage, but it is not yet known whether and to what extent altered AM function contributes to the initiation of the process, or simply results from it.

In this regard the significance of local macrophage proliferation which accompanies chronic lung inflammation (24) in relation to overall AM function remains to be determined.

In conclusion our studies substantiate alterations of AM subpopulations in patients with pulmonary sarcoidosis. 25F9+ AM are characteristic for pulmonary sarcoidosis. They are suggested to be responsible for enhanced Interleukin-1 production and release which results in T-lymphocyte and fibroblast proliferation resulting in granuloma formation and eventually lung fibrosis.

Address of author:

Heinrich Klech MD FCCP
2nd Med.Dept.Wilhelminenspital
Montleartstraße 37
A - 1171 Vienna, Austria

REFERENCES

1.   Holt PG (1986) .Down-regulation of immune responses in the lower respiratory tract: the role of alveolar macrophages.Clin.exp.Immunol.63:261-270

2.   Mackaness GB (1971).The induction and expression of cell-mediated hypersensitivity in the lung. Am.Rev.Respir.Dis 104:813

3.   Hunninghake GW (1984).Release of Interleukin-1 by Alveolar Macrophages of Patients with Active Pulmonary Sarcoidosis.Am.Rev.Respir.Dis.129:569-572

4.   Hunninghake GW (1987).Immunoregulatory Functions of Human Alveolar Macrophages. Am.Rev.Respir.Dis.136:253-254

5.   DuBois RM (1985). The alveolar macrophage.Thorax 40:321-327

6.   Toews GB,Lem VM,Weissler JC,Nunez-Ollero G, Ball EJ, Stastny P,Lipscomb MF (1986). Antigen Presentation by Alveolar Macrophages in Patients with

Sarcoidosis. Ann.NY Acad.Sci.465:74-81.

7. Pinkston P,Bitterman PB,Crystal RG (1983).Spontaneous release of interleukin-2 by lung T lymphocytes in active pulmonary sarcoidosis.N Engl J Med 308:793-800

8. Hunninghake GW,Gadek JE,Young RC,Kawanami O,Ferrans VJ,Crystal RG (1980). Maintenance of granuloma formation in pulmonary sarcoidosis by T-lymphocytes within the lung. N Engl J Med. 302:594-8

9. Rennard SI,Hunninghake GW,Bitterman PB,Crystal RG.(1981).Production of fibro-nectin by the human alveolar macrophage:mechanism for the recruitment of fi-broblasts to sites of tissue injury in interstitial lung diseases. Proc Natl. Acad Sci USA 78:7147-51

10.Bitterman PB, Adelberg S,Crystal RG (1983).Mechanisms of pulmonary fibrosis: spontaneous release of the alveolar macrophage-derived growth factor in the interstitial lung disorders.J Clin Invest 72:1801-13

11.Zwadlo G, Schlegel R,Sorg C.(1986).A Monoclonal Antibody to a Subset of Hu-man Monocytes found only in the Peripheral Blood and Innflammatory Tissues. J Immunol.137:512-518

12.Zwadlo G,Bröcker EB,v.Bassewitz DB,Feige U,Sorg C.(1985). A Monoclonal Anti-body to a Differentiation Antigen Present on Mature Human Macrophages and Ab-sent from Monocytes. I Immunol.134:1487-1492

13.Köck A,Danner M,Stadler BM,Luger TH.(1986). Cahracterization of a Monoclonal antibody directed against the Biologically Active Site of Human Interleukin-1 J Exp Med 163:463-468

14.Köller U,Majdic O,Liszka K,Stockinger H,Pabinger-Fasching I,Lechner K,Knapp W. (1985).Lymphocytes of haemophilia patients treated with clotting factor con-centrates display activation-linked cell-surface antigens. Clin.exp.Immunol. 59:613-621

15.Reese TS,Karnovsky MJ (1967).Fine structural localisation of a blood-brain barrier to exogenous peroxidase.J.Cell.Biol. 34:207-217

16.Conover WJ (1980).Practical non parametric statistics.2nd edn.J.Wiley,New York

17.Monick M,Glazier J,Hunninghake GW.(1987).Human Alveolar Macrophages Suppress Interleukin-1 (IL-1) Activity Via the Secretion of Prostaglandin E_2 Am Rev Respir Dis 135:72-77

18.Rich EA,Tweardy DJ,Fujiwara H,Ellner JJ.(1987).Spectrum of Immunoregulatory Functions and Properties of Human Alveolar Macrophages.Am Rev Respir Dis136: 258-265

19.Hunninghake GW,Crystal RG (1981).Pulmonary sarcoidosis:a disorder mediated by excess helper T-lymphocyte activity at sites of disease activity.N Engl J Med 305:429-34.

20.Hunninghake GW,Glazier AJ,Monick MM,Dinarello CHA.(1987).Interleukin-1 Is a Chemotactic Factor for Human T-Lymphocytes.Am Rev Respir Dis 135:66-71

21.Venet A,Hance AJ,Saltini C,Robinson BWS,Crystal RG (1985).Enhanced alveolar macrophage mediated antigen induced T-lymphocyte proliferation in sarcoidosis J.clin.Invest. 75:293

22.Kleinhenz ME,Fujiwara H,Rich EA.(1986).Interleukin-1 Production by Blood Mono-cytes and Bronchoalveolar Cells in Sarcoidosis. Ann.NY Acad Sci.465:91-97

23.Hance AJ,Douches S,Winchester RJ,Ferrans VJ,CrystalRG (1985).Characterization of mononuclear phagocyte subpopulations in the human lung by using monoclonal antibodies.J.Immunol.134:284

24.Bitterman PB,Saltzman LE,Adelberg S,Ferrans VJ,Crystal RG(1984).Alveolar Macro phage Replication.One Mechanism for the expansion of the mononuclear phagocyte population in the chronically inflamed lung.J.clin.Invest.74:460

© 1988 Elsevier Science Publishers B.V. (Biomedical Division)
Sarcoidosis and other granulomatous disorders
C. Grassi, G. Rizzato, E. Pozzi, editors

REGULATION OF NEUTROPHIL MOBILITY BY ALVEOLAR MACROPHAGES FROM PATIENTS WITH SARCOIDOSIS.

Yves SIBILLE, William W. MERRILL, Stephen B. CARE, Gary P. NAEGEL, J. Allen D. COOPER Jr. and Herbert Y. REYNOLDS.

Pulmonary Section, Yale University Medical School, New Haven, CT 06510, USA.

INTRODUCTION

Although lung infiltration by polymorphonuclear neutrophils (PMN) is uncommon in pulmonary sarcoidosis these cells are found more frequently among the lavage cells of patients with advanced and fibrotic disease (1). However, whether PMN contribute to lung injury or merely collect in already damaged lungs is unknown. Furthermore, an increased percentage of PMN in BAL is also found occasionally in some non fibrotic patients with radiological stage I and stage II disease (2).

Alveolar macrophages (AM) can secrete in vitro chemotactic factors for PMN (3) and activated AM recovered from patients with idiopathic pulmonary fibrosis spontaneously release more chemotaxins in culture than AM from normals (4). Although AM from patients with sarcoidosis are activated in vivo, little information is available about the ability of sarcoid cells to release chemotactic factors for PMN. The present study was designed to investigate the profile of PMN chemotaxins released in vitro by AM from patients with pulmonary sarcoidosis and the relationship between this release and the PMN infiltration of alveolar structures as assessed by BAL.

MATERIAL AND METHODS

Study population and bronchoalveolar lavage :

Fourteen normal non smokers and twenty one non smoking patients with sarcoidosis were recruted for this study. Twelve patients were radiographically stage I sarcoidosis, 6 were stage II and 3 had stage III.

After informed consent, a bronchoalveolar lavage (BAL) procedure was performed following a well described protocol (5).

Cell culture

After a 10 min centrifugation at 500 g, BAL cells were separated from the BAL fluid and were resuspended ($1 \times 10^6/1.8ml$) in modified Mc Coy's 5a medium and incubated for various time at 37°C, 5 % CO_2. After one hour adherence step. Supernatant containing unattached cells was removed and replaced with 1.0 ml Mc Coy's. Further studies were performed on culture supernatants.

PMN CHEMOTAXIS

Peripheral blood PMN were isolated from heparinized venous blood by using a one step centrifugation using a Hypaque-Ficoll gradient (6) and PMN chemotaxis was assayed in a 48 well microchemotaxis chamber (7). Data were expressed as a percent of the maximal FMLP-induced chemotaxis.

HPLC studies

AM culture supernatants were separated by molecular sieve HPLC columns (I-60) separating compounds of molecular weight between 50,000 to less than 1,000 daltons. Eluting fractions were tested for their effect on PMN migration.

Assay for leukotriene B_4 (LTB_4), Interleukin-1 (IL-1) and C_{5a}

The presence of LTB_4 in supernatants was tested by reverse phase (C_{18}) HPLC and radioimmunoassay (8). IL-1 activity was tested by the incorporation of (^3H) thymidine into C3H/HeJ mouse thymocytes (9). C_{5a} release in culture was investigated by radioimmunoassay (10).

RESULTS

BAL cell data and PMN chemotaxis :

BAL cell counts and differentials are given in table 1. After an adherence step, BAL cells from sarcoid patients released spontaneously in short term culture (4 h) more chemotactic activity for PMN (68.8 ± 35.1 %, expressed as percentage of the chemotaxis induced by 10^{-7} M. FMLP) than corresponding cells from normals. The same pattern was observed after long term cultures (18 h) and no difference related to disease stage was noticed. This increased chemotactic activity released by sarcoid AM correlated with the presence of PMN in the alveolar space as assessed by BAL neutrophilia ($r = 0.71$, $p < 0.01$).

Characterisation of the chemotactic activity

After HPLC molecular sieve separation of the AM culture supernatants, the elution points of the chemotactic activity were distributed into 3 major peaks (15.000 - 10.000 daltons, 8 - 10,000 d and below 1,000 daltons). In addition to these peaks, we also observed a peak of inhibitory activity on PMN mobility, mostly in the low molecular weight range (< 1.000 d) of the HPLC chromatogram. None of these peaks appear to correspond to either C_{5a} or LTB_4. In contrast, IL-1 was found increased in culture supernatants from sarcoid AM (2.4 ± 0.5 U/ml) as compared to normal AM (0.5 ± 0.2 U/ml) ($p < 0.05$).

DISCUSSION

The present study demonstrates that adherent BAL cells from patients with pulmonary sarcoidosis release in culture more chemotactic activity for PMN than respiratory cells from normals. This appears to represent one additional marker of macrophage activation in sarcoidosis. A correlation was observed between the percentage of PMN recovered by BAL and the PMN chemotactic activity released into culture. These data suggest that in vitro chemotactic factor release by AM is an accurate reflection of this in vivo function. From the different know PMN chemotaxins we tested, only IL-1 may account at least in part for the increased chemotactic activity observed in sarcoid AM culture supernatants. This is in agreement with previous reports demonstrating that sarcoid AM release in vitro more IL-1 than normal AM (11, 12).

Finally, we also observed that respiratory cells from both normals and sarcoid patients could release in vitro factor(s) with inhibitory activity on PMN mobility and this may explain, at least partially the low PMN count usually observed in these individuals.

In conclusion, through the release of both chemotaxins and inhibitory factor(s), AM have the capability to regulate the PMN traffic within alveolar structures of patients with pulmonary sarcoidosis.

TABLE 1

Lavage cell counts and differentials in normal and sarcoidosis patients

	Total cell counts $BALx10^6/100ml$ of recovered BAL	Differential cell count mean $\pm$ SD (ranges)			
		AM	Lymphocytes	Neutrophils	Eosinophils
Normals (n = 14)	11.8 ± 4.3	89.6 ± 4.9	9.5 ± 4.7	0.8 ± 1.3	0.1 ± 0.3 0.
Sarcoidosis patients (n = 21)	31.4 ± 23.5*	64.6 ± 19.6*	33.0 ± 18.9*	1.5 ± 2.0	0.6 ± 1.7

* p < 0.05, between sarcoidosis patients and corresponding values from normals.

REFERENCES

1. ROTH C., HUCHON G.J., ARNOUX A., STANISLAS-LEGUERN G., MARSAC J.H., CHRETIEN J.
   Bronchoalveolar cells in advanced pulmonary sarcoidosis.
   Am. Rev. Respir. Dis., 1981; 124 : 9-12.

2. TONNEL A.B., VOISIN C., LAFITTE J.J., RAMON P., AERTS C.
   Variation des populations cellulaires recueillies par lavage bronchoalvéolaire en fonction de la topographie des lésions et de l'étage exploré.
   Institut National de la Santé et de la Recherche Médicale, Paris, 1979; 84 : 271-279.

3. MERRILL W.W., NAEGEL G.P., MATTHAY R.A., REYNOLDS H.Y.
   Alveolar macrophage-derived chemotactic factor for neutrophils-Kinetics of "in vitro" production and partial characterization.
   J. Clin. Invest. 1980; 66 : 268-276.

4. HUNNINGHAKE G.W., GADEK J.E., FALES H.M., CRYSTAL R.G.
    Human alveolar macrophage derived chemotactic factor for
    neutrophils.
    J. Clin. Invest. 1987; 79 : 319-326.

5. REYNOLDS H.Y., NEWBALL H.H.
    Analysis of proteins and respiratory cells obtained from human
    lungs by bronchial lavage.
    J. Lab. Clin. Med., 1974; 84 : 559-573.

6. FERRANTE A., THONG H.Y.
    A rapid one-step procedure for purification of mononuclear and
    polymorphonuclear leukocytes from human blood using a modification
    of the Hypaque-Ficoll technique.
    J. Immunol. Meth. 1978; 24 : 389-393.

7. FALK W., GOODWIN R.H., Jr. LEONARD E.J.
    A 48-well micro chemotaxis assembly for rapid and accurate
    measurement of leukocyte migration.
    J. Immunol. Meth., 1980; 33 : 239-247.

8. ROKACH J., HAYES E.C., GIRARD Y., LOMBARDO D.L., MAYCOCK A.L.,
    ROSENTHAL A.S., YOUNG R.N., ZAMBONI R., ZWEERINK H.J.
    The development of sensitive and specific radioimmunoassays for
    leukotrienes.
    Prostagl. Leukot. Med. 1984; 13 : 21-25.

9. MELTZER M.S., OPPENHEIM J.J.
    Biodirectional amplification of macrophage-lymphocyte interactions
    : enhanced lymphocyte activation factor production by activated
    adherent mouse peritoneal cells.
    J. Immunol. 1977; 118 : 77-82.

10. HUGLI T.E., CHENOWETH D.E.
    Biologically active peptides of complement : techniques and
    significance C_{3a} and C_{5a} measurement. (ED) RM Nakamura. In
    "Future perspectives in clinical laboratory immunoassays" New York,
    ALAN R LiSS Inc. 1980 pp.430-460.

11. HUNNINGHAKE G.W.
     Release of Interleukin-1 by alveolar macrophages of patients with
     active pulmonary sarcoidosis.
     Am. Rev. Respir. Dis. 1984; 129 : 569-572.

12. KORETZKY G.A., ELIAS J.A., KAY S.L., ROSSMAN M.D., NOWELL P.C.,
     DANIELE R.P.
     Spontaneous production of interleukin-1 by human alveolar
     macrophages.
     Clin. Immunopathol. 1983; 29 : 443-450.

THE EFFECT OF ANGIOTENSIN II(A-II) ON THE ACCESSORY FUNCTION OF BALF
MACROPHAGES - A POSSIBLE AUTOSTIMULATORY MECHANISM OF T LYMPHOCYTE
ALVEOLITIS IN SARCOIDOSIS -

SONOKO NAGAI, TAKATERU IZUMI, MINORU TAKEUCHI, KAZUHIKO WATANABE, SHUNSAKU OSHIMA
Chest Disease Research Institute, Kyoto University, Kyoto, Japan

INTRODUCTION

Most cases of sarcoidosis show spontaneous regression but there are some cases
of a long duration. Therefore, it is reasonable to assume that some factors
induce a state of continuous activation of macrophages to maintain T lymphocyte
alveolitis, because activated macrophages can present antigens to T cells or
can help the response of T cells to mitogens.

It has been reported that elevated SACE levels are correlated with disease
activity in sarcoidosis[1] and reflect their production by activated macrophages
in granulomatous lesions.[2,3] In the pathogenetic process, ACE converts
angiotensin I(A-I) to A-II, which may activate macrophages (via binding to A-
II receptors on macrophages[4]), and enhance these accessory functions, resulting
in a significant increase of lung T cells.[5] Therefore, we investigated the
effect of A-I/A-II, which was added exogenously, on the accessory function
of blood monocytes and BALF macrophages in T cell proliferation under the
stimulation of anti-OKT-3 antibody (OKT3-Ab), which mimicks antigenic action
to antigenic receptors on T cells.[6]

MATERIALS AND METHODS
Study population

In our study, we examined only non-smoking healthy individuals and sarcoidosis
patients.

Healthy controls: All eight individuals showed no signs of infection or
allergic diseases roentogenologically, physically and from their laboratory data.

Sarcoidosis: We selected active cases with abnormal chest X ray's findings
and elevated SACE levels. Active cases were divided into two groups: new cases
detected within 6 months by abnormal chest X ray's findings (stage I n=7) and
prolonged patients with sarcoidosis for more than 5 years (stage I n=2, stage III
n=5). No patient had been treated by corticosteroid within the past 6 months.
Methods

Bronchoalveolar lavage: We lavaged all cases performed using sterilized
warm saline (50 ml x 6) in the right middle lobe. The recovered fluid (BALF)
was filtered by gauze and centrifuged to obtain BALF cells.[7]

Blood mononuclear cells: These cell fractions were prepared by the

Ficoll-Pacque centrifugation method.

Autologous mixed cell cultures for evaluating the accessory function: We further fractionated both BALF cells and blood mononuclear cells by the E rosette method to obtain the E rosette forming cell fraction (E_4^+ cells: Tp (blood T cells), T_B(BALF T cells)) and non-E rosette forming cell fraction (E_4^- cells: mo (blood monocytes), Mϕ (BALF macrophages)). E_4^+ cells could be purified to 95% of T cells and E_4^- cells with the purity of 95% mo/Mϕ.

Tp cells (1 x 10^6/ml in 10% human AB serum-RPMI) and mo/Mϕ (1 x 10^6/ml in 10% human AB serum-RPMI) inactivated by 3000 rad radiation were mixed at a ratio of 4 to 1 in 96 well microplates (Corning 25860, flat bottom), and cultured for 72 hours under stimulation with OKT3-Ab (Ortho Pharmaceutial Corp, Raritan, N.J.). ^{3}H-thymidine incorporation during the last 18 hours was measured by a liquid scintillation counter.

A-I/A-II (Sigma, St. Louis, Mo.) was added from the start of culture. The effect of A-II/A-I was expressed as the stimulation index

$$(S.I.) = \frac{\Delta cpm \ (Tp + mo/M\phi + OKT3-Ab + AII/A-I)}{\Delta cpm \ (Tp + mo/M\phi + OKT3-Ab)}$$

Statistics: The mean ± S.E. of each experiment within the patient and control groups was determined. Comparisons of these values were performed using Student's t test.

RESULTS

Accessory functions of BALF macrophages and blood monocytes in autologous T cell proliferation (Fig. 1): No significant accessory function of mo/Mϕ was detected without stimulation of OKT3-Ab in the patients or the healthy controls. Under stimulation by OKT3-Ab at the final concentration of 25 ng/ml, maximal accessory function was detected with Tp cells. This accessory function of BALF macrophages in the cases of sarcoidosis was similar to that in the healthy controls.

As to T_B cells, similar results were found. The findings of the accessory function of mo with T_B being greater than that with Tp may be due to the presence of Mϕ in T_B fractions.

The effect of A-II/A-I on the accessory function in T cell proliferation (Figs 2, 3, 4, 5): No A-II/A-I had effect on Tp cell proliferation in the absence of accessory cells or on the accessory function in Tp cell proliferation in the absence of OKT3-Ab (data not shown).

We evaluated the concentrations of A-II/A-I (1.9 x 10^{-9}M, 1.9 x 10^{-7}M, 1.9 x 10^{-5}M) in culture. The average ± S.E. of S.I. showed no dose-response relationships between the concentration of A-II/A-I added and the Tp cell

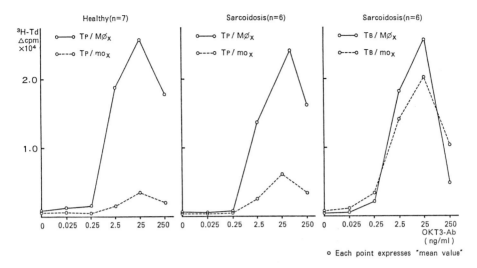

Fig. 1. Accessory function of BALF macrophages/blood monocytes in autologous T cell proliferation of Tp (blood T cell) or T_B (BALF-T cell): 1 x 10^5/well + Mϕ (BALF macrophage) or mo (blood monocyte) 2.5 x 10^4/well in 10% human AB serum-RPMI, cultured to 72 hrs at 37°C under 5% CO_2 with various doses of a OKT3-Ab.

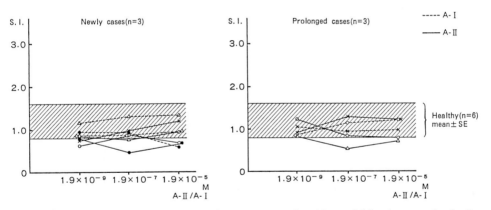

Fig. 2. The effect of A-II/A-I on the accessory function of blood monocyte in Tp cell proliferation. Solid lines: addition of A-II; dotted lines: addition of A-I; shaded area: mean ± S.E. of healthy controls (n=7).

proliferation supported by the accessory cells under the stimulation of OKT3-Ab (25 ng/ml) in any cases tested.

No enhancement by A-II was observed when monocytes were used as the accessory cells in any cases studied (Fig. 2). However, the accessory function of BALF macrophages was enhanced by A-II at the concentrations added exogenously in the prolonged cases of sarcoidosis. (Fig. 3.)

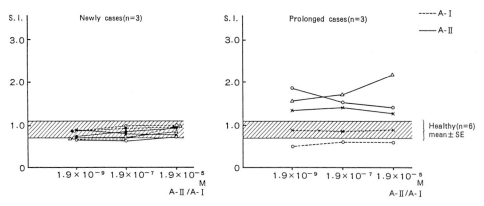

Fig. 3. The effect of A-II/A-I on the accessory function of BALF macrophages in Tp cell proliferation. Solid lines: addition of A-II; dotted lines: addition of A-I; shaded area: mean ± S.E. of healthy controls (n=7).

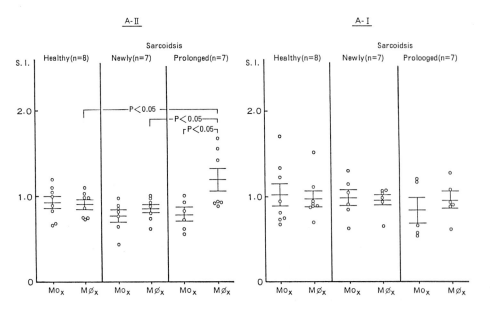

Fig. 4. The effect of A-II/A-I on the accessory function in blood T cell proliferation.

We selected the A-II concentration of 1.9×10^{-7}M to evaluate its effects on the accessory function in Tp cell proliferation, based on the no dose-response relationships. Figure 4 summarizes the effect of A-II/A-I.

To evaluate the specificity of the effects of A-II, we performed the same experiments using A-I added exogenously.

We found significant enhancement by A-II of the accessory function of Mφ in the prolonged cases, compared to both in the healthy controls and the newly detected cases. These findings were also observed in the experiments using T_B cells as responder T cells (Fig. 5), though not significant.

In the prolonged cases, the A-II-induced enhancement was significant on the accessory function by Mφ, not by mo. These findings were also observed in the experiment using T_B as responder T cells (Fig. 5).

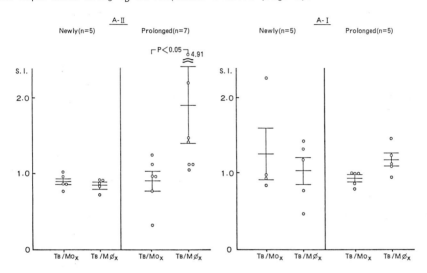

Fig. 5. The effect of A-II/A-I on the accessory function in BALF-T cell proliferation.

DISCUSSION

Immunological processes have been implicated in the pathogenesis of pulmonary sarcoidosis. Therefore, it is necessary to examine the factors responsible for maintainance of T lymphocyte alveolitis that leads to the formation of epithelioid cell granuloma.

We used OKT3-Ab which mimics some antigens in one-way mixed cell culture as the stimulatory substance because there is no information on the etiological agents in sarcoidosis.

The enhanced accessory function of BALF macrophages compared to blood monocytes was detected both in healthy controls and active sarcoidosis. It should be stressed that the accessory function of BALF macrophages may be determined by various factors including the ratio of accessory cells to T cells, a characteristics of the antigen and mitogen and any other stimulatory or inhibitory factors. However, in our culture conditions, we found that A-II enhanced rather specifically the accessory function of BALF macrophages in both

134

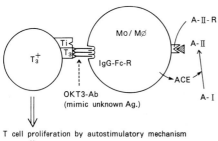

T cell proliferation by autostimulatory mechanism

Maintainance of MØ-T lymphocyte alveolitis

Fig. 6. Maintainance of Mφ-T lymphocyte
        alveolitis

blood and BALF T cell proliferation
in the non-smokers with active
sarcoidosis of a long duration.
These findings suggest that T
lymphocyte alveolitis is maintained
in sarcoidosis of a long duration
by an autostimulatory mechanism
whereby A-II is endogenously produced by ACE, which is derived from
activated macrophages.

Whether this autostimulatory
mechanism is mediated by receptors
to A-II remains to be elucidated
(Fig. 6).

SUMMARY

   There are some patients with sarcoidosis of a long duration who has elevated
SACE levels. It has been reported that ACE was released from activated macrophages at the lesions. We hypothesized that this enzyme could convert A-I
to A-II, which could enhance the accessory function of BALF macrophages in
T cell proliferation. We found that A-II enhanced this accessory function
in the cases of sarcoidosis with longer duration. These findings suggest that
T lymphocyte alveolitis is maintained in sarcoidosis of a long duration by an
autostimulatory mechanism whereby A-II is endogenously produced by ACE, which
is derived from activated macrophages.

REFERENCES

1. Lieberman J (1975) Am J Med 59: 365-372

2. Grönhagen-Riska C, Fyhrquist F, von Willebrand E (1986) Annals NY
    Acad Sci 465: 242-249

3. Hinman LM, Stevence C, Matthay RA, Gee JBL (1979) Science 205: 202-203

4. Thomas DW, Hoffman MD (1984) J Immunol 132: 2807-2812

5. Weinstock JV, Blum AM (1985) Cell Immunol 94: 558-567

6. Bolhuis RL, Gravekamp C, van de Griend RJ (1986) Clinics in immunol
    and allergy 6: 29-90

7. Nagai S, Fujimura N, Hirata T, Izumi T (1984) Eur J Respir Dis 67: 1-9

ACKNOWLEDGEMENT

   We thanks to Dr. Mio T, Dr. Emura M, Dr. Kitaichi M for their help in the
bronchoalveolar lavage. We also thank Mrs. Tanioka F for her technical help
in performing our experiments.

MAST CELLS IN SARCOIDOSIS

P. ROTTOLI, L. ROTTOLI, M.G. PERARI,°C. VINDIGNI, A. COLLODORO,°M. CINTORINO, S. BIANCO

Institutes of Respiratory Diseases and °Pathology, University of Siena, Italy

INTRODUCTION

Sarcoidosis, a multisystem disease, still provides a very interesting study model, given the complexity of its immunological and inflammatory reactions. Although the main pathogenetic mechanisms seem to be understood, many aspects are still not clear. It is possible that, as well as lymphocytes and macrophages, which play a major role in the pathogenesis of this disease, other cells are important in inducing alterations of the immune reaction. For example, mast cells (MC) may be involved in the pathogenesis of pulmonary fibrosis, as suggested by recent data obtained in experimental models and in some interstitial lung diseases (1,3,5,8). The proliferation of MC, or rather of their subpopulation, seems dependent on a T lymphocyte product IL_3 (4). In sarcoidosis, the number of lymphocytes is greatly increased and they spontaneously release lymphokines. It is possible that among these there is also the growth factor for MC. It has also recently been suggested (11) that the activation of H2-R bearing $CD8^+$ lymphocytes and HI-R bearing $CD4^+$ lymphocytes to produce LCF and Ly MIF may be induced by antigen or histamine released from MC and might be one mechanism by which $CD4^+$ cells are recruited to and immobilized at granuloma sites. This suggests a possible role of MC in the formation of granulomas. At present, there is a great deal of interest in studying the possible role of MC in inflammatory and immunological reactions as well as in IgE-mediated reactions (2). Very little research has been carried out on MC in sarcoidosis. However, recently, research workers have begun to study them in bronchoalveolar lavage (BAL) and their presence has been reported in sarcoidosis, extrinsic allergic alveolitis, cryptogenic fibrosing alveolitis and asthma (6,9,10).

The aim of the present study was to evaluate the number of MC in the BAL of patients with sarcoidosis and other lung diseases and to consider their relationship with other immunocompetent cells. Mast cells were also studied in bronchial biopsies performed at the time of BAL.

PATIENTS AND METHODS

Patients

Thirty-eight patients with sarcoidosis (19 males; mean age 43 yrs), 8 of whom were smokers, were studied. The diagnosis was based on a positive biopsy, in addition to the presence of typical clinical features and laboratory data. No patient was receiving steroids at the time of BAL.   On the basis of chest x-ray, the patients were classified as follows: 8 patients with stage 1, 27 with stage II, 3 with stage III.   According to clinical and laboratory findings 28 were considered active forms.   Eight patients with lung cancer, undergoing fibroscopy for diagnostic purposes (6 males; mean age 60.5 yrs, range 43-72, all smokers) were also studied together with 10 patients with chronic bronchitis (CB)(7 males; mean age 62 yrs) 6 of whom were smokers.   The control group consisted of 5 non-smoking subjects (3 males; mean age 55 yrs) with normal respiratory function and no evidence of lung disease.

Methods

  Bronchoalveolar lavage (BAL) and cell population counts were performed as previously described (7). Slides were stained with toluidine blue 0.5% in HCl 0.5N for 30 minutes for identification of MC.   Two thousand or more consecutive cells were counted.   E rosette and monoclonal antibody techniques (OKT_3, OKT_4, OKT_8; Ortho Pharmaceutical Corp.) were used to identify the lymphocyte subpopulations.

  Statistical analysis was performed using Student's t test and correlation coefficient.

Bronchial biopsies were fixed in Carnoy and 5 serial ($4 \pm 0.5 \mu$ thick) sections were stained with haematoxylin/eosin for histological diagnosis and with toluidine blue (0.1%) for MC detection.   Five high magnification (400 x) fields were considered in every section to count MC and their number per mm^2 of area of tissue section was calculated.

RESULTS

  BAL cells with an affinity for toluidine blue were identified as MC because of their morphology.   The cells varied in shape from oval to round and in size. Sometimes, it was possible to see partially degranulated MC and clusters of granules outside the cell membrane.   Our data show that MC are present in BAL, although in lower percentages compared to lymphocytes (Table 1).   The % of MC varied greatly in patients with sarcoidosis from 0.001 to 0.8% with a mean value of ($M \pm SE$) 0.21 ± 0.03.   Considering MC as the number of cells/ml of recovered BAL, they were between 3.5 and 2792/ml of BAL recovered (438 ± 98 M $\pm$ SE). There was a significant difference with the control group both as percentage and as no. of cells/ml (mean values of controls - 0.09 ± 0.02% and 141 ± 42 cells/ml). A highly significant difference was found between active and inactive sarcoidosis both in % (0.27 vs 0.054) and as no. of cells/ml of BAL recovered (578 vs 73) ($p \angle 0.01$).   There was no difference in the quantity of fluid recovered between the two groups.   The significant difference between the number of MC in active and inactive disease suggests a possible relationship between MC and

TABLE I Lymphocytes and MC recovered in BAL from patients with sarcoidosis, chronic bronchitis, lung cancer and controls (M $\pm$ SE)

	No.	Ly/ml recovered BAL	MC/ml recovered BAL
Sarcoidosis	38	77,900 $\pm$ 17,300	438 $\pm$ 98
Active	28	99,500 $\pm$ 22,300	578 $\pm$ 28
Inactive	10	25,500 $\pm$ 11,300	73 $\pm$ 28
CB	10	48,200 $\pm$ 16,000	525 $\pm$ 165
Cancer	8	22,200 $\pm$ 11,400	241 $\pm$ 129
Controls	5	11,000 $\pm$ 3,100	141 $\pm$ 42

lymphocytes which are usually increased in sarcoidosis.

The following highly significant correlations were found: between mast cells/ml of recovered BAL and: 1) Ly/ml ($r = 0.64$, p $/0.001$); 2) E rosette forming cells ($r = 0.63$, p $/0.001$); 3) CD_3^+ lymphocytes ($r = 0.51$, p $/0.001$); 4) CD_4^+ lymphocytes ($r = 0.89$, p $/0.001$). A weak but significant correlation was found between MC and CD_8^+ lymphocytes ($r = 0.44$, p $/0.05$). The % of MC in the group with CB varied from 0.07 to 0.5% (M $\pm$ SE = 0.24 $\pm$ 0.04) and from 43.3 to 1320 as number of cells/ml of recovered BAL (525 $\pm$ 165, M $\pm$ SE). In the group with lung cancer the % of MC varied from 0.02 to 1.3 (0.23 $\pm$ 0.11, M $\pm$ SE) and from 4.3 to 834 as number of cells/ml of recovered BAL (M $\pm$ SE = 241 $\pm$ 129). The correlation between the number of MC/ml and the lymphocytes/ml was highly significant also in these groups ($r = 0.81$ for CB and $r = 0.93$ for lung cancer).

Bronchial biopsies: the presence of MC in bronchial biopsies was investigated in 27 patients with active sarcoidosis and in 8 patients with CB. The number of MC/mm^2 of tissue in sarcoidosis varied greatly from 0 to 79 and the mean value was 14.8 $\pm$ 3.5 (M $\pm$ SE). In the patients with CB the range was between 6 and 44 and the mean value was 24.3 $\pm$ 4.6. There was no significant difference between the two groups of patients.

Dividing the sarcoidosis patients into two groups on the basis of the presence or absence of granulomas in the biopsies, we did not find any significant difference, even if there were greater values in the group without granulomas. Generally, there were no MC inside the granulomas, whereas they were found in the periphery.

The biopsies without granulomas were divided into three groups according to histological pattern: with inflammatory cells (lymphocytes, neutrophils, etc), with normal picture and with fibrosis. The lowest numbers of MC were found in the group with fibrosis in the biopsy.

138

DISCUSSION

Our results in BAL demonstrate an increase of MC in active sarcoidosis, chronic bronchitis and lung cancer. These data confirm previous reports (6,8,9).

The correlation between Ly and MC found in sarcoidosis, CB and lung cancer requires confirmation with functional studies, but suggests that MC are involved in many inflammatory reactions, probably with different functions. The correlation found in sarcoidosis with CD_4^+ lymphocytes could indicate a relationship between the MC present in the alveoli and T helper/inducer lymphocytes. No other authors have found a relationship between MC and lymphocytes in sarcoidosis, but this may depend on different expressions of the results. The reported increase of anti-IgE induced histamine released from bronchoalveolar cells of sarcoidosis patients with more than 20% of lymphocytes is, in our opinion, in agreement with our findings.(6)

The MC in bronchial biopsies were studied to see if they were also present at different levels in the lung of patients with sarcoidosis. The data so far obtained have shown that MC are present, but in lower numbers than in CB. In sarcoidosis, no difference was found between the various morphological patterns of the biopsies, even where they have no evident pathological appearances. It is difficult at present, to confirm whether MC are increased in sarcoidosis because of the problem of finding normal controls for bronchial biopsies.

It is possible that MC are involved in many immunological reactions and a functional study on the release of mediators, perhaps differing according to the type of activation and/or to the MC subpopulation involved, could provide data to clarify their role in the pathogenesis of sarcoidosis as well as other inflammatory diseases.

REFERENCES

1. Agius RM, Horwarth PH, Church MK et al (1986) In: Befus AD et al (eds) Mast Cell Differentiation and Heterogeneity. Raven Press, New York.
2. Bienenstock J, Befus AD, Denburg JA (1983) In: Befus AD et al (eds) Mast Cell Differentiation and Heterogeneity. Raven Press, New York.
3. Claman HN (1985) Immunology Today 6: 192
4. Ezeamuzie IC, Assem ES (1984) Agents Actions 13: 223
5. Faulkner CS, Connelly KS (1973) Lab Invest 28: 545
6. Flint KC, Leung KBP, Hudspith BN et al (1986) Thorax 41: 94
7. Lenzini L, Heather CJ, Rottoli P, et al (1978) Respiration 36: 145
8. Kawanami O, Ferrans VJ, Fulner JD, Crystal RG (1979) Lab Invest 40: 717
9. Rottoli L, Rottoli P, Perari MG et al (1986) Eur J Resp Dis 49: A142
10. Wardlaw AJ, Cromwell O, Celestino D et al (1986) Clin Allergy 16: 163
11. Berman JS, Beer DJ, Bernardo J et al (1986) Ann NY Acad Sci 465: 98

© 1988 Elsevier Science Publishers B.V. (Biomedical Division)
Sarcoidosis and other granulomatous disorders
C. Grassi, G. Rizzato, E. Pozzi, editors

CUTANEOUS GRANULOMATA IN RESPONSE TO INJECTION WITH AUTOLOGOUS BRONCHOALVEOLAR
LAVAGE CELL PREPARATIONS IN SARCOIDOSIS PATIENTS

JOHN F. HOLTER, YASH P. KATARIA, H. KIM PARK
Department of Medicine and Department of Clinical Pathology and Diagnostic Medicine, East Carolina University School of Medicine, Greenville, NC 27858 (USA)

Mononuclear leukocytes are thought to be the building blocks of the granuloma
in sarcoidosis. Early in the course of the disease, open lung biopsies reveal a
diffuse mononuclear cell alveolitis. Later, noncaseating granulomata appear as
the alveolitis wanes (1,2). This temporal sequence of mononuclear cell influx
followed by granuloma formation has also been demonstrated by Kataria and Park
(3) in serial biopsies of Kveim-Siltzbach skin test sites. The mononuclear cell
influx in the skin and the alveolitis in the lung are both comprised of T-helper
lymphocytes and monocyte-macrophages.

Because the mononuclear cells of the sarcoid alveolitis are the cellular
precursors of granulomata, they may harbor a Kveim-like granulomagenic activity.
In this study, mononuclear cells harvested by bronchoalveolar lavage were
assessed for granulomagenic activity by intracutaneous injection and subsequent
skin biopsy analogous to the Kveim test.

MATERIALS AND METHODS

Subjects. Eighteen sarcoidosis patients and 8 normal volunteers were lavaged.
All sarcoidosis patients met the following inclusion criteria: 1) a clinical
picture compatible with pulmonary sarcoidosis; 2) histologic demonstration of
noncaseating granulomas; and, 3) no concurrent corticosteroid therapy. Control
subjects consisted of healthy volunteers.

Bronchoalveolar Lavage. The procedure was performed as previously described
(4), using a 4.9 mm diameter fiberoptic bronchoscope (Model BF-4B2 Olympus
Corporation of America, New Hyde Park, N.Y.). Sterile saline at room temperature
was instilled into the right middle lobe in ten aliquots of 20 ml each. Under
low continuous suction, fluid was aspirated into a 250 ml flask primed with 50 ml
of Hanks' Balanced Salt Solution without calcium or magnesium (HBSS), which
contained penicillin 500 units/ml and streptomycin 500 ug/ml.

Lavage Fluid Processing. Mucus was removed from the fluid by filtration
through 2 plys of sterile gauze. The cells were pelleted (270 x g, 20 min),
washed twice (in HBSS containing 100 u/ml penicillin and 100 ug/ml streptomycin),
and counted by hemacytometer.

Autologous Lavage Cell Preparation. With minor modification, processing was
patterned after Chase's (5) procedure for preparation of Kveim-Siltzbach antigen

from sarcoidal spleen. Two centrifugations (5500 x g, 20 min) on day 1 were
followed by heating (58° C., 75 minutes) and freezing (-80° C.) on three successive days. Sterility was evaluated by aerobic, anaerobic, fungal, and viral
cultures. After these inoculations, preparations were suspended in phosphate
buffered saline (pH 7.2) containing 0.25% phenol and kept at 4° C. until use.

Skin Testing. Each study subject underwent two intracutaneous injections:
one with the autologous lavage cell preparation, and one with validated Kveim-
Siltzbach antigen (6). Punch biopsies (4 mm) of both sites were obtained at 4-5
weeks, and examined after routine hematoxylin/eosin staining.

Skin Biopsy Interpretation. The requirement for a granuloma-positive biopsy
was well-defined nodular aggregates of epithelioid cells interspersed with
lymphocytes, with or without Langhans' giant cells. A granuloma-negative biopsy
included any or all of the following: 1) scattered epithelioid cells or macrophages, 2) isolated foreign body type giant cells, or 3) focal perivascular
mononuclear infiltrate. All biopsies were examined closely for the presence of
foreign body material, including inspection by polarized light microscopy.

When both biopsies revealed noncaseating granulomas, they were further compared
using monoclonal antibodies (Leu-1, Leu-2a, Leu-3a, Leu-7, Leu-14, Leu M3,
anti-lysozyme, and anti-Interleukin 2 receptor) with a previously described
avidin-biotin-immunoperoxidase staining technique (3).

Statistical methods. Significant difference of means ($\pm$ SD) was at $P<0.05$
using Wilcoxon's rank sum test for independent samples (7). P=NS indicates not
significant.

RESULTS

Fourteen sarcoidosis patients and 5 normal volunteers were injected respectively with 14.2 $\pm$ 6.0 (range 6.8-25.4) and 10.7 $\pm$ 5.0 (range 5.4-19.2) million
autologous lavage cells (ALC) at one site (P=NS), and with Kveim-Siltzbach
antigen at another site. Four sarcoid patients and 3 normal volunteers were not
injected because their cell preparations were found to be contaminated with
oropharyngeal bacteria.

Table I shows the skin biopsy results. All 14 sarcoid patients had granulomas
at the Kveim biopsy site. Of these, 6 (43%) also had noncaseating granulomas at
the ALC site. There was no significant difference in the number of cells
injected into ALC positive (12.7 $\pm$ 5.4 x 10^6) and ALC negative (15.3 $\pm$ 6.3 x 10^6)
sarcoid patients. Two of the 6 positive ALC biopsies contained significant
foreign body material. Of the remaining 4, two had no detectable foreign material and 2 had insignificant foreign material, i.e., very small or peripherally
located. None of the normal volunteers formed granulomas at the ALC site. One
volunteer had a positive Kveim-Siltzbach skin test.

TABLE I

SKIN BIOPSY RESULTS

SARCOIDOSIS PATIENTS n = 14		Kveim-Siltzbach Antigen Biopsy (-)	(+)	NORMAL VOLUNTEERS n = 5		Kveim-Siltzbach Antigen Biopsy (-)	(+)
Autologous Lavage Cell Biopsy	(-)	0	8	Autologous Lavage Cell Biopsy	(-)	4	1
	(+)	0	6		(+)	0	0

Figure 1 is an example of a pair of positive biopsies from the same sarcoidosis patient. Both the Kveim-Siltzbach site (Fig. 1A) and the autologous lavage cell site (Fig. 1B) reveal characteristic noncaseating epithelioid granulomatous inflammation. Neither biopsy contained foreign material.

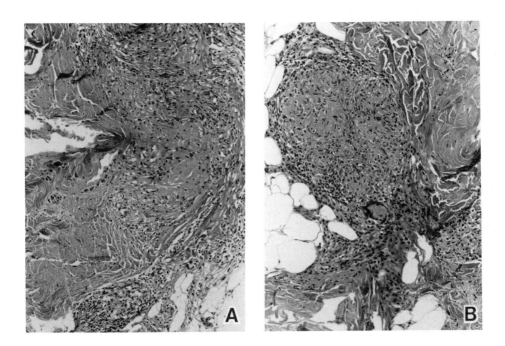

Fig. 1. Skin biopsies from the same sarcoid patient. A) Kveim-Siltzbach site. B) Autologous lavage cell site. Hematoxylin/eosin stain.

Kveim-Siltzbach and ALC epithelioid granulomas contained similar subsets of mononuclear cells. In biopsies of both, lymphocytes were almost exclusively

T cells (Leu-1 positive), and the vast majority of these were T-helper cells (Leu-3a positive). Occasional lymphocytes bearing Interleukin-2 receptors were seen. Epithelioid cells stained positively with Leu-M3 and anti-lysozyme.

DISCUSSION

Autologous lavage cells from sarcoidosis patients but not those from normal volunteers can induce epithelioid granulomas in the respective host. These granulomas are histologically similar to those induced by Kveim-Siltzbach antigen, both on routine hematoxylin/eosin staining and when mononuclear cell subtypes of the granulomas are compared. The foreign material encountered is not likely to have an etiologic role since significant foreign body material was not detected in 4 of the 6 ALC granulomas. Foreign body granulomas have a distinctive giant cell reaction limited to the area of the foreign body, and lack the immune-mediated inflammatory amplification characteristic of the sarcoid granulomatous response (8). Moreover, epithelioid cells are not a feature of foreign body granulomas. The ALC granulomas of the sarcoid patients contained aggregates of epithelioid cells interspersed with lymphocytes, and Langhans' type giant cells.

In conclusion, nonviable autologous bronchoalveolar lavage cells have granulomagenic activity similar to Kveim-Siltzbach antigen in sarcoidosis patients. No such activity was found in normal control autologous lavage cells. In sarcoidosis, a factor capable of inducing granulomas is associated with the mononuclear cells from which the granulomas evolve.

ACKNOWLEDGEMENTS

Funding for this project was provided in part by the Pitt County United Way and the American Lung Association of North Carolina.

REFERENCES

1. Rosen Y, Athanassiades TJ, Moon S, Lyons HA (1978) Chest 74:122-125

2. Bernaudin JF, Lacronique J, Soler P, Lange F, Kawanami O, Bassett F (1981) Bull Europ Physiopath Resp 17:27-64

3. Kataria YP, Park HK (1986) Ann NY Acad Sci 465:221-232

4. Hunninghake GW, Gadek JE, Kawanami O, Ferrans VJ, Crystal RG (1979) Am J Path 97:149-206

5. Chase MW (1961) Am Rev Resp Dis 84:86-88

6. Kataria YP, Sharma OP, Israel H, Rogers M (1980) In: Williams WJ, Davies BH (eds) Eighth International Conference on Sarcoidosis and Other Granulomatous Diseases. Alpha Omega, Cardiff, pp 660-667

7. Snedecor GW, Cochran (1980) Statistical Methods. The Iowa State University Press, Ames, p 144

8. Boros DL (1978) Prog Allergy 24:183-267

PATHOGENESIS OF GRANULOMA FORMATION IN LYMPH NODES WITH SARCOIDOSIS

EISHI Y, TAKEMURA T[*], MATSUI Y[**], and HATAKEYAMA S

Dept. of Pathology, Tokyo Medical & Dental University, 5-45, 1-chome, Yushima, Bunkyo-ku, Tokyo 113, Japan   Dept. of Pathology(*) and Internal Medicine(**), Japan Red Cross Medical Center, Hiroo, Shibuya-ku, Tokyo 150, Japan

INTRODUCTION

In sarcoidosis no causative agent has so far been defined, even though immunological processes are thought to be involved in the formation of the granuloma. We have examined lymph nodes from cases of sarcoidosis in an attempt to define the cause of the granulomatous condition.

The study was initially motivated with an observation that IgA and/or IgM immunoglobulins were bound to a phagocytosed material in sinus macrophages of the lymph nodes with sarcoidosis. This observation suggested that immune complexes in macrophages were generated outside the lymph node and carried to the nodes, and that the phagocytosed substance is refractory to digestion and persisting within macrophages.

As it was assumed that such refractory substances for macrophages might be derived from either Mycobacterium tuberculosis (M.t) or Proponibacterium acnes (P.a), we attempted to examine the extent of involvements of these bacteria or bacterial components in sarcoidosis granuloma. We have identified in these granulomas an indigestible bacterial cell wall component, muramyl dipeptide (MDP) which has already been shown to cause granuloma formation when administrated experimentally[1].

MATERIAL AND METHODS

Immunohistochemical procedures:

An indirect peroxidase method was used for the detection of immunoglobulins (IgG, IgA, and IgM) and the PAP method was used to detect MDP, in either formalin-fixed paraffin tissue sections after appropriate trypsin digestion[2] or in PLP-fixed cryostat sections for electronmicroscopy. The ABC method was used to detect lymphocyte subset markers in aceton-fixed cryostat sections.

Preparation of antiserum specific to MDP:

Antiserum was produced in rabbits immunized with MDP-BSA, and purified by the absorption of its anti-BSA activity with a BSA-binding sepharose gel. The specificity of the antiserum was confirmed by absorbing with MDP-BSA-binding sepharose gel. This absorption resulted in a loss of anti-MDP activity of the serum and the simultaneous abolition of the specific

144

Table 1:   Purification and Specificity of the Antiserum to MDP

		Staining Results		Antibody Activity to		
	Absorbent	BKG	Positivity	MDP	BSA	HSA
1	None	+	+	+	+	+
2*	HSA	–	+	+	+	–
3*	BSA	–	+	+	–	–
4	MDP–BSA	–	–	–	–	–

BKG: Background staining   1: Crude serum   2: Human Serum
Albumin * 3. Bovine Serum Albumin   4: The serum purified
in above* was used here for absorption with MDP–BSA

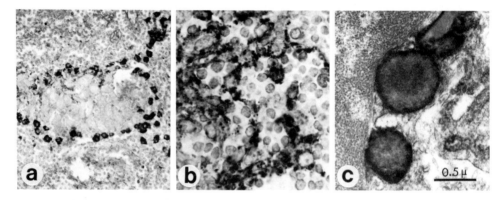

Fig. 1:   Localization of Immunoglobulins in Lymphnodes with Sarcoidosis
(a) IgG-containing plasma cells around the granuloma
(b) IgA-positive granules in macrophages of the hyperplastic sinuses
(c) IgA-positive granules in sinus macrophages (electron-microscopy)

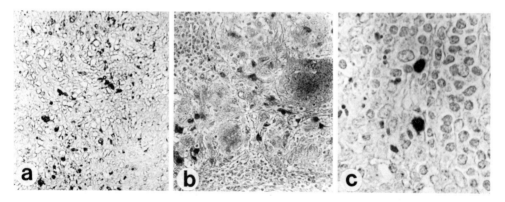

Fig. 2:   Localization of MDP in Tuberculosis and Sarcoidosis
(a) MDP-positive epithelioid cells in tuberculous granulomas
(b) MDP-positive epithelioid cells and Langhans giant cells in sarcoidosis
(c) MDP-positive granules in sinus macrophages of lymph nodes with sarcoidosis

staining reaction in sections treated with this absorbed serum (Table 1).

Measurement of antibody activity to MDP, HSA and BSA:

Peroxidase conjugated MDP-lysine (Px-MDP) was prepared by the method of Wilson and Nakane[3]. The binding activity of Px-MDP with rabbit anti-MDP antibody, captured by anti-rabbit IgG antibody coated onto ELISA plates, was measured to detect anti-MDP antibody activity. Antibody activity against HSA or BSA, was detected indirectly on ELISA plates coated with each protein.

RESULTS

We have examined lymph nodes taken by Daniels biopsy from 50 cases of sarcoidosis. In 42% of the nodes we have demonstrated abundant immunoglobulin (Ig) granules of IgA and/or IgM, mainly in macrophages within the hyperplastic sinuses with or without accompanying granuloma (Fig. 1b). No Ig granules were detected in lymph nodes biopsied from patients with other diseases such as tuberculosis and sinus reticulosis.

These IgA and/or IgM granules were located in the phagolysosomes of the macrophages in electron-microscopy (Fig. 1c). Occasionally the phagolysosomes resembled pleomorphic chromogens named Hamazaki-Wesenberg (H-W) bodies, a kind of inclusion body in which interest has recently been revived in connection with sarcoidosis[4], and there were transitional structures intermediate between Ig-positive lysosomes and H-W bodies. No IgG granules were detected in the macrophages, even though there were abundant IgG plasma cells intermingled with Leu-1 (pan T) and Leu-3 (Helper) positive lymphocytes, closely associated with granuloma (Fig. 1a). IgA and/or IgM plasma cells were sparsely distributed through the tissue and had no association with granuloma.

These observations led us to the speculation that insoluble antigenic substance coupled with IgA and/or IgM were generated outside the lymph node, phagocytosed by macrophages and persisting within these cells without further degradation. If it is the case, M.t and P.a were assumed to be most suspective as the antigen.

Immunohistochemical examinations was carrried out with antibodies raised against M.t and P.a to clarify the nature of the Ig-binding antigenic substance and H-W bodies. It resulted, however, in negative reactions. Further, there was no correlation between the number of H-W bodies in the lymph nodes and the numbers of P.a cultivated from the nodes.

In contrast, positive results were obtained immunohistochemically with a conventional antiserum against the bacterial cell wall component, MDP, in cases of sarcoidosis (lymph nodes and Kveim-Siltzbach granuloma) and tubersulosis (lymph nodes and pulmonary), but not in cases from control diseases including

146

foreign body granulomas such as berylliosis, except for a few cases of the skin lesion with infected epidermal inclusion cyst.

In tuberculous granulomas, vacuolar or coarse-granular positive stainings were observed in epithelioid cells located in the outer margin of caseous necrosis and in macrophages around the granuloma (Fig. 2a). In lymph nodes with sarcoidosis, MDP was demonstrated not only in the granulomas (epithelioid cells and Langhans giant cells) but also in sinus macrophages (Fig. 2b and 2c). Some of the positive staining within macrophages was associated with H-W bodies

This anti-MDP antiserum could detect bacteria or their degradated components in macrophages on histological sections when either M.t or P.a was injected into rat footpads and examined on 8 days after the injection.

DISCUSSION

It is unresolved at the moment whether the persistence of the material in macrophages is due to the nature of the material itself or to an impaired function of lysosomal digestion by the macrophages.

The demonstration of the presence of the bacterial cell wall component MDP in sinus macrophages, epithelioid cell and Langhans giant cells, suggested that the phagocytosed material in these cells might be derived from the bacteria which possess indigestible bacterial cell wall containing MDP, such as M.t and P.a. MDP positivity in the skin lesion with infected epidermal cysts might reflect an conventional residence of P.a in the skin of normal subjects.

Finally we would suggest that these bacteria could be associated with pathogenesis of granuloma formation in lymph nodes with sarcoidosis, while further examination would be needed to address a mechanism of granuloma formation in sarcoidosis, in connection with these bacteria.

REFERENCES
1. Tanaka A, Emori K, Nago S (1982) Epithelioid granuloma formation requiring no T cell function. Am J Pathol 106:165
2. Eishi Y, Hatakeyama S, Takemura T, Hajikano H, Hirokawa K (1981) Demonstration of various antigens on paraffin sections of formalin-fixed tissues; Trypsin-treated indirect peroxidase-labelled antibody technique. The Bulletin of Tokyo Medical and Dental University 28:27
3. Wilson MB, Nakane PK (1978) "Immunofluorescence and Related Techniques" ed. by Knapp W et al, Elsevier, Holland, 1978, p.215
4. Edward A. Moscovic (1978) Sarcoidosis and Mycobacterial L-forms, A critical reappraisal of pleomorphic chromogenic bodies (Hamazaki corpuscles) in lymph nodes. Pathology Annual part 2, p.69

© 1988 Elsevier Science Publishers B.V. (Biomedical Division)
Sarcoidosis and other granulomatous disorders
C. Grassi, G. Rizzato, E. Pozzi, editors

ANTIGEN PRESENTING CAPACITY IN SARCOIDOSIS

YASUTAKA INA, SATOFUMI SADO, MASAHIKO YAMAMOTO, KATSUTOSHI TAKADA, MUNEHIKO MORISHITA*, MANABU ASAI, KEIKI ARAKAWA AND MASAHARU NODA

Second Dept. of Internal Medicine, Nagoya City Univ. Medical School, Mizuho-cho, Mizuho-ku, Nagoya 467, Japan.
*Second Dept. of Internal Medicine, Aichi Medical Univ., Nagakute Aichi 480-11, Japan.

INTRODUCTION

Recently activated T-lymphocytes are considered to play a major role in the development of sarcoidosis. However, the mechanism of T-lymphocyte activation is not well-known[1, 2]. By the way, it is generally accepted that T-lymphocytes activate and proliferate in response to antigens presented by antigen presenting cells (APC) in association with HLA class II antigens[3].

Therefore we studied the antigen presenting capacity (APCC) of peripheral blood monocytes and alveolar macrophages in sarcoidosis, using purified protein derivatives (PPD) as the antigen.

MATERIALS AND METHODS

Materials

Nine patients with sarcoidosis (4 men and 5 women with an average age of 48.1 ± 14.3yr) and 9 normals (5 men and 4 women with an average age of 50.2 ± 14.2yr) were studied. None was taking medication at the time of study and all showed positive PPD skin tests (PPD-s).

Methods

Preparation of lung and blood effector cells.

Lung mononuclear cells were obtained using bronchoalveolar lavage. The cells recovered by lavage were immediately centrifuged (600 g, 5 min), washed sequentially and resuspended in RPMI-1640 medium (Gibco Laboratories, Grand Island, New York) containing 10% fetal calf serum (FCS, Gibco). Blood mononuclear cells were purified from heparinized peripheral blood obtained by a density gradient centrifugation using Ficoll-Conray, washed sequentially, and resuspended in RPMI-1640 medium containing 10% FCS.

Purification of alveolar macrophages (AM), blood monocytes (Mo) and T-lymphocytes.

Lung and blood mononuclear cells were incubated in plastic culture dishes (Falcon 1005, Oxnard, CA) at 37°C in a humidified atmosphere of 5% CO_2 in air to permit attachment of macrophages and monocytes. After 1 hr of incubation, the cells were washed vigorously to remove nonadherent cells. Adherent cells were removed from the dishes by gently scraping with a rubber policeman. This procedure increased the numbers of cells morphologically compatible with macrophages and monocytes to greater than 95%.

Nonadherent cells from plastic culture dishes were passed through a nylon-wool column to remove

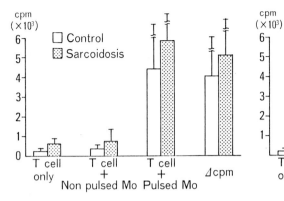

Fig. 1. Antigen presenting capacity
by monocytes

Fig. 2. Antigen presenting capacity
by alveolar macrophages

TABLE 1.
COMPARISON OF APCC TO LUNG
VERSUS BLOOD T-LYMPHOCYTES.

TABLE 3.
HLA-DR ANTIGENS ON MONOCYTES
AND ALVEOLAR MACROPHAGES.

Culture condition*	n	cpm*
BT cell alone	5	394±196
+Mo	5	4527±1558
+AM	5	3213±2366
LT cell alone	4	220±37
+Mo	4	2099±1655
+AM	4	793±163

※ BT : blood T-lymphocyte　　* mean±S.D.
　 LT : lung T-lymphocyte

		DR Antigen (MFI*)		
	n	Monocytes	n	Macrophages
Normal	8	57±16	4	142±56
Sarcoidosis	13	66±16	4	140±52

*MFI : mean fluorescence intensity

TABLE 2. ALLOGENEIC APCC

T-cell	(HLA-DRtype)	APC	PPD Nonpulsed	PPD Pulsed	Δcpm
Control	(2, w8)	Control	569±4	3400±289	2831
		Sarcoidosis	312±108	2928±1151	2616
Sarcoidosis	(4, w8)	Control	207±115	177±107	−30
		Sarcoidosis	52±10	171±68	119

B-lymphocytes and then T-lymphocytes were purely obtained.

Assay for APCC by Mo and AM.

To pulse the adherent cells with antigens, adherent cells (1×10^6/ml) were incubated for 60 min at $37°C$ in the presence of PPD ($100 \mu g$/ml) and mitomycin-C (MMC; $50 \mu g$/ml,). Control (nonpulsed) adherent cells were treated only with MMC. The treated cells were washed and adjusted to the appropriate cell concentration (2×10^5/ml, unless otherwise stated) in RPMI-1640. Co-culture of antigen-pulsed adherent cells with column-purified T-lymphocytes was carried out in triplicate in the wells of round bottom microtiter plates. The cultures were incubated for 5 days at $37°C$ in a humidified atmosphere of 5% CO_2 in air. To quantify T-lymphocyte proliferation, 16 to 18 hours prior to harvesting, $0.2 \mu Ci$ of [^3H] thymidine was added to each well. Triplicate samples were harvested using a multiple sample harvester and counted in a liquid scintillation counter. APCC was expressed as Δ cpm (cpm in PPD-pulsed APC-cpm in nonpulsed APC).

Quantification of alveolar macrophages and blood monocytes expressing HLA-DR surface antigens.

The expression of DR antigens on Mo and AM was analysed by the indirect immunofluorescence method, using FACS III (Becton Dickinson) as described elsewhere[4].

RESULTS AND DISCUSSION

Antigen presentating capacity (APCC).

Blood monocytes from normals showed APCC to autologous blood T-lymphocytes. To evaluate the dependence on the relative numbers of T-lymphocytes and monocytes, these T-lymphocytes were cultured with various numbers of PPD-pulsed monocytes. When the monocyte to T-lymphocyte ratio was 1:5, APCC was optimal (Fig. 1). Therefore, APCC was determined in the condition of APC to T-lymphocyte ratio of 1:5.

As shown in Fig. 1, Mo from both normal controls and sarcoidosis showed APCC to autologous T-lymphocytes. Mo from sarcoidosis functioned more efficiently as APC than that from controls, but not significant.

As reported previonsly[5,6], AM from normal controls was hardly capable of functioning as APC. However, AM from sarcoidosis showed APCC to autologous T-lymphocytes ($P < 0.05$ as compared with normal controls) (Fig. 2).

Table 1 shows the comparison of APCC by Mo or AM to lung versus blood T-lymphocytes. APCC by autologous Mo or AM to lung T-lymphocytes was not significantly different from that to blood T-lymphocytes.

To evaluate APCC by Mo in PPD-s negative patients with sarcoidosis, T-lymphocytes from PPD-s positive normal control were co-cultured with Mo from PPD-s negative patients, sharing at least one HLA-DR antigen, resulting that allogeneic APCC was observed between them (Table 2). However, no significant difference in APCC was observed between PPD-s positive and negative patients with sarcoidosis.

HLA-DR antigens on the surface of Mo and AM.

150

To assess whether the enhancement of APCC by AM in sarcoidosis is caused by the increased expression of HLA-DR antigens on AM, HLA-DR antigen expression was analysed. But the density of HLA-DR antigens on Mo or AM in sarcoidosis was not significantly different from that of normals (Table 3), suggesting that the possibility is little.

Effect of IFN-γ or Interleukin-1 (IL-1) on APCC.

To examine the effect of IFN-γ on APCC, APC was precultured in the presence of IFN-γ for 24 hr and then APCC was assayed. To study the effect of IL-1 on APCC, IL-1 was added to the co-culture of APC and T-lymphocytes and APCC was determined. Neither IFN-γ nor IL-1 induced any APCC in controls (Data not shown).

Together with these results, Mo and AM from patients with sarcoidosis functioned as an efficient APC, as reported previously[5, 6], suggesting that T-lymphocyte activation in sarcoidosis might partially caused by the enhanced APCC. However, the mechanism which enhances APCC in sarcoidosis is now unclear.

REFERENCES

1. Hunninghake, G.W., Fulmer, J.D., Young, R.C., Gadek, J.E. and Crystal R.G. 1979. Localization of the immune response in sarcoidosis. Am. Rev. Respir. Dis. 120: 49-57.

2. Hunninghake, G.W. and Crystal R.G. 1981. Pulmonary sarcoidosis: A disorder mediated by excessive helper T-lymphocyte activity at sites of disease activity. N. Engl. J. Med. 35: 429-434.

3. Koide, Y., Awashima, F., Yoshida, T.O., Takenouchi, T., Wakisaka, A., Moriuchi, J. and Aizawa, M. 1982. The role of three distinct Ia-like antigen molecules in human T cell proliferative responses: Effect of monoclonal anti-Ia-like antibodies. J. Immunol. 129: 1061-1069.

4. Ball, E.D., Guyre, P.M., Glynn, J.M., Rigby, W.F.C. and Fanger, M.W. 1984. Modulation of class I HLA antigens on HL-60 promyelocytic leukemia cells by serum-free medium: Re-induction by γ-IFN and 1, 25-dihydroxyvitamin D_3 (calcitriol). J. Immunol. 132: 2424-2428.

5. Venet, A., Hance, A.J., Saltini, C., Robinson, B.W.S. and Crystal R.G. 1985. Enhanced alveolar macrophage-mediated antigen-induced T-lymphocyte proliferation in sarcoidosis. J. Clin. Invest. 75: 293-301.

6. Lem, V.M., Lipscomb, M.F., Weissler, J.C., Nunez, G., Ball, E.J., Stastny, P. and Toew, G.B. 1985. Bronchoalveolar cells from sarcoid patients demonstrate enhanced antigen presentation. J. Immunol. 135: 1766-1771.

IN-VITRO SARCOID GRANULOMAS - DIFFERENCES BETWEEN ACTIVE AND INACTIVE DISEASE

B.B. MISHRA, S.M. PHILLIPS, H. PATRICK AND H. ISRAEL
Temple University Hospital, University of Pennsylvania School of
Medicine, Jefferson Medical College, Philadelphia USA.

INTRODUCTION

The lack of a satisfactory animal model in sarcoidosis has been a serious
obstacle to the understanding of the mechanism of sarcoid granuloma formation.
The failure to model the multisystem spontaneous growth of granulomas and
their subsequent spontaneous regression has been a major drawback, but the
development of the in-vitro antigen coated bead granuloma model[1](IVG) may
overcome this problem. The in-vitro granulomas (IVGs) exhibit many features
which are characteristic of hypersensitivity type granulomas[1,2], while
reproducing in-vitro many of the events of the in-vivo granulomatous response.
This may allow peripheral blood cells of patients to be tested for fluctuations in their in-vitro reactivity as the intensity of the in-vivo granulomatous response varies with the activity of sarcidosis.

METHODS

Symptomatic and asymptomatic patients with sarcoidosis who had not been on
immunosuppressive therapy in the previous three months were studied after
informed consent. Sarcoidosis had been diagnosed on the basis of clinical
features and laboratory or pathological evidence of multisystem granulomas.
Normal volunteers and untreated symptomatic patients with other
diseases constituted the controls.

In vitro granulomas were cultured using antigen coated or plain poly-
acrylamide beads, as described previously[1]. Briefly, ficoll-hypaque
separated peripheral blood mononuclear cells were cultured in triplicate in
24-well culture plates with the beads. The medium used was RPMI 1640 with
10% fetal calf serum, glutamine and gentamycin. Tetanus toxoid coated
beads were used because all subjects in the study had been immunised with
tetanus toxoid. The grading of the in-vitro granulomas and the calculation
of the Granuloma Index (G.I.) has been described before[1].

RESULTS

Twelve patients with acute symptoms and ten asymptomatic or chronically
symptomatic patients with sarcoidosis were studied.

Based on the size of the collections of cells that were adherent to plain

beads and to tetanus coated beads, the patients could be divided into two
groups. One group consisted of patients whose G.I. was significantly higher
than that of simultaneously studied normal controls (p<0.005 with tetanus
coated beads and p<0.025 with plain beads; Tetanus -L and Plain - L,
respectively, in Fig.2.) Except one, all patients in this group were symptomatic due to active sarcoidosis or had presented due to recently discovered
abnormal chest X-ray. The single exception was a patient who had had
inactive sarcoidosis for 15 years, and had presented with palpitation due
to dysrrhytmias, but, who did not have clinical evidence of active sarcoidosis at the time of the study. In this group of patients, there was a
positive correlation (correlation coefficient:0.4) between the level of the
serum angitensin converting enzyme (SACE), and the patients granuloma rank
with tetanus coated beads; the granuloma rank was based on the significance
of the difference (p value) between the patient's G.I. and the paired
normal control's G.I. The patient with the most significant difference had
the highest rank. There was also a positive correlation between the Kvein
reactivity rank and the G.I. rank (coefficient of correlation:0.6). The

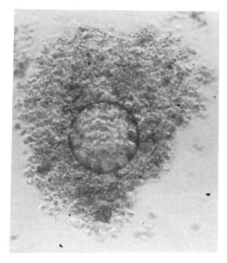 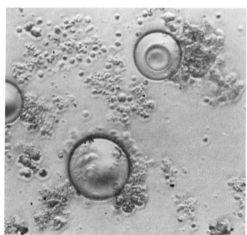

Fig 1a   Fig 1b

Fig.1a. Large in-vitro granuloma, grade 7: Active sarcoid mononuclear cells
with tetanus toxoid coated bead. Fig 1b. paired normal control in-vitro
granuloma with tetanus toxoid coated beads. Both subjects were tetanus-immune

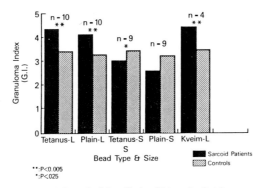

DIFFERENCE BETWEEN SARCOID G.I.
& PAIRED CONTROLS: ANALYSIS BY SIZE OF G.I.
& TYPE OF ANTIGEN ON BEADS

Tetanus-L: Tetanus Toxoid Coated Beads — G.I. Larger than Control
Plain-L: Plain Beads — G.I. Larger than Control
Tetanus-S: Tetanus Toxoid Coated Beads — G.I. Smaller than Control
Plain-S: Plain Beads — G.I. Smaller than Control
Kveim-L: Kveim Antigen Coated Beads — G.I. Larger than Control
n: Number of Patients & Paired Controls in each Group

Fig. 2

Kveim reactivity rank was based on the diameter of the Kveim reaction in
these subjects.

   The G.I. of the second group of patients was significantly smaller than
that of paired normal controls (Tetanus -S in Fig.2). The results were not
significantly different between this group of subjects and matched controls
for the G.I. calculated with plain beads (Plain-S in Fig. 2). Three of
the ten patients in this group had presented with acute symptoms and active
sarcoidosis, but had been symptomatic for more than two months and none
required immunosuppressive therapy.

DISCUSSION
   The correlation between high SACE levels and a high G.I. rank
demonstrates that the in-vitro reactivity correlates with clinical
disease activity, because of the correlation that exists between the
SACE level itself and disease activity. The correlation also suggests a link between the expression of ACE genes and the expression
of genes that regulate lymphocyte adhesion in the in-vitro granulomas.
   The Kveim reaction is a model and a measure of in-vivo granuloma
formation[5]. Therefore the correlation between the G.I. rank and the
Kveim reactivity is supportive evidence that the in-vitro granulomas
reflect the in-vivo granulomatous response in patients with sarcoidosis.

154

The granuloma index (G.I.) is a measure of intercellular and cell-bead adhesion and has been shown to correlate in an antigen specific manner with the development of in-vivo delayed type hypersensitivity reaction in response exposure to a sensitising antigen on the antigen coated beads[1,3,4,6]. In this study, the antigen specific nature of the in-vitro granulomatous response, is apparently contradicted by the formation of large IVGs around plain, antigen free beads by cells from subjects with acute sarcoidosis (Fig.2 Plain-L). But the presence or absence of antigen on the beads would be inconsequential if the antigens are carried by the antigen presenting cells[7]. This study suggests indirectly that the antigen presenting cells from patients with acute sarcoidosis are able to circulate while primed with an antigen. Alternative mechanisms of macrophage and lymphocyte activation may also be responsible for the same observation.

The G.I. with tetanus coated beads is lower in tetanus-immune chronic inactive sarcoid patients than in normal controls. This phenomenon is analogous to antigen specific granuloma modulation described in studies of chronic human schistosomiasis[3]. The in-vivo analogue is the presumed reduction in size of tissue granulomas which accounts for the improvement in clinical laboratory indices of disease without treatment in sarcoidosis and in chronic schistosomiasis.

The in-vitro granuloma model is the closest to an assay of the activity of in-vivo sarcoid granulomas and it may facilitate the study of the mechanism of growth and regression of sarcoid granulomas, as well as the testing of potential therapeutic agents.

REFERENCES

1. Bentley AG, Phillips SM, Kaner RJ, Theodorides VJ, Linette GP, Doughty BL (1985) J Immunol 134: 4163-4169

2. Boros DL (1978) Prog Allergy 24: 183-267

3. Doughty BL, Ottesen EA, Nash TE, Phillips SM (1984) J Immunol 133: 993-997

4. Bentley AG, Doughty BL, Phillips SM (1982) Am J Trop Med Hyg 31: 1168-1180

5. Mishra BB, Poulter LW, Janossy G, Geraint James D (1983) Clin Exp Immunol 54: 705-715

6. Lammie PJ, Linette GP, Phillips SM (1985) J Immunol 134: 4170-4175

7. Unanue ER, Allen PM (1987) Science 236: 551-557

MONOCYTES DERIVED MULTINUCLEATED GIANT CELLS: IMMUNOPHENOTYPE AND FUNCTIONAL ANALYSIS

H. KREIPE, H.J. RADZUN, P. RUDOLPH, J. BARTH*, K. HEIDORN, W. PETERMANN*, M.R. PARWARESCH

Depts. of Pathology and Internal Medicine*, University of Kiel, FRG

INTRODUCTION

Since first described by Langhans as a common feature of tuberculosis, multinucleated giant cells (MGC) have been observed in many other granulomatous diseases. The exact functional significance of macrophage forming syncytia, however, remains unclear (1). In the present study MGC produced in vitro from cultured blood monocytes (BM) were investigated with respect to their immunophenotype, interleukin-1 production, cytostatic activity, and release of oxygen free radicals.

MATERIAL AND METHODS

Lymphokine rich supernatants from Concanavalin A stimulated blood lymphocytes were used to induce giant cell formation in separated cultured BM from healthy donors. Immunophenotyping was performed by immunocytochemistry with a panel of monocyte/macrophage specific monoclonal antibodies of the Ki-M series (2). Functional analysis included a murine thymocyte proliferation assay for measuring interleukin-1 secretion of MGC and two assays for screening factor bound as well as cell-mediated cytostatic activity of MGC using human tumor cell lines (K-562, BJAB, Hela) as targets. Release of oxygen free radicals of MGC was registered after addition of zymosan by chemiluminescence.

RESULTS AND DISCUSSION

Formation of MGC in vitro

MGC occured within 48 hours after onset of stimulation of BM and could be enriched to a purity of greater than 90% due to their adhesion to the ground of the culture vessel. On the average 20 nuclei could be observed in MGC with up to 150 nuclei in some syncytia.

Immunophenotype of MGC in vitro and in vivo

Cultured MGC as well as their in vivo counterparts such as foreign body giant cells exhibited a strong reactivity with the monoclonal antibodies Ki-M6 and Ki-M8, whereas the Ki-M1, Ki-M2 and Ki-M4 antigens were reduced or missing. The proliferation associated antigen Ki-67 could not be detected, indicating that MGC in vitro and in vivo were generated by fusion of non-dividing cells. The immunophenotype of MGC resembled that of mature macrophages like alveolar macrophages. Antigens specific for immune accessory cells such as Ki-M1 and Ki-M4 recognizing dendritic cells were missing.

Interleukin-1 secretion

Compared with unfused cultured BM from the same donors, MGC did not show an enhanced interleukin-1 secretion, indicating that the release of this inflammatory mediator is not a specific function of MGC.

Cytostatic activity

As MGC of monocytic origin can be observed in a variety of neo-plasias, we analysed factor bound as well as cell mediated cytostatic activity of MGC in comparison to unfused cultured BM. In neither assay did MGC prove to be more efficient than unfused macrophages. Hence, it seems unlikely that MGC occuring in malignant tumors play a signifi-cant role in host defense.

Chemiluminescence response

Measuring the production of oxygen free radicals in response to zymo-san, we found a 20-30 fold increase in MGC when compared with unfused macrophages. Although this increase results mainly from summing up the activity of single cells that underwent cell fusion, the functional sig-nificance of MGC formation could lie in the synchronization and concen-tration of oxygen-free radical release.

In conclusion MGC as generated in this study represent mature macro-phage derivations possibly engaged in host defense in infectious diseases.

REFERENCES
1. Schlesinger L, Musson RA, Johnston RB (1984) J Exp Med 155:168-178
2. Kreipe H, Radzun HJ, Parwaresch MR (1986) Histochem J 18:441-450

© 1988 Elsevier Science Publishers B.V. (Biomedical Division)
Sarcoidosis and other granulomatous disorders
C. Grassi, G. Rizzato, E. Pozzi, editors

DECREASED   PHOSPHATIDYLETHANOLAMINE   METHYLTRANSFERASE   (PMT)   ACTIVITY   IN
T LYMPHOCYTES IN SARCOIDOSIS : AN INDICATOR OF T CELL IMMATURITY

Y. PACHECO*, F. GORMAND*, P. FONLUPT**, M. DUBOIS**, M. PERRIN-FAYOLLE*,
H. PACHECO**

* Service de Pneumologie du Pr PERRIN-FAYOLLE, Centre Hospitalier Lyon-Sud,
   69310 Pierre-Bénite, France

** UNITE INSERM 205, I.N.S.A., 69100 Villeurbanne, France

INTRODUCTION

Oligoclonal helper T lymphocytes accumulation at the sites of sarcoidosis disease plays probably an important role in macrophage activation and granuloma formation (1). We have previously shown that alveolar T cell percentage involved in S (G_2 + M) phase of cell cycle were higher in sarcoidosis patients than in normal controls (2). But we could not answer if this result correlate with cell activation or cell differentiation. To clarify this problem we studied membrane PMT activity in T cells, because the activities of PMT alter as cells and tissues differentiate or develop and phospholipid methylation and subsequent turnover of methylated lipids in the membrane might be related to initiating programms of the cellular differentiation (3). PMT plays an important regulatory role in membrane signal transmission (4).

MATERIAL AND METHODS

PMT activity was measured in blood and alveolar T lymphocytes in 8 patients who presented with pulmonary sarcoidosis (for clinical data see table) and 8 normal controls. Blood and alveolar T lymphocytes were prepared as described in (2).

N°	Age	Sex	Smoking	Chest X-Ray type	Extrapulmonary localisation	TST	Histological diagnosis
1	30	W	NS	II	0	–	M
2	39	W	NS	IIIa	0	–	M
3	20	W	NS	II	Kidney	–	M
4	35	M	NS	II	Spleen	–	TB
5	45	M	NS	IIIa	0	–	GG
6	34	M	NS	II	0	–	M
7	40	M	NS	IIIa	0	–	TB
8	42	M	S	II	0	–	TB

TST = Tuberculin skin test ; histological diagnosis. M : Mediastinoscopy.
TB Transbronchial biopsy. GG : peripheral lymphnode biopsy.

Enzyme activity was determined with measure of tritiated methyl group incorporation from tritiated S Adenosyl-Methionine in membrane phospholipid methylation according to (5).

RESULTS

Membrane phospholipid methylation in peripheral blood T lymphocytes was lower in sarcoidosis patients than in normal controls. PMT activity was lower in alveolar T lymphocytes than in blood T lymphocytes in patients (PMT activity is expressed in Fmol/mg protein).

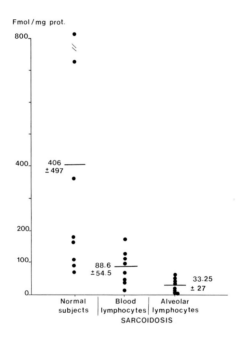

COMMENTS

These results can be compared with a recent study carried out by our group on B cells of leukemia and lymphoma, in which a close relation was observed between PMT activity, cell maturity and percentage of cells in S phase of cell cycle (6). In these diseases the lower PMT activity the higher immaturity and percentage of cells in S phase of cell cycle were. We hypothesize that decreased PMT activity in blood and alveolar T lymphocytes in sarcoidosis could be an indicator of T cell immaturity.

REFERENCES

1. Muller-Quernheim J, Saltini C, Sondermeyer P, Crystal RG (1986) J. Immunol., 137:3475-3483

2. Pacheco Y, Cordier G, Perrin-Fayolle M, Revillard JP (1982) Am. J. Medicine, 73:82-88

3. Hirata F, Hatanaka M, Wano Y, Matsuda K (1986) In: Borchardt RT, Creveling CR, Per Magne Ueland (Eds) Biological methylation and drug design. Humana Press, Clifton New Jersey pp 67-74

4. Hirata F, Axelrod J (1980) Science, 209:1082-1090

5. Fonlupt P, Rey C, Pacheco H (1981) Biochemical Biophysical Res. Commun 100:1720-1726

6. Pacheco Y, Magaud JP, Dubois M, French M, Fonlupt P, Prigent AF, Rey C, Germain D, Pacheco H (1985) C.R. acad. Sc. Paris 301:711-716

ISOLATION OF CELL WALL-DEFECTIVE ACID-FAST BACTERIA FROM SKIN
LESIONS OF PATIENTS WITH SARCOIDOSIS

DAVID Y. GRAHAM, DIANE C. MARKESICH, DEBRA C. KALTER, HAROLD H.
YOSHIMURA

Departments of Medicine and Dermatology, VA Medical Center and
Baylor College of Medicine, Houston, Texas (U.S.A.)

INTRODUCTION

Sarcoidosis is a multisystemic chronic granulomatous disease
of unknown etiology. Over the years, a variety of etiologies
have been postulated ranging from infection with cell wall-
defective mycobacteria through a reaction to inhaled pine
pollen. The search for the still-elusive persisting antigen
continues and the similarities between sarcoidosis and chronic
mycobacterial infections continue to intrigue investigators.

Recently, mycobacteria have been isolated (initially as cell
wall-defective forms called spheroplasts) from tissues of
patients with another chronic granulomatous disease of unknown
etiology, Crohn's disease (1-3). Because of our success (3) in
isolating spheroplasts from intestinal tissues of patients with
Crohn's disease, chronic ulcerative colitis, and from an
occasional normal person, we decided to apply our culture
techniques to skin biopsies obtained from patients with
sarcoidosis. We have been successful in obtaining spheroplasts
of acid-fast bacteria from skin biopsies from sarcoid patients
but not from skin biopsies from patients without sarcoidosis.

MATERIALS AND METHODS

Sarcoid tissue was obtained by punch biopsy (3 to 6 mm) of
the skin. Approximately one-half of the skin biopsy was
processed for culture; the remainder was submitted for
histological examination. Tissue specimens for culture were
homogenized in a glass homogenizer of the ten Broeck or Dounce
type in 2 ml of 0.1% hexadecylpyridinium chloride. The
homogenate was decontaminated overnight (up to 24 h) at room
temperature and 0.15 ml of suspension was inoculated onto a

minimum of 4 slants of Herrold's Egg Yolk medium (HEYM)
containing 4.1 g/l of sodium pyruvate and 2 mg/l mycobactin J
(Allied Labs, Ames, IA). When the inoculum had dried, the tubes
were sealed and incubated indefinitely. Cultures were examined
with a dissecting microscope once per week for the first month
and at least monthly thereafter. Bacterial colonies that
appeared on HEYM slants were subcultured to HEYM and "MG3" liquid
medium which consisted of veal infusion broth, 1% yeast extract,
10% horse serum, 0.3M sucrose, 0.2% $MgSO_4$, 0.1% ferrous ammonium
sulfate, 0.1% sodium citrate, and mycobactin J; pH 5.0 to 5.5.

RESULTS

Punch skin biopsies were obtained from 9 sarcoid patients
and 5 controls. In addition, an endoscopically obtained lung
biopsy was obtained from 2 patients with sarcoidosis.
Spheroplasts have been isolated from 6 of 9 skin biopsies from
patients with sarcoidosis compared to 0 of 5 controls ($p = 0.05$,
Fisher's Exact Test). Bacterial colonies were small, clear,
moist and glistening and required from 3 to 12 months to appear
(median time 7 months). Three of the 6 spheroplast isolates have
also grown in subculture; we detected colonies after 3 months on
HEYM and significant sediment and turbidity in MG3 medium after 1
month.

Ziehl-Neelson stains failed to reveal any identifiable acid-
fast forms in smears of primary isolates. The presence of
microorganisms was confirmed by staining with acridine orange
(4). Subcultures were shown to contain a few acid-fast rods and
pleomorphic forms after staining by Kinyoun's procedure (which
uses a 4% carbolfuchsin solution). Numerous acid-fast rods were
seen after oxidation of smears with 10% periodic acid before
acid-fast staining (5).

DISCUSSION

Previous studies attempting to prove a relationship between
sarcoidosis and mycobacteria, especially cell wall-defective
mycobacteria, have been either anecdotal or could not be
replicated (reviewed in 6-8). For example, in 1964, Mankiewicz
and Beland (9) reported that mycobacteria infected with

mycobacteriophages caused a condition similar to human sarcoidosis after inoculation into guinea pigs. Bowman and co-workers were unable to confirm this report (10). Most recently, the possible association of mycobacteria and sarcoidosis has fallen into disfavor as illustrated by the fact that there were no papers concerning a possible mycobacterial etiology of sarcoidosis published as part of the proceedings of the Tenth International Conference on Sarcoidosis and Other Granulomatous Disorders.

Our study again calls attention to mycobacteria as a prime suspect for the etiologic agent for sarcoidosis. If subsequent studies confirm this speculation, the path for future research will be clearer. Our further examination of this hypothesis will include continued culture and identification of the acid-fast organisms.

ACKNOWLEDGMENTS

This study was supported by the research program of the Veterans Administration and by a grant from the National Foundation for Ileitis and Colitis.

REFERENCES

1. Chiodini RJ, Van Kruiningen HJ, Thayer WR, Merkal RS, Coutu JA (1984) Possible role of mycobacteria in inflammatory bowel disease. I. An unclassified Mycobacterium species isolated from patients with Crohn's disease. Dig Dis Sci 29:1073-9.

2. Chiodini RJ, Van Kruiningen HJ, Thayer WR, Coutu JA (1986) Spheroplastic phase of mycobacteria isolated from patients with Crohn's disease. J Clin Microbiol 24:357-63

3. Graham DY, Markesich DC, Yoshimura HH (1987) Mycobacteria and inflammatory bowel disease: Results of culture. Gastroenterology 92:436-42.

4. Chattman MS, Mattman LH, Mattman PE (1969) L-forms in blood cultures demonstrated by nucleic acid fluorescence. Am J Clin Path 51:41-50.

5. Nyka W (1967) Method for staining both acid-fast and chromophobic tubercle bacilli with carbolfuchsin. J Bact 93:1458-60.

6. Thomas PD, Hunninghake GW (1987) Current concepts of the pathogenesis of sarcoidosis. Am Rev Respir Dis 135:747-60.

7. Moscovic EA (1982) Sarcoidosis and mycobacterial L-forms:
    histologic studies. In: Domingue GJ (ed) Cell wall-deficient
    bacteria. Basic principles and clinical significance.
    Addison-Wesley, Reading, MA, pp 299-320.

8. Mitchell DN, Rees RJW (1983) Some diseases of possible
    mycobacterial etiology. In Ratledge C and Stanford J (eds)
    The biology of the mycobacteria. Volume 2. Immunological and
    environmental aspects. Academic Press, London, pp 525-36.

9. Mankiewicz E, Beland J (1964) The role of mycobacteriophage
    and of cortisone in experimental tuberculosis and
    sarcoidosis. Am Rev Resp Dis 89:707-20.

10. Bowman BU, Amos WT, Geer JC (1972) Failure to produce
    experimental sarcoidosis in guinea pigs with Mycobacterium
    tuberculosis and mycobacteriophage DS6A. Am Rev Resp Dis
    105:85-94.

© 1988 Elsevier Science Publishers B.V. (Biomedical Division)
Sarcoidosis and other granulomatous disorders
C. Grassi, G. Rizzato, E. Pozzi, editors

IMMUNE-RESPONSE OF PERIPHERAL T LYMPHOCYTES TO SCW ANTIGEN AND CIRCULATING IMMUNE
COMPLEXES LEVELS AS PROGNOSTIC FACTORS IN PATIENTS WITH ACTIVE SARCOIDOSIS

KATSURO YAGAWA, SHINICHIRO HAYASHI, NOBUHIRO KAMIKAWAJI, KENICHI OGATA,
KENICHI MATSUBA AND NOBUAKI SHIGEMATSU
Research Institute for Diseases of the Chest, Faculty of Medicine, Kyushu
University, 3-1-1 Maidashi, Higashiku, Fukuoka 812 (Japan)

INTRODUCTION

Sarcoidosis is a disease characterized by non-caseous granuloma formation in
multiple-organs. The precise mechanism for the granuloma formation is still
unclear. However, the immunological-reaction is thought to play some roles for
the incidence of this disease. Increase in population of a subset of thymus-de-
rived lymphocytes, more specifically, a subset identified by the OKT-4(helper/
inducer) phenotype is usually observed in BALF of sarcoidosis patients (1).
These lymphocytes release several important regulatory proteins, such as IL-2,
which promotes expansion of lymphocyte pool, and a monocyte chemotactic factor,
which promote granuloma formation (2).

Circulating immune complex(CIC) is detected in about one-half of patients with
sarcoidosis. Those patients have been found to have better prognosis, and the
activation of T suppressor cells by CIC is thought to be responsible for the
better prognosis (3). The present study was undertaken to know whether the prognosis in patients with active sarcoidosis is related with the in vitro immune
-response of peripheral T-lymphocytes to streptococcal antigen and CIC levels.

MATERIALS AND METHODS

Cases

Patients include 66 cases with active sarcoidosis who admitted to or visited
Dept. of Respiratory Disease, Kyushu Univ. Medical School. Diagnosis of the
disease was made in all cases by pathological examination of biopsy specimens of
lung, lymphnodes or skins. Chest X-ray examinations and measurements of serum
ACE activity were repeated in one to two months intervals, and Ga-scintilation of
lung was performed in six months intervals to follow the disease activity.

Among 66 cases, 42 were followed for at least 2 years. Those 42 cases were
separated according to their prognosis into two groups of improved and not improved cases. The dicision of the improvement was made when cases fulfill the
following criteria; reduced or no uptake of Ga into lung, normalization of serum
ACE level and disappearance or reduction of hilar lymphadenopathy.

The measurement of T cell response

Membrain protein(M-protein) purified from cell wall fragments of A-group streptococcus(SCW-fragments) is a kind gift from T. Sasazuki(Kyushu Univ. Medical School) and is used as the stimulating antigen for the measurement of T cell response (4). Mononuclear cells were separated from peripheral blood by Ficall-gradient centrifugation. The cells were incubated with 1 ug/ml of the antigen. On the 7th incubation day, radiolabelled thymidin was added and further incubated for 24 hrs. Then, the radioactivity incorporated into the cells was counted.

Measurement of circulating immune complexes(CIC)

CIC levels were measured by complement consumption activity of polyethylene glycol absorbed immune complexes.

RESULTS AND DISCUSSION

Distribution of the T cell response to SCW antigen in healthy controls, the sarcoidosis cases with low or not detectable CIC levels, and those with high CIC levels are shown in Figure 1.

The cases were separated into high and low responder groups at the cut off point of 9.6 according to the reports by T.Sasazuki who first found that normal population are separated into high and low responder groups by the intensity of T cell response to the SCW antigen and which is genetically controlled (4). More than 70% in healthy controls and the sarcoidosis cases with low or not detectable CIC levels belonged to high responder group. On the other hand, less than 50% in the sarcoidosis cases with high CIC levels was high responders to the antigen. These data may indicate that the T cell response is modulated by CIC in some sarcoidosis cases.

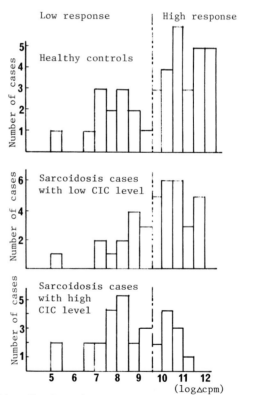

Distribution of T cell response to SCW-Antigen

Fig. 1. In Vitro T Cell Response to SCW-Antigen

To know whether the significant correlation exists between the prognosis and the immune response to the SCW antigen or CIC levels, 42 cases with active sarcoidosis who have been followed more than 2 years were separated according to their prognosis into improved and no change or worsened cases. As shown in Fig.2 about 60% among 27 improved cases were low responders to the SCW antigen. On the contrary, only 5 among 15 no change or worsened cases, were low responders.

Relation between the CIC levels and the prognosis of each sarcoidosis cases was shown in Fig.3. High CIC levels were found in 45% among 27 improved cases and, in 27% among 15 no change or worsened cases, respectively.

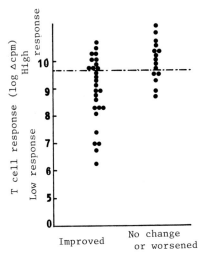

Fig.2. T Cell Response to SCW
-Antigen and Prognosis

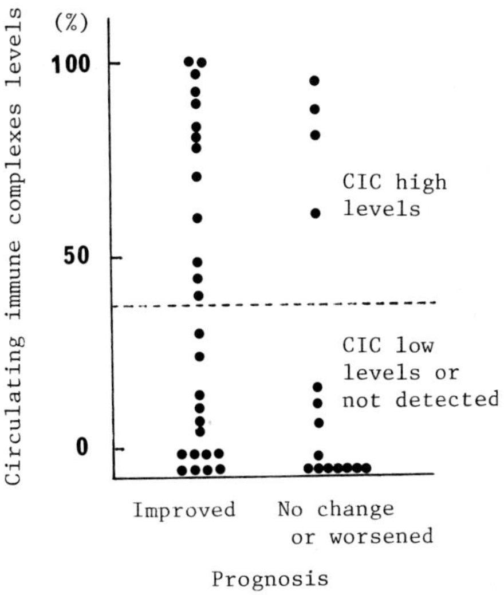

Fig.3. Circulating Immune
Complexes Levels and Prognosis

The data presented here are summarized in Table I. 10 among 12 cases with active sarcoidosis who showed low T cell response to the SCW antigen and high CIC levels measured at the onset of the disease improved or became disease-free within 2 years. On the other hand, the disease activity remained unchanged or progressed in more than 50% of cases with the high T cell response and low CIC levels. These results may indicate that both T and B cell dependent immune response play a role for the regulation of disease activity in sarcoidosis.

TABLE I.   T CELL RESPONSE, CIC LEVELS AND PROGNOSIS

T cell response	CIC level	Prognosis		% Improved cases
		Improved	No change or worsened	
High	High	3	2	60%
High	Low	7	8	47%
Low	High	10	2	83%
Low	Low	7	3	70%

Hepatosplenic Schistosomasis are also characterized by granuloma formation. Recent study by T.Sasazuki et al revealed that granuloma formation is only formed in those cases who show high responsiveness to the antigens derived from the worm, whereas, the low responder cases became disease free without formation of granuloma (5). He also found that the immune responsiveness to the antigens is genetically regulated by HLA-linked Ir gene. The present study revealed that the immune responsiveness of peripheral T lymphocytes to the antigen derived from streptococcus cell wall is well related with the prognosis of sarcoidosis. This result may indicate that persistent presence of mass of streptococcal bacteria or its derivative in upper airways plays some roles for the incidence of sarcoidosis, maybe working as causative agent. This concept might be more hightened by the following observations, 1)epitheroid cell granuloma is formed in animal models by injection of cell wall fragments of streptococcus which are collected from tonsilla of sarcoidosis patients, 2)poor prognosis is often observed in those sarcoidosis cases who carry local infections such as chronic tonsillitis, dental caries and/or sinusitis, 3)normalization and disappearance of BHL are often followed after tonsillectomy in chronic type of sarcoidosis cases who carry chronic tonsillitis.

Recent study indicates that some of HLA-Dr gene product are predominantly manifested in sarcoidosis case, which suggests that incidence and/or prognosis of this diseases are genetically controlled (6). A study is now in progress to clarify whether prognosis of sarcoidosis is related with a selective manifestation of some HLA-Dr gene products.

REFERENCES

1. Hunninghake,G.W., Crystal,R.G.: Pulmonary sarcoidosis - A disorder mediated by excess helper T-lymphocyte activity at sites of disease activity (1981) N Engl J Med 305:429-434

2. Hunninghake,G.W., Bedell,G.N., Zavala,D.C., Monick,M., Brady,M.: Role of interleukin-2 release by lung T-cells in active pulmonary sarcoidosis (1983) Am Rev Respir Dis 128:634-638

3. Daniele,R.P., McMillan,L.J., Dauber,J.H., Rossman,M.D.: Immune complexes in sarcoidosis - A correlation with activity and duration of disease (1978) Chest 74:261-264

4. Sasazuki,T., Kaneoka,H., Nishimura,Y., Kaneoka,R., Hayama,M., Ohkuni,H.: An HLA-linked immune suppression gene in man (1980) J Exp Med 152:297s-313s

5. Ohta,N., Nishimura,Y., Iuchi,M., Sasazuki,T.: Immunogenetic analysis of patients with post-schistosomal liver cirrhosis in man (1982) Clin Exp Immunol 49:493-499

6. Kunikane,H., Abe,S., Tsuneta,Y., Nakayama,T., Tajima,Y., Misonou,J., Wakisaka, A., Aizawa,M., Kawakami,Y.: Role of HLA-Dr antigen in Japanese patients with sarcoidosis (1987) Am Rev Respir Dis 135:688-691

ANERGY: A CORRELATE OF GRANULOMATOUS INFLAMMATION IN SARCOIDOSIS

MARY ELLEN KLEINHENZ, M.D.

Department of Medicine, Case Western Reserve University and University
Hospitals of Cleveland, Cleveland, Ohio, USA 44106

INTRODUCTION

Anergy on skin-testing with recall antigens is a frequent occurrence in
patients with sarcoidosis and was initially recognized as absence of
tuberculin reactivity (1). Subsequent studies have demonstrated that anergy
in sarcoidosis extends to other recall antigens (2) and is associated with a
failure to acquire delayed-typed hypersensitivity to new antigens(3).
Longitudinal studies in tuberculin-reactive sarcoidosis patients suggest that
anergy is acquired during sarcoidosis (4) and recovery of in vivo antigen
reactivity with remission of sarcoidosis has been observed (1). Despite
these observations, the relationship of anergy to the immunopathologic
processes underlying other clinical manifestations of sarcoidosis remains
uncertain. To examine this question, delayed hypersensitivity to a battery
of recall antigens was evaluated in a series of sarcoidosis patients in whom
lymphocytic alveolitis or cutaneous lesions provided clear evidence of active
granulomatous inflammation.

METHODS

Human Subjects. Forty-five patients with sarcoidosis and 20 healthy
volunteers participated in this study. Informed consent was obtained from
each subject. In 41 patients, the diagnosis of sarcoidosis was established
histologically; 4 asymptomatic patients, had bilateral hilar lymphadenopathy
for greater than 1 year as their only sign of sarcoidosis. Active
granulomatous inflammation was defined as lymphocytic alveolitis with greater
than 15% E-rosetting T cells on bronchoalveolar lavage or as new or
progressive cutaneous granulomata. Inactive sarcoidosis was defined as the
complete resolution of all signs of sarcoidosis or, in the asymptomatic
patient, radiographically stable, nonprogressive disease for more than 12
months.

The duration of sarcoidosis was estimated from the clinical history.
Spirometry and diffusing capacity for carbon monoxide were performed in the
Adult Pulmonary Function Laboratory of University Hospitals of Cleveland and
compared with values predicted by Morris (5) and Burrows (6) respectively.

Skin Testing. A battery of four commercially available skin test reagents
was applied to each subject: mumps antigen (Connaught Laboratories, Inc.,
Swiftwater, PA); purified protein derivative of tuberculin, 5TU, (Connaught
Limited, Willowdale, Ontario Candana); candida albicans allergenic extract,
Center Laboratories, Port Washington, NY) and trichophyton allergenic extract
(Center Laboratories). Test suspensions were innoculated intradermally and
sites inspected and palpated at 48 and 72 hours. A reaction ≥ 5 mm induration
was recorded as a positive result.

Characterization of blood T cells. T cells were separated from a sample of
heparinized whole blood by Ficoll Hypaque density gradient sedimentation and
a two-step depletion of adherent mononuclear cells (7). Fractions of T cells
reacting with monoclonal antibodies to T helper (Leu 3a) and T suppressor
(Leu 2a) cells were assayed by indirect immunofluorescence.

Statistical Analysis. Results were analyzed with Microstat, software
program published by Ecosfsot, Inc.,1985

RESULTS

Patients with sarcoidosis were segregated into 2 groups reflecting the
evidence of granulomatous inflammation; essential clinical features of the
two patient groups are presented in Table 1. Patients with active
sarcoidosis did not differ in age and sex distribution, lung function, or
duration of sarcoidosis. Twenty-four patients were identified as having
active sarcoidosis by lymphocytic alveolititis; not surprisingly, the mean
number of bronchoalveolar cells recovered at lavage from these patients was
greater than in the patients with inactive sarcoidosis. The mean
bronchoalveolar T cell fraction in patients with active sarcoidosis was
$33\pm15\%$.

Fifteen patients with sarcoidosis failed to respond at any skin test site;
1 anergic patient however was receiving cortisteroids and was excluded from
data analysis. Since at least 1 postive skin test was observed in each
healthy subject, the frequency of anergy was significantly increased in the
sarcoid patient population (X^2=6.012, p=0.01). Thirteen anergic patients
had active sarcoidosis and a significant correlation between evidence of
granulomatous inflammation and anergy was established (X^2=4.19, p=0.04).
The anergic and antigen-reactive sarcoidosis patients did not differ in
age,sex, or duration of sarcoidosis. Anergy was not correlated with
disturbances in lung function or the intensity of lymphocytic alveolitis
graded by the number of cells recovered at bronchoalveolar lavage or by the

fraction of T cells present in the bronchoalveolar cell fraction. Three anergic patients recovered skin test reactivity with corticosteroid treatment or spontaneous remission of sarcoidosis.

The distribution of T cell subpopulations in nonadherent blood T cells from anergic and antigen-reactive sarcoidosis patients was not different from controls (Table 2).

TABLE 1

FEATURES OF PATIENTS WITH SARCOIDOSIS

	Active Sarcoidosis	Inactive Sarcoidosis
n	34	11
age (yrs)	34 ± 10*	37 ± 11
Bronchoalevolar Cells (x10^6)	42 ± 32*	14 ± 5
FVC**	73 ± 16	91 ± 21
DLCO**	78 ± 18	90 ± 19
Anergy (n)	13	1

*data are presented as mean ± 1SD
**data are presented as mean percent of predicted ± 1SD

DISCUSSION

In this study, anergy on skin testing with a battery of common recall antigens was more frequent in patients with sarcoidosis than in healthy volunteers; among sarcoidosis patients anergy was observed more commonly in individuals with objective evidence of current granulomatous inflammation. An association of anergy with age, sex, corticosteroid therapy, radiographic extent and duration of sarcoidosis, or disturbance of lung function was not observed. Neither the intensity of lymphocytic alveolitis or maldistribution of circulating T cell subpopulations were determinants of anergy in these patients with sarcoidosis. This suggests that anergy results directly from the immunopathologic processes which initiate and maintain granuloma formation rather than as a consequence of organ dysfunction or damage. The recovery of antigen skin reactivity with corticosteroid treatment or spontaneous resolution of sarcoidosis as documented in 3 patients in this study, has been observed previously (8) and further supports this notion. While the basis for anergy in sarcoidosis remains to be determined, this study establishes anergy as a correlate of active granulomatous inflammation which underlies other clinical manifestations of sarcoidosis.

TABLE 2

T CELL REACTIVITY WITH MONOCLONAL ANTIBODY

	Leu 3a	Leu 2a
Healthy Subjects	68 ± 11*	31 ± 13
Antigen Reactive Sarcoidosis	69 ± 6	29 ± 7
Anergic Sarcoidosis	67 ± 18	31 ± 15

*mean percent $\pm$ 1 SD

REFERENCES

1. Nitter L (1953) Acta Radiologica (Supple) 105:1-202
2. Friou GJ (1952) Yale J Biol Med 24:533-539
3. Sharma OP, James DG, Fox RA (1971) Chest 60:35-37
4. Turiaf J, Menault M, Battesti JP (1970) Ann Med Interne (Paris) 121:117-134
5. Morris JF, Koski A, Johnson LC (1971) Am Rev Respir Dis 103:57-67
6. Burrows BJ, Kasik JE, Niden AH, Barclay WR (1961) Am Rev Respir Dis 84:798-806
7. Kleinhenz ME, Ellner JJ (1987) J. Lab Clin Med 110:31-40
8. Citron KM, Scadding JB (1957) 26:277-289

AUTOLOGOUS MIXED LYMPHOCYTE REACTIONS PROBE MACROPHAGE FUNCTION IN SARCOIDOSIS

MONICA SPITERI & L W POULTER

Department of Thoracic Medicine & Immunology, Royal Free Hospital, Hampstead
London, NW3

INTRODUCTION

It is well established that the inflammation associated with pulmonary
sarcoidosis involves a lymphocyte alveolitis, as observed by the lymphocytosis
in bronchoalveolar lavage (BAL) of such patients, as well as the histological
appearance of non-caseating granulomata involving macrophage - like cells
(1-3). So far, activation of these lymphocytes has been demonstrated 'in
vitro'; such activity being dependent on the macrophage - like cell population.

In the following study, we set out to investigate the intrinsic reactivity
between the macrophage and lymphocyte populations as occurs 'in vivo' (without
any manipulation by either exogenous mitogen or antigen) in the lung and
peripheral blood of patients with sarcoidosis and healthy volunteers.

SUBJECTS

The study population consisted of 9 patients with biopsy-proven sarcoidosis:
6 males, 3 females; mean age 38 years; 8 non-smokers, 1 smoker (1 pack/day).
All had their diagnosis for at least 1 year; 7 patients had not received
any prior treatment, while 2 patients had stopped their systemic corticosteroids
at least 18 months before. All 9 patients had unequivocal bilateral parenchymal
shadowing in their lung fields (grade 3 chest x-ray) in addition to a
restrictive ventilatory defect.

A control population of 9 healthy medical students, all non-smokers;
8 males, 1 female; mean age 22 years, were recruited into the study following
formal consent. All had normal chest x-ray and pulmonary function tests.
None had a past history of lung disease or a history of viral illness in
the preceding 2 weeks.

METHODS

BAL was performed in all sarcoid patients and normal volunteers by using
a total of 180 ml of 0.9% normal saline; each time the right middle lobe
was lavaged. Bronchoalveolar cells (BAC) were separated from lavage fluid
by centrifugation; the cell pellet was washed twice in RPMI 1640 and then
resuspended in culture medium (RPMI 1640 + glutamine, streptomycin and
penicillin). All recruits had 20 ml of peripheral blood taken; peripheral

blood mononuclear cells (PBM) were separated out initially on lymphoprep, then washed twice in Hanks' solution, and resuspended in culture medium. BAC and PBM were respectively counted in a hemacyometer, following which each cell suspension was adjusted to a concentration of 1×10^6 cells/ml. Mitomycin - C(M) was used to treat some samples of BAC and PBM respectively (BACM, PBMM). The 4 cell suspensions (BAC, BACM, PBM, PBMM) were then separately incubated at 36.4 °C for 45 minutes in a humidified CO_2 incubator, following which autologous mixed lymphocyte reaction (AMLR) were set up, using 1×10^5 cells of each cell suspension in each microtitre well. These were then harvested for 4 days, after which tritiated thymidine (3_{HT}, $1 \mu Ci$.) was added to each well, and cell uptake counted after 18 hours.

RESULTS

The results of our study are seen in Tables I and II, where each figure represents the mean and standard deviation of counts per min from incorporated 3_{HT} that has resulted from AMLR in PBM and BAL cell suspensions respectively.

<table>
<tr><td colspan="3">Table I</td><td colspan="3">Table II</td></tr>
<tr><td colspan="3">Reactivity in Blood</td><td colspan="3">Reactivity in BAL</td></tr>
<tr><td></td><td>Normal</td><td>Sarcoid</td><td></td><td>Normal</td><td>Sarcoid</td></tr>
<tr><td>BLOOD</td><td>1111 ± 193</td><td>290 ± 37.2</td><td>BAL</td><td>178 ± 22.5</td><td>223 ± 45.8</td></tr>
<tr><td>BLOODM</td><td>159 ± 24.4</td><td>193 ± 46.7</td><td></td><td></td><td></td></tr>
<tr><td>BLAM</td><td>187 ± 43.2</td><td>169 ± 32.2</td><td>BALM</td><td>187 ± 43.2</td><td>169 ± 32.2</td></tr>
<tr><td>BLOOD</td><td>567 ± 159</td><td>301 ± 41.7</td><td></td><td></td><td></td></tr>
</table>

NB: BACKGROUND CONTROL 16 ± 2.02

Table I shows that AMLR in sarcoid patients' peripheral blood is significantly suppressed when compared to the normal. The normal shows an 8 to 9 - fold increase over mitomycin treated controls, while in sarcoid patients less than 1 to 2 - fold increase is seen. When mitomycin treated BAL samples were used to stimulate PBM, no effect was seen in sarcoid samples in contrast to the normal where BAL inducers(ie the macrophage - like population) suppressed the level of stimulation in the blood AMLR. Table II shows that when using BAC, no stimulation was recorded in normal or sarcoid lavage.

DISCUSSION

Lymphocytes can be stimulated by antigen presented by macrophages. The antigen stimulated response initiated by such macrophages represents an amplification of the baseline stimulation normally present when macrophages meet autologous lymphocytes. The AMLR is therefore a baseline reactivity which can be easily measured by the uptake of DNA precursors in any lymphocyte - macrophage suspension, even when no addition of antigen or mitogen is made. Addition of mitomycin C to a specific cell population will effectively block cell division therin: this will thereby force a one-way interaction if PBM and BAC suspensions are mixed together. Thus, on analysing the results shown in Table I, the implication arises that not only are alveolar macrophages poor inducers as has been reported previously (4), but they also inhibit lymphocyte reactivity. In addition, Table II confirms that there is an inherent reduced reactivity in the lung when compared to the peripheral blood.

It could be justifiably argued that the above results may be influenced by gross differences in lymphocyte proportions, as lymphocytosis is generally present in sarcoid BAL. Infact, differential cell counts of our BAC and PBM showed far fewer lymphocytes in normal BAL, while proportionately more lymphocytes were present in normal blood (Table III).

MEAN DIFFERENTIAL COUNTS IN AMLR

	M$\emptyset$ (x10^5/ml)	LY (x10^5/ml)
NORMAL		
BAL	9.1 ± 0.18	0.8 ± 0.15
BLOOD	2.9 ± 0.25	7.1 ± 0.25
SARCOID		
BAL	6.7 ± 0.59	2.9 ± 0.56
BLOOD	5.4 ± 0.54	4.6 ± 0.54

AMLRs were therefore set up using a titration of normal lymphocytes (0.5 - 8.0 x 10^5/ml) against a constant proportion of macrophages (6.0 x 10^5/ml); the selected range covering the extremes previously seen in test samples. This showed that AMLR was directly proportional to the numbers of lymphocytes present. Using this information, we were able to predict isotope incorporation in AMLRs of our test cultures, and compare these figures with actual results obtained (Table IV).

Table IV

	EXP	ACT
SARCOID		
BAL	375 ± 35	233 ± 46
BLD	500 ± 50	290 ± 37
	(p < 0.01)	
NORMAL		
BAL	150 ± 15	178 ± 23
BLD	900 ± 100	1100 ± 200

Interestingly it was found that the actual results obtained using normal PBM or BAC were the same as the predicted values; in contrast to the sarcoid samples where the actual results obtained were significantly lower than the predicted results. This implies that patients with sarcoidosis do *not* have increased lymphocyte activation in their lung 'in vivo'; in addition, there is also a suppression of AMLR in the blood of such patients. Our results also imply that there are aberrations of function both in the lymphocyte and macrophage populations of the lung in sarcoidosis.

REFERENCES

1 HUNNINGHAKE G W, CRYSTAL R G. 1981 pulmonary sarcoidosis: A disorder mediated by excessive helper T-lymphocyte activity at sites of disease activity. N ENGL J MED 35: 429

2 HUNNINGHAKE G W, GADEK J E, et al 1980 maintenance of granuloma formation in pulmonary sarcoidosis by T-lymphocytes within the lung. N ENGL J MED 302: 594

3 VENET A, HANCE A J et al 1985 enhanced alveolar marcophage-mediated antigen-induced T-lymphocyte proliferation in sarcoidosis. J CLIN INVEST 75: 293

4 LEM V M, LIPSCOMB M F et al 1985 bronchoalveolar cells from sarcoid patients demonstrate enhanced antigen presentation. J IMMUNOL 135: 1986

ACKNOWLEDGEMENT

We would like to thank Drs Clarke, du Bois, and Noble for their support, and Miss M O'Malley for her secretarial assistance.

OCULAR MANIFESTATIONS OF SARCOIDOSIS PRECEEDING SYSTEMIC
MANIFESTATIONS

C. STEPHEN FOSTER, M.D., FACS
Harvard Medical School, Immunology Service, Massachusetts Eye
and Ear Infirmary, Boston, Massachusetts

INTRODUCTION

One of the many systems which may be affected by the
granulomatous inflammation characteristic of sarcoidosis is the
eye. Ocular involvement in generalized sarcoidosis is common,
with 25-50% incidence of ocular manifestations reported in
large sarcoidosis surveys. Conversely, 3% of uveitis patients
in large surveys have systemic sarcoidosis.

Less well recognized is the fact that ocular involvement
may preceed, by several years, non-ocular detectable signs of
sarcoidosis. The purpose of this report is to emphasize this
fact and to present data supporting the idea that ocular
manifestations of sarcoidosis may preceed the subtlest
diagnostic manifestations by at least four years.

METHODS AND MATERIALS

New patients referred to the Immunology Service of the
Massachusetts Eye and Ear Infirmary between January 1, 1983 and
December 31, 1983 form the basis of this report. The patients
were evaluated prospectively for underlying systemic disease as
a basis of diverse forms of inflammatory eye disease. Repeat
evaluations have been conducted every six to twelve months for
those patients for whom inconclusive data suggesting an occult
systemic disorder were obtained. June 30, 1987 was arbitrarily
chosen as the final date for definitive establishment of the
diagnosis of sarcoidosis in any of the patients initially
evaluated during the calendar year of 1983 for the purpose of
this report.

The patient population was subsequently stratified into
uveitis and non-uveitis subpopulations. The uveitis patients
with sarcoidosis were further substratified into two groups:
patients in whom the diagnosis of sarcoidosis was established
during the initial evaluation on our Service; and patients in

whom the diagnosis of sarcoidosis was subsequently established, some time between initial presentation to us and June 30, 1987.

Our diagnostic criteria for sarcoidosis included clinical manifestations compatible with that diagnosis and a positive biopsy showing non-caseating epithilioid granulomas. Ancillary data, including elevated angiotensin converting enzyme assay, positive gallium scan, elevated serum and urine calcium, and anergy to ubiquitous skin test antigens, were not employed as diagnostic criteria, but rather as supportive evidence.

RESULTS

Eight hundred twenty eight new patients were referred to the Immunology Service in 1983 for evaluation of ocular or adnexal inflammation. Most (545) of these referrals were for reasons other than uveitis. Eight of these 545 patients were discovered to have sarcoidosis. Two presented with chronic conjunctivitis, one with a conjunctival granuloma, three with tear insufficiency, and two with lacrimal gland enlargement.

Uveitis referrals numbered 283 patients. Biopsy-proven systemic manifestations of sarcoidosis were discovered in six of these individuals, and in an additional eight, such manifestations eventually developed. The demographic characteristics of this group of 14 patients are shown in Table 1.

TABLE 1
DEMOGRAPHIC CHARACTERISTICS OF UVEITIS PATIENTS WITH SARCOIDOSIS

Sex		Race		Age (years)	
Male	Female	Black	Caucasian	Average	Range
6	8	5	9	34.5	9-69

The interval from onset of uveitis to diagnosis of sarcoidosis was 9 months to 4 years (average 2.2 years).

The ocular manifestations of the potentially blinding inflammation are shown in Tables 2 and 3.

TABLE 2
ANTERIOR OCULAR MANIFESTATIONS

Pathema	# of cases
Anterior uveitis	5
Band keratopathy	2
Synechiae	6
Iris nodules	3
Cataract	10
Glaucoma	3

TABLE 3
POSTERIOR OCULAR MANIFESTATIONS

Pathema	# of cases
Intermediate uveitis	4
Vitritis	9
Retinal vasculitis	8
Chorioretinitis	4
Papillitis	4
Macular edema	11
Subretinal neovascularization	2

The biopsy site establishing the diagnosis was lung in seven cases, lymph node in one, kidney in one, skin in three, nerve and synovium in one, and conjuctiva in one.

All patients were treated with systemic, topical, and periocular steroids prior to and following establishment of the diagnosis. Six patients received TP-5 and two were treated with Cyclosporine. Therapeutic complications were limited to corticosteroid side-effects (Table 4).

TABLE 4
COMPLICATIONS FROM CORTICOSTEROID USE

Complication	# of cases
Cataract	12
Glaucoma	4
Hip necrosis	1
Peptic ulcer	2

The visual acuity in the 28 eyes of these 14 patients with ocular sarcoidosis as of June 30, 1987 is shown in Table 5.

TABLE 5
VISUAL ACUITY IN 28 EYES OF 14 PATIENTS WITH SARCOIDOSIS

Visual acuity	# of eyes
20/20-20/40	13
20/50-20/100	8
20/200 or less	7

It is important, however, to consider what proportion of these patients are legally blind (i.e., visual acuity of 20/200 or less in the better eye) or visually handicapped (i.e., visual acuity between 20/50 and 20/100 in the better eye). The data in Table 6 show that 12.5% of the patients with sarcoid uveitis became legally blind, and that another 12.5% were visually handicapped.

TABLE 6
VISUAL FUNCTION IN THE BETTER EYE

Visual acuity	# of patients
20/20-20/40	8
20/50-20/100	3
20/200 or less	3

DISCUSSION

The data from this study underscore several important, underrecognized points. First, ocular inflammation secondary to sarcoidosis may represent the presenting manifestation of sarcoidosis. Our findings suggest that close collaboration between the ophthalmologist and sarcoidosis specialist might disclose occult systemic sarcoid earlier than is presently the case; six of our cases were diagnosed during the initial systemic evaluation. It must be achnowledged, however, that an appropriate evaluation earlier in these six patients would probably have been non-diagnostic, at least soon after the onset of the uveitis. The second point of emphasis from our data relates to this, in that we personally evaluated a cohort of patients longitudinally and repeatedly, and eventually discovered evolving systemic manifestations of sarcoidosis in eight patients, all of whom had previously shown no diagnostic evidence of sarcoid. This finding emphasizes the importance of periodic re-evaluation of patients with "granulomatous" uveitis compatible with the ocular manifestations of sarcoidosis in whom the diagnosis cannot initially be established.

A third point of emphasis from this study is the fact that 12.5% of the sarcoid uveitis patients are blind and another 12.5% are visually handicapped. Glaucoma, destruction of retina, and optic nerve damage were responsible for the loss of ocular function in these patients. Clearly, ocular involvement in sarcoidosis is a medically, sociologically and economically important consideration in our care of patients with this disease.

And the final point of emphasis from this study relates to the issue of loss of visual function. Current therapeutic strategies for ocular sarcoidosis are clearly imperfect and are basically unchanged from 30 years ago. Not only are some patients losing sight in spite of conventional corticosteroid therapy, but also significant ocular and extraocular complications from such therapy are occasionally encountered. These limitations of steroid therapy are not trivial. Additional safe, effective treatment for sarcoid uveitis is desperately needed.

© 1988 Elsevier Science Publishers B.V. (Biomedical Division)
Sarcoidosis and other granulomatous disorders
C. Grassi, G. Rizzato, E. Pozzi, editors

CHARACTERIZATION OF ALVEOLAR MACROPHAGES FROM SARCOIDOSIS PATIENTS USING DIFFERENT MONOCLONAL ANTIBODIES OF THE KI-SERIES

J. BARTH, W. PETERMANN, P. ENTZIAN, H. KREIPE[*], H.J. RADZUN[*], M.R. PARWARESCH[*]
Department of Medicine and [*]Department of Pathology, University of Kiel, D 2300 Kiel (W. Germany)

INTRODUCTION

According to lymphocyte differentiation using lymphocyte specific monoclonal antibodies, phenotypic differentiation of alveolar macrophages may help evaluate further data concerning the recognition of different variations of the mononuclear phagocyte system. The immunophenotype of resident alveolar macrophages could be characterized and differentiated from monocytes. The purpose of this study was to evaluate the antigen pattern of alveolar macrophages from patients with sarcoidosis II. Further under investigation was whether markers of cellular activity would be expressed by alveolar macrophages from patients with sarcoidosis II.

PATIENTS AND METHODS:

Patients. 12 patients with histologically proven pulmonary sarcoidosis (radiographic stage II)

Control subjects. a) 8 healthy volunteers. Heparinised blood was drawn to isolate monocytes. b) 8 patients with small peripheral lung nodes. Middle lobe or lingula of the non-affected lung was taken for broncho-alveolar lavage.

Alveolar macrophages. Alveolar macrophages were obtained by bronchoalveolar lavage with 5 x 20 ml of physiologic saline after centrifugation with 300 g for 10 min.

Blood monocytes. Mononuclear cells from heparinised blood were isolated by Ficoll-Hypaque-gradient centrifugation. The separation of the monocyte fraction was performed by adherence to glass culture dishes.

Monocyte/macrophage specific monoclonal antibodies. Ki-M 1 reacts with blood monocytes,macrophages and interdigitating reticulum cells. Ki-M 2 and Ki-M 3 react with a membrane-associated antigen. Ki-M 6 and Ki M 8 react with an intracytoplasmic antigen (1,2).

Monoclonal markers of activity. Ki-67 reacts with a nuclear antigen associated to cell proliferation. Ki-1 reacts with activated lymphocytes and Sternberg-Reed cells. Anti-TAC reacts with the IL-II receptor.

Immunostaining of cytospin preparations. a) A three-step immuno-peroxidase method using peroxidase-labelled secondary and tertiary antibodies.
b) An alkaline phosphatase -antialkaline phosphatase method (APAAP).

184

RESULTS

Immunostaining with monoclonal antibodies of the Ki-M series revealed phenotypic differences between blood monocytes and alveolar macrophages. In contrast
to blood monocytes, alveolar macrophages from normal subjects did not express
the Ki-M 2 or Ki-M 3 antigen, whereas Ki-M 8 showed a higher degree of immunoreactivity in alveolar macrophages than in blood monocytes. The monoclonal
marker of activity Ki-1 and the monoclonal antibody Ki-67 did not show
immunoreactivity with monocytes and alveolar macrophages from control subjects.
Even no reactivity we could found in monocytes and alveolar macrophages from
control patients after staining with anti-Tac.
Different changes in the phenotypic staining pattern of alveolar macrophages
from patients with sarcoidosis II could be observed. The Ki-M 8 antigen showed
a decreased expression, whereas a minor part of the alveolar macrophages from
sarcoidosis patients expressed the Ki-M 2 and Ki-M 3 antigen as opposed to
normal alveolar macrophages.
Furthermore we could confirm the recent observation of anti-Tac positivity
of a small alveolar macrophage fraction taken from patients with sarcoidosis (3).
A minor number of alveolar macrophages from sarcoidosis patients showed Ki-1
reactivity. Also a small part of alveolar macrophages from sarcoidosis patients
($4.8^{\pm}1,2$ %) exhibited Ki-67 immunoreactivity, whereas no positivity could be
found in alveolar macrophages from control subjects.

CONCLUSIONS

The differences observed in the expression of Ki-M 2 and Ki-M 8 antigens
indicate a different maturity stage for monocytic alveolar macrophages taken
from control subjects compared to alveolar macrophages from sarcoidosis patients.
A small fraction of alveolar macrophages from patients with sarcoidosis express
markers of cellular activity possibly indicating functional activation including the readiness to proliferation.

REFERENCES

1. Parwaresch MR, Radzun HJ, Kreipe H, Hansmann ML, Barth J (1986)
    Monocyte/macrophage-reactive monoclonal antibody Ki-M 6 recognizes an
    intracytoplasmic antigen. Am J Pathol 124: 141-151

2. Radzun HJ, Kreipe H, Bödewadt S, Hansmann ML, Barth J, Parwaresch MR (1987)
    Ki-M 8 monoclonal antibody reactive with an intracytoplasmic antigen of
    monocyte macrophage lineage. Blood 69: 1320-1327

3. Hancock WW, Kobzik L, Colby AJ, O'Hara CJ, Cooper AG, Godleski JJ (1986)
    Detection of lymphokines and lymphokine receptors in pulmonary sarcoidosis.
    Immunohistologic evidence that inflammatory macrophages express the IL-2
    receptor. Am J. Pathol 123: 1-8

© 1988 Elsevier Science Publishers B.V. (Biomedical Division)
Sarcoidosis and other granulomatous disorders
C. Grassi, G. Rizzato, E. Pozzi, editors

CORRELATION BETWEEN PGE_2 PRODUCTION AND SUPPRESSOR CELL ACTIVITY OF ALVEOLAR MACROPHAGES IN INTERSTITIAL LUNG DISEASES.

E. FIREMAN[*], S.BEN EFRAIM[+], J. GREIF[*], A. ALGUETTI[#], D. AYALON[#] AND M. TOPILSKY[*]
[*]Institute of Pulmonary Diseases, [#]Inst. of Reproductive Endocrinology, Tel Aviv Medical Center, [+]Microbiology Department, Tel Aviv University, Israel.

INTRODUCTION

Alveolar macrophages (AM) are known to play a central role in the regulation of immune responses of the lung. Among these functions, AM have enhancing and suppressing effects on antigen and mitogen stimulated T cell proliferation. The most common products implicated in these down regulation activity are prostaglandins. Both exogenous administration of E series of PGs and endogenous production of PGE_2 by mononuclear phagocytes have been shown to suppress several important lymphocyte and macrophage functions, such as N.K. activity, monokine release and Ia and HLA-DR expression. This suppressive cell activity (SA) has been demonstrated in AM from smokers (1), asthmatics (2) and patients suffering from Interstitial Lung Diseases (ILD) (3). The aim of this study was to analyze the mechanism of suppression of alveolar cells in diverse diseases of the lung.

MATERIAL AND METHODS

Population study. Three groups of patients were studied: a) 5 Controls (CO); b) 8 Lung cancer (CA); c) 11 Interstitial Lung Diseases (ILD), subdivided according to the predominating cell type in BAL. The first group (7) showed a lymphocytic pattern (Sarcoidosis >31% lymphocytes in BAL) and the second group(4) had a neutrophilic pattern (IPF >12% neutrophils in BAL).

Methods. AM were co-cultured with autologous peripheral lymphocytes (1:1 concentrations) for 72 hrs in supplemented medium. Suppression was calculated by the conventional formula. PGE_2 was assayed by radioimmunoassay from culture fluids recovered from adherent AM cultured for the same period of time as the suppressor cell activity assay.

RESULTS

Effect of AM on blastic proliferation. AM of patients of the CA, CO and ILD groups suppress lymphocytic proliferation by $0.46 \pm 18.8\%$, $12.6 \pm 14.2\%$ and $71.9 \pm 1.5\%$ respectively ($p < 0.001$ ILD compared to CO and CA groups).

PGE2 production of AM in correlation to SA. Low SA (<40%) correlates well with low secretion of PGE_2 (0.233 ± 0.004 mg/ml/10^5 cells) in the CA and CO group (Fig.1). In patients with ILD, only in the neutrophilic pattern the high SA correlated with an elevated secretion of PGE_2 (1.51±0.26 mg/ml/10^5 cells). In Sarcoidosis there was no correlation between suppression and PGE_2 secretion since AM secreted low levels of PGE_2 (0.413±0.22 mg/ml/10^5 cells). Suppression of lymphocytic proliferation was achieved by 10^{-4} – 10^5 M of exogenous PGE_2 but unfractioned supernatants recovered from highly suppressive AM achieved the same effect by a much lower concentration (10^{-9} – 10^{-10} M) (Fig. 2). Further studies are necessary to identify factors, other than PGE_2 that down a regulate immuno response.

Fig. I

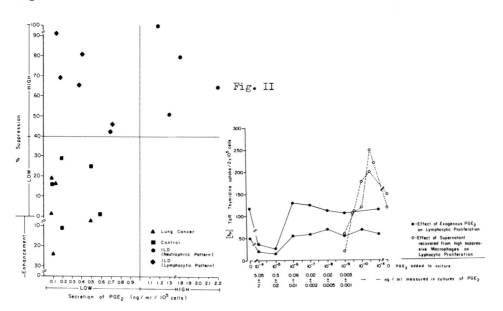

Fig. II

REFERENCES

1. Deshazo RD, Bank SD, Dieem JE et al (1983) BAL cell-lymphocyte interactions in normal nonsmokers and smokers. Am Rev Respir Dis 128:516-522
2. Anbas P, Cosso B, Godard F et al (1984) Decreased suppressor cell activity of alveolar macrophages in bronchial asthma. Am Rev Respir Dis 130:875-878
3. Fireman E, Ben Ephraim S, Greif J et al (1987) Suppressor cell activity of alveolar macrophages in ILD. Clin Exp Immunol. Submitted for publication.

© 1988 Elsevier Science Publishers B.V. (Biomedical Division)
Sarcoidosis and other granulomatous disorders
C. Grassi, G. Rizzato, E. Pozzi, editors

A GENOTYPIC AND PHENOTYPIC ANALYSIS OF T CELLS PROLIFERATING IN THE LUNG OF PATIENTS WITH ACTIVE SARCOIDOSIS

ZAMBELLO R, TRENTIN L, CASORATI G, SIVIERO F, MASCIARELLI M, TOMMASINI A, AGOSTINI C.

Departments of Clinical Medicine and Pneumology, Padua University; Department of Genetic, Turin University; Clinical Pathology, Cittadella Hospital, Padua, Italy.

INTRODUCTION

Active pulmonary sarcoidosis is characterized by the accumulation in the lung of CD4+ lymphocytes with a consequent disorganization of the normal parenchymal structure (1). These cells have been demonstrated to proliferate in situ and to produce different lymphokines, namely Interleukin-2 and γ-Interferon, which are considered to sustain and enhance the inflammatory processes (2,3).

It is not established whether CD4+ lymphocytes accumulating in the lung are restricted to a specific population of clonal origin. To test this possibility, taking advantage of the recently developed methodologies of molecular biology, we have evaluated the organization of the T rearranging gamma gene locus (TRG-γ) and the T cell receptor beta-gene region (TCR-β) in cells recovered from bronchoalveolar lavage (BAL) of patients with active pulmonary sarcoidosis. In addition, the phenotypic expression of different epitopes of the CD4 molecule, which is involved in the binding site for some viral infections, has been studied with a panel of monoclonal antibodies (MoAbs), referred to as the T4 A-F series, to investigate whether a particular CD4 epitope-bearing population was selected.

MATERIALS AND METHODS

Patients. 10 patients with biopsy-proven sarcoidosis were studied. Disease activity was evaluated according to clinical and laboratory criteria, as previously reported (4). All patients were non smokers and had not received therapy at the time of the study.

Gene rearrangement study. DNA was extracted from BAL T cells and peripheral blood mononuclear cells (PBMC), digested with Bam HI and Eco RI restriction endonucleases, size fractionated through 0.6 gel electrophoresis and hybridized to the Jγ1 segment of the gamma locus and to the β2 constant region gene (Cβ2) probes, as previously described in detail (5).

Phenotypic analysis. A panel of MoAbs recognizing distinct epitopes of the CD4 molecule and named T4, T4A, T4B, T4C, T4D, T4E and T4F (provided by Ortho Diagnostic) was used. Analysis was performed using the indirect immuno fluorescence technique and a flow cytometer (Ortho Cytofluorograph IIs).

RESULTS AND DISCUSSION

In all cases, TRG-γ analysis with both Bam HI and Eco RI restriction enzymes showed multiple rearranged Jγ1 gene containing segments which are characteristic of the polyclonal T cells. TCR-β analysis following both restriction enzymes, documented a reduction of the germ line band intensity, pointing out that the majority of the BAL cells are polyclonally rearranged. However, a faint novel band of identical size (13 Kb) was noted in BAL cells but not in PBMC from all sarcoid patients after Bam HI digestion (Fig. 1). According to the intensity, the latter band could not account for more than 10% of the total cell population.

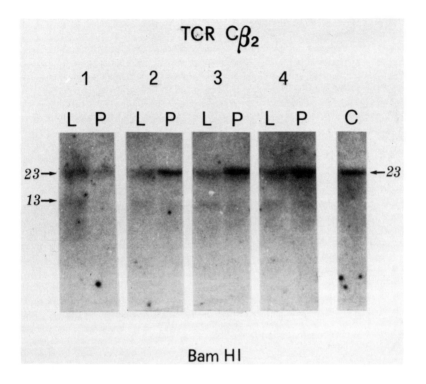

Fig. 1. Southern blot analysis of four representative DNA samples of BAL lymphocytes (L) and PBMC (P) from four patients with active sarcoidosis, following digestion with Bam HI and hybridization to the $C\beta 2$ probe. Note that in all cases a faint new band of 13 Kb is shown in BAL cells. Lane C represents unrearranged control DNA (fibroblasts).

Phenotypical analysis showed that the frequency of cells positive for MoAbs belonging to the T4 A-F series was similar to the T4 baseline value without a preferential positivity to any of the above quoted reagents (Fig. 2).

In conclusion, we have shown that the majority of BAL T cells are polyclonally rearranged at the TCR gamma and beta loci. It must be pointed out that we have observed a not completely random rearrangement at the TCR-β region. In fact, a small percentage of cells (probably less than 10%) showed a consistent β-gene reorganization in all BAL samples. However, the nature and the possible functional role of this subpopulation deserves further investigation. The non-selective expression of CD4 epitopes is neither consistent with the evidence of a preferential polymorphic expression of these epitopes (7) in sarcoid patients, nor with the possibility that a specific agent utilizes discrete epitopes of the CD4 molecule for binding site, as recently demonstrated for Human Immunodeficiency Virus infection (8).

Further studies, in particular those involved in the identification of inciting antigen(s), will contribute in clarifying the activation pathways of lung T cells in sarcoid patients.

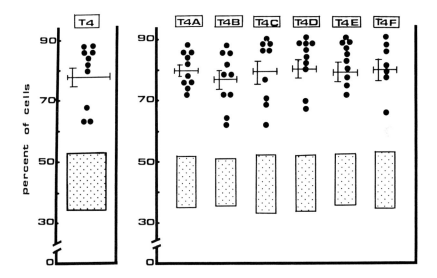

Fig. 2. Expression of CD4 epitopes on lymphocytes recovered from BAL of 10 patients with active sarcoidosis. Shaded areas represent the control range.

REFERENCES
1. Crystal RG, Bitterman PB, Rennard SI, Hance AJ, Keogh BA (1984) N Engl J Med 310:235
2. Pinkston P, Bitterman PB, Crystal RG (1983) N Engl J Med 308:793
3. Robinson BWS, McLemore T, Crystal RG (1985) J Clin Invest 75:1488
4. Agostini C, Trentin L, Zambello R, Luca M, Cipriani A, Pizzolo G, Semenzato G (1985) Clin Immunol Immunopathol 37:262
5. Foa R, Casorati G, Giubellino MC, Basso G, Schirò R, Pizzolo G, Lauria F, Lefranc MP, Rabbitts TH, Migone N (1987) J Exp Med 165:879
6. Rogozinski L, Bass A, Glickman E, Talle MA, Goldstein G, Wang J, Chess L, Thomas Y (1984) J Immunol 132:735
7. Karol RA, Eng J, Dennison DK, Faris E, Marcus DM (1984) J Clin Immunol 4:71
8. Sattentau QJ, Dalgleish AG, Weiss RA, Beverley PCL (1986) Science 234:1120

© 1988 Elsevier Science Publishers B.V. (Biomedical Division)
Sarcoidosis and other granulomatous disorders
C. Grassi, G. Rizzato, E. Pozzi, editors

SUPPRESSION OF LOCAL IMMUNOGLOBULIN PRODUCTION IN ACTIVE PULMONARY SARCOIDOSIS
BY ORAL PREDNISONE THERAPY.

MARIO SPATAFORA, ANGELA MIRABELLA, ANNA BONANNO, LOREDANA RICCOBONO,
ANNA MERENDINO, VINCENZO BELLIA, GIOVANNI BONSIGNORE

Consiglio Nazionale delle Ricerche, Istituto di Fisiopatologia Respiratoria,
Via Trabucco 180, I-90146 Palermo (Italy)

INTRODUCTION

In active pulmonary sarcoidosis (PS) most of lung T cells, as recovered by
bronchoalveolar lavage (BAL) are of the helper-inducer subset, so that the local
ratio to suppressor-cytotoxic cells is markedly increased (1). The latter imbalance may be responsible, at least in part, for activation of B cells to produce
immunoglobulins (Ig's); in this context increased proportions of Ig-secreting
cells (2) and elevated IgG and IgA levels have been detected in BAL fluid of
patients with active PS (3).

Corticosteroids represent the most widely used therapy for PS; although some
debate remains about their effects upon the ultimate prognosis, recent investigations have shown that steroids are able to reduce the activity of the alveolitis by lowering T cells percentage in BAL and ^{67}Gallium (^{67}Ga) lung uptake (4).
The present study was carried out to evaluate the effects of prednisone therapy
upon Ig levels in the epithelial lining fluid of patients with active disease.

PATIENTS AND METHODS

Twelve patients (5 M, 7 F; aged 38.5 $\pm$ 4.3 years (mean $\pm$ SEM)) with biopsy proven active PS (BAL T lymphocytes 30%; positive ^{67}Ga lung scan) were studied.
Patients evaluation was performed before and after 6 months of oral prednisone
therapy (0.75 mg/kg body weight for 6 weeks; then dosage tapered 2.5 mg each week
to a daily dose of 0.25 mg/kg) by measuring: 1) percentage of T lymphocytes in
BAL; 2) ^{67}Ga lung scan indexes; 3) IgG, IgA and IgM concentrations in BAL fluid.
See reference 3 for details.

RESULTS

Prednisone therapy significantly lowered percentages of T lymphocytes in BAL (baseline 42.3 $\pm$ 3.1; after therapy 20.9 $\pm$ 2.7; p 0.01) and ^{67}Ga lung scan indexes (baseline 147 $\pm$ 13.8; after therapy 89 $\pm$ 12.3; p 0.01). Biochemical analysis of BAL showed a significant therapy-induced decrease of IgG and IgA local production, as assessed by comparisons of IgG/albumin and IgA/albumin ratios, albumin being considered as a marker of alveolar capillary membrane permeability (IgG/Alb: baseline 1.32 $\pm$ 0.18; after therapy 0.42 $\pm$ 0.15; p 0.001) (IgA/Alb: baseline 0.51 $\pm$ 0.06; after therapy 0.17 $\pm$ 0.04; p 0.001). In contrast, comparisons of IgM/albumin ratios did not show any change over the study period (IgM/alb: baseline 0.06 $\pm$ 0.02; after therapy 0.07 $\pm$ 0.03; p 0.2).

DISCUSSION

The present study demonstrates that oral prednisone therapy is effective in reducing IgG and IgA levels in the epithelial lining fluid of patients with active PS. Moreover, in agreement with previous reports (4), it provides evidence that steroids can reduce the number and state of activation of inflammatory cells in the lower respiratory tract, as demonstrated by BAL and ^{67}Ga lung scan data.

The role played by local Ig synthesis in the pathogenesis of PS is still unclear. Although Ig's and immune complexes have been shown to be present in sarcoid granulomata within the lungs (5), lack of complement components (6) suggests that B cells activation is not a "key-mechanism" and merely reflects elevation of cell-mediated immune processes. Therefore, the effects of steroid-induced reduction of local Ig levels upon the course of the disease, as demonstrated in the present study, need to be further studied.

REFERENCES

1. Hunninghake GW, Crystal RG (1981) N Engl J Med 305:429-434

2. Rankin JA, Naegel GP, Schrader CE et Al (1983) Am Rev Respir Dis 127:442-448

3. Spatafora M, Mirabella A, Rossi GA et Al (1985) Respiration 48:127-135

4. Rossi GA, Bernabò di Negro G, Balzano et Al (1985) Lung 163:83-93

5. Ghose T, Landrigan P, Asif A (1974) Chest 66:264-268

6. Semenzato G, Pezzutto A, Pizzolo G et Al (1984) Clin Immunol Immunopathol 30:29-40

OUTLOOK

TAKATERU IZUMI
Chest Disease Research Institute, Kyoto University, Sakyo-ku, Kyoto 606 (JAPAN)

The outlook on the session, "Sarcoid granuloma formation-immunology" will be described from the following 3 aspects. The first aspect is the history and goal of the immunological studies of sarcoidosis. The second is additional information on the pathogenesis of sarcoidosis obtained through this session. The third is the necessity of international immunological study of this disease.

1. History and goal of immunological studies of sarcoidosis

A small-scale international symposium was held in Nara 8 years ago in 1979. The introduction for the Session of Immunology is shown in the following.

The history of immunologic studies on sarcoidosis began in 1913, when Jadassohn reported that many sarcoidosis patients were tuberculin-negative. Numerous studies have been carried out since then, and the history of this research can be divided into three periods.

The first period begins with Jadassohn's description of tuberculin negative conversion and Salvesen's report on increased serum gamma globulin (1935) and ends in 1970. There were many reports of abnormal immunologic responses in sarcoidosis patients, but there was no exact analytical study of the mechanism. Important work from this period include a review by Chase (1965) and a monograph by Chrétien (1970).

The second period covers the first half of the 1970s, when interest was focused on the activites of T- and B-cells as a central theme of clinical immunology. It was found that, in sarcoidosis, T-cells increased and B-cells decreased in the peripheral blood, but the cause of this phenomenon remained unknown.

In the third period, the latter half of the 1970s, progress in the field of basic immunology brought a diversity in the research methods of clinical immunology. There have been new findings from T-cell population studies and an increased understanding of the function of monocyte-macrophages. One of the most interesting research subjects in sarcoidosis is the relationship among three types of monocyte-macrophages: 1) the type with an accessory cell function, 2) the type with a suppressor function, and 3) the type which receives a stimulus and progresses to epethelioid cells and then to sarcoid granulomas.

Problems of immunoregulatory substances in the serum have also received considerable attention in the last few years.

Another recent development in the field of immunologic research on sarcoidosis of particular interest is the finding that, in addition to peripheral blood

194

cells, bronchoalveolar lavage cells can now easily be used as a productive material.

We anticipate that much of the current data in from the latter half of the 1970s will be presented at this symposium. One of the most important questions that still remain in the immunology of sarcoidosis is why the tuberculin test exhibits a negative reaction and why the serum gamma globulin is elevated. I would like to suggest that the solution of these problems will bring us closer to an understanding of the process by which sarcoidosis occurs, which is the objective of immunologic research on sarcoidosis.

(Izumi,T)

The introduction summarized the history of immunological studies on sarcoidosis since the report on conversion from positive to negative of tuberculin reaction observed in patients with sarcoidosis by Jadassohn in 1913 and referred to the generalization of the technique of bronchoalveolar lavage (BAL) since the report by Reynolds and Newball in 1974. Since this symposium in Nara, we have obtained much information on the pathogenesis of sarcoid granuloma formation by applying the BAL technique. A brilliant investigation by Crystal and colleagues (NIH) deserves special attention, and the important portion of this study was reported at the 9th International Conference on Sarcoidosis and Other Granulomatous Disorders in Paris in 1981.

There are three goals for the immunological studies of sarcoidosis. The first goal is clarification of the mechanisms of sarcoid granuloma formation, in other words an explanation of the pathogenesis of sarcoid granuloma as a result of immune responses. The second is an elucidation of the mechanism by which immunological symptoms such as conversion to negative tuberculin reaction and hypergammaglobulinemia develop in sarcoidosis patients. The third is clarification of the association between the sarcoid granuloma formation and development of these immulogical symptoms, i.e., complete understanding of the immunological phenomena in sarcoidosis patients.

2. Pathogenesis of sarcoidosis - What we learned from the presentations in this session -

This session lasted for more than 7 hours. It included a total of 34 presentations consisting of 19 oral presentations, 55 poster presentations, and 10 poster displays and discussions. It is impossible for me to review and introduce all of them. Therefore, I would like to select some interesting topics.

My understanding of the pathogenesis of sarcoid granuloma formation is shown in Fig. 1.

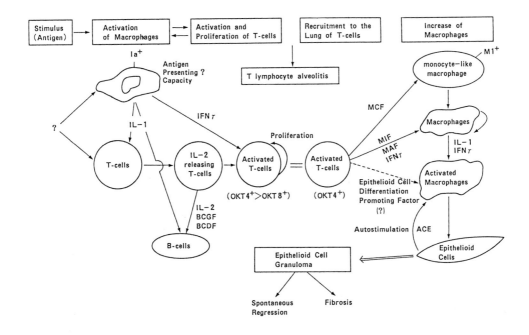

Fig. 1 Pathogenesis of sarcoid granuloma formation

Sarcoidosis is induced by an unknown causative agent. Most of the
granulomas regres spontaneously, but some progress to fibrosis.

Identification of the causative agent of sarcoidosis is the most important
problem. The report by Holter et al. (Greenville) was of great interest. They
reported that non-viable BAL cell preparation has the ability to form granuloma
that is similar to the ability of the Kveim antigen. Further studies are
needed, and the evaluation of the effective substance in the cell preparation
may produce excellent results. Graham et al. (Houston) also presented an
interesting report. Mycobacteria has been long suspected as the cause of
sarcoidosis. They isolated spheroplast of acid-fast bacteria from sarcoid
tissues but not from controls. Further examinations are awaited.

Evaluation of monocytes and macrophages using monoclonal antibodies were
performed by Neuchrist et al. (Münster), Ainslie et al. (London), Agostini et
al. (Padua), and Barth et al. (Kiel). The problem in these studies is whether
the macrophages are antigen-presenting cells, suppressor cells, or cells in the
process of differentiation to epithelioid cells. At present, a definite marker
for epithelioid cells remains to be identified.

O'Connor et al. (Dublin) showed increases of IL-1 in the BAL fluids (BALF) of sarcoidosis patients. They measured IL-1 by the RIA method. This method has an advantage over the conventional bioassay in that it excludes the effects of biological inhibition. Increases in IL-1 were observed only in 29% of patients even in the active stage and, therefore, the data can be also interpreted to show a range of sarcoidosis activity.

The mechanism by which T lymphocytes especially OKT4$^+$ cells selectively increase in the lung of sarcoidosis patients includes local proliferation and recruitment from the blood. Ikeda et al. (Kumamoto) showed the presence of a lymphocyte chemotactic factor in BALF. Saltini et al. (Bethesda) reported that the unbalanced activation of the helper T-cell population in the sarcoid lung is not due to a generalized suppressor of T-cell defect.

A number of regulatory mechanisms are involved in the formation, development, regression, and fibrosis of sarcoid granuloma. Fireman et al. (Tel Aviv) demonstrated no association between the suppressive activity of macrophages and PGE$_2$ production. Jones et al. (Cardiff) reported an inhibitor of lymphocyte transformation reaction in the BALF of patients with high intensity alveolitis.

The general prognosis of sarcoidosis is good. However, some cases result in poor outcomes. Of 275 patients we have observed for 5 years or more in Kyoto, more than 75% showed complete regression of the disease. The cause of persistent lesions in a part of sarcoidosis patients is an unsolved puzzle. Nagai et al. (Kyoto) showed enhancement of accessory function of alveolar macrophages by angiotensin II in patients with prolonged course. The finding suggests the possibility of the presence of autostimulatory mechanisms by ACE produced by activated macrophages or epithelioid cells in the development of T lymphocyte alveolitis in sarcoidosis patients.

3. Necessity for international studies on immunology of sarcoidosis

The clinical picture of sarcoidosis varies greatly among patients and populations. A number of excellent reports have been made by Crystal and colleagues. We have carried out supplemental studies. The results showed both similar and different BALF cell findings in sarcoidosis patients between Bethesda and Kyoto. The increases in the BALF cell number, lymphocytes, and OKT4$^+$/OKT8$^+$ ratio were similar between Bethesda and Kyoto. Sontaneous release of IL-1, γ-IFN, and IL-2 was not observed in the patients in Kyoto. However, production of cytokines following stimulation of cells with mitogens such as PHA and LPS was observed also in Kyoto. The explanation for these differences in BALF cell findings remains unknown. Of course, technical problems should always be considered, in addition to the differences due to disease activity and stage. Most of our patients in Kyoto had only BHL, but no symptoms, and the disease was detected in a health survey. Although, the pathology of sarcoidosis should be the same, population differences should be taken into consideration. The differences in BALF cell findings might affect the clinical features and outcomes.

I hope that population differences in immunological findings will be discussed in the XII World Congress on Sarcoidosis and Other Granulomatous Disorders in Kyoto (1991).

PANEL DISCUSSION:
THE CELLULAR ORIGIN OF SACE AND THE VARIOUS
FACTORS IN REGULATING ITS PRODUCTION

THE CELLULAR ORIGIN OF ANGIOTENSIN CONVERTING ENZYME (ACE) AND THE VARIOUS
FACTORS REGULATING ITS PRODUCTION (INTRODUCTION TO A PANEL DISCUSSION)

RICHARD A. DeREMEE, M.D.
Professor of Medicine, Mayo Medical School, Consultant in Thoracic Diseases
and Internal Medicine, Mayo Clinic, Rochester, Minnesota 55905, USA

It was paper number 48[1] given the afternoon of Wednesday, October 8, 1975.
The event was the VII International Conference on Sarcoidosis chaired by the
late Louis Siltzbach. The place was the Barbizon Plaza Hotel, New York City.
Many of us in this room, myself included, listened with fascination as the
speaker concluded, "A measure of serum angiotensin converting enzyme is an
effective way for confirming a diagnosis of active sarcoidosis and for judging
the disease's activity or control by steroid therapy." Of course, that
speaker was Dr. Jack Lieberman, whose observation opened a vast arena of
research. To sarcoidologists, Jack can truly be considered the "Father of
SACE." Immediately after Jack's paper, Emanuel Silverstein[2] presented data
suggesting cells in sarcoid lymph nodes were producing ACE. Since these
papers, the literature on ACE, particularly as it pertains to sarcoidosis, has
exploded with many new names coming to prominence in the field.

Today I am pleased to chair this panel officially entitled "The Cellular
Origin of Angiotensin Converting Enzyme and the Various Factors Regulating its
Production." It is good to have Father Lieberman back to present his
interesting data on ACE inhibitors. Dr. Carola Grönhagen-Riska will, among
other things, discuss her work with malignant monocytes. My colleague and
coworker, Dr. Michael Rohrbach, will present results of his work on ACE
induction. Finally, Dr. Philippe Delaval will bring us all back to less
rarified atmosphere to the realm of clinical practice presenting his extensive
data from bronchoalveolar lavage and gallium scanning, correlating these
results with serum angiotensin converting enzyme (SACE). We hope he will
resolve the question of which test for "activity" is the one we should be
using in evaluating our patients with sarcoidosis.

It is not my intention in the course of this brief introduction to preempt
any of the speakers, but I would like to make two predictions and ask a
question which may or may not be approached by our panelists. The first
prediction is that ACE will ultimately be found to play an important role in
immune regulation. Secondly, ACE inducing factor (AIF) will be similar or the
same as the putative cytokine that stimulates monocytes to convert vitamin D
substrates into 1,25-dihydroxy vitamin D. My question is can we develop a

test to detect the specific form of ACE produced by monocytes and thereby more easily identify the patient with sarcoidosis?

REFERENCES

1. Lieberman J (1976) Ann NY Acad Sci 278:488-497
2. Silverstein E, Friedland J, Lyons HA (1976) Ann NY Acad Sci 278:498-513

ACE IN PHYSIOLOGIC AND PATHOLOGIC CONDITIONS

C Grönhagen-Riska, V Koivisto, H Riska, E von Willebrand & F Fyhrquist

Minerva Institute for Medical Research, P.O.Box 819, 00101 Helsinki, Finland, IIIrd and IVth Dept. of Medicine, Transplantation Laboratory, University of Helsinki, and Mjölbolsta Hospital

INTRODUCTION

Angiotensin I-converting enzyme (ACE), also called kininase II (EC 3.4.15.1) is a membrane-bound and freely circulating glycoprotein and enzyme. Its molecular weight is about 160,000 dalton and about 25% of the molecule consists of sugar moieties (1). It is mainly situated in vascular endothelial cells in the lungs, but also in the kidneys, testes, placenta and umbilical cord and in epithelial cells of intestines or proximal tubules and in neuroepithelial cells of the brain (2-4). Freely circulating ACE is probably shed from membranes, the mechanism behind the shedding is unknown. The most important physiologic functions of ACE is to activate angiotensin I into angiotensin II (AII), which is the active component of the renin-angiotensin system, and to inactivate bradykinin, a very strong vasodilator and inflammatory mediator. Bradykinin is also inactivated by another enzyme and bradykinin accumulation has not been shown in association with ACE inhibitor treatment of hypertension.

Cells of the monocytic cell line may also produce ACE and increased amounts have been observed in peripheral monocytes of patients with sarcoidosis (5), but mainly in granulomatous epithelioid cells of that disease, in which serum ACE (SACE) activity is increased, too, due to shedding of ACE from macrophages (6,7). Other granulomatous diseases in which increased SACE activity has been reported are, e.g., leprosy, atypical mycobacterial infections, and a limited number of mainly miliary cases of tuberculosis. Other macrophage-involving diseases that may appear with high SACE are, e.g., asbestosis and silicosis (for detailed references, see 8).   An immunologic mechanisms for ACE production in macrophages, mainly the existence of a lymphokine, which induces ACE synthesis has been indicated (9). On the other hand, non-organic induction of ACE in macrophages, e.g., by silicate or asbestosis particles, or by ACE inhibitors (see below) does not corroborate this notion.

The present review will briefly deal with ACE synthesis by monocytic cells involved in granulomatous or other inflammatory reactions. The second part of the paper deals with regulation of ACE in cells and serum, and how this is affected by endogenous or exogenous factors, such as age, thyroid hormones, glucocorticosteroids and ACE inhibitors. Original papers will be referred to, original data will be presented in detail.

ACE IN MONOCYTIC CELLS

General comments

The mechanisms behind increased ACE production by cells of monocytic origin have not been clearly elucidated, but a certain degree of maturity of the cells seems to be required; ACE values are high in histiocytic medullary reticulosis, but normal in monocytic leucaemia, the malignant monocytic cell line U-937 expresses ACE only after induction and development into a more macrophage-like cell (10,11). Many immunologically or infectiously induced granulomatous conditions vary with respect to ACE production by epithelioid cells and macrophages, the most notable example   being TB,   in   which   disease SACE is   nearly always normal. These discrepancies may, of course, be due to quantitative differences considering, e.g., the systemic nature of sarcoidosis and the usually local foci of TB and other granulomatous disorders.

ACE in some granulomatous disorders.

We have looked for the presence of ACE in different types of granulomas. An anti-ACE antiserum developed in rabbits after immunization with purified human lung ACE (11, 12) was used. Granulomatous tissue was snap frozen in liquid nitrogen and stored in -80°. Cryostat sections, 5 um, were fixed in acetone, -20°, for 15 min., and then brought into room temperature before labelling with the anti-ACE antiserum (1:50 dilution) and consequent staining with an indirect immunoperoxidase technique (13).

Epithelioid cells and macrophages in sarcoid granulomas obtained from conjunctiva stained strongly positively, whereas corresponding cells of chalazion granulomas were ACE negative (14). Liver samples were obtained from a patient who had died of miliary TB. None of the cells of the tuberculous granulomas stained positively for ACE.

Pleural ACE in rheumatoid arthritis.

We also measured pleural fluid ACE (PACE) in patients with pleurisy of various aetiology, among others in19 patients with tuberculous pleurisy. Other diseases studied were cancer, 16, pneumonia,12,   rheumatoid arthritis (RA),9,   and systemic lupus erythematosus (SLE), 5. Nine patients with hydrothorax from uncompensated congestive heart failure were "controls". PACE values were complemented with simultaneously measured SACE. Only the RA patients had a significantly increased mean PACE value compared with controls, p < .01., values varied from 20-100 U/ml, but did not overlap with either those of controls or of SLE patients. Overlapping between the other groups was seen. Similar results were obtained when PACE/SACE ratios of the patient groups were calculated. RA patients had a significantly higher mean ratio and there was hardly any overlapping with SLE patients, or with controls. None of the patients had increased SACE activity (Riska et al., submitted for publication).

A rheumatic pleural nodule was obtained by thoracoscopy from the patient with the highest PACE value of our series. Tissue was handled and immunoperoxidase stained with anti-ACE antiserum as described above. Normal rabbit IgG was used as control. Rheumatic nodules mainly consist of histiocytic cells and an outer layer of lymphocytes and granulation tissue (15,16). Nodular histiocytes stained positively for ACE, whereas control stains were negative.

In conclusion, a new group of patients with increased local production of ACE was found and the source was identified as rheumatic nodular cells of monocytic origin. The finding may be used as a means of differentiating between patients with pleurisy caused by RA or SLE. The possible pathogenetic importance of ACE production in rheumatic nodules remains open.

ACE during renal transplant rejection

We have also observed the versatility of ACE production within another context, i.e., ACE-positive macrophages obtained by fine-needle aspiration biopsy (FNAB) from a renal transplant during rejection episodes (17). Rejection is an exponent of cell-bound immune reaction, blast cells and "activated" lymphocytes in FNAB indicate acute rejection, the presence of monocytes and/or macrophages in the aspirate indicates serious, destructive inflammation (17). Most of our renal transplant patients have received Cyclosporine A in combination with methylprednisolone for immunosuppression and there have been only slight fluctuations within normal limits (< 40 U/ml) of the patients' SACE. However, in some patients who received Cyclosporine monotherapy SACE increments were observed in association with rejection diagnosed by clinical means and by FNAB (see example in Fig. 1). As methylprednisolone was initiated SACE decreased, while the FNAB cytological score indicated reversal of rejection. Immunoperoxidase staining of cytocentrifuged FNAB samples with our anti-ACE antiserum indicated ACE positive macrophages in the kidney during rejection. Increased SACE may have reflected shedding by these, but possibly also by circulating monocytes, which were mobilized to the transplant. Usually SACE cannot be used as a means for detection of rejection as most patients

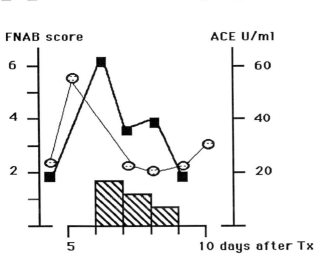

Figure 1. FNAB cytological score (17) before, during and after rejection of cadaver kidney transplant, and corresponding SACE values. Methylprednisolone (initially 180 mg) was given for 3 days starting on day 6 (indicated by striped columns). Upper normal limit for FNAB score is 2, and for SACE 40 U/ml. Tx = transplantation.

receive daily methylprednisolone, which inhibits SACE fluctuations.

Thus, ACE synthesis by monocytic cells may vary both in granulomatous and in other mechanical or inflammatory reactions involving macrophages. Obviously these cells must reach a certain degree of maturity before ACE may be expressed, on the other hand the triggering mechanism may be of both a specific, immunologic, or of an unspecific nature.

Some results have proposed immunologic functions of ACE itself. These hypothetical properties of ACE have not been identified. They may be associated with the oligosaccharide moiety of the molecule, which would suggest specific receptors of other leucocytes, on the other hand, they may be associated with the enzymatic action of ACE.

REGULATION OF ACE SYNTHESIS

Age.

High SACE has been reported in children under 16 years of age (18,19). Values above upper normal limit of adults appear in about 22% of these, and mean value is about 30% higher. There are no detectable age dependent variations of SACE in adults (19).

Thyroid function.

High and low SACE in association with hyper- and hypothyroidism, respectively have been reported (20,21). We found a significantly increased mean value in hyperthyroid patients with Graves' disease, about 50% of them had values above the normal upper level. The same, but to a lesser degree was observed in treated thyroid cancer patients substituted with high thyroxine doses and kept on a high euthyroid level (22). Patients on regular thyroxine substitution who were "normal euthyroids" had slightly lower ACE levels than healthy controls. Hypothyroid patients had a significantly decreased mean. Particularly in hyper- and hypothyroid patients there were strong positive correlations between SACE values and serum thyroxine (T4) (r=0.86), or serum triiodothyronine (T3) (r=0.93).

Monodeiodination of T4 to T3 is thought fundamental for thyroid hormone activity, but this conversion varies in different tissues, and serum concentrations of thyroid hormones, particularly during T4 treatment, may not adequately reflect peripheral hormonal effects . SACE values were often on a subnormal level in clinically adequately substituted hypothyroid patients who had normal T3 values. However, high T4 suppression to cancer patients, during which T3 was close to levels measured during ordinary substitution therapy, brought SACE to normal, or even elevated levels. Thus, SACE may prove a more specific probe than hormone measurements for monitoring peripheral response both to endogenous and to exogenously administered thyroid hormone.

Increased SACE in conjunction with high lysozyme (LZM) concentration usually indicates predominant macrophage or epithelioid cell origin of these enzymes. No such correlation was observed in this study, which indicates that ACE was either produced in excess by endothelial cells or metabolized more slowly than usually. Hypothetical induction of ACE synthesis may be associated with the biological action of thyroid hormone, which may induce synthesis of many enzymes, e.g., carboxypeptidase A and B and NAPDH-dehydrogenase (23). Silverstein and coworkers (24) did not observe any effect on ACE synthesis of alveolar mouse macrophages or peripheral human monocytes subjected to T3 in culture. However, these negative observations do not exclude a possible effect of thyroid hormone on endothelial cells, or even monocytes *in vivo*.

Glucocorticosteroids.

Decreased SACE after steroid treatment in sarcoidosis is a well known phenomenon. However, in the early days of clinical ACE investigations the same was observed in healthy volunteers and in patients with originally normal SACE levels and diseases other than sarcoidosis, who were treated with steroids (25,26). This finding was recently challenged by results which showed no immediate effect of steroids on SACE activity in healthy volunteers (27). However, the studies were not quite comparable, since the earlier investigations evaluated the effect of prolonged steroid administration.

Dexamethasone has been shown to cause increased ACE synthesis in human monocytes in culture (28). The increase became apparent after 3-5 days in culture, and was inhibited by cycloheximide. Other experimental results have indicated the same. When rats were given dexamethasone, 40 ug/day, ACE contents of pulmonary cell membrane fractions increased by about 75%, while serum levels remained unchanged (29). Dexamethasone, 10 nmol/l induced ACE production in cultured human endothelial cells, too, immunofluorescence stains with our anti-ACE antiserum indicated both increased intracellular and membrane-bound amounts (29).

Taken all together, results of steroid effects on cellular, tissue and serum ACE are compatible with increased cellular synthesis of, stabilization of membrane-bound, and consequently decreased or unchanged amounts of serum ACE.

Glycemic control.

Increased SACE in about 20% of patients with diabetes mellitus has been reported (30). A correlation between diabetic angiopathy and endothelial damage and increased SACE was suggested. We offer another explanation on the basis of results obtained from ten insulin dependent diabetics (mean age 27 years, all men) studied during continuous subcutaneous insulin infusion (CSII). One of the patients had intermittent albuminuria, none of the others had any evidence of diabetic neuro-, nephro- or retinopathy. Patients remained hospitalized during the whole experiment and blood samples were obtained on the third day of conventional insulin treatment, which preceded the CSII, and on day 7 and 14 of the insulin infusion. Some of the data are presented in table 1. During pump therapy mean diurnal glucose levels were reduced to close to normal, and HbA1 declined by 14%. ACE was initially normal, but decreased in all CSII patients, being 20% below normal mean after 14 days. The fall in ACE was closely related to the decline in HbA1 ($r = 0.91$, $p < .001$).

208

Table 1. Mean values (± SEM) of diurnal blood glucose (BG), plasma free insulin (IRI) and of HbA1 and SACE in diabetic patients before and during continuous subcutaneous insulin infusion. Controls were 8 healthy age and weight matched subjects (58 persons for SACE).

	DIABETICS			CONTROLS
	conventional	pump 7 days	pump 14 days	
BG (mmol/l)	9.4 ± 0.7	6.4 ± 0.7*	5.6 ± 0.5**§	4.1 ± 0.1
HbA1 (%)	11.6 ±0.6	11.0 ±0.5	10.2 ±0.4*§§	8.3 ± 0.1
plasma free IRI (uU/ml)	35.2 ± 4.4	25.2 ±1.5*	19.8 ± 1.4*§§	11.5 ± 0.6
SACE (U/ml)	30.6 ±2.8	26.7 ± 2.0***	23.5 ± 1.7***§§	28.1 ± 0.8

*, ** &*** = $p < .05$, $< .005$ & $< .001$ compared with conventional therapy
§ & §§ = $p < .05$ & $< .001$ compared with controls

In another study, we followed a 46 year old woman with previous type II diabetes and extreme obesity. In 1980 she presented with hypoglycemia and inappropriately high insulin levels and with marked Acanthosis nigricans of her neck and axillae. Pancreatic angiography revealed a tumour, which was extirpated and benign insulinoma was confirmed. Fig. 2. depicts SACE, HbA1, and glucose values before and after extirpation of the tumour, and the results indicate close relation between these variables.

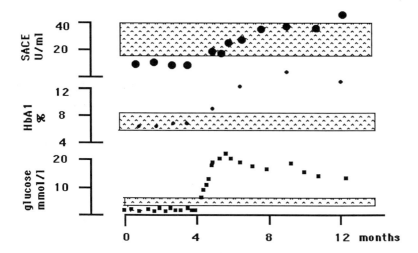

Figure 2. Changes in blood levels of ACE, HbA1 and glucose before and after (at 4 months) removal of insulinoma. Shaded areas indicate normal variation of controls.

Simultaneous and quantitatively similar SACE and HbA1 changes as glucose levels fluctuate suggest similar mechanism(s) affecting their concentrations. A high glucose environment in diabetes causes nonenzymatic glycosylation of and increased erythrocyte concentrations of HbA1.

We suggest that nonenzymatic glycosylation (31) of ACE decreases metabolic clearance of this glycoprotein as a consequence of diabetic hyperglycaemia. The hepatic asialoglycoprotein receptor responsible for removal of many circulating glycoproteins cannot discriminate between D-galactosyl and D-glucosyl-terminated glycoproteins (32). Thus, increased concentrations of glycosylated proteins after/during hyperglycaemia may overload these receptors, and, e.g., cause decreased removal of ACE. Reduction of glucose during insulin infusion or low levels in an insulinoma patient would have the opposite effect.

Effect of ACE inhibitors on ACE synthesis.

We were the first to report increased ACE in serum and lungs of rats treated with the ACE inhibitors captopril and enalapril (33,34). The same has been observed for SACE in humans treated for hypertension (35) or congestive heart failure (36) with ACE inhibitors. SACE increments may be covered by the presence of the inhibitor in analyzed samples. Captopril may be removed by, e.g., chloramine T treatment, which probably oxidates the functionally important SH-group of captopril, or by prolonged storage, the enalapril effect can be eliminated by dialysis (37).

Experiments with cultured human endothelial cells from umbilical cord showed that addition of an ACE inhibitor, captopril 0.2- 1.0 ug/ml, to the culture medium caused a dose dependent increase of ACE synthesis, which was inhibited by cycloheximide. ACE was identified and quantitated both with our anti-ACE antiserum which was stained with fluorescein-coupled anti-human IgG goat antiserum (38), and with a labelled specific ACE inhibitor, Substance 351A* (Merck Sharp & Dohme) (39) and results indicated more than 50% more ACE in endothelial cells exposed to captopril than in controls (29).

351A* was also used to quantitate the effect on ACE synthesis in human macrophages by ACE inhibitors, alone, and with *E. coli* lipopolysaccharide (LPS) which activates macrophages. Treatment with captopril resulted in a significant (close to 50%) increase of ACE contents. LPS treatment did not induce ACE synthesis, but combined treatment with LPS and captopril, and also with LPS and enalapril caused marked ACE increases, about two- and fourfold, respectively, compared with controls (29).

Thus, ACE inhibitors cause increased ACE synthesis in endothelial cells and macrophages and in macrophages LPS has an additive effect, although ineffective alone. Increased cellular synthesis is associated with increased SACE activity, which is easily detectable when the ACE inhibitor has been eliminated from samples to be analyzed. Induction of ACE by its inhibitors has not been shown to delete the antihypertensive effect of these drugs even during long-term treatment. The effect of ACE inhibitors, when experimentally administered to study the possible immunologic functions of ACE (40-42) should be evaluated against this knowledge.

210

Concluding remarks.

ACE is produced both by endothelial and some epithelial cells, and during certain conditions by cells of the monocytic cell line, which have reached a certain stage of maturity. Mechanism(s) which initiate ACE production in macrophages are unknown, in some granulomatous conditions, such as sarcoidosis, they might be dependent on activated T-helper cells. In rheumatic nodule histiocytes and in macrophages contributing to kidney transplant rejection the mechanism might be similar, although this has not been unequivocally shown to be so.

ACE synthesis in "non-immunological" conditions is regulated by such variables as age, thyroid hormones, glucocorticosteroids, glycemic control and the use of ACE inhibitors. Children have higher mean SACE activity than adults, endo- or exogenously induced thyroid hormone changes cause corresponding SACE fluctuations, and glucocorticosteroids appear to induce ACE production in cells, but to decrease shedding of ACE from membranes, which results in slightly decreased SACE levels. Hyperglycemia induces SACE increments and vice versa, probably due to non-enzymatic glycosylation and changes in metabolic clearance by hepatic lectins. ACE inhibitor treatment induces ACE synthesis in cells and SACE increments, which may be initially masked in samples, if the inhibitor has not been removed either by chemical destruction, prolonged storage or dialysis. When evaluating possibly immunologically induced SACE changes all these factors should be borne in mind.

References

1. Hartley, JL, Soffer RL (1978) Biochem Biophys Res Comm 83:1545-1552

2. Depierre D, Bargetzi JP, Roth M (1978) Biochim Biophys Acta 523:469-476

3. Bruneval P, Hinglais N, Alhenc-Gelas, F (1986) Histochemistry 85:73-80

4. Defendini R, Zimmerman EA, Weare JA, et al. (1983) Neuroendocrinology 37:32-40

5. Okabe T, Yamagata K, Fujisawa M, et al. (1985) J Clin Invest 75:911-914

6. Silverstein E, Friedland J, Lyons HA, et al. (1976) Proc Natl Acad Sci USA 73:2137-2141

7. Pertschuk LP, Silverstein E, Friedland J (1981) Am J Clin Pathol 75:350-354

8. Grönhagen-Riska C (1980) Acad. Dissert, Univ of Helsinki, ISBN 951-99272-0-4, 1-98

9. Rohrbach, MS (1984) Biochem Biophys Res Comm 124:843-849

10. Grönhagen-Riska C, Klockars M, Selroos O (1983) N Engl J Med 308-283-284

11. Grönhagen-Riska C, Fyhrquist F, von Willebrand E (1986) Ann NY Acad Sci 465:242-249

12. Grönhagen-Riska C, Fyhrquist F (1980) Scand J Clin Lab Invest 40:711-719

13. Grönhagen-Riska C, Honkanen E, von Willebrand E, et al. (1987) Clin Exp Immunol (in press)

14. Immonen I, Friberg K, Grönhagen-Riska, et al. (1986) Acta Ophthalmol 64:519-521

15. Beumer HM, van Belle CJ (1972) Respiration 29:556-564

16. Schneider PJ, Ehrlich GE (1972) Chest 62:747-749

17. von Willebrand E (1980) Clin Immunol Immunopathol 17:309-322

18. Lieberman J (1975) Am J Med 59:365-372

19. Grönhagen-Riska C (1979) Scand J Respir Dis 60:83-93

20. Yotsumoto H, Imai Y, Kuzuya N, et al. (1982) Ann Intern Med 96:326-328

21. Smallridge RC, Rogers J, Verma PS (1983) JAMA 250:2489-2493

22. Grönhagen-Riska C, Fyhrquist F, Välimäki M, et al. (1985) Acta Med Scand 217:259-264

23. Greengaard O (1970) In: Biochemical Actions of Hormones, Ed. Litwack G, Acad Press NY, pp 53-87

24. Silverstein E, Schussler GC, Friedland J (1983) Am J Med 75:233-236

25. Turton CWG, Grundy E, Firth G, et al. (1979) Thorax 34:57-62

26. Grönhagen-Riska C, Selroos O, Niemistö M (1980) Eur J Respir Dis 61:113-122

27. Thompson PJ, Kemp MW, McAllister AC, et al. (1986) Am Rev Respir Dis 134:1075-1077

28. Friedland J, Setton C, Silverstein E (1978) Biochem Biophys Res Comm 83:843-849

29. Fyhrquist F, Grönhagen-Riska C, Hortling L, et al. (1983) Clin Exp Hypert A5(7&8)1319-1330

30. Lieberman J, Sastre A (1980) Ann Intern Med 93:825-826

31. Bunn HF, Gabbay KH, Gallop PM (1978) Science 200:21-27

32. Stowell CP, Lee YC (1978) J Biol Chem 253:6107-6110

33. Fyhrquist F, Forslund T, Tikkanen I, et al. (1980) Eur J Pharmacol 67:473-475

34. Forslund T, Fyhrquist F, Grönhagen-Riska C, et al. (1980) Eur J Pharmacol 80:121-125

35. Grönhagen-Riska C, Forslund T, Hortling L, et al. (1983) Acta Med Scand S677:110-114

36. Fyhrquist F, Hortling L, Forslund T, et al. (1982) In: ACE inhibition in congestive heart failure; from principle to practise, Ed. Cohn JN, Biomedical Information Corp NY, pp 51-62

37. Fyhrquist F, Grönhagen-Riska C, Hortling L, et al. (1983) J Hypert 1(S1):25-30

38. Fyhrquist F, Hortling L, Grönhagen-Riska C (1982) J Clin Endocrinol 55:783-786

39. Fyhrquist F, Tikkanen I, Grönhagen-Riska C, et al. (1984) Clin Chem 30:696-700

40. Weinstock JV, Boros DL, Gee JB (1981) Gastroenterology 81:48-53

41. Schrier DJ, Ripani LM, Katzenstein Al, et al. (1982) J Clin Invest 67:931-936

42. Martin MFR, McKenna F, Bird HA, et al. (1984) Lancet i:1325-1328

© 1988 Elsevier Science Publishers B.V. (Biomedical Division)
Sarcoidosis and other granulomatous disorders
C. Grassi, G. Rizzato, E. Pozzi, editors

ANGIOTENSIN CONVERTING ENZYME INDUCING FACTOR (AIF): A POTENTIAL MEDIATOR OF
THE INCREASED ANGIOTENSIN CONVERTING ENZYME LEVELS IN SARCOIDOSIS

MICHAEL S. ROHRBACH, ULRICH SPECKS, ZVEZDANA VUK-PAVLOVIC, AND A. KELLY CONRAD

Thoracic Diseases Research Unit, Mayo Clinic/Foundation, Rochester, MN 55905
(USA)

INTRODUCTION

Circulating peripheral blood monocytes are the basic building blocks for the
formation of epithelioid cell granulomas. The monocytes are attracted to the
site of granuloma formation in response to the lymphokine, monocyte chemotactic
factor, secreted by T-lymphocytes at the granuloma site (1). Once at the
inflammatory site, the monocytes mature to macrophages and ultimately into
epithelioid cells. In some granulomatous diseases, such as sarcoidosis, this
maturation of monocytes into epithelioid cells is accompanied by the induction
of angiotensin converting enzyme (ACE)(2).

We have postulated that this induction of ACE is due to the action of a
soluble angiotensin converting enzyme inducing factor (AIF). We report here the
results of our studies on the in vitro generation of AIF in co-cultures of monocytes and T-lymphocytes as well as the detection of AIF present in vivo in the
cell-free bronchoalveolar lavage (BAL) fluid and serum of sarcoidosis patients.

METHODS

Cell Isolation and Culture

Human peripheral blood monocytes and T-lymphocytes were isolated from the
buffy coats of normal healthy adult donors obtained from the Mayo Blood Bank by
a combination of Ficoll-Hypaque gradient centrifugation, sheep red blood cell
rosette formation and Percoll gradient centrifugation as previously described
(3,4). Monocytes were cultured in 16 mm wells in 24 well Co-Star tissue culture
plates at 6×10^5 cells/well. Each well contained 1 mL of a 1:1 mixture of
Media 199 and RPMI 1640 supplemented with 2 mM glutamine, 100 U/mL penicillin
and 100 mcg/mL streptomycin. Cultures were carried out for six days in a fully

humidified atmosphere of 5% CO_2:95% air. Cultures were terminated by centrifugation at 1000 xg, removal of media and lysis by the addition of 0.15 mL of 2%
Triton X-100. ACE activity in the lysates was assayed as previously described
(5).

To study the induction of monocyte ACE by several agents, cultures were
prepared that in addition to the monocytes also contained 4 x 10^6 autologous
T-lymphocytes/well, 10% heat-inactivated BAL fluid that had been concentrated
10-fold by ultrafiltration with a YM5 filter or 10% heat-inactivated serum.

RESULTS AND DISCUSSION

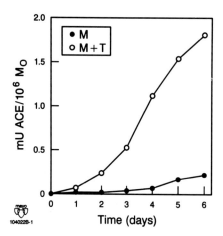

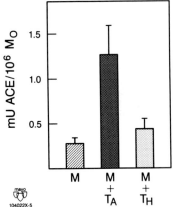

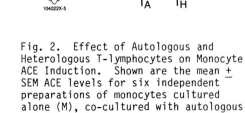

Fig. 1. Time Dependence for
Monocyte ACE Induction. Shown
are the mean ACE levels for
monocytes cultured alone (O, N=4)
and co-cultured with autologous
T-lymphocytes (O, N=4).

Fig. 2. Effect of Autologous and
Heterologous T-lymphocytes on Monocyte
ACE Induction. Shown are the mean +
SEM ACE levels for six independent
preparations of monocytes cultured
alone (M), co-cultured with autologous
T-lymphocytes (M+T_A) and co-cultured
with heterologous T-lymphocytes (M+T_H).

ACE Induction by T-lymphocytes

Freshly isolated human peripheral blood monocytes have little or no detectable
ACE activity. When cultured, however, these cells mature into macrophages over
a period of several days and synthesize ACE at a level normally found in

resident alveolar macrophages, i.e. approximately 0.2 mU ACE/10^6 monocytes.
Inclusion of T-lymphocytes during the culture period increased the level of
monocyte ACE up to 10-fold (Fig. 1). Previous studies have demonstrated that
this T-lymphocyte dependent increase in monocyte ACE was due to a significant
increase in the rate of ACE synthesis by the monocytes and that the newly
synthesized enzyme was incorporated into the monocyte plasma membrane as an
ecto-enzyme (6). The amount of monocyte ACE was nearly linearly dependent upon
the number of T-lymphocytes present in the culture up to a concentration of 4 to
6 million T-lymphocytes/well, a concentration that produced maximal induction of
ACE. Although autologous T-lymphocytes were capable of inducing monocyte ACE,
the presence of heterologous T-lymphocytes during the culture period did not
increase monocyte ACE levels above those observed in monocytes cultured alone
(Fig. 2). This observation indicates that self-recognition is an essential
component in the T-lymphocyte dependent induction of monocyte ACE.

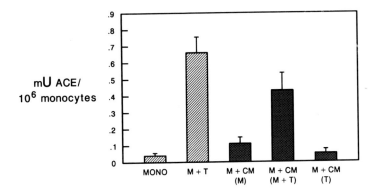

Fig. 3. Cellular Requirements for the Production of AIF. The two bars
on the left hand side represent the control ACE values obtained after six
days of culture for monocytes alone (MONO) and monocytes co-cultured with
autologous T-lymphocytes (M+T). The three bars on the right represent
the ACE induced in the monocytes when cultured with the conditioned media
from monocytes alone (M), monocytes + T-lymphocytes (M+T) or T-lymphocytes
alone (T). Data are the mean ± SEM (N=5) (Reprinted with permission of
the American Review of Respiratory Disease).

216

This T-lymphocyte dependent induction of monocyte ACE was due to the action of a soluble factor (AIF) generated during the co-culture period (4). As shown in Figure 3, the cell-free conditioned media from monocyte and T-lymphocyte co-cultures was able to induce nearly the same level of ACE in freshly isolated monocytes as were autologous T-lymphocytes. In contrast, the conditioned media from either monocytes or T-lymphocytes cultured alone induced little or no ACE. In addition, conditioned media from monocytes and heterologous T-lymphocytes also failed to induce ACE (data not shown). These results indicated that a specific interaction between monocytes and T-lymphocytes was required for the production of AIF.

Since monocyte/macrophages and T-lymphocytes are in intimate contact in the sarcoid granuloma, we sought to determine if AIF was also present in the cell-free BAL fluid and serum of sarcoidosis patients.

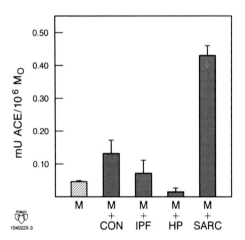

Fig. 4. Effect of BAL Fluid on Monocyte ACE Induction. Shown are the mean ± SEM ACE values for monocytes cultured alone (M; N=3) or co-cultured with cell-free BAL fluid from control subjects (M+CON; N=4), idiopathic pulmonary fibrosis patients (M+IPF; N=4), hypersensitivity pneumonitis patients (M+HP; N=4) or sarcoidosis patients (M+SARC; N=8). ACE levels differed statistically (p<0.05) from monocyte alone ACE values only for co-cultures with sarcoidosis BAL fluid.

ACE Induction by BAL Fluid

Addition of cell-free BAL fluid from patients with active, untreated sarcoidosis to cultured monocytes produced a statistically significant ($p<0.05$) induction of ACE over a six-day culture period (Fig. 4). In contrast, BAL fluid from control subjects or patients with idiopathic pulmonary fibrosis or hyper-sensitivity pneumonitis did not significantly increase ACE levels above those obtained in monocytes cultured alone.

The BAL fluid AIF remains active after heating to 56° for 1 hour and has a molecular weight greater than 5000 daltons as judged by ultrafiltration. Attempts to obtain a more precise molecular weight by gel filtration have resulted in the complete loss of activity. Without a physio-chemical charac-terization of AIF, it is impossible to exclude the possibility that AIF activity is merely a previously undescribed function of one of the many lymphokines and monokines known to be secreted by cells in the sarcoid granuloma. We have, however, eliminated one of the most likely lymphokines from consideration. Gamma-interferon, also known as macrophage activating factor, when added to cultured monocytes produces a dose dependent suppression of ACE activity (data not shown). Thus, gamma-inferferon is not likely to be responsible for AIF activity.

ACE Induction by Serum

The presence of AIF activity in BAL fluid suggested that it may also be present in serum since AIF released at the granuloma site would be expected to diffuse to all adjacent compartments. Examination of the sera of ten patients with active untreated sarcoidosis revealed the presence of AIF activity in 5 out of the 10 sera as judged by the ability of the sera to promote at least a two-fold induction of monocyte ACE (Fig. 5). Under the same conditions several independent samples of serum from normal healthy subjects did not induce ACE (Fig. 6). Like BAL fluid AIF, serum AIF activity was stable to heating at 56° for 1 hour.

218

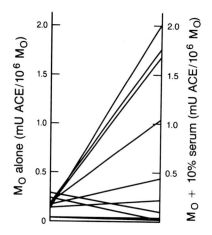

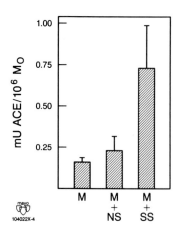

Fig. 5. Effect of Sarcoid Serum on Monocyte ACE Induction. Shown are the ACE levels for monocytes cultured alone for six days or in the presence of 10% heat-inactivated serum from ten individual patients with sarcoidosis.

Fig. 6. Comparison of Monocyte ACE Induction by Normal and Sarcoid Serum. Shown are the mean ± SEM ACE levels for monocytes cultured alone (M; N=10) or in the presence of normal AB+ serum (M+NS; N=10) or sarcoidosis serum (M+SS; N=10).

The detection of AIF activity in both the BAL fluid and serum of patients with active sarcoidosis provides encouraging support for our hypothesis that the induction of ACE in the sarcoid granuloma epithelioid cells is regulated by a soluble factor. Several questions remain to be answered, however, before we can assert with certainty that AIF plays a role in ACE induction in sarcoidosis. First, we need to know if AIF in BAL fluid and serum are physiochemically the same. Second, we need to know how AIF activity correlates with the clinical status of the disease over time. Third, we need to define the specificity of the presence of AIF for sarcoidosis. Studies designed to answer these questions are currently underway in our laboratory.

ACKNOWLEDGEMENTS

This work was supported in part by NIH grant HL-28482 and by funds from the Mayo Foundation.

REFERENCES

1. Hunninghake GW, Gadek JE, Young RC, Kawanami D, Ferrans J, Crystal RG (1980) N Engl J Med 303:594-598

2. Silverstein E, Pertshuk LP, Friedland J (1979) Proc Natl Acad Sci USA 76:6646-6648

3. Tracy PB, Rohrbach MS, Mann KG (1983) J Biol Chem 258:7264-7267

4. Conrad AK and Rohrbach MS (1987) Am Rev Resp Dis 135:396-400

5. Rohrbach MS (1978) Analyt Biochem 84:272-276

6. Rohrbach MS (1984) Biochem Biophys Res Comm 124:843-849

COMPARISON OF AN INTRINSIC SERUM-ACE INHIBITOR TO CAPTOPRIL AND ENALAPRIL IN MAN.

JACK LIEBERMAN, ADRIANA SASTRE, FARIS ZAKRIA
Respiratory Disease and Endocrinology Divisions, Veterans Administration Medical Center, Sepulveda, California, USA, 91343, and
the UCLA School of Medicine.

INTRODUCTION

The serum ACE test for the evaluation and diagnosis of sarcoidosis can be affected by ACE-inhibitor medication used for the
treatment of hypertension and congestive heart failure, and by
an intrinsic spontaneous ACE inhibitor present in approximately
25% of blood specimens submitted for ACE testing (1). The purpose
of this study was to compare the inhibitory characteristics of
the spontaneous vs the medicinal inhibitors, and to determine
simple means for identifying the presence of inhibitor.

MATERIAL AND METHODS

Serum ACE Assay

Serum ACE levels were measured by our modification of the spectrophotometric assay of Cushman and Cheung (2). This method may
be somewhat insensitive in comparison to newer methods developed,
but, as will become apparent from this presentation, is most useful
for detection of the intrinsic ACE inhibitor and the effect of
medicinal inhibitors.

Detection of an Intrinsic ACE Inhibitor

ACE activity was measured with both undiluted and a 1:8 dilution
of serum (diluted with physiological saline). Presence of an ACE
inhibitor was manifest by a rise in ACE activity (corrected for
dilution) of more than 10 units/ml above that of the undiluted
serum. The actual serum dilution occurring in the assay was 1:1.67
with undiluted serum and 1:9.36 for the 1:8 dilution (1).

RESULTS

The Intrinsic ACE Inhibitor

Prevalence. An ACE inhibitor was detected in 71 (25.4%) of 280
sera tested. Of the 280 sera, 154 had normal ACE levels (<30
units/ml) with undiluted sera; of these, 11 (7.04%) developed elevated levels (>35 units/ml) with the 1:8 dilution. Of 44 sera with

"borderline elevated" values (30-35 units/ml), the level became elevated upon dilution in 22 (50%), and of 82 sera with elevated levels, activity rose to even higher values in 38 (47%).

The presence of inhibitor appeared to be most common in sera with elevated ACE levels. The majority of sera with elevated ACE levels were from patients with sarcoidosis, either with or without an ACE inhibitor (77 & 78% respectively). Seventeen of 74 samples with the inhibitor had diagnoses other than sarcoidosis, including some conditions reported previously as being associated with elevated serum ACE, such as diabetes mellitus, cirrhosis of the liver, Lennert's lymphoma and antitrypsin deficiency.

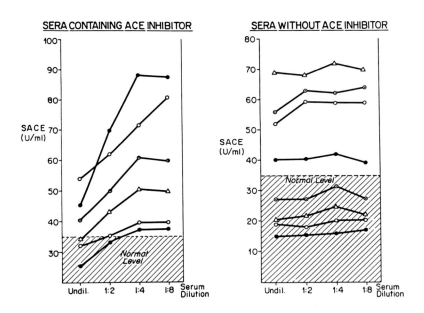

Figure 1. Effect of serum dilution on ACE activity of sera with and without the intrinsic ACE inhibitor

ACE inhibitor vs linearity of the ACE assay. This ACE assay is linear to a maximum of 70 units/ml with undiluted serum. Sera with activity over 70 units show an increase in activity upon dilution, making it difficult to distinguish between an inhibitor effect and alinearity of the assay at this level. This problem was clarified by examining the effect of serum dialysis (against 0.85% saline) on ACE activity and the subsequent effect of dilution.

Effect of dialysis. Five sera showing putative effects of an

ACE inhibitor were dialyzed overnight with one change of dialysis
fluid (1 liter) at 1 hour. Dialysis caused a reduction in the maximum ACE activity attainable through dilution to approximately
that of the undiluted serum, suggesting that inhibition had become
irreversible. After dialysis, any increase in activity with dilution reflects alinearity of the assay rather than the presence of
inhibitor (Figure 2).

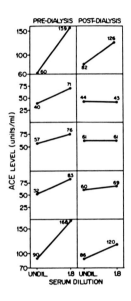

Fig. 2. Effect of serum-dialysis upon serum ACE activity of undiluted and 1:8 diluted sera.

Preliminary 8-fold dilution of serum prior to dialysis, and subsequent re-concentration to the original volume, prevented the
appearance of irreversible inhibition, in that the rise in activity
continued to appear with a 1:8 dilution of the dialyzed serum.
Effect of serum dilution in the ACE assay. Another method for
measuring serum ACE (Fugizoki method (3)) involves a 1:6 dilution
of the serum with substrate (0.1 ml serum + 0.5 ml substrate).
The effect of serum dilution was studied with this assay as compared to the same assay with less dilution of serum (0.3 ml serum
+ 0.3 ml substrate)(1:2 final dilution). With the 1:6 dilution-
assay no increase in activity occurred when a 1:8 dilution of serum
with saline was used, whereas the modified 1:2 dilution-assay prod-

uced 26% enhancement of activity with 1:8 serum pre-dilution. This experiment shows that the intrinsic ACE inhibitor will not be detected if the assay itself involves excessive dilution of the serum. Thus, future studies of the intrinsic ACE inhibitor to learn its significance and biological effect must utilize an assay that does not require more than a two-fold dilution of serum.

Medicinal ACE Inhibitors

The two most commonly used ACE inhibitors in the USA are enalapril and captopril. Both are rapidly absorbed orally, though the duration of ACE inhibition is much longer for enalapril (4). We have detected other differences between the actions of these two ACE inhibitors.

Rates of onset of ACE inhibition. Ten mg enalapril were given orally to 6 hypertensive subjects, and blood samples were obtained at 30 minute intervals for 4 hours. Five subjects showed a maximum decline in serum ACE activity by 1-2 hours, whereas the appearance of ACE-inhibition was much delayed in the 6th subject with maximum effect by 4 hours. Tests of serum ACE activity prior to ingestion of the enalapril revealed that the slow-responding subject's serum contained the intrinsic ACE inhibitor (causing a 14 unit/ml rise of ACE activity with a 1:8 serum dilution). This observation raises the question of whether the presence of intrinsic ACE inhibitor may slow the onset of action of medicinal ACE inhibitor.

Ingestion of 25 mg captopril by one subject caused a more rapid onset of ACE inhibition with maximum effect by 30-60 minutes. This difference between enalapril and captopril may be due to the need for enalapril to be converted by the liver to the active compound enalaprilate, whereas captopril itself is the active ACE inhibitor.

Spontaneous loss of captopril inhibition in stored serum. Blood was drawn from ten subjects 30 minutes after ingestion of 25 mg captopril. ACE activity was assayed 1 hour after serum retrieval; serum was then stored at 4°C, and ACE was re-assayed daily. Approximation of half-life values for the ACE inhibition by captopril revealed that some patients were rapid metabolizers of captopril with half-lives of 1 to 4 days, whereas 3 of the 10 patients were slow metabolizers with half-lives from 10 to 17 days. These observations suggest that the dosage and frequency of captopril administration could vary for different subjects dependent upon their rate of metabolization of captopril inhibition.

Effect of serum dilution on ACE levels in the presence of medicinal inhibitors. Table 1 shows the mean ± S.D. for ACE activity of undiluted and 1:8 dilutions of serum in patients receiving enalapril or captopril, plus controls. ACE levels were generally much lower with enalapril inhibition, and inhibitor reversal by serum dilution was more apparent with captopril than with enalapril. Serum dilution caused a rise of ACE activity into the normal range in 9 of 10 patients receiving captopril. None of the sera from those receiving enalapril showed a rise of ACE activity into the normal range with a 1:8 serum dilution. Control sera with normal ACE levels and no intrinsic inhibitor showed no change of ACE activity with dilution of the sera.

TABLE I

EFFECT OF SERUM DILUTION ON ENALAPRIL AND CAPTOPRIL INHIBITION OF SERUM ACE.

Drug	Serum ACE (Mean ± S.D.)		Change in ACE Level
	Undiluted	1:8 Dilution	
Enalapril	1.67 ± 0.83	6.1 ± 2.76	4.43 units
(n = 7)	(0.8 - 3.3)	(0 - 10.8)	
	P = .02		
Captopril	9.13 ± 2.6	20.2 ± 6.5	11.07 units
(n = 10)	(3.4 - 16.0)	(7.2 - 32.0)	
	P < .001		
Control	21.8 ± 4.7	23.1 ± 5.7	1.3 units
(n = 20)	(12.8 - 33.6)	(14.8 - 34.0)	
	P = N.S.		

Effect of serum dialysis. Sera from 8 patients receiving 25 mg captopril by mouth one hour prior to blood drawing were dialyzed overnight, then tested for ACE activity in comparison to non-dialyzed sera. All dialyzed sera showed a rise of ACE activity up to the baseline level known for each subject, indicating total loss of ACE inhibition by captopril following dialysis. In contrast, ten sera from subjects receiving enalapril showed no significant loss of ACE inhibition following dialysis.

226

CONCLUSIONS

1. An intrinsic ACE-inhibitor is present in approximately 25% of sera submitted for ACE assay.
2. Seventy-seven percent of sera containing the inhibitor are from patients with sarcoidosis.
3. The inhibitory effect can be eliminated by a 1:8 dilution of serum, either prior to assay, or within the assay.
4. Presence of the intrinsic ACE-inhibitor may delay onset of ACE inhibition from enalapril or captopril.
5. The inhibitory effect of enalapril is only minimally reversed by serum dilution, whereas that of captopril is reversed more significantly.
6. The effect of captopril is lost during serum storage at 4°C, although the rate of loss is variable in different individuals (i.e. 1-4 day half-life vs 10-17 day half-life).

SPECULATION

1. An intrinsic ACE inhibitor may play a protective role in man. Does it help regulate blood pressure? Is it protective in patients with sarcoidosis?
2. Presence of the intrinsic inhibitor may delay the effect of ACE-inhibitor medication.
3. Both the intrinsic ACE-inhibitor and ACE-inhibitor medication can interfere with the diagnostic value of the serum ACE assay for sarcoidosis.
4. Future studies to detect the intrinsic ACE-inhibitor must use an ACE assay with a relatively high serum:substrate ratio, since excessive dilution of serum will eliminate the inhibitory effect.

ACKNOWLEDGEMENTS

This research was supported by the Medical Research Service of the Veterans Administration.

REFERENCES
1. Lieberman J, Sastre A (1986) Chest 90:869-875.
2. Lieberman J (1975) Am J Med 59:365-372 (Erratum:60:A23,1976).
3. Kasahara Y, Ashihara Y (1981) Clin Chem 27:1922-1925.
4. Fyhrquist F (1986) Drugs 32 (Suppl. 5):33-39.

SACE RELATED TO OTHER MARKERS, AS CLINICAL PERSPECTIVE.

Ph DELAVAL, B DESRUES, P BOURGUET, C PENCOLE, JP L'HUILLIER
Hopital Pontchaillou, Centre Hospitalier Universitaire. Rennes cedex 35033 France

INTRODUCTION

Since 1975, serum Angiotensin Converting Enzyme (SACE) has been proposed as a biological marker of sarcoidosis, especially of the granulomatous phase. 12 years later, the place of SACE in the management of sarcoidosis is still debated because of conflicting results regarding its significance in term of diagnosis value, marker of activity, predictive value and follow-up tool.

SACE AS A DIAGNOSIS TOOL ?

SACE levels are elevated in many patients with sarcoïdosis. Data from the literature show that high SACE values are observed in 50 to 75 % of the patients with sarcoïdosis, especially in the clinically active forms (1-2-3-4). It is accepted that SACE is not specific for sarcoidosis and may be elevated in other diseases , particularly other granulomatous diseases, such as pneumoconiosis, primary biliary cirrhosis, hypersensitivity Pneumonitis, Histoplasmosis (5-6-7-8-9). Despite the lack of specificity of SACE measurement, high values does aid to diagnosis together with clinical, radiological, and histological data. On the reverse, for Klech (10),normal SACE levels together with negative [67]GA scan have a high predictive value for exclusion of active sarcoidosis. But, we must keep in mind that SACE level reflects only the activity of the producing cells and not necessarily the activity of the disease.

SACE AND CHEST ROENTGENOGRAPH

The majority of authors accepts the fact that although the lowest SACE levels tend to occur in patients with radiological stage I and the highest in stage II and III, there is no significant statistical difference (3-11-12). This can be easily explained by the fact that SACE is not only produced in thoracic sites of the disease but also in extra-thoracic localisations. Moreover, as it has been outlined by Gronhagen-Riska , the ACE producing cells of the monocytoid cell line must reach a certain degree of maturation before they express this glycoprotein(13). In other words SACE levels probably express the capacity of secretion of the producing cells.

SACE RELATED TO OTHER BIOLOGICAL "MARKERS"

Conflicting results have been reported these last ten years, when authors try to compare SACE to other markers mainly [67]Gallium scan and bronchoalveolar lavage cells. SACE and [67]Gallium scan are supposed to explore the same pathologic phase of the disease,i-e, the granulomatous phase. If we compare thoracic [67]Gallium uptake and SACE most often no correlation can be found whatever method you choose to appreciate the degree of [67]Gallium uptake. Even with an absolute quantitation of thoracic [67]Gallium uptake that we have previously reported (14), which gives us precise values and not a grade classification, no correlation can be found. However, in 89 cases of our

serie, we found a significant correlation between SACE levels and number of [67]Gallium uptake sites, the latter reflecting spread of the disease over five sites (thoracic and extra-thoracic) examined (15). Even if an ACE inhibitor in the serum of patients can be, in part, the cause of these discrepancies, this reinforces the idea that SACE likely provides information regarding the total body granuloma burden of the disease(16-17) and not only pulmonary involvement; sarcoidosis beeing by definition a multisystemic disease.

The same reasons may explain conflicting results observed in comparing SACE levels and Bronchoalveolar lavage (BAL) cells, especially T. lymphocytes cells. Because SACE does not correlate with BAL T. lymphocytes expressed either in percentage or in absolute number, elevated SACE does not predict which patient will have elevated proportion of lavage T.Lymphocytes and is a poor predictor of the intensity of the alveolitis as assessed by Crystal in sarcoidosis, based on T. lymphocytosis alveolitis and [67]Gallium thoracic uptake(18). SACE is neither sensitive nor specific enough for high risk of intensity alveolitis (19), although BAL-ACE activity correlates well with the number of alveolar macrophages in controls (20). However, RC-DTPA which is supposed to assess respiratory epithelial permeability (thus damage) correlates well with SACE (21). In fact, in sarcoidosis we have to deal with alveolitis which probably preceeds granuloma and fibrosis. Each of the markers cited may represent the activity of these stages. In individual patients, discrepancies between them may be clearly explained by the fact they are not present at the same time and degree and that some markers are the expression of one localization of the disease like alveolitis, and other the expression of thoracic and extra-thoracic localisations.

SACE AND PROGNOSIS

Initial SACE determinations do not discriminate between progressive and non progressive forms (22-23-24-25-26), thus we cannot take the decision of treatment on the basis of SACE determination. In our group, we have followed 37 patients, mainly stage I and II on the chest X-Ray, for a mean period of 3 years. The initial SACE values were not different between the group of patients who deteriorated and the group of patients who improved (27). This is in agreement with the majority of the authors. In chronic sarcoidosis patients observed for many years, Israel (28) noted that this marker and other may remain elevated without evidence of spread or progression indicating that the evidence of cellular activity is not by itself a reliable guide for the need of treatment. Moreover, Turner-Warwick (24) has recently shown that clinical improvement could still occur in some patients when all the new markers might be interpreted as indicating no disease activity. But the reverse has also been reported (29)

However, under steroid therapy, SACE determinations may be useful because we may expect to bring SACE level down to normal range as clinical control of the disease is obtained (3-12-30-31) even if there is no correlation between the pretreatment SACE level and response to therapy (32)

The european survey reported in 1986 shows that steroids suppress SACE levels more than [67]Gallium uptake and [67]Gallium uptake more than BAL Lymphocytes, suggesting that the time course of the SACE level rebounds seems quicker than the [67]Gallium uptake rebound (33). As SACE occasionally antedated changes in clinical status in individuals, its main value remains the monitoring of response to steroids and detection of relapse before clinical or radiological signs occur (34).

SACE reflects only the activity of monocytoid cells, their capacity to secrete this glycoprotein , but it does not tell us clearly if the disease is active or not

Even if these new markers of cells activity help us to better understand this fascinating disease, we still have to behave as clinicians in the care and management of sarcoidosis patients.

REFERENCES

1. Lieberman J. (1975). Elevation of serum angiotensin-converting enzyme level in sarcoidosis. Am J Med 59: 365-372

2. Rohrbach MS, DeRemee RA. (1979). Serum angiotensin-converting enzyme activity in sarcoidosis as measured by a simple radiochemichal assay. Am Rev Respir Dis 119: 761-767

3. Larzul JJ, Le Treut A, Couliou H, Beaumont D, Delaval Ph, Sapene M, de Labarthe B. (1981). Taux serique de l'enzyme de conversion de l'angiotensine dans la sarcoïdose. Nouv Presse Med 9: 675-678

4. Sandron D, Lecossier D, Grodet A, Basset G, Battesti JP. (1984). Intérêt diagnostique, pronostique et évolutif de l'enzyme de conversion de l'angiotensine serique dans la sarcoïdose. Ann Med Interne 135: 46-50

5. Studdy P, Bird R, James DG, Sherlock S.(1978).Serum angiotensin-converting enzyme (SACE) in sarcoidosis and other granulomatous disorders. Lancet 2: 1331-1334.

6. Davis SF, Rohrbach MS, Thelen V, Kuritsky J, Gruninger R, Simpson ML, DeRemee RA.(1984). Elevated serum angiotensin-converting enzyme (SACE) activity in acute pulmonary histoplasmosis. Chest 85:307-310.

7. Grivaux M, Pieron R, Lancastre F, Beneteau B, Baumann. (1986).Augmentation du taux de l'enzyme de conversion de l'angiotensine au cours de la schistosomose. Presse Med 15: 664

8. Coetmeur D, Larzul JJ, Delaval Ph, Le Rest R, Le Treut A (1983). Activité sérique de l'enzyme de conversion de l'angiotensine I dans les alvéolites allergiques extrinsèques. 12: 362-363

9. Huuskonen MS, Järvisalo J, Koskinen H, Kivistö H. (1986). Serum angiotensin-converting enzyme and lysosomal enzymes in tobacco workers. Chest 89: 225-228

10. Klech H, Kohn H, Kummer F, Mostbeck. (1982) Assessment of activity in sarcoidosis: sensitivity and specifity of [67]gallium scintigraphy, serum ACE levels, chest roentgenography, and blood lymphocyte subpopulations. Chest 82:732-738

11. Derveaux L, Demedts M, Lijnen P, Amery A. (1983). Plasma angiotensin converting enzyme in the diagnosis and monitoring of disease activity in sarcoidosis. Eur J Respir Dis 64:197-206

12. Sharma OP. (1986). Markers of sarcoidosis activity. Chest 90: 471-473

13. Grönhagen-riska C, Fyhrquist F, Von Willebrand E. (1986). Angiotensin I-converting enzyme: a marker of highly differentiated monocytic cells. Ann N Y Ac Sc 465:242-249

14. Bourguet P, Delaval Ph, Herry JY. (1986). Direct quantitation of thoracic gallium-67 uptake in sarcoidosis. J Nucl Med 27: 1550-1556

15. Beaumont D, Herry JY, Sapene M, Bourguet P, Larzul JJ, de Labarthe B. (1982). Gallium-67 in the evaluation of sarcoidosis: correlations with serum angiotensin-converting enzyme and bronchoalveolar lavage. Thorax 37: 11-18

16. Thomas PD, Hunninghake GW. (1987). Current concepts of the pathogenesis of sarcoidosis. Am Rev Respir Dis 135:747-760

17. Junod AF. (1983). Les marqueurs des populations cellulaires du poumon profond. Rev Fr Mal Resp 11: 285-291

18. Schoenberger CI, Line BR, Keogh BA, Hunninghake GW, Crystal RG.(1982). Lung inflammation in sarcoidosis: a comparison of serum angiotensin-converting enzyme levels with bronchoalveolar lavage and gallium-67 scanning assessment of T.lymphocyte alveolitis. Thorax 37:19-25

19. Cohen RD, Bunting PS, Meindok HO, Chamberlain DW, Rebuck AS. (1985). Does serum angiotensin converting enzyme reflect intensity of alveolitis in sarcoidosis? Thorax 40: 497-500

20. Eklund A, Blaschke E. (1986) Relationship between changed alveolar-capillary permeability and angiotensin converting enzyme activity in serum in sarcoidosis. Thorax 41: 629-634

21. Dusser DJ, Collignon MA, Stanislas-leguern G, Barritault LG, Chretien J, Huchon GJ. (1986). Respiratory clearance of [99m]TC-DTPA and pulmonary involvement in sarcoidosis. Am Rev Respir Dis 134: 493-497

22. Rust M, Bergmann L, Kuhn T, Tuengerthal S, Bartmann K, Mitrou PS, Meier-sydow J. (1985). Prognosis value of chest radiograph, serum angiotensin-converting enzyme and T helper cell count in blood and in bronchoalveolar lavage of patients with pulmonary sarcoidosis. Respiration 48: 231-236

23. Bjermer L, Bâck O, Roos G, Thunell M. (1986). Mast cells and lysozyme positive macrophages in bronchoalveolar lavage from patients with sarcoidosis: valuable prognostic and activity marking parameters of disease? Acta Med Scand 220: 161-166

24. Turner-Warwick M, McAllister W, Lawrence R, Britten A, Haslam PL.(1986). Corticosteroid treatment in pulmonary sarcoidosis: do serial lavage lymphocyte counts, serum angiotensin converting enzyme measurements, and gallium-67 scans help management? Thorax 41:903-913

25. Finkel R, Terstein AS, Levine R, Brown LK, Miller A. (1986). Pulmonary function tests, serum angiotensin-converting enzyme levels, and clinical findings as prognostic indicators in sarcoidosis. In: Johnson Johns C (eds) Tenth international conference on sarcoidosis and other granulomatous disorders. Ann N Y Acad Sci 465: 665-671

26. Choudat D, Stanislas-Leguern GM, Mordelet-Dambrine MS, Chretien J, Huchon GJ. (1983). Serum activity of angiotensin converting enzyme and pulmonary radiography as prognosis criteria in sarcoidosis. Eur J Respir Dis 64: 355-359

27. Delaval Ph, Pencole C, Bourguet P, Genetet N, Desrues B, Dassonville J, Kernec J. (1987). Predictive value of serum angiotensin converting enzyme, bronchoalveolar lavage T.lymphocyte subsets and gallium-67 lung scan in pulmonary sarcoidosis. In: Stam J, Siebelink J, Vanderschueren R, Wagenaar J (eds). The lung and the environment. 6th congress of the european society of pneumology. 83 (abstract)

28- Israel HL, Sperber M, Steiner RM. (1983). Course of chronic hilar sarcoidosis in relation to markers of granulomatous activity. Invest Radiol 18: 1-5

29. Robbins PS, Patrick H, Maurer HH, Fewell JW. (1983). Effect of corticosteroid therapy on objective gallium scoring of pulmonary sarcoidosis. Am Rev Respir Dis 127(suppl.): 76

30. DeRemee RA, Rohrbach MS. (1984). Normal serum angiotensin converting enzyme activity in patients with newly diagnosed sarcoidosis. Chest 85:45-48

31. Roulston JE, O'Malley GI, Douglas JG. (1984). Effects of prednisolone on angiotensin converting enzyme activity. Thorax 39: 356-360

32. Baughman RP, Fernandez M, Bosken CH, Mantil J, Hurtubise P. (1984). Comparison of gallium-scanning, bronchoalveolar lavage, and serum angiotensin-converting enzyme levels in pulmonary sarcoidosis. Am Rev Respir Dis 129: 676-681

33. Rizzato G, Blasi A. (1986) A european survey on the usefulness of ^{67}Ga lung scans in assessing sarcoidosis: experience on 14 research centers in seven different countries. In: Johnson Johns C (eds) Tenth international conference on sarcoidosis and other granulomatous disorders. Ann N Y Acad Sci 465: 463-478

34. Lieberman J, Schleissner LA, Nosal A, Sastre A, Mishkin FS. (1983). Clinical correlations of serum angiotensin-converting enzyme (ACE) in sarcoidosis. Chest 84: 522-528

PATHOLOGY FROM GRANULOMA TO FIBROSIS

SARCOIDOSIS - FROM GRANULOMA FORMATION TO FIBROSIS. STATE OF THE ART

FRANCOISE BASSET, PAUL SOLER, ALLAN J. HANCE

INSERM U.82, CHU Xavier Bichat, Paris (France)

INTRODUCTION

Sarcoidosis is a multisystem granulomatous disease defined by Scadding (1), after Williams (2), as "a chronic inflammatory response in which cells of the mononuclear phagocyte series are prominent, usually forming focal aggregations". These focal aggregations are classically described as noncaseating, epithelioid and giant cell granulomas. Sarcoid granulomas usually affect the lung parenchyma, upper respiratory tract and lymph nodes, but other organs (e.g., liver, spleen, skin, eyes, salivary glands, bone, joints, nervous system) are often involved in this systemic disease. Granulomas constitute the pathological hallmark of sarcoidosis. However, although granulomas must be identified at sites of active sarcoid lesions to confirm the diagnosis, they are not specific, and sarcoid-like granulomas have been described in many other pathological conditions. Therefore, sarcoid granulomas must be placed in a compatible clinical and pathological context which confers on them their full diagnostic value.

The purpose of this presentation is to discuss some important pathological features of sarcoidosis which are useful in establishing this diagnosis. Specifically, we will: 1) Describe the structure of sarcoid granulomas and compare their structure with that of granulomas present in other interstitial lung diseases; 2) Discuss other pathological features of lung tissue from patients with sarcoidosis, that is, the pathological context within which the granulomas are found; and 3) Evaluate the late pathological features of sarcoidosis, emphasizing the factors which result in the progression of "granulomatous" lesions to fibrosis.

THE GRANULOMA

The sarcoid granuloma

The sarcoid granuloma consists typically of a well defined, usually rounded, collection of epithelioid cells, with variable numbers of multinucleate giant cells, which are often located centrally. The periphery of this collection of epitheloid cells may be formed by a rim of lymphocytes or by a fibrotic area, both of variable width. Granulomas are often aggregated into masses that can replace normal tissue in the affected areas.

The main component of the sarcoid granuloma appears to be, at least numerically, epithelioid cells. Epithelioid cells are large, pale stained cells with abundant cytoplasm and clear, eccentric nuclei which are usually kidney shaped. Epithelioid cells have poorly defined cell limits, a highly characteristic feature which is explained by their ultrastructural appearance. On electron micrographs, the plasma membrane of epithelioid cells forms elongated filopodia which interdigitate with those of adjacent cells, producing the fuzzy cell contours seen with light microscopy (3-5). Other ultrastructural characteristics of epithelioid cells are the presence of numerous cytoplasmic vesicles with finely granular content, which are probably modified lysosomal structures (3-5). The vesicles often have communications with each other and, much more rarely, with the plasma membrane. The nucleus is richer in euchromatin than in heterochromatin, a feature perhaps related to cell activation (6). Nuclear bodies of several types are frequently observed (4).

The above features are those of mature epithelioid cells forming the bulk of most florid granulomas. However, other morphologically distinct cells can also be seen. Some resemble macrophages; others have features intermediate between macrophages and mature epithelioid cells (7,8). Finally, some cells have dilated cisterns of rough endoplasmic reticulum resulting in a plasmacytoid or fibroblastoid appearance. Some of these populations have been described as separate types of epithelioid cells. However, they may also correspond to evolutionary stages in the maturation of epithelioid cells (7), or may represent plasma cells and/or fibroblasts interspersed with epithelioid cells (8).

In addition to epithelioid cells, sarcoid granulomas contain variable numbers of multinucleate giant cells. Multinucleate giant cells are usually of the Langhans type, with numerous peripheral nuclei forming a circle or an arc around a granular cell center. Giant cells sometimes contain characteristic (but non-specific) inclusion bodies, referred to as asteroid, conchoid, and crystalline inclusion bodies, the nature, significance and histogenesis of which remain unknown. Multinucleate giant cells appear to be formed by coalescence of epithelioid cells, after fusion and desintegration of their surface interdigitations (4). Their ultrastructural characteristics are similar to those of epithelioid cells. In addition, large cytoplasmic osmiophilic lamellar bodies that may result from the degenerated cell membranes (4,5,8) and/or multiple centrioles (5) may be present.

Lymphocytes are often interspersed with epithelioid and giant cells, but their predominant location is peripheral, forming a complete rim around the aggregate of epithelioid cells. Labelling with monoclonal antibodies shows that a large majority of these lymphocytes are T-lymphocytes. T4 positive cells predominate within granulomas and in the inner area of the peripheral rim, and T8 positive cells predominate at the outer margin of this rim (9). B lymphocytes usually form compact clusters at the margins of the granulomas.

By definition, the sarcoid granuloma is noncaseating; this feature is an important difference as compared to the tuberculous granuloma, which has similar cell components but typically has a central area of caseous necrosis. However, a minority of sarcoid granulomas also show small central areas of acidophilic, fibrinoid necrosis, sometimes containing a few lymphocytes or cell debris.

All granulomas generally have a similar appearance in a given sample. This seems to indicate that their development and evolutionary changes (prominence of lymphocytic infiltration or of fibrosis) occur simultaneously in the course of the disease.

Sarcoid-like granulomas

The granulomas present in other granulomatous diseases are composed of similar constituents to those described above for sarcoid granulomas. However, these other granulomatous diseases can be distinguished from sarcoidosis either because of differences in the structure of the granulomas per se or because of the presence of other associated pathological abnormalities. Tuberculous granulomas have been mentioned previously. Similarly, there are other diseases caused by mycobacteria (e.g. leprosy); fungi; parasites; bacteria (e.g., brucellosis, tularemia, syphilis, lymphogranulomia inguinale) and viruses (e.g., varicella) in which granuloma formation may be present (1). Most of these lesions have a prominent necrotic tendency. In addition to these classical differential diagnoses, sarcoid-like noncaseating granulomas can also participate in complex histopathological pictures such as those observed in Wegener's granulomatosis and its variants (10), chronic eosinophilic pneumonia (11), primary biliary cirrhosis and lymphangioleiomyomatosis (FB: unpublished). Sarcoid-like granulomas are also well known to occur as satellite lesions in the vicinity of primary or metastatic tumors, including lymphomas (12).

Sarcoid-like granulomas also exist in other circumstances, in which their pathological differential diagnosis can be very difficult. This is the case in chronic berylliosis, the granulomas of which may be strictly identical to sarcoid granulomas (13). While the lymphocytic alveolitis is usually more intense in chronic berylliosis than in sarcoidosis, this finding is often equivocal, and the differential diagnosis often rests primarily on clinical and biological data.

Silicotic lesions may also raise difficult problems of interpretation, since typical silicotic nodules can be associated with typical sarcoid granulomas. We found this association in 11 out of 43 open lung biopsy samples that we have reviewed. This association has rarely been emphasized in the literature (14), although the association between silicosis and tuberculosis is well known.

Lastly, granulomas of hypersensitivity pneumonitis must be considered among the differential diagnoses of sarcoidosis, although their pathological aspect rarely takes a real sarcoid-like appearance (10). Despite their similar cell components, granulomas in hypersensitivity pneumonitis differ from sarcoid granulomas by their smaller size, their more prominent lymphocytic component, the rarity of giant cells, and by differences in the topography of lesions, which will be discussed below.

The differential diagnosis between sarcoid-like and real sarcoid granulomas is especially difficult in small tissue samples, such as those obtained by transbronchial biopsies, which may contain only satellite sarcoid-like lesions. In open lung biopsies, which normally provide relatively large samples, it is usually easier to analyse the pathological context, and to evaluate the significance of the granulomas in this light.

THE PATHOLOGICAL CONTEXT OF SARCOID GRANULOMAS

Although the nature of the granulomas per se, is an important aspect of the pathology of sarcoidosis, other pathological feature of involved tissue (the "pathological context" of the granulomas) are often equally important in establishing whether granulomas are likely to result from sarcoidosis or other diseases. Two important aspects of this pathological context, the nature of the alveolitis and the topographical distribution of the granulomas, are discussed below.

Alveolitis

A important feature of the pathological context of pulmonary sarcoid granulomas is the accompanying alveolitis. In sarcoidosis, the alveolitis has both mural and luminal components, but their intensity is variable. Mural alveolitis is characterized by the presence of variable numbers of inflammatory cells, mainly lymphocytes, in the alveolar walls. In the luminal alveolitis variable numbers of alveolar macrophages and lymphocytes are usually the predominant cell types present. A direct relationship between the intensity of alveolitis and the severity of the respiratory function impairment has been shown by Carrington (13).

The frequency of non-granulomatous interstitial pneumonitis was stressed by Rosen (15), who found it as a predominant or prominent feature in 62% of 128 pulmonary granuloma-containing open lung biopsy specimens from patients with sarcoidosis. From this study, the authors drew the conclusion that alveolitis (especially the mural cell infiltrate, according to their description) was an early or an initial lesion preceding granuloma formation. This cell infiltrate consisted of macrophages and lymphocytes. It appeared focally distributed, but no apparent selective perivascular or peribronchial localization was noted. Luminal alveolitis was mild or absent.

We were able to confirm most of Rosen's statements. In a semi-quantitative study we showed an inverse relationship between the intensity of alveolitis and the profusion of granulomas (16). However, although mural alveolitis, mainly lymphocytic, appeared predominant, the intraalveolar component of alveolitis was sometimes important in our material and consisted of both alveolar macrophages and lymphocytes. The histological observation of this luminal alveolitis in sarcoidosis is in agreement with the findings obtained with bronchoalveolar lavage (17). It seems only surprising that alveolitis was so long ignored in sarcoidosis, probably because the whole histological picture was dominated by the presence of granulomas.

Lymphocytic alveolitis is not specific of sarcoidosis. In fact, lymphocytic infiltrates are often more abundant and more widely distributed in other granulomatous disorders, especially chronic berylliosis and hypersensitivity pneumonitis, than in sarcoidosis. Conversely, as already mentioned, the granulomatous component is usually less developped in these diseases than in sarcoidosis, reinforcing the impression that there is an inverse relationship between granulomas and alveolitis, as was found with sarcoidosis (13,15,16).

It must be stressed that $T4^+$ T-lymphocytes are the predominant lymphocytic population present in the sarcoid cell infiltrates, which is not necessarily the case in other diseases in which a lymphocytic alveolitis is present. For example, $T8^+$ T-lymphocytes may predominate is some, but not all, patients with hypersensitivity pneumonitis.

Another important characteristic of sarcoid alveolitis is its tendency to represent a transient phenomenon, which regresses, at least in great part, when granuloma formation progresses, as suggested by Rosen's comments (15) and by our own semiquantitative study (16). This regressive tendency of the alveolitis has two important consequences: Firstly, it may explain why septal interstitial fibrosis is relatively infrequent in sarcoidosis. Secondly, this regressive tendency is consistent with the finding that only few and mild destructive

changes of alveolar walls are seen in lung samples of patients with sarcoidosis
examined with the electron microscope.

Topographical distribution of granulomas

The topographical distribution of pulmonary sarcoid granulomas has been
evaluated in several studies. By counts performed on numerous sections of 43
pulmonary biopsies, it was shown that 75% of the sarcoid granulomas were located
in the peribronchovascular, subpleural and interlobular connective tissue
sheaths (16), all sites which contain lymph vessels. Only 25% appeared to be
located in alveolar tissue, and even in this location, they were often found in
association with arterioles or venules. Similar counts have not been performed
on tissue containing sarcoid-like granulomas, because these samples rarely
contain sufficient numbers of granulomas to make such comparisons possible.
However, Carrington reported similar findings in a comparative study of
berylliosis and sarcoidosis (13) concluding that no distinction could be made
between the two diseases as regards the topographical distribution of
granulomas. In hypersensitivity pneumonitis granulomas are usually much less
numerous than in sarcoidosis, and they usually have no tendency to become
aggregated. Unlike other authors (10), we failed to observe a selective
peribronchiolar and perivascular, distribution of granulomas in hypersensitivity
pneumonitis; in a study of 18 pulmonary biopsies from patients with this
disease we found small granulomas mainly in alveolar walls or at the
intersection of alveolar walls (18). Therefore, we consider the peribronchiolar
and perivascular location of granulomas more suggestive of sarcoidosis than of
hypersensitivity pneumonitis.

Vascular involvement

Vascular involvement has been mentioned sporadically in descriptions of
sarcoid lesions (10,12). The most detailed study was made by Rosen et al. (19),
who found a granulomatous angiitis in 69% of 128 open lung biopsies from
patients with sarcoidosis. Venous involvement was prominent, but associated or
even isolated arterial involvement was also observed. As controls, Rosen
studied samples taken at autopsy or surgery from 113 patients with pulmonary
tuberculosis, and found pulmonary granulomatous angiitis in less than 2%.
Carrington et al., in a comparative study of sarcoidosis and chronic berylliosis
(13), reported the presence of angiitis involving pulmonary arteries, veins, or
both, in 42% of 47 specimens from sarcoidosis patients. This angiitis was
sometimes severe, with obliteration and destruction of blood vessels. In
contrast, angiitis was found only in 1 of the 13 specimens from patients with
berylliosis.

From these two studies, it appears that pulmonary granulomatous angiitis, although not specific of sarcoidosis, is observed very frequently in this disease, and is not characteristic of all granulomatous disorders. We have made similar findings in our material. We found vascular involvement by sarcoid granulomas in a large majority of our samples from patients with sarcoidosis. In contrast, we did not find any vascular involvement by granulomas in biopsies from patients with hypersensitivity pneumonitis (18). Vascular involvement by granulomas was sometimes observed in biopsies from patients with pulmonary Langerhans' cell granulomatosis (histiocytosis X), but fibrotic obliteration was the most frequent vascular change in this disease; more rarely, vessel walls were thickened and infiltrated by a few inflammatory cells. Both changes suggested that the vascular involvement in Langerhans' cell granulomatosis was a passive phenomenon due to topographical contiguity of vessels to lesions. Granulomatous angiitis similar to that seen in sarcoidosis was never present (20).

The vascular changes in sarcoidosis can take different forms, most of which were described by Rosen (19) and by Carrington (13). The most characteristic aspect is the development of transmural granulomas with segmental erosion or destruction of elastic laminae. Another frequent finding is that of small vessels closely apposed to or located within apparently fresh granulomas. In fibrotic areas, mainly between aggregated and/or involuted granulomas, vessels completely obliterated by fibrous and/or inflammatory tissue are often present. Other changes are detectable only when specific stains for elastin are used, such as granulomatous phlebitis between confluent granulomas (19), or the presence of elastic remnants circumscribing small isolated granulomas (FB, unpublished). All these different forms of vascular involvement by sarcoid granulomas suggest that the relationship between the vessels and the sarcoid process is not fortuitous, and that granulomatous vasculitis is an important feature in sarcoidosis.

An entity described in 1973 by Liebow (21) as distinct from sarcoidosis was called "necrotizing sarcoidal granulomatosis", sometimes referred to as "necrotizing sarcoidal angiitis" (12,22). As expressed by these two eponyms, the main pathological features in this entity are confluent sarcoid-like granulomas, granulomatous vasculitis and varying degrees of necrosis. Originally, it seemed that clinical features were not identical to those of the usual forms of sarcoidosis. For example, hilar lymph node and extrapulmonary involvement were reported to be absent. More recent published series showed that these differences have not always been confirmed, and the clinical course

and prognosis of this disease are similar to those of sarcoidosis. In light of
the knowledge that granulomatous angiitis is a common feature in sarcoidosis,
and that fibrinoid necrosis may be present in granulomas, our impression is that
the entity described as "necrotizing sarcoidal granulomatosis" deserves to be
integrated in sarcoidosis, and may represent only a pathological variant with
prominent vascular changes and necrosis.

FIBROTIC CHANGES IN SARCOIDOSIS

There is no precise data concerning the frequency of "pulmonary fibrosis" in
sarcoidosis, and its frequency would probably be evaluated differently in terms
of clinical, pathological or pulmonary function test data.

However, there is a general agreement that sarcoid granulomata in the lungs
resolve spontaneously without sequelae in the majority of patients, roughly 70%
according to M. Turner-Warwick (23). In an additional subset of patients,
resolution is obtained under steroid therapy. In some individuals, widespread
granulomata appear to persist for long periods of time without compromising
pulmonary function and without radiographic evidence of distortion of lung
architecture. By contrast, in a minority of patients, 10 to 15% according to
M. Turner-Warwick (23), less than 5% according to Dalquen (24), there is a
progression to irreversible distortion of the lung architecture, occurring over
varying lengths of time. The mechanisms which determine these different modes
of evolution are unknown.

From the pathologist's viewpoint, the progression from granulomas to fibrosis
is perhaps easier to understand than the possibility of complete resolution of
the granulomatous process. From our previous analysis of the main pathological
components of the sarcoid lung lesions, one could anticipate that fibrosis might
be associated with alveolitis, granulomas, vascular lesions, or with a
combination of several factors.

As already mentioned, alveolitis is an early and often transient phenomenon,
which regresses, at least partly, when granulomas develop (15,16). In addition,
sarcoid alveolitis usually does not have a marked destructive tendency, as shown
by the rarity of epithelial necrosis and of intraluminal septal cell migration.
Therefore, migration of fibroblasts and inflammatory cells through gaps in the
alveolar lining is seen only exceptionally in sarcoidosis, while it is observed
much more frequently in other interstitial disorders (25). Evaluation of
pathological specimens from other diseases suggests that such alveolar damage is
often an initial event in the subsequent thickening of alveolar walls or
remodeling of the alveolar architecture. Thus, these features of sarcoid

alveolitis explain why widespread interstitial fibrosis is not frequent in
sarcoidosis, and why architectural remodeling by intraluminal fibrosis is
exceptional in areas distant from granulomas. However, persistent alveolitis,
when present, may aggravate or induce fibrotic changes in non granulomatous
areas, and results in variable degrees of interstitial fibrosis (30). As judged
by cell counts performed on samples of bronchoalveolar lavage, the alveolitis of
patients with long standing sarcoidosis contains elevated numbers of
neutrophils, and these potent inflammatory cells may play a role in inducing
epithelial injury and subsequent fibrosis (31).

Vascular involvement remains to be studied in more detail. From what is known
of sarcoid involvement of the eye and the central nervous system, vascular
lesions appear to have a segmental distribution along blood vessels (28) and to
be sometimes reversible. Therefore, except in the rare and late occurrence of
obliteration of relatively large arteries in the lung, fibrosis does not seem to
be related primarily to vascular lesions.

In contrast, several lines of evidence suggest that fibrosis in sarcoidosis
occurs at the sites of prior granuloma formation. First, sarcoid granulomas are
sometimes surrounded by a fibrotic or hyalinotic ring which progresses
centripetally (29). Sarcoid lesions in lymph nodes exhibit particularly well
the different steps of this evolution.

Secondly, sarcoid lesions, especially in the lung, have a marked tendency to
aggregate. They sometimes form large consolidated areas in which few or no
preserved alveolar structures remain visible. These aggregated granulomas are
sealed to each other, and the whole mass is surrounded by fibrotic tissue. The
fibrotic tissue is sometimes loose and infiltrated by variable numbers of
inflammatory cells, or can also be compact, poorly cellular, or even hyalinotic.

Furthermore, the distribution of fibrotic changes seems to coincide with that
of granulomas. Granulomas, and especially aggregated granulomas forming large
fibrotic masses, are located mainly in subpleural, peribronchial and
interlobular connective tissue sheaths. Sarcoid granulomas are also frequently
present in the submucosa of bronchi (30). According to a radiologist's
viewpoint, "pulmonary fibrosis can only be diagnosed with certainty from the
chest radiograph when there are changes of upper lobe shrinkage with elevation
of the hila, tenting of the diaphragm and upper zone linear opacities" (31).
These radiological changes seem to correspond well to what can be expected from
the late evolution of granulomatous areas, since peribronchial and subpleural
apical fibrotic masses undergo retraction and may become coalescent. This
retraction and bronchial involvement may account for elevation of the hila,

telescoping of airways and severe distortion of bronchial architecture, which may be present in end-stage sarcoid lesions (12). Similarly, linear opacities may correspond to thickened and fibrotic interlobular septa, which contain only small residual granulomas, isolated multinucleate giant cells, or even residual calcified conchoid bodies, without cellular remnants. The reasons why these changes predominate in the upper parts of the lung are unclear.

Interstitial fibrosis sometimes develops in areas contiguous to fibrotic masses or thickened interlobular septa. In end stage lesions, extensive pulmonary fibrosis can be observed, but it differs from that of idiopathic pulmonary fibrosis by the presence of thin-walled cystic spaces (12). Infectious processes may complicate these massive fibrotic changes. Not unusually, Aspergillus fungus balls develop in such cystic spaces.

An additional factor may play a role in the development of pulmonary fibrosis in sarcoidosis. As mentioned already, typical silicotic nodules were seen in proximity of typical sarcoid granulomas in 11 out of 43 open lung biopsies that we reviewed. These nodules were usually small, rounded, composed of hyaline concentric lamellae with little or no necrosis, and they were practically acellular. These hyaline nodules were variably distant from granulomas, and were sometimes contiguous to fibrotic or hyalinotic areas surrounding aggregated granulomas. Birefringent particles were often present in these nodules, but usually in small numbers. Occupational or environmental reports obtained from these patients disclosed an exposure to mineral particles in most of them, but generally of short duration and slight intensity. Although the presence of hyaline nodules was mentioned previously in some descriptions of fibrotic changes in sarcoidosis (1,12,22), their silicotic nature was rarely discussed (14). We do not intend to suggest that silicosis plays a causative role in sarcoidosis; however, our impression is that a slight, moderate or transient exposure to mineral particles may induce or worsen the occurrence of fibrotic changes in this disease. The reasons for that belief are the following: First, the preferential involvement of the upper pulmonary zones in sarcoid fibrosis is reminiscent of that observed generally in pneumoconioses. Second, the development of sarcoid lesions at the site of subcutaneously deposited mineral particles is a well known phenomenon, which suggests that a relationship can exist between the two processes, as has been demonstrated in the skin in certain cases (14). Third, the striking similarities which exist between pulmonary lesions of sarcoidosis and of berylliosis demonstrate that inhaled foreign particles are able to induce or exacerbate sarcoid-like lesions. In conclusion, sarcoid fibrosis appears to occur predominantly at the sites of prior granuloma formation, at least in its localized, limited forms. The induction of extensive interstitial fibrosis may require additional factors, such as persistent alveolitis and/or inhalation of noxious foreign particles.

REFERENCES

1. Scadding JG, Mitchell DN (1985) In: Sarcoidosis; 2nd edition. Chapman and Hall, London, pp 13-25

2. Williams GT, Williams WJ (1983) Granulomatous inflammation – A review. J Clin Path 36:723-733

3. Hirsch JG, Fedorko ME, Dwyer CM (1967) The ultrastructure of epithelioid and giant cells in positive Kveim test sites and sarcoid granulomata. In: Turiaf J, Chabot J (eds) La sarcoïdose. IV Conf Intern. Masson, Paris, pp 59-70.

4. Kalifat SR, Bouteille M, Delarue J (1967) Etude ultrastructurale des altérations cellulaires et extracellulaires dans le granulome sarcoïdosique. In: Turiaf J, Chabot J (eds) La sarcoïdose. IV Conf Inter. Masson, Paris, pp 71-88

5. Basset F, Collet A, Chrétien J, Normand-Reuet C, Turiaf J (1967) Etude ultramicroscopique des cellules de la réaction de Kveim. In: Turiaf J, Chabot J (eds) La sarcoïdose. IV Conf Intern. Masson, Paris, pp 89-109

6. Danel C, Dewar A, Corrin B, Turner-Warwick M, Chrétien J (1983) Ultrastructural changes of bronchoalveolar lavage cells in sarcoidosis and comparison with tissue granulomas. Am J Pathol 112:7-17

7. Soler P, Basset F, Bernaudin JF, Chrétien J (1976) Morphology and distribution of the cells of a sarcoid granuloma: ultrastructural study of serial sections. Ann NY Acad Sci 278:147-160

8. Wanstrup J (1967) On the ultrastructure of granuloma formation in sarcoidosis. In: Turiaf J, Chabot J (eds) La sarcoïdose. IV Conf Intern Masson, Paris, pp 110-116

9. Semenzato G, Agostini C, Zambello R, Trentin L, Chilosi M, Angi MR, Ossi E, Cipriani A, Pizzolo G (1986) Activated T cells with immunoregulary functions at different sites of involvement in sarcoidosis. Ann NY Acad Sci 465:56-73

10. Katzenstein ALA, Askin FB (1982) Surgical pathology of non neoplastic lung disease. W.B. Saunders Co. Philadelphia, London, pp 152-165

11. Carrington CB, Addington WW, Goff AM, Madoff IM, Marks A, Schwaber JR, Gaensler EA (1969) Chronic eosinophilic pneumonia. N Eng J Med 280:787-798

12. Cole SR, Johnson KJ, Ward PA (1983) Pathology of sarcoidosis, granulomatous vasculitis and other idiopathic granulomatous diseases of the lung. In: Fanburg BL (ed) Sarcoidosis and other granulomatous diseases of the lung. Marcel Dekker NY Basel pp 149-202

13. Carrington CB, Gaensler EA, Mikus JP, Schachter AW, Burke GW, Goff AM (1976) Structure and function in sarcoidosis. Ann NY Acad Sci 278:265-283

14. Uehlinger E (1967) La sarcoïdose réactionnelle ou symptomatique. In: La sarcoïdose. IV Conf Intern Masson, Paris, pp 15-23

15. Rosen Y, Athanassiades TJ, Moon S, Lyons HA (1978) Non granulomatous interstitial pneumonitis in sarcoidosis. Relationship to development of epithelioid granulomas. Chest 74:122-125

16. Lacronique J, Bernaudin JF, Soler P, Lange F, Kawanami O, Saumon G, Georges R, Basset F (1983) Alveolitis and granulomas: sequential course in pulmonary sarcoidosis. In: Chrétien J, Marsac J, Saltiel JC (eds) Sarcoidosis and other granulomatous disorders. Pergamon Press, Paris, pp 36–42

17. Crystal RG, Roberts MC, Hunninghake GW, Gadek JE, Fulmer JD, Line BR (1981) Pulmonary sarcoidosis: a disease characterized and perpetuated by activated lung T-lymphocytes. Ann Intern Med 94:73–94

18. Kawanami O, Basset F, Barrios R, Lacronique JG, Ferrans VJ, Crystal RG (1983) Hypersensitivity pneumonitis in man. Light and electron microscopic studies of 18 lung biopsies. Am J Pathol 110:277–291

19. Rosen Y, Moon S, Huang CI, Gourin A, Lyons HA (1977) Granulomatous pulmonary angiitis in sarcoidosis. Arch Pathol Lab Med 101:170–174

20. Basset F, Corrin B, Spencer H, Lacronique J, Roth C, Soler P, Battesti JP, Georges R, Chrétien J (1978) Pulmonary histiocytosis X. Am Rev Respir Dis 118:811–820

21. Liebow AA (1973) The J Burns Anderson lecture: pulmonary angiitis and granulomatosis. Am Rev Respir Dis 108:1–18

22. Katzenstein ALA, Askin FB (1982) Surgical pathology of non neoplastic lung disease. WB Saunders Co. Philadelphia, London, pp 166–202

23. Turner-Warwick M (1986) Pulmonary fibrosis in sarcoidosis: who, why, when, how. Sarcoidosis 3:128–129

24. Dalquen P (1986) Pulmonary fibrosis in sarcoidosis. Help from the pathologist. Sarcoidosis 3:129

25. Basset F, Ferrans VJ, Soler P, Takemura T, Fukuda Y, Crystal RG (1985) Intraluminal fibrosis in interstitial lung disorders. Am J Pathol 122:443–461

26. Crystal RG, Hunninghake GW, Gadek JE, Keogh BA, Rennard SI, Bitterman PB (1983) State of the art: the pathogenesis of sarcoidosis. In: Sarcoidosis and other granulomatous disorders. Chrétien J, Marsac J, Saltiel JC (eds). Pergamon Press, Paris, Oxford, pp 13–35

27. Arnoux A, Danel C, Stanislas-Leguern G, Marsac J, Huchon G, Saltiel JC, Dufat R, Chrétien J (1979) Données cellulaires concernant 65 lavages bronchoalvéolaires effectués au cours de sarcoïdoses. In: Le lavage bronchoalvéolaire chez l'homme. INSERM, Paris, 84:289–297

28. Caplan L, Corbett J, Goodwin J, Thomas C, Shenker D, Schatz N (1983) Neuro-ophtalmologic signs in the angiitic form of neurosarcoidosis. Neurology 33:1130–1135

29. Uehlinger E (1964) The sarcoid tissue reaction. Acta Med Scand 176 (suppl. 425):7–13

30. Turiaf J, Marland P, Rose Y, Sors C (1952) Le diagnostic bronchoscopique et bronchobiopsique des formes pulmonaires de la sarcoïdose de BBS. Bull Mem Soc Med Hop Paris 30–31:1098–1116

31. Flower CDR (1986) Pulmonary fibrosis in sarcoidosis. Help from the radiologist. Sarcoidosis 3:131

© 1988 Elsevier Science Publishers B.V. (Biomedical Division)
Sarcoidosis and other granulomatous disorders
C. Grassi, G. Rizzato, E. Pozzi, editors

ISOLATION AND PREPARATION OF ACELLULAR SARCOID GRANULOMA (SARCOID MATRICIAL COMPLEX, SMC)

CHRISTINA TAKIYA*, **, ALETH CALLE**, LUIZ EDUARDO CARDOSO**,
SIMONE PEYROL**, JEAN-FRANCOIS CORDIER***, JEAN-ALEXIS GRIMAUD**

* Departamento de Patologia, Faculdade de Medicina UFRJ, Rio de Janeiro (Brazil)
** Laboratoire de Pathologie Cellulaire, CNRS UA 602, Institut Pasteur, 77 rue Pasteur, 69365 Lyon cedex 7 (France)
*** Hôpital Cardiovasculaire et pneumologique Louis Pradel, 28 avenue du Doyen Lépine, 69374 Lyon (France)

INTRODUCTION

The extracellular matrix (EM) acts not only as a structural support but has also an important role in the control of cell functions (1, 2, 3, 4).

The biochemical composition and the structural arrangement of the extracellular matrix seem to contribute to these functions as demonstrated in different in vitro systems (2, 5, 6, 7, 8). Moreover, to simulate the in vivo extracellular environment, methods have recently been developed to obtain a system for culturing cells on these extracellular matrix (9, 10, 11).

In the present study, we describe the preparation of acellular sarcoid granulomas with preservation of its major morphological and biochemical characteristics. The availability of these acellular matrices as substratum is demonstrated here, allowing the verification of the effect of this polymorphic matrix on morphology and differentiation of connective tissue cells.

MATERIAL AND METHODS

Obtention of acellular sarcoid granulomas (SMC)

Granulomas were isolated from frozen pieces of spleen obtained from a sarcoid patient submitted to splenectomy. The tissue was homogenized in a Sorvall Omni-mixer for 5 minutes in an intermittent fashion and in an ice bath to prevent enzymatic digestion of extracellular matrix proteins. The homogenate was subsequently filtered in a sintered glass filter (porosity 40-60 μm) under vacuum and washed with distilled water containing antiproteases (leupeptin (Sigma) at 1 μg/ml and soybean trypsin inhibitor (Sigma) at 10μg/ml). When the filtrate became clear the retentate was collected and centrifuged at 400 g for 15 minutes allowing the separation of an almost pure fraction of granulomas from debris (mostly splenic connective matrix framework), which remained in suspension.

The subsequent steps to remove cells are shown in table I, consisting of a modified procedure already described for schistosomal acellular granulomas (12).

Table I : Obtention of acellular SMC

Granulomas

> Osmotic lysis - 1 h at 4°C
> 1 g of tissue in 15-20 vol. distilled water + antiproteases
>
> Centrifugation

Granulomas
(pellet)

> 3 % Triton X 100 in distilled water (15-20 vol./g tissue) +
> antiproteases overnight at 4°C, constant agitation
>
> Centrifugation

Granulomas
(pellet)

> Wash 3 times (1 h each) with distilled water + antiproteases
> 15-20 vol/g tissue
>
> Centrifugation

Granulomas
(pellet)

> Incubation with 50 ml distilled water + 1 mg DNase + 5 mg
> RNase + 5 mg $CaCl_2$/3g tissue
> 1 h at 20°C
> Wash 3 times (1 h each) with distilled water + antiproteases
>
> Centrifugation

Granulomas

> 4 % sodium deoxycholate in distilled water (15-20 vol./g tissue)
> overnight at 4°C, constant agitation
> Wash extensively - several baths of distilled water (15-20 vol./g
> tissue)
>
> Centrifugation

acellular granulomas

Assessment of the acellularity and biochemical preservation of the EM

Light and electron microscope (TEM and SEM) analysis of Bouin's fixed, paraffin-embedded sections stained with connective tissue stains (Masson's trichrome, Picro-sirius red, silver impregnation and periodic acid-Schiff techniques). For EM osmic tetroxyde-cacodylate buffer fixative was used.

Immunolabeling of connective tissue proteins in snap-frozen sections and using polyclonal antibodies against collagen isotypes (I, III, IV), type III procollagen and fibronectin. Preparation of immune reagents and the staining technique were carried out as previously described (13). Cross-reactivity and monospecificity of antibodies were controlled by ELISA techniques.

Biochemical assays. Tissue samples were treated with acetone (two changes of 24 hours each at 4°C), dried, weighted and used for the following assays : **hydroxyproline** : performed according to the method of Bergman and Loxley (14); **glycosaminoglycans** (GAG) : total GAG were isolated from samples of about 19 mg by papain (Boehringer) digestion using a modification of the procedure of Wagner and Salisbury (15). Uronic acid was assayed by the method of Bitter and Muir (16) with glucuronolactone (Sigma) as the standard, and the sulfated GAG were identified by agarose gel electrophoresis (17).

Cell culture. Human skin fibroblasts were obtained from explants of foreskin, grown in Dulbecco's medium supplemented with 10 % foetal calf serum, penicillin (50 U/ml) and streptomycin (50 μg/ml). Cells were subcultured by trypsinization and used in passages 3 to 6. Fibroblasts (50.000) were seeded and cultivated on acellular SMC in plates of 96 wells coated with silicone (Serva). After 72 hours of culture in the same medium, cultures on SMC and control cultures of fibroblasts on glass coverslips were fixed and routinely treated for scanning and transmission electron microscopy.

RESULTS

Morphological study of acellular SMC

With the treatment applied, single and confluent (the majority) fibrotic granulomas were obtained, with the almost complete disappearance of the cellular components.

The classical connective tissue methods for light microscopy exhibited only a slight bleaching of its staining characteristics (fig. 1). In transmission electron microscopy, some membrane debris were rarely observed and the extracellular matricial network exhibited collagen fibers organized in a loose or dense pattern with its characteristic periodicity. The importance of the microgranular component of the connective matrix of sarcoid granuloma was evident (fig. 4). Moreover, the clearness of the trabecular architecture of this matrix was shown by the scanning electron microscopical analysis (fig. 2).

250

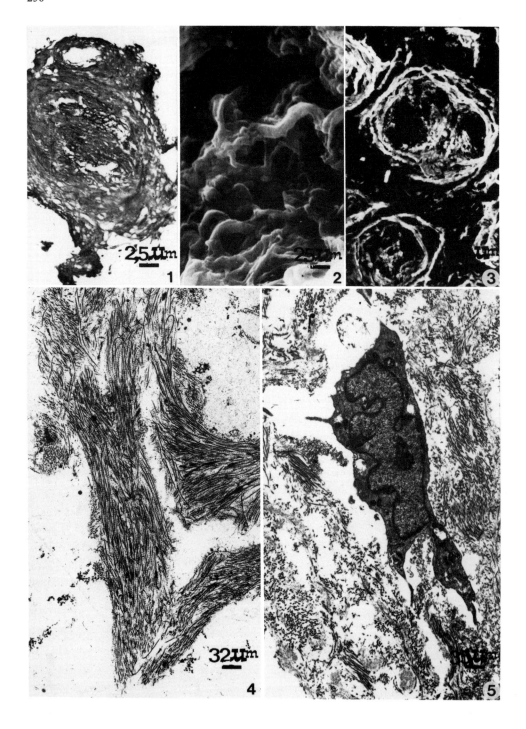

Preserved immunoreactivity of types I, III and IV collagens, fibronectin and laminin was demonstrated by immunofluorescence (fig. 3). After repopulation in vitro fibroblasts have the same morphological appearance than those observed in tissue (fig. 5).

Biochemical assays

The total collagen and GAG contents are shown in table II. Dermatan sulfate was the only sulfated GAG detected (results not shown).

TABLE II

TOTAL HYDROXYPROLINE (OH-pro) AND URONIC ACID (UA) CONTENTS OF SARCOID GRANULOMAS

Results are expressed as micrograms per milligram of dry tissue

SMC	OH-pro	UA
cellular	24.69	1.04
acellular	69.73	3.96

DISCUSSION

Since the influence of the substratum of cell culture on the proliferation and phenotypic modulation of cells have been demosntrated, studies have been carried out on this topic. The use of individual or complex components of the extracellular matrix as cell culture substratum has long been assayed (4, 18, 19, 20, 21, 22, 23). These studies emphasized not only the importance of the different components of the extracellular matrix but also the necessity of a tri-dimensional support to give cells the optimal conditions to express their functions and their differentiated state (6, 7, 8, 11, 24, 25, 26, 27, 28). More recently, procedures to obtain tri-dimensional acellular extracellular matrix obtained from tissues have been described. The basic aim of these studies is to give cells conditions closer to the in vivo ones (10, 12, 29, 30, 31). The procedure presently described is similar to these methods (10, 32) based on a detergent action. The morphological and immunoreactivity integrity of the remaining extracellular matricial proteins was demonstrated. The detergents do not affect the different components during the time of procedure (32). However the diminution of the staining properties of the connective matrix could be due to a solubilization of a part of these components as the proteoglycans associated to cell membranes. Nonetheless, the major components of the acellular SMC are still present as demonstrated by immunohistological and biochemical methods.

The polymorphic and loose aspect of the SMC, distinct from the classical reparative fibrosis (33) provides a very interesting model for the analysis of these matricial mediated cell interactions. This type of matrix allows an easy diffusion pathway for inflammatory cells and secreted chemical mediators contributing to the maintainance of the inflammatory process, as it has been largely demonstrated one of the characteristics in sarcoidosis. Furthermore, the continuous presence of these mediators could exert selective effects on different connective cell populations involved in the turnover of the connective tissue in inflammatory processes (34).

ACKNOWLEDGEMENTS

This work was supported by a grant from Fonds Spécial des Comités Départementaux contre les Maladies Respiratoires et la Tuberculose and a fellowship of Société d'Hépatologie Expérimentale.

REFERENCES

1. Meier S, Hay ED (1974) Dev Biol 38:249-270

2. Gospodarowicz D, Delgado D, Vlopavsky I (1980) Proc Natl acad Sci USA 77:4094

3. Kleinman HK, Klebe RJ, Martin GR (1981) J Cell Biol 88:473-485

4. Tseng SCG, Savion N, Gospodarowicz D, Stern R (1983) J Cell Biol 97:803-809

5. Vlodavsky I, Levi A, Lax I, Fuks Z, Schlesinger J (1982) J Dev Biol 93:285

6. Chambard M, Gabrion J, Mauchamp J (1981) J Cell Biol 91:157-166

7. Montesano R, Mouron P, Amherdt M, Orci L (1983) J Cell Biol 97:935-939

8. Hall HG, Farson DA, Bissell MJ (1982) Proc natl acad Sci USA 79:4672-4676

9. Hixson DC, Chesner J, Walborg Jr EJ (1980) J Cell Biol 87:121a

10. Rojkind MZ, Gatmaitan S, Mackensen M, Giambrone P, Reid L (1980) J Cell Biol 87:255-263

11. Wicha MS, Lowrie G, Kohn E, Bagavandoss P, Mahn T (1982) Proc natl acad Sci USA 79:3213-3217

12. Takiya C, Lenoir J, Grimaud JA (1986) Cell mol Biol 32:647-653

13. Grimaud JA, Druguet M, Peyrol S, Chevalier O, Herbage D, El Badrawy N (1980) J Histochem Cytochem 28:1145-1156

14. Bergman I, Loxley R (1963) Anal Chem 35:1961

15. Wagner WD, Salisbury BGJ (1978) Lab Invest 39:322-328

16. Bitter T, Muir H (1962) Anal Biochem 4:330-334

17. Dietrich CP, Dietrich SMC (1976) Anal Biochem 70:645-647

18. Emmerman JT, Pitelka DR (1977) In vitro 13:328-346

19. Dunn GA, Ebendal T (1978) Exp Cell Res 111:475-479

20. Campbell A, Wicha MS (1985) J Clin Invest 75:2085-2090

21. Fridman R, Alon Y, Doljanski F, Fuks Z, Vlodavsky I (1985) Exp Cell Res 158 : 461-476

22. Scott-Burden T, Bogenmann E, Jones PA (1986) Exp Cell Res 156:527-535

23. Thivolet CH, Chatelain P, Nicoloso H, Durand A, Bertrond J (1985) Exp Cell Res 159:313-322

24. Bellows CG, Melcher AH, Aubin JE (1981) J Cell Sci 50:299-314

25. Schor SL, Schor AM, Bazil GW (1981) J Cell Sci 48:301-314

26. Nusgens B, Merrill C, Lapiere C, Bell E (1984) Coll Rel Res 4:351-364

27. Wilde CJ, Hasan HB, Mayer RJ (1984) Exp Cell Res 151:519-532

28. Parry G, Lee EYH, Farson D, Koval M, Bissel MJ (1985) Exp Cell Res 156:487-499

29. Hixson DC, Ponce ML, Allison JP, Walborg EF (1984) Exp Cell Res 152:402-414

30. Kaecher-Djuricic V, Staubli A, Meyer JM, Ruch JV (1985) Differentiation 29:169-175

31. Lwebuga-Mukasa JS, Ingbar DH, Madri JA (1986) Exp Cell Res 162:423-435

32. Meezan EJ, Huelle T, Brendel K, Carson EC (1975) Life Sci 17:1721-1732

33. Peyrol S, Takiya C, Cordier JF, Grimaud JA (1986) Ann NY Acad Sci 465:268-285

34. Narayanan AS, Page RC, Kuzan F (1978) Lab Invest 39:61-65

IMMUNOHISTOCHEMICAL ANALYSIS OF SARCOID GRANULOMAS: EVIDENCE OF
PROLIFERATING LYMPHOCYTES AND PRESENCE OF CELLS WITH CYTOPLASMIC
INTERLEUKIN-1 (IL-1).

MARCO CHILOSI, PAOLA CAPELLI, MAURIZIO LESTANI, LICIA MONTAGNA,
GIOVANNI PIZZOLO (#), ANGIOLO CIPRIANI (^), CARLO AGOSTINI (*),
LIVIO TRENTIN (*), RENATO ZAMBELLO (*), GIAMPIETRO SEMENZATO (*).

Istituto di Anatomia Patologica, and Cattedra di Ematologia (#),
University of Verona; Istituto di Medicina Clinica (*) and
Divisione di Pneumologia (^), University of Padova, Italy.

INTRODUCTION

The main characteristic feature of sarcoidosis deals with an
accumulation of activated T-cells with the "helper phenotype"
(CD4), and activated macrophages at all sites of ongoing inflam_
mation (1-3). Several lines of evidence demonstrated that two
types of mechanisms are involved in this cellular accumulation
i.e. an enhanced recruitment of immunocompetent cells from the
peripheral pool via specific chemotactic factors (4) and/or a
local proliferation (5,6). In this study we have analyzed
lymphocyte and macrophage cell heterogeneity in inflamed tissues
of sarcoidosis patients with a panel of reagents including the
monoclonal antibody Ki67 which reacts with cells in the
proliferative phases G1, G2, M and S (7).

MATERIAL AND METHODS

Mediastinal lymph nodes. Fresh frozen tissue samples were
obtained from five patients with active sarcoidosis at surgery.

Bronchoalveolar lavage (BAL) samples were obtained from 16
untreated sarcoid patients. 10 patients were affected by active
disease.

Enzyme-histochemical and Immunohistochemical studies The numbers
of Ki67-positive lymphocytes and macrophages, were assessed by
counting cells exhibiting Ki67 nuclear staining associated with
membrane-bound reactivity for CD3 (Leu-4) and/or cytoplasmic

reactivity for alpha-naphthyl acetate esterase (ANAE). More than 500 cells were evaluated on each cytospin preparation using a 40x objective. The alkaline-phosphatase anti-alkaline phosphatase (APAAP) and avidin-biotin peroxidase (ABC) techniques were used in combination for revealing nuclear Ki67 antigen together with differentiation antigen on cell membranes (8). For Ki67/ANAE double-staining technique the immunochemical demonstration of Ki67 was performed first, using the APAAP technique, followed by the ANAE reaction. The anti IL-1 antibody was a rabbit antiserum specific for recombinat interleukin-1 (Cistron, NJ)

RESULTS

In sarcoid lymph nodes the epithelioid granulomas were surrounded by cells mainly characterized by the CD4+ "helper/ inducer" phenotype. A variable number of Ki67+ cells were seen around granulomas, scattered or in small foci. Double marker analysis with Ki67 and membrane differentiation antigens defined these cells as T lymphocytes (CD3+), predominantly expressing the CD4 "helper/inducer" phenotype. A number of Ki67+ T-cells could be demonstrated also within granulomas.

Macrophages The double marker techniques (Ki67 plus ANAE or other macrophage-related markers) could not demonstrate the presence of replicating macrophages within or around sarcoid granulomas in any sample studied. BAL preparations from all patients with active disease contained a large number of lymphocytes (28%-53%; mean 38+7). In all cases most lymphocytes (mean 88%+9) were of T origin (CD3+) and exhibited the "helper/inducer" phenotype (CD4+/CD8 ratio: 8.2+2.3). In all samples from patients with active disease a proportion of Ki67+ replicating lymphoid-looking cells were detectable (4%-10%; mean 6.2+ 2.2). Double-staining techniques showed that we are actually dealing with ANAE-, CD3+, CD4+ cells. The lymphocytes were absent or scanty in the samples obtained from patients with inactive disease and Ki67 positive lymphocytes in these preparations were never observed.

Variable numbers of Ki67+/ANAE+ macrophages were seen in all BAL samples from patients with sarcoidosis. The proportions of replicating macrophages ranged between 2% and 14% (mean 6.5+3.7) (active: mean 6.8+3.48; nonactive: mean 6.0+4.51) and did not appear significantly related to disease activity.

Reactivity with anti-IL-1 antibody: An evident immunoreactivity for IL-1 could be demonstrated in all sarcoid lymph node samples. This was confined to cells forming epithelioid granulomas. The reactivity appeared evenly distributed in the cytoplasm of epithelioid cells.Giant cells were mainly devoid of IL-1 reactivity, with the exception of a thin, rather intense rim of staining at the membrane edge. In BAL preparations most alveolar macrophages (70-95%) exhibited cytoplasmic immunoreactivity for IL-1. IL-1 content and cell-distribution were similar in samples from both active and non-active disease patients.

DISCUSSION

Ki67+/CD4+ lymphocytes were found in BAL samples from most active sarcoid patients, as well as in particular areas in lymph node samples. Our analysis confirms and extends previous observations suggesting that an enhanced cell proliferation takes place at sites of ongoing inflammation in sarcoidosis. We observed that the presence of proliferating CD4+ lymphocytes is a common feature of different affected tissues. A proportion of Ki67+ macrophages could be also demonstrated in all BAL preparations of our series, unexpectedly irrespective of the activity. Another interesting observation in our study was the peculiar distribution of the replicating cells in affected lymph nodes. As expected, CD4+ T-lymphocytes were the main cell-population with replicating capability. These cells were mainly seen in extra-granulomatous T-cell areas, and to a lesser extent within granulomas. Granuloma macrophages never expressed features of replication activity in our study, despite a careful search on many granulomas with the Ki67/ANAE combined method.

In this study we also provide evidence that alveolar macrophages in sarcoid BAL contain a large amount of IL-1 related molecules, thus confirming their activated status. Nevertheless this feature does not appear to be related with the activity of the disease. Furthermore, epithelioid macrophages in lymph node granulomas expressed strong cytoplasmic immunostaining with anti-IL-1 antibody. Interestingly, giant cells were mainly devoid of the IL-1 molecule. These data suggest that in sarcoidosis the accumulation and proliferation of IL-1 laden phagocytes at sites of disease activity is not sufficient to induce inflammation phenomena and that a cooperative signal from activated CD4+ lymphocytes is needed for triggering the release of mediator molecules and consequent tissue damage.

REFERENCES

1. Hunninghake GW, Crystal RG (1981) N Engl J Med 305:429-434
2. Semenzato G, Pezzutto A, Chilosi M, Pizzolo G (1982) N Engl J Med 306:48-49
3. Semenzato G, Agostini C, et al.(1986) Ann NY Acad Sci 465:56-73
4. Beer DJ, Crulshank WW, Kornfeld H, Berman JS (1985) Am Rev Respir Dis 131:A14
5. Venet A, Hance AJ, et al. (1985) J Clin Invest 75:293-301
6. Bitterman PB, Saltzman LE, et al. (1984) J Clin Invest 74:460-469
7. Gerdes J, Lemke H, et al. (1984) J Immunol 133:1710-1715
8. Chilosi M, Menestrina F, et al. (1986) Bas Appl Histochem 30:55 (Abstr.)

FIBRONECTIN (FN) IN SARCOIDOSIS: EVALUATION OF PLASMA LEVELS AND DISTRIBUTION IN LUNG TISSUE.

*CARLO ALBERA,**LAURA VIBERTI,*BRUNO BARTONE,*PAOLO GHIO,*FRANCO BARDESSONO,
*GIORGIO SCAGLIOTTI,*FELICE GOZZELINO,*LUIGI PESCETTI AND*GIOVANNI PESCETTI.

University of Turin, Pulmonary Diseases Departement * and Pathology Service **
S.Luigi Gonzaga Hospital, 10043 Orbassano (Torino, Italy).

INTRODUCTION

Sarcoidosis is a systemic granulomatous disease characterized by an accumulation of inflammatory, immunocompetent cells within the alveolar stuctures, leading either to a complete resolution or to lung fibrosis (1). Fibronectin (FN)is a glyco-protein of molecular weight 440 000 daltons, involved in the interaction of cells with extracellular matrix playing a role in the dynamic balance of the lung cellular and extracellular integrity and topography (2). Furthermore FN was been identified, as well as other substances, in the number of mediators released by activated mononuclear cells in pulmonary sarcoidosis (3); these substances are involved in the lung injury mechanisms as well as in its reparative process. Some of these substances may be detected in peripheral blood, in BAL fluid, in tissues and on cells surface.(1)

In this context, the present study was designed to evaluate FN plasma levels and FN distribution in lung tissue in sarcoidosis patients with different disease stages, different disease activity and during steroid therapy.

PATIENTS AND METHODS

Were studied 35 patients (15 males, 20 females, mean age 41.5) having biopsy proven sarcoidosis; 10 were smokers; the disease duration was ranging from 1 to 60 months; the chest X ray stage was: 2 stage 0, 10 stage I, 21 stage II and 2 stage III (parenchimal lesions in 23/35 cases); 8 patients were on steroids. As control population was used a group of 13 normal individuals (6 males, 8 females, mean age 37, 7 smokers) and 4 subjects with other lung diseases: 2 cases of miliary tubercolosis and 2 cases of ILD Progressive Systemic Sclerosis (PSS) associated; all these patients were non smokers females with mean age 37 years and were not on steroids. Bronchoalveolar lavage (BAL) and 67 Ga scan were performed and evaluated as previously described (4).

Plasma FN level was determined using the immuno-turbidimetric assay(Boehringer, Mannheim)in peripheral blood samples collected with EDTA, reading the absorbance at 365 nm in a Varian DMS 90 spectrophotometer; the results are expressed as FN μg/ml; (normal range = mean value in healthy controls $\pm$ 2 sd.) Tissue FN was detected in fixed, parafine embedded biopsy specimens by immuno-reaction using policlonal rabbit antibody against both, plasma and tissue FN with peroxidase-antiperoxidase method (PAP)(Bio Genex laboratories). Statistical evaluation was performed with t Student's test for unpaired data.

RESULTS

Results obtained in our study are showed in figure n.1. Plasma FN was high in 13/35 (37.4%) sarcoidosis patients and low in 5/35 (14.2%). The mean value in sarcoidosis and in healthy were respectively 366.9 $\pm$ 131.5 and 328.3 $\pm$ 37.7 μg/ml. (p=ns). Three of 4 patients with other lung disease showed an hig FN plasma level. In 8 sarcoidosis patients on steroid therapy FN plasma levels were lower (mean values) (280 $\pm$ 147.71 μg/ml) than those measured in the 27 untreated cases (386.66 $\pm$ 122.33 μg/ml) with statistically significative difference ($p < 0.05$).

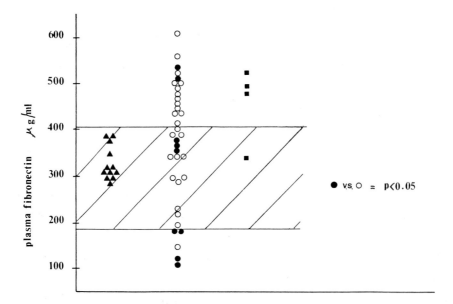

fig. n. 1 : fibronectin plasma levels in
o sarcoidosis ($\bullet$ on steroid)
$\blacksquare$ other lung diseases
$\blacktriangle$ healthy controls

FN plasma levels were examined in 4 groups of sarcoidosis patients differing for: disease duration (1–12/13–60 months), parenchimal involvement at the chest X ray (yes/no), 67 Ga lung scan (+/−), and BAL lymphocites ($\geqslant$30% /$\leqslant$ 30%). The results in these groups were respectively: 390+121.5/312.5+147.5; 385+145/332+96.8; 399.5+112/310+140.5; 370.3+102.6/331+172.8; p= ns in all groups.

Tissue FN was detected in 15/23 (62.2%) lung biopsy specimens from sarcoidosis patients. FN immunoreactivity localizes in macrophages as well as in extracellular matrix and within endothelial structures; was no evidence of positive reaction in granulomas. Positive reaction localizes with the same pattern in biopsies from tuberculosis and ILD PSS associated (more evident positive reaction in endothelial structures in PSS). FN plasma levels was 345+112.12 in cases with positive tissue reaction and 298+157.3 in case with negative tissue FN (p=ns).

DISCUSSION

Some authors referred that: A) an early evidence of FN in alveolar structures during experimental paraquat lung fibrosis (5), B) high FN serum levels (6) or decreased circulating FN accompained by acquisition of surface FN and enhanced expression of a FN receptor on alveolar macrophages (7) in hyperoxic pulmonary injury. Moreover alveolar macrophages from patients with Idiopathic Pulmonary Fibrosis (IPF) show higher FN secretion than those from healthy controls (8); alveolar macrophages from patients with ILD PSS associated show the same characteristics (9).

On the other hand, Rennard and coll.(2) observed that, plasma FN levels were within the normal range in 20 sarcoidosis patients as in other interstitial or non interstitial lung diseases without any relationship with prednisone therapy, and FN in BAL fluid was increased in ILD. The authors conclude that, FN in BAL may be either produced or concentrated locally or more slowly removed.

From the above referred data it is clear that, the mechanisms involved in the modification of FN levels in plasma and tissues, and the relationship between plasma FN and lung tissue FN, are multiple and not completely understood.

In our study FN plasma levels show no significative difference in studied subjects in agreement with the results obtained by Rennard and coll. (2)

The difference in treated patients, which in our study showed lower FN plasma levels, may be related either to an aspecific reduction of protein synthesis or to a specific action on the ativated macrophages in sarcoidosis patients.

The FN tissue distribution observed in examined cases, seems to be related to

FN secreting cells as well as to FN (plasma FN?, FN from macrophages?) extracellular deposition.

In conclusion further data, particularly FN localisation in tissues, FN levels in plasma and in BAL fluid, FN and FN receptors on cell surface, must be evaluated to completely understand the role of fibronectin in the developement of lung fibrosis in pulmonary sarcoidosis.

REFERENCES

1. Hunninghake GW, Garrett KC, Richerson HB, Fantone JC, Ward PA, Rennard SI, Bitterman PB, Crystal RG.(1984) Am Rev Respir Dis 130:476–496

2. Rennard SI, Crystal RG.(1981) J Clin Invest 69:113–122

3. Saltini C, Crystal RG.(1985) Int Archs Allergy appl Immun suppl 1 92–100

4. Albera C, Ghio P, Besso P, Pescetti G, Bardessono F, Scagliotti G, Gozzelino F, Aversa S, Viberti L, Giuliano.(1986) Lotta contro la Tubercolosi e le malattie polmonari sociali. 56:107–115

5. Fukuda Y, Ferrans VJ, Schoenberger CI, Rennard SI, Crystal RG.(1985) Am J Pathol 118:452–475

6. Glass M, Kaplan JE, Macarak E, Aukberg SJ, Fisher AB.(1984) Am Rev Respir Dis 130:237–241

7. Kradin RL, Zhu Y, Hales CA, Bianco C, Colvin RB.(1986) Am J Pathol 125:349–357

8. Bitterman PB, Adelberg S, Crystal RG.(1983) J Clin Invest 72:1801–1813

9. Rossi GA, Bitterman PB, Rennard SI, Ferrans VJ, Crystal RG.(1985) Am Rev Respir Dis 131:612–617

GENERATION OF SUPEROXIDE ANION BY ALVEOLAR MACROPHAGES IN
SARCOIDOSIS .

M.A. CASSATELLA*, G. BERTON*, C. AGOSTINI[+], R. ZAMBELLO[+],
L.TRENTIN[+], A. CIPRIANI& AND G. SEMENZATO[+]
*Institute of General Pathology, University of Verona; [+]Department
of Clinical Medicine, 1st Medical Clinic and Clinical Immunology
Branch, and &Department of Pneumology, University of Padua; Italy

INTRODUCTION

There is a general agreement that the interaction between

lymphocytes and macrophages plays a central role in the

pathogenesis of sarcoidosis (1,2). Since molecules derived from the

reduction of oxygen are well known as mediators of lung injury (3),

the activation of the macrophage capability to produce toxic

oxygen molecules by lymphocytes-derived factors could be

responsible for the development of the tissue damage in sarcoid

lung.

We present here results of studies on the oxygen metabolism of

macrophages recovered from the bronchoalveolar lavage (BAL) of

patients with sarcoidosis. We show that alveolar macrophages (AM)

from sarcoid patients produce higher amounts of superoxide anion

(O_2^-) upon triggering and that there is a good correlation between

capability to metabolize oxygen and the state of the disease.

MATERIAL AND METHODS
__Study population.__ A total of 43 patients (23 men, 20 women; mean
age 36.6+11) were studied. On the basis of percentage and absolute
numbers/ml of T lymphocytes recovered from the BAL and, when
available, the positivity of ^{67}Ga scan, the following groups of
patients were defined: i) 23 patients with active sarcoidosis: high
intensity lymphocytic alveolitis($>$ 28%, $>$50x10^3 lymphocytes in
the BAL) and ^{67}Ga scan positivity; ii) 20 patients with inactive
sarcoidosis: low intensity lymphocytic alveolitis ($<$ 12%, $<$
25x10^3/ml lymphocytes in the BAL) and ^{67}Ga scan negativity.
    Isolation and cultivation of alveolar macrophages. BAL mono-
nuclear cells were obtained and depleted of T lymphocytes as

previously described (4). AM were suspended in Krebs ringer phosphate buffer containing calcium and glucose (KRPCaG, 5) when they were assayed immediately for O_2^- production. For cultivation, AM were suspended in RPMI containing 50U/ml penicillin, 50μg/ml streptomycin and 10% heat inactivated foetal calf serum. AM were plated at a density of 2.0×10^5 cells/well in a volume of 0.5 ml in 24 wells trays.

O_2^- production. AM were assayed immediately after the isolation in 24 wells trays as described in reference 6. Assays of AM monolayers were performed as described in references 5 and 6.

Proteins. These were assayed in AM monolayers as described in reference 5.

RESULTS AND DISCUSSION.

Figure 1 shows O_2^- production by AM obtained from BAL of sarcoid patients and assayed immediately after isolation. AM produced a low but consistent amount of O_2^- also spontaneously and this was likely

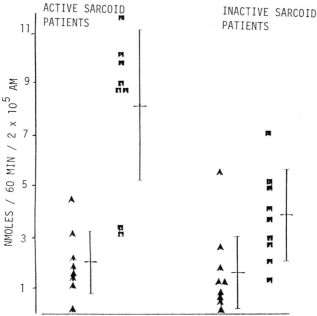

Figure 1. O_2^- production by sarcoid AM assayed immediately after the isolation. Triangles: spontaneous activity. Squares: activity in the presence of 100 ng/ml PMA. The mean results of duplicate assays of each independent experiment and the means ± SD are reported. The difference between the spontaneous activity of active and inactive sarcoid AM was not significant. For the PMA-stimulated activity p was <0.01.

due to adherence and spreading to the tissue culture plasic used

for the incubation of the cells (6). This unstimulated production

was comparable in AM of active and inactive sarcoid patients. PMA

simulated the O_2^- production by AM, but in AM of active sarcoid

patients this was two times higher than in AM of inactive sarcoid

patients.

Figure 2 shows data of O_2^- production by AM of sarcoid patients

after two days of cultivation. The O_2^- production by AM of healthy

subjects is reported for comparison. The spontaneous O_2^- production

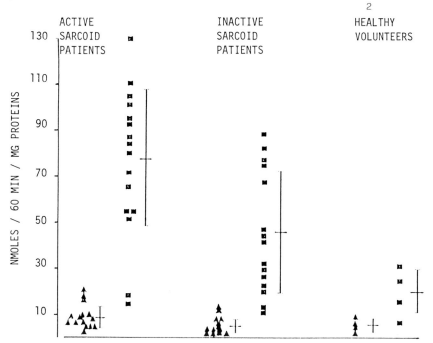

Figure 2. O_2^- production by sarcoid and normal AM after two days of
cultivation. Triangles: spontaneous activity. Squares: activity in
the presence of 100 ng/ml PMA. The results of duplicate assays of
each independent experiment and the means + SD are reported. The
differences between the spontaneous activity of the three
population tested were not significant. For the PMA-stimulated
activity, p was < 0.001 when the mean values obtained with inactive
sarcoid AM were compared either with healthy volunteers or active
sarcoid patients.

by AM after two days of cultivation was negligible. The production of O_2^- was effectively stimulated by PMA but to a different extent in the three population tested. AM of sarcoid patients produced more O_2^- in response to PMA than control AM. In sarcoid AM the production of O_2^- was correlated with the state of the disease since AM isolated from BAL of patients with active sarcoidosis produced higher amounts of O_2^- in response to PMA.

In conclusion, the results presented in this paper show that in patients with sarcoidosis AM are activated in their capability to metabolize oxygen with production of O_2^-. In the active state of the disease, when T lymphocytes accumulate in the alveolus this capability is enhanced in comparison with the inactive state when alveolitis is of low intensity.

ACKNOWLEDGEMENTS
   Supported in part by grants from C.N.R., " Gruppo Immunologia"(N. 86.00478.04) and from University of Padova(N. 12.01.4689).

REFERENCES
1. Hunninghake GW, Garrett KC, Richerson HB; Fantone JC, Ward PA, Rennard SI, Bitterman PB, Crystal RG (1984) Am Rev Resp Dis 130:476-496

2. Semenzato GP (1986) Sem Respir Med 8:17-29

3. Fantone JC, Ward PA (1984) Am Rev Resp Dis 130:484-491

4. Semenzato GP, Agostini C, Zambello R, Trentin L, Chilosi M, Angi MR, Ossi E, Cipriani A, Pizzolo G (1986) Ann NY Acad Sci 465:56-73

5. Berton G, Cassatella MA, Cabrini G, Rossi F (1985) Immunology 54:371-379

6. Berton G, Gordon S (1983) Immunology 49:693-704

EFFECTS OF MURAMYLDIPEPTIDE AND INDOMETHACIN ON SCHISTOSOME EGG-INDUCED GRANU-
LOMATOUS INFLAMMATION IN THE LUNG

SEM H. PHAN, STEVEN L. KUNKEL

Department of Pathology M0602, University of Michigan Medical School, Ann
Arbor, MI 48109-0602, USA.

INTRODUCTION

Lung granulomatous inflammation in sarcoidosis can progress and result in
pulmonary fibrosis. The macrophage appears to play a key role in the fibrotic
process. There is evidence that the macrophage in granulomatous lesion is
activated (1,2) and thus likely to be releasing a multitude of mediators, and
whose release are modulated by certain agonists and arachidonate metabolites
(3,4). Muramyldipeptide (MDP) stimulates mediator release, while endogenous
prostaglandin E_2 (PGE_2) is an inhibitor of mediator release (3,4), and of
fibroblast proliferation and collagen synthesis (5,6). In this study, MDP and
indomethacin (an inhibitor of endogenous PGE_2 production) were administered to
animals with schistosome egg-induced lung granulomatous inflammation to examine
if pulmonary fibrosis could be induced by such attempts at enhancing macrophage
mediator release.

MATERIALS AND METHODS

Animals and Induction of Model. Female CBA/J mice weighing 20-25 mg were used
throughout this study. Schistosome egg-induced lung granulomatous inflammation
was induced as previously described (7). Egg-treated animals were treated with
5 mg/kg indomethacin intraperitoneally (i.p.) daily, 5 mg/kg MDP i.p. daily,
or both. Control groups consisted of untreated animals, and animals treated
with the above-indicated agents, but without receiving schistosome eggs. All
treatments started at day 0, and at days 9 and 15, animals were sacrificed for
the determination of mean lung granuloma size and lung collagen synthesis and
deposition.

Morphometry and Lung Collagen Metabolism. Measurements of lung granuloma
areas, collagen synthesis and hydroxyproline content were done as previously
described (7,8).

Statistics. Mean values of treatment groups were compared with that of control
or other treatment groups using the Student's t-test when comparing two groups

at a time. A p-value <0.05 was considered to be statistically significant.

RESULTS

Control animals administered schistosome eggs alone had a mean granuloma size of 26258 ± 1259 μm^2 (Table I) on day 15. Concomitant treatment with indomethacin did not significantly increased the mean granuloma size. In contrast, treatment with MDP caused a dose dependent increase in granuloma size up to as high as 134% of control (p<0.001) at a dose of 5 mg/kg, and decreasing to 113% of control which was not statistically significant. Concomitant treatment with both MDP and indomethacin caused no further significant increase above those levels caused by the corresponding doses of MDP alone.

TABLE I EFFECTS OF SCHISTOSOME EGGS, MDP AND INDOMETHACIN ON LUNG GRANULOMA SIZE.

Treatment	Dose mg/kg	Granuloma Size μm^2	Significance(p)*
(SE)**	-	26258+/-1259	-
(SE) + MDP	2.50	32282+/-1416	<0.002
(SE) + MP	5.00	35198+/-1587	<0.001
(SE) + MDP	10.00	29582+/-1582	>0.05(NS)
(SE) + INDO	5.00	28320+/-1537	>0.05(NS)
(SE) + MDP+ INDO	2.50 5.00	31474+/-1875	<0.02
(SE) + MDP+ INDO	5.00 5.00	33278+/-1729	<0.002
(SE) + MDP+ INDO	10.00 5.00	31237+/-1690	<0.02

*Compared to schistosome eggs alone.
**Abbreviations used were SE, schistosome eggs; and INDO, indomethacin.

Analysis of lung collagen synthesis and deposition revealed no significant enhancement above the respective control levels, except for the group treated with both MDP and indomethacin at the 15 day time point (Tables II and III). A 30% increase (p<0.005 vs. schistosome eggs alone) in total lung collagen (Table II) was present in the group receiving eggs, indomethacin and 5 mg/kg MDP at the 15 day time point. Histologic examination of lung tissue revealed that the increase in collagen was primarily in around the granulomas, with no evidence of significant interstitial pattern of fibrosis. All other treatment or control groups show no significant increase in lung collagen content when compared to the control, untreated group.

TABLE II

EFFECTS OF SE, MDP AND INDOMETHACIN ON TOTAL LUNG COLLAGEN CONTENT

TREATMENT	LUNG COLLAGEN CONTENT[1]	
	DAY 9	DAY 15
SE	93 ± 5	95 ± 4.4
SE + INDO[2]	95 ± 2.2	91 ± 7.6
SE + MDP[2]	88 ± 7.1	110 ± 8.0
SE + INDO + MDP[2]	108 ± 2.8	130 ± 5.63[3]

[1]Data expressed as mean ± SE, N = 4-7. Data calculated as μg hydroxy-proline per lung, and expressed as % of control (untreated) mean value.
[2]Indo and MDP does were 5 mg/kg and 5 mg/kg, respectively.
[3]p <0.01 vs. control (untreated mean and p<0.005 vs. SE mean.

This increase in lung collagen deposition is due to a net increase in lung collagen synthesis as shown by the data in Table III. Thus, animals treated with eggs, MDP and indomethacin showed a greater than two-fold increase in collagen synthesis at the 15 day time point when compared to untreated controls. This increase was significant at $p < 0.001$ versus untreated controls, and at $p < 0.02$ versus controls receiving eggs only.

TABLE III

EFFECTS OF SE, MDP AND INDOMETHACIN ON LUNG COLLAGEN SYNTHESIS

TREATMENT	LUNG COLLAGEN SYNTHESIS[1]	
	DAY 9	DAY 15
SE	108 ± 14.5	150 ± 28
SE + INDO[2]	ND	78.6 ± 10.3
SE + MDP[2]	103 ± 13.5	142.5 ± 15.2
SE + INDO + MDP[2]	70 ± 8.7	238 ± 10.5[3]

[1]Data expressed as means ± SE with N = 4-7 after conversation as % of control (untreated mean value. ND implies not determined.
[2]Indomethacin and MDP doses were 5 mg/kg and 5 mg/kg, respectively.
[3]p<0.001 when compared vs. control (untreated) mean, and p<0.02 vs. SE mean.

DISCUSSION

Based on previous data showing the inhibitory effects of the cyclooxygenase product, PGE_2, and the stimulatory effects of lipopolysaccharide and MDP on macrophage mediator production, this study was undertaken to see if enhancement of such mediator release by administration of the cyclooxygenase inhibitor indomethacin, and MDP could enhance lung granulomatous inflammation and induce pulmonary fibrosis. The results show that MDP alone could stimulate lung granulomatous inflammation, and that the addition of indomethacin had no further enhancing effect. On the other hand, the combination of MDP and indomethacin was needed to cause a significant increase in lung collagen deposition and synthesis. These data would suggest that the mere stimulation of macrophage mediator release by MDP is not sufficient to induce a fibrotic response in the lung. It would appear that removal of the inhibitory effects of PGE_2 on macrophage mediator release and/or fibroblast proliferation and collagen synthesis would also be required to achieve fibrosis. Even then the fibrosis remains circumscribed, and it may be that another factor(s) is required to achieve more extensive interstitial fibrosis. However, this model may be useful as the basis for the development of a more useful of sarcoidosis or lung granulomatous disease with potential for progression to pulmonary fibrosis.

ACKNOWLEDGEMENTS

This work was partially supported by grants HL28737, HL31237 and HL31963 from the NIH. Drs. Phan and Kunkel are Established Investigators of the American Heart Association. We would like to thank Kathleen Atkins for her superb editorial assistance and, Bridget McGarry for excellent technical asssistance.

REFERENCES

1. Kunkel SL, Chensue SW, Plewa M, Higashi GI (1984) Am J Pathol 114:240-249
2. Kunkel SL, Chensue SW, Mouton C, Higashi GI (1984) J Clin Invest 74:514-524
3. Kunkel SL, Chensue SW, Phan SH (1986) J Immunol 136:186-192
4. Phan SH, McGarry BM, Loeffler KM, Kunkel SL (1987) J Leuk Biol 42:106-113
5. Baum BJ, Moss J, Breul SD, Crystal RG (1978) J Biol Chem 253:3391-3397
6. Elias JA, Zurier RB, Schreiber AD, Leff JA, Daniele RP (1985) J Leuk Biol 37:15-21
7. Chensue SW, Kunkel SL, Ward PA, Higashi GI (1983) Am J Pathol 111:78-87
8. Phan SH, Kunkel SL (1986) Am J Pathol 124:343-352

© 1988 Elsevier Science Publishers B.V. (Biomedical Division)
Sarcoidosis and other granulomatous disorders
C. Grassi, G. Rizzato, E. Pozzi, editors

RELATIONSHIP BETWEEN MARKERS OF MACROPHAGE AND FIBROBLAST ACTIVITY IN
BRONCHOALVEOLAR LAVAGE FLUID IN SARCOIDOSIS.

ELEONORA BLASCHKE[1], ANDERS EKLUND[2], ROGER HÄLLGREN[3], ROINE HERNBRAND[1],
ÅKE HANNGREN[2].
[1]Clinical Chemistry Dept; [2]Thoracic Medicine Dept, Karolinska Hospital,
Stockholm; [3]Internal Medicine Dept, University Hospital, Uppsala, Sweden.

INTRODUCTION

Elevated fibronectin in the BAL fluid (L-Fn) in sarcoid patients, possibly
derived from alveolar macrophages, may be a link in the development of fibrosis
by chemoattraction of fibroblasts (1). Elevated hyaluronan in the BAL fluid
(L-HA) of sarcoids reflects probably an activation of fibroblasts (2). We
examined therefore the relationships between L-Fn, L-HA and signs of alveolitis.

PATIENTS AND METHODS

Seventy-four patients with histologically proven sarcoidosis (mean age 39 $\pm$
11 yrs, 44 women, 12 smokers) and 57 healthy volunteers (mean age 30 $\pm$ 11 yrs,
32 women, 33 smokers) were lavaged (3) with 5 x 50 ml saline (mean recovery 63 $\pm$
12 %). After centrifugation of the BAL fluid at 400 g for 5 min differential
cell counts were made and the supernatant analyzed for albumin (L-Alb) and ACE
(3). L-Fn was assayed with a double-sandwich ELISA developed in our laboratory,
using normal and HRP-labelled antifibronectin antisera (Dakopatts). The lower
limit of sensitivity was 10 ug/L, the coefficient of variation 3.7 %. L-HA was
analyzed with a Pharmacia research kit (2). The Mann-Whitney test and Spearman's
correlation coefficient were used for statistics.

RESULTS

L-Fn was significantly (p < 0.001) elevated in sarcoids (median Fn 280, inter-
quartile range 100 - 602 ug/L) compared to controls (43, 24 - 72 ug/L). Similarly, L-HA was significantly higher (p < 0.001) in sarcoids (median 39, 28 - 71
ug/L) than in controls (25, 16 - 30 ug/L). Also L-Alb was significantly (p <
0.001) increased in sarcoids (74, 46 - 106 mg/L) compared to controls (36, 30 -
43 mg/L).

L-Fn correlated significantly (p < 0.001) with L-HA and L-Alb (Fig 1a-b) and
to a lesser degree with L-ACE (r = 0.66, p < 0.001) and the percentage of L-
lymphocytes (r = 0.38, p < 0.001). It did not correlate with the number of
alveolar macrophages.

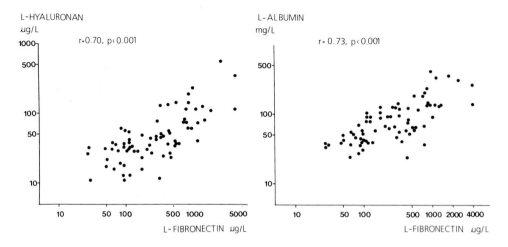

Fig. 1a-b.   Correlation between L-Fn and L-HA (a) and L-Albumin (b).

Eleven patients were lavaged at two consecutive occasions. L-Fn, L-HA
and L-Alb increased concomitantly in 4 and decreased concomitantly in 5 of the
patients. Lymphocyte percentages and L-ACE varied more.

CONCLUSIONS

1) The elevated levels and the close relationship of L-Fn and L-HA suggest that
    fibronectin in sarcoidosis may function as a mediator between alveolar macro-
    phages and fibroblasts.

2) As the correlation between L-Fn and L-ACE indicates, the fibronectin may
    originate in activated alveolar macrophages.

3) A prerequisite for an increased production of fibronectin in macrophages may
    be an alveolar inflammatory process characterized by an injured alveolar-
    capillary membrane, as the high L-Alb and the strong correlation of L-Fn and
    L-Alb indicate.

4) Fibronectin may be a chemoattractant for fibroblasts which in turn produce
    hyaluronan, but fibronectin and hyaluronan could also serve, possibly
    together with fibrin, as matrix for subsequent cell migration, leading to
    fibrosis.

REFERENCES

1) Rennard SI & Crystal RG (1982) J Clin Invest 69:113-122.
2) Hällgren R et al. (1985) Br Med J 290:1778-1781.
3) Eklund A & Blaschke E (1986) Thorax 41:629-634.

© 1988 Elsevier Science Publishers B.V. (Biomedical Division)
Sarcoidosis and other granulomatous disorders
C. Grassi, G. Rizzato, E. Pozzi, editors

PATHOLOGY FROM GRANULOMA TO FIBROSIS : OUTLOOK

A.BLASI - Naples - Italy.

This Session on the Pathology from granuloma to fibrosis foca-
lized some aspects on this topic, whose interest is not only
concerning the pathological point of view, but also the related immunological, physiopathological and clinical questions.
Some of this questions were pointed from the participants-as
speakers- at our Session.
The pathological reconstruction presented by Françoise Basset
gave us a complete view of the movement leading from granuloma
to fibrosis.
Fibrosis is - indeed - a potential risk for all,or fast all
the granulomatous disorders of the lung.

The fibrosing risk in Sarcoidosis:
In the Sarcoidosis the fibrosing risk is actually realizing
in the 10-15% of all the cases of intrathoracic involvement.
It is singular that in the Sarcoidosis the histological movement towards the fibrosis is realizing in the lung, but is
very poor in the glands and never present in the liver and eye
lesions.In this connection -I think so- it is to consider that
in the liver and in the eye it is no present, in the granuloma, the participation of the activated alveolar macrophages,
whose roll is determinant for the release of the principles
producing fibrosis.
As it was stressed in our Session by Basset, the pathological
steps induced in the lung by the sarcoid movement are marked
by:
- mural or luminal alveolitis
- isolated or aggregated granulomas with
possible vascular involvement
- fibrosis.
The derangement of the alveolar structures induced by alveolitis and the maintenance of the alveolitis,are thedeterminant
factors for the formation of the granuloma and fibrosis.
Although the ultrastructural investigations have the incontro-
vertible aptitude to detail all the morpho-functional charac-

ters of the activated effector cells (macrophages and lymphocytes); and although the bronchial lavage permits to collect
the cellular population related to the different phases of the
lung open biopsy and the traditional optic microscopy is,still
now, the best and the more suggestive way to follow-up the
steps and the mutual relationship from alveolitis, granuloma,
fibrosis,until the "end stage" of pulmonary sarcoidosis.

The "long" and the "short" way from sarcoid granuloma to fibrosis.
The appearance of a collagenous extracellular matrix is a early
morphological announcement of the incoming fibrosis.
I should like now to ask: it is possible the movement from alveolitis to fibrosis without the granuloma formation?
I think that in the majiority of cases the steps are:alveoli-
tis - granuloma - fibrosis; but it is also possible a"short
way" of the sarcoid fibrosis: persistent alveolitis - fibrosis.

Reversibility of sarcoid fibrosis.
An other question is concerning the reversibility of the fibrosis.
In personal observations, I have some cases of sarcoidosis in
stage III, with general and functional compromissions, in which
the lung open biopsy demonstrates - in the histological specimens - a sarcoid granulomatous disorder with an evident collagenous networks. After steroid therapy, a persistent clinical
recovery was obtained, with return to the radiological and physiological normality.
According to G.James and W.Jones Williams, it is to presume
that some forms of collagen (Type III perhaps) are completely
reversible.

Final clinical remark.
The traditional Stage III of intrathoracic Sarcoidosis,inclu-
des many cases of lung involvement which really have different overlapping radiological changes -micronodular,nodular,
reticular,reticulo-nodular- and also different clinical cha-
racters and different destiny: sometime with a complete and
definitive recovery, sometime with persistent radiological

changes and irreversible disability.

So it is convenient and justifiable-according to the opinion
of our Colleague Om P.Sharma- to enrol in Stage III the cases
with X ray abnormality of diffuse pulmonary infiltration or
micronodular or reticulo-nodular interstitial pattern and with
evident respondence to steroid therapy; and to add a Stage IV
to include the situations in which fibrosis reached advanced
radiological changes and irreversible disabiliting steps.

In this way, the Stage IV would be corresponding to the pathological "end stage" of Sarcoidosis,in which massive fibrosis
and hialinosis induce the loss of the alveolar unit.

REFERENCES

1.James G.Jones Williams W. (1985) Sarcoidosis and other granulomatous disorders.W.B.Saunders Company,London.

2.Sharma O.P. (1975) Sarcoidosis - A Clinical Approach
Charles Thomas,Publisher,Springfield.

EPIDEMIOLOGY

EPIDEMIOLOGY OF SARCOIDOSIS   STATE-OF-THE-ART

YUTAKA HOSODA

Radiation Effects Research Foundation (RERF) Hiroshima, Japan

INTRODUCTION

Sarcoidosis detected and undetected

Epidemiology is defined as the science of occurrence of diseases in human populations (A. Ahlbom and S. Norell). Sarcoidosis is detected in various ways; patients' complaints, incidental X-rays or periodical mass X-rays. There are also some cases which cannot be detected even by annual mass X-rays because their BHL develops and then disappears asymptomatically during the interval between the annual mass surveys. In the Japanese working population in which sarcoidosis notification has been made since 1960, 90% of the cases were detected by annual mass X-rays and the remaining 10% by complaints. When progress of the disease is taken into account, a high resolution rate is observed during the first two years after onset, followed by a lowered rate, especially beyond five years after onset. The rate of persistent cases ranges from 10% to 30%, depending on the means by which the cases were detected.[1] Except for acute onset cases, the so-called "insidious cases" may be the remnants of asymptomatic cases. There may be several cases undetected for each insidious symptomatic case. When disease frequency is discussed, these should be taken into consideration.

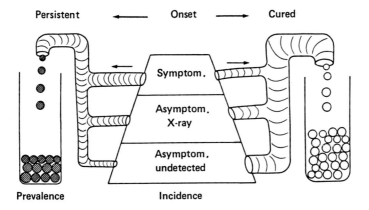

Figure 1   Sarcoidosis, detected and undetected

Standardization

In any epidemiological study, standardization of methodology is vital. Two topics in this regard will be discussed below.

Diagnostic criterion   There is general agreement that this disease should be diagnosed by both clinical and histological evidence. The most reliable method of case collection is to deal with only histologically proven cases. However, true sarcoidosis cases will be included even among histologically unproven cases. If such cases are excluded, the frequency of the disease may be considerably underestimated. In 1960, the Washington Conference on Sarcoidosis proposed four diagnostic criteria; histologically proven cases as groups I, II and III and histologically unproven cases as group IV, with a note that group IV is acceptable for study under special circumstances as in some epidemiologic investigations. The Conference, however, did not specify a clinical criterion for group IV. Inquiries on group IV were made internationally to famous sarcoidologists by the author. Twenty replies have so far been received. Histologically unproven sarcoidosis was unconditonally accepted by one and conditionally by 14 and was not accepted by five. Those who responded with conditional acceptance had a common view of group IV: 1) presence of BHL, 2) complimentary evidence such as negative tuberculin, elevated ACE, positive Ga scan, and lymphocytosis in BALF, 3) exclusive evidence of other diseases such as tuberculosis, fungus diseases, and tumors, 4) extra-pulmonary involvements compatible with sarcoidosis, and 5) clinical course for a certain duration, perhaps 6 months or longer. When this criterion is applied to Japanese cases in regard to sex and age distribution, comparability was demonstrated between histologically proven and unproven cases, convincing us to accept the above-mentioned criterion. Diseases to be differentiated from sarcoidosis may vary from one country to another. In Japan, more than 97% of 223 biopsied BHL cases were caused by sarcoidosis, 3 of tuberculosis and 2 of pneumoconiosis.[26]

Table 1   Majority view on diagnostic criteria of histologically unproven cases for epidemiologic study

1)   Presence of BHL

2)   Complimentary evidence such tuberculin, ACE, Ga scan, BAL, etc

3)   Exclusive evidence of other diseases

4)   Extra-pulmonary involvements, if any

5)   Clinical course for a certain duration

In epidemiological studies, case collection is made several months or even longer after the patients' hospital visit. There is thus a great time difference between clinicians who are requested to make an immediate diagnosis and epidemiologists who want to collect cases much later. If cases are carefully collected, the histologically unproven cases will be an important addition to the frequency of histologically proven sarcoidosis.

Serum ACE Measurements Four methods have been available for serum ACE measurement; methods of 1) Cushman & Cheung modified by Liebermann, 2) Friedland-Silverstein, 3) Fujirebio Kasahara and 4) Boehlinger Mannheim Yamanouchi Neels. It was revealed[3a] that the Cushman & Cheung method gives little variance for intra-laboratory measurements, but not for inter-laboratory measurements. From these results, inter-laboratory comparisons should be made carefully. On the other hand, the last two subsequently developed methods gave a smaller variation than the old method. In every case, ACE reports should have attached the method employed.

FREQUENCY

Recent morbidity

Extensive epidemiological reviews of this disease have been published in 1983[4] and 1985.[5] Here, subsequent data will be presented.

Table 2 Recent world morbidity of sarcoidosis (1980s)

	Place (Reporter)	Rate per 10^5	n	M/F	Peak Age M	Peak Age F	Main Involv.	Secular Trend	Survey	Year
Incidence Rate	Isle of Man S.A. Parkes	14.7	66	0.8	35-39	30-34	EN or BHL 64%	unchanged	Hospital & General Pract.	1977-82
	N. Sweden M. Thunell	14.0	175	0.8	20s	50s	EN and Heerfordt 23%		New admission	1978-83
	German Democrat Republic Th. Scharkoff	8.1 ≀ 10.2	1575	0.7	20s	20s		unchanged	Registry mass X-ray	1961-84?
	Quebec G. Renzi	4.3	256						Hospital	1984
	Japan Jap. S. Commit. Hosoda et al	0.7	382	0.8	20s	20s 50s	BHL 90%	unchanged	Hospital (18 pref.)	1984
Prevalence Rate	Wales Hosp. Activity Analysis	5.0							Admission	1984
	Japan Jap S. Commit. Hosoda et al	1.7	1969	0.6	20s	20s 50s	BHL 90%	slight increase	Nation-wide survey	1984
	China Yu et Luo	(0.1) Beijin	64	0.6	20s 30s	50s	BHL 83%	increase	Univ. hospital	1985

It was once supposed that the Chinese people might have a low susceptibility to sarcoidosis. This hypothesis was not true. Bovornkitti of Bangkok made a personal visit to China in 1979 and reported that the total number of patients may exceed 300. Four hundred and eleven cases of sarcoidosis were reported among the Chinese in 1986[8b] and then the number was increased to 564[9] in 1987. In 1985, in a 17-university joint survey 64 cases, 25 males and 39 females, were collected, of which 59 were histologically confirmed and 57 were detected by symptoms, 70% by respiratory symptoms, 18% by symptoms of the skin, 7% by symptoms of the eye, and 43% by superficial lymph adenopathy. X-ray examinations revealed 50% of them to have BHL, 22%, BHL plus pulmonary mottling, 6%, lung mottling only, and 6%, other types. Serum ACE was elevated beyond 41 μ ml in 39 of 49 cases examined (Liebermann method). The prevalence rate per 100,000 among Beijing inhabitants was 0.1.

Table 3   Incidence rate of sarcoidosis in Japan; A prospective
cohort study (20 to 54 years of age)

	N. observed Person Years (Age 20-54)	N. cases	per 100,000 Person Years
1960-65	68,330	8	2.3
1965-69	71,463	8	2.2
1970-74	73,622	7	1.9
1975-79	77,312	7	1.8
1980-84	75,180	11	2.9

All X-rayed annually
(Hosoda, Saitoh and Odaka)

In addition to Table 1, secular trends have been revealed by two sourses of information. In the German Democratic Republic,[30] incidence rates per 100,000 in 1970, 1975, 1980 and 1985 were 7.3, 8.8, 10.6, and 7.1, respectively, in males and 8.7, 10.0, 11.7 and 9.1, respectively, in females. Prevalence rates per 100,000 in the respective years were 27.6, 38.5, 47.6 and 46.3 in males and 35.3, 46.1 58.9 and 58.5 in females. In Japan, a prospective cohort study[29] has been made on a working population (20 to 54 years of age) since 1960 and incidence rates per 100,000 person years by five year periods from 1960 to 1984 have been reported; 2.3 in 1960-65, 2.2 in 1965-69, 1.9 in 1970-79 and 2.9 in 1980-84. The incidence rates showed no secular changes in either country and prevalence rates showed an increase in the two countries.[31]

In Japan and the German Democratic Republic, mass chest X-rays have been extensively conducted to detect a large number of asymptomatic cases. The age distribution is different between mass survey-detected cases and symptom-detected cases. Mass X-ray surveys usually show the age peak to be in the 20s in males and in the 20s and/or 50s in females, forming a bimodal curve in some surveys. It is speculated that those females whose involvements are discovered in middle age might have had the initial asymptomatic disease long before clinical manifestation. As BHL is regarded to be a relatively early manifestation, age-specific incidence rate of BHL was investigated. Of 799 incidence cases, 678 had BHL. The age distribution of the 799 cases and the 678 cases of BHL showed nearly the same pattern, suggesting the female cases in the 50s occurring in recent years are not the remnants of old involvements which were not detected in their youth.[10a)]

Mortality

A few mortality reports of this disease have been made for the USA[11)] and other countries of the world.[10b)] Recently, Mortality Statistics of Intractable Diseases in the World, which include sarcoidosis, was published[10d)] (Tables 5a & 5b). Sex difference in mortality is not large, though more females tend to die than males. Age-specific rates rise with age, but the rates beyond the 70s tend to decline in most countries. Secular trend has not changed much between the two five year periods in most countries. In the USA, the mortality rates have gradually increased since 1950. The rise continued until 1960 followed by a stable trend thereafter, except for non-white females whose rate showed a further rise until 1970. The rate is almost unchanged in England & Wales and Japan.

Table 4   World Mortality of Sarcoidosis

| | | Asian Pacific | | | | | American Continent | | | | |
| | | New Zealand | Australia | | Japan | | Canada | U.S. White | | U.S. Nonwhite | |
Sex	Age	1971-78	1968-71	1973-77	1968-72	1973-78	1974, 76,77	1968-72	1973-78	1968-72	1973-78
Male	0- 4	–	–	–	–	0.00	–	–	–	–	–
	5-14	–	–	0.02	0.00	–	–	–	–	–	–
	15-24	–	0.02	0.03	0.00	0.00	0.01	–	–	–	–
	25-34	0.06	0.03	0.02	–	0.02	–	–	–	–	–
	35-44	0.08	0.10	0.23	0.01	0.02	0.05	–	–	–	–
	45-54	0.24	0.21	0.15	0.03	0.04	0.19	–	–	–	–
	55-64	0.51	0.28	0.18	0.07	0.06	0.14	–	–	–	–
	65-74	0.95	0.34	0.29	0.09	0.14	0.35	–	–	–	–
	75+	0.75	0.72	0.28	0.09	0.15	0.23	–	–	–	–
	n	18	25	31	40	85	22	231	273	243	351
	Crude rate	0.15	0.10	0.09	0.02	0.03	0.06	0.05	0.05	0.40	0.44
	Adjust rate	0.15	0.10	0.09	0.02	0.02	0.06	–	–	–	–
Female	0- 4	–	–	–	–	–	–	–	–	–	–
	5-14	–	–	–	0.01	0.00	–	–	–	–	–
	15-24	–	0.02	–	0.01	0.00	–	–	–	–	–
	25-34	–	–	0.06	0.01	0.01	0.04	–	–	–	–
	35-44	0.24	0.03	0.13	0.02	0.03	0.05	–	–	–	–
	45-54	0.33	0.32	0.19	0.03	0.03	0.19	–	–	–	–
	55-64	0.86	0.41	0.34	0.06	0.09	0.37	–	–	–	–
	65-74	1.20	0.82	0.34	0.10	0.17	0.40	–	–	–	–
	75+	2.16	0.42	0.23	0.10	0.10	0.15	–	–	–	–
	n	35	36	35	61	103	33	357	414	372	702
	Crude rate	0.29	0.15	0.10	0.02	0.03	0.10	0.08	0.07	0.56	0.79
	Adjust rate	0.24	0.13	0.09	0.02	0.03	0.08	–	–	–	–

(N. Hayakawa and M. Kurihara. Tables rearranged by Y. Hosoda according to regions and mortality rate)

Table 5   World Mortality of Sarcoidosis

Sex	Age	Scandinavia							Ireland and Britain					European Continent						
		Denmark		Sweden		Norway		Finland	Ireland		N Ireland	England & Wales		Germany F.R.		Netherlands	Belgium		France	Italy
		1969-73	1975-78	1969-74	1975-80	1969-74	1975-80	1974-79	1968-72	1973-78	1968-78	1968-72	1973-78	1968-72	1973-74,76	1976-78	1969-73	1974-77	1968-70	1974
Male	0-4																			
	5-14																			
	15-24		0.05			0.05		0.05	0.09			0.01	0.02	0.00	0.01					
	25-34	0.11	0.06	0.14	0.10			0.04		0.17		0.06	0.04	0.04	0.02	0.03	0.03		0.01	0.03
	35-44	0.50	0.50	0.36	0.23	0.24	0.16	0.06	0.78	0.21	0.33	0.11	0.16	0.16	0.15	0.08	0.03	0.08	0.03	0.08
	45-54	1.09	0.27	0.42	0.53	0.68	0.38	0.31	0.62	0.53	0.46	0.23	0.17	0.26	0.22	0.23	0.07	0.12	0.12	0.06
	55-64	1.58	0.47	0.72	0.80	0.78	0.96	0.09	0.69	1.37	0.52	0.27	0.27	0.39	0.30	0.33	0.20	0.06	0.14	0.20
	65-74	2.04	1.28	1.79	1.89	0.92	0.95	0.59	1.01	1.12	0.98	0.28	0.25	0.47	0.38	0.24	0.38	0.27	0.23	0.25
	75+	2.55	0.97	1.84	2.30	1.08	1.14	-	-	0.96	2.15	0.20	0.45	0.27	0.25	0.44	0.24	0.56	0.07	0.12
	n	77	29	104	118	37	35	14	22	31	21	131	164	204	102	20	20	14	30	17
	Crude rate	0.63	0.29	0.43	0.48	0.32	0.29	0.10	0.30	0.32	0.25	0.11	0.11	0.14	0.11	0.10	0.08	0.07	0.06	0.06
	Adjust rate	0.48	0.22	0.29	0.30	0.24	0.21	0.09	0.28	0.29	0.22	0.09	0.09	0.12	0.09	0.09	0.06	0.05	0.05	0.05
Female	0-4																			
	5-14																			
	15-24										0.08			0.02	0.02					
	25-34	0.12	0.06		0.03	0.07	0.11				0.10			0.05	0.10	0.06				
	35-44	0.28	0.08	0.18	0.07	0.16	-		0.26	0.11	0.32	0.05	0.06	0.18	0.05	0.08	0.02	0.05	0.02	0.05
	45-54	0.73	0.17	0.64	0.60	0.14	0.46	0.12	0.62	0.43	0.53	0.21	0.28	0.18	0.14	0.18	0.10	0.12	0.06	0.19
	55-64	1.76	1.06	1.27	0.94	0.88	1.11	0.45	1.42	1.14	0.81	0.40	0.41	0.42	0.43	0.90	0.07	0.25	0.11	0.14
	65-74	2.22	1.47	2.18	2.13	1.31	1.38	0.83	0.36	0.58	1.16	0.47	0.45	0.58	0.57	1.12	0.25	0.55	0.46	0.16
	75+	3.09	1.72	1.91	2.45	1.18	0.97	0.59	0.58	0.45	0.99	0.22	0.30	0.23	0.36	1.13	0.07	0.23	0.12	0.34
	n	86	41	144	146	39	48	24	21	26	29	197	254	288	165	55	14	22	39	23
	Crude rate	0.69	0.40	0.59	0.59	0.33	0.39	0.16	0.29	0.27	0.34	0.16	0.17	0.18	0.17	0.26	0.06	0.11	0.08	0.08
	Adjust rate	0.44	0.23	0.35	0.31	0.20	0.24	0.10	0.24	0.25	0.27	0.11	0.11	0.12	0.11	0.18	0.04	0.07	0.05	0.06

Autopsy

A unique autopsy registration system was established in 1959 in Japan and 26 volumes of data have been published until 1984, providing such information as institution, autopsy number, age, sex, address, clinical diagnosis, occupation, main pathological findings and other associated lesions of the pathological diagnosis. The average autopsy rate of the deceased was around 4%; the number of autopsy cases from 1974 to 1983 being 313,533 out of 7,086,598 deaths. During this period, there were 289 sarcoidosis deaths reported by death certificates,[10e] but 114 cases with pathological findings of sarcoidosis were reported during the same period.[10f] Of the 114 cases, two thirds had no ante-mortem diagnosis, of which one-half died of sarcoidosis and the other half of diseases other than sarcoidosis. The direct cause of death of the sarcoidosis cases was frequently cardiac involvement. These results suggest that a large number of overlooked sarcoidosis cases are not included in deaths shown by death certificates or cases detected by morbidity surveys (Iwai et at, 1987, Milan). The secular trend has been nearly unchanged during the past decade in regard to the number of deaths, sarcoidosis deaths and autopsied sarcoidosis cases, but autopsy cases have increased in number.

INVESTIGATIONS ON RISKS

Risk factors have been studied through descriptive and analytic epidemiological methods, mainly in the United States[13,14,15] and Japan.[10c] The case-control study made by the author was focussed on the hypothesis of impaired cellular immunity in sarcoidosis popular in the 1970s, but the BALF study revealed that this disease has an activated macrophage-monocyte condition. Sarcoidosis may be a rare disease whose immunological interpretation has been completely altered in recent years. Further studies should be attempted on the basis of a new hypothesis. In the following items investigated by case-control study, "s" designates sarcoidosis cases and "c," controls. If sarcoidosis cases have a higher, lower or similar rate in comparison with controls, the results are simplified as either s>c, s<c, or s=c.

Host-related factors

Patient factors

1. Ethnic groups: A high risk in non-whites[14] and Puerto Ricans[17] in the United States in morbidity and in mortality.[12a] Londonites who were born in Ireland and British Caribbeans showed a higher prevalence rate of intrathoracic sarcoidosis than those born in UK.[4]

2. Age: A high risk in the 20s in males and in the 50s in females. Mass X-rays may reveal another female peak in the 20s (Table 1).

3. Sex: A slightly higher risk in females with a male/female ratio of 0.6 to 0.8 (Table 1).

4. Genetic factors: (a) Blood type: Type A dominant[18] or no association.[10c] (b) HLA:[16] Some reports support an association with HLA phenotype, but others do not. HLA is likely to be associated with the sites involved, but not with the development itself.

5. Physiques: s=c for body mass index prior to onset[10c]

6. Previous health: (a) Previous illness: s=c in tuberculosis[13,10c] and other diseases[10c] such as eye diseases, rheumatic fever, measles, mumps, chicken pox, herpes zoster and simplex, and asthma in childhood. (b) Surgery: s=c in tonsillectomy, appendectomy and sinusitis operation.[10c] (c) Immunology: Previous BCG vaccination showed no association.[17] s=c by BCG scar observation.[10c] A similar onset rate in the historical cohort study among tuberculin-positives and tuberculin-negatives prior to onset by medical records.[22]

7. Present illness: s=c in habitual tonsillitis, chronic sinusitis, bronchial asthma, urticaria, eczema, drug rash, skin hypersensitivity to chemicals and keloid[10c] and hay fever.[13]

Family Factors

1. Illness, present and past (1) Tuberculosis: s>c[21] and s=c,[13] (2) Other diseases: Rheumatoid fever s=c,[10c] syphilis s=c[13] eczema, urticaria, bronchial asthma, hay fever and drug rash,[13] (3) Surgery: Appendectomy s=c.[10c]

2. Number of deaths and family members: Family members and deaths s=c[10c]

Socio-economic factors

1. Income: s>c (p>0.05)[15]
2. Education: s=c[15]
3. Occupation, professional: s>c[17,10c]

Environmental factors (Time and space)

1. Secular trend:

It was controversial whether this disease was overlooked among a large number of tuberculous cases and whether the disease has really increased or not. In an FRG child sanatorium, out of about 70,000 tuberculous children hospitalized for a 20-year period from 1940 to 1959,[19] 1,158 had unilateral lymphadenopathy and 53 had BHL. Tuberculin-positive BLH cases numbered 10, 8, 14 and 8 in the four five-year periods, while tuberculin-negative BHL cases numbered 0, 1, 4 and 8 during the same four periods, respectively, showing a gradual increase. Some of them were diagnosed as having "Lungenwurzeltuberkulose bei zur Zeit Tuberkulinreaktion negativem Kinder." On the other hand, in a large Japanese working population, in which all have been X-rayed every year since 1941, tuberculin negatives were tuberculin tested every three months until the 1950s.[20] Clinical features of tuberculosis changed along with a decrease in tuberculosis mortality in the general population. In 1941-45, 45% of 911 primary tuberculous cases presented hilar node tuberculosis, while in 1947-50 only 4% of 289 showed it. Among hilar node tuberculosis cases, BHL was found in 2%. Then, in the 1950s, a few tuberculin-negative BHL cases were detected among the previous tuberculin positives, but no hilar node tuberculosis was detected among the fresh converters.

These data suggest a likelihood of increase in the number of sarcoidosis cases during a long range of time, though sarcoidosis may have been overlooked due to poor interest of the physicians. In the recent 10 or 20 years, the secular trend has likely not changed.

2. Seasonal variation:

Erythema nodosum has been reported to occur most frequently in winter in Finland.[12] In Japan, 678 symptomatic BHL cases were found in 1963-72, the rates of May-June and July-August being significantly higher (test for uniformity was not uniform, $p < 0.001$). Besides, in cold areas, the peak months were later than in the warm areas.[28] In the 1987 Milan Conference, two abstracts showed a seasonal variation of occurrence. In Barcelona, the period from April to June showed the peak occurrence of Lofgren syndrome ($p < 0.01$ Baardinas 1987, Milan) and in France, the period was from March to June when that syndrome was most frequently found (Maffre J. Ph, 1987, Milan). Further investigations should be made on etiological factors possibly related to seasonal variations.

3. Climate: In regard to morbidity and mortality, the northern areas have a high frequency in the world except for the USA. Attention should again be directed to the climate zones, as the author emphasized.[28]

The Oxford seasonal climate consists of summer and winter in combination. To simplify the matter, three zones are designated by three names; (1) cold zone for cool summer combined with a) cold or b) mild winter, (2) warm zone for full summer combined with cold winter, and (3) very warm zone for full summer combined with mild winter.

In Europe, Scandinavian countries and European countries belong to the cold zone (1^a) and Britain and west France to the cold zone (1^b). In the American continent, Canada belongs to the cold zone, north US to the warm zone and south US to the very warm zone. In Italy, the central mountainous area belongs to the cold zone, the north to the warm zone and the south to the very warm zone. In Japan, there are three climate zones from the north to the south. In the United States, the southeast has been reported to be dominant in frequency by many authors. The reasons should be further investigated.

4. Birth place and lifetime residence: Predominant in rural area $s > c$[13] or $s = c$[10c]

5. Local outbreaks: Except for Furano area, Hokkaido, Japan,[10] no local outbreaks have been reported.

6.   Housing: Residence in wooden or ferro-concrete structure, residence on the ground floor or 1st floor or above s=c[10c)

7.   Heating system of the house: Kerosene, coal, steam s=c[10c)

8.   Pets: Pet feeding s=c[15,10c), presence of rats in the house s=c[10c)

9.   Hair sprays: s=c[15)

10.   Plants near the house: Pine, cedar, gingko trees s=c[10c)

Habits

1.   Unprescribed drugs: s c Buck, Bresnitz s<c Hosoda

2.   Smoking: S>c Terris,[25) Comstock[26) s=c Hosoda,[10c) Bresnitz[15)

3.   Foods: s=c[10c) intake (no, rarely, sometimes, frequently) of rice, bread, noodles, chicken, pork, beef, whale, ham or sausage, sea fish, river fish, shell, prawn or crab, squid or octopus, soft roe, egg raw or cooked, cow milk, yogurt, miso soup

Others

1.   Infectious agents.   Many infectious agents have been suggested as etiological factors.   One mentioned in recent hypotheses is propionibacterium acnes[23,24) which was isolated from the lymph nodes of sarcoidosis patients at a high frequency and concentration. A double blind study on recent BHL cases was attempted using cephalexin. No difference in BHL regression was found after one year between the drug and placebo groups, suggesting no causal association with this bacterium.[22)

2.   Immigration.   The highest frequency of this disease has been reported in Hokkaido, Japan, where the majority of people are decendents of immigrants who moved there more than 100 years ago. Therefore, residents of Hokkaido may have been exposed to environmental and seasonal factors related to the occurrence of this disease. Racial factors may be ignored in this island.[22)

3.   Family clustering. Family clustering has been generally accepted.[5) This clustering is due to genetic factors or common exposure.   The clustering was frequently observed in blood-related persons, but no difference has been found between blood-related persons and married couples.[27)

4.   Time space relationship.   No study has been made except for a report, which was negative for time-residence and time-work-place relationship in Kyoto and Sapporo.[28)

CONCLUSION

1.   In epidemiological studies of sarcoidosis, the method of case detection, diagnostic criteria and measurements of specimens should be standardized.

2.   Secular trend of this disease has hardly changed during the past one or two decades.

3. The risk of occurrence of sarcoidosis has been reported in association with ethnic groups, age, sex, family, immigration, climatic zones and seasonal variations. In the search for possible etiological agents, these factors should be considered as well.

4. The immunological state of the patients may be after all the result of the disease. Epidemiologists should direct attention to the immunological state prior to disease onset in these patients or in individuals blood related to these patients in attempting to detect persistent markers.

5. Case-control study should be pursued based on a new hypothesis, since the disease is interpreted as having activated   macrophage-monocyte system. In the old concept it was a disease of impaired cellular immunity.

6. Genetic epidemiology is concerned with interaction of environmental and genetic determinants in common diseases. Epidemiology and genetics should be coordinated in the near future.

ACKNOWLEDGMENT

The author wishes to extend his thanks to Drs. M. Odaka, N. Saitoh, Y. Hiraga, and S. Mizuno for their assistance and cooperation in this study.

REFERENCES

1. Hosoda Y, Hashimoto T, Odaka T (1971) Lung and Heart 18, 46-56

2a. Hiraga Y, Hosoda Y (1981) In: Sarcoidosis, University of Tokyo Press, Tokyo pp 373-377

2b. Hosoda Y, Saito N (1981) Ibid pp 399-408

2c. Yanagawa Y, Hosoda Y (1981) Ibid pp 355-372

3a. Yotsumoto, H et al (1980) In: Eighth Int'l Conf. Sarc. Alpha Omega Pub, Cardiff pp 277-282

3b. Hosoda Y, Saito M, Odaka M et al (1980) Ibid pp 237-244

4. James DG, Jones Williams W (1985) Sarcoidosis, WB Saunders, London

5. Bresnitz EA, Strom BL (1983) Epid. Rev. 51, 124-156

6. Parkes AS, Baker SD, Bourdillon RE (1985) Thorax 40, 284-87

7. Thunell M (1987) Umea Univ. Med. Dis. New Series 190, Umea

8a. Renzi G (1987) Jap J. Chest Dis. 46, 518-21

8b. Y. RJ (1987) Ibid 513-517

9. Luo WC (1987) Abstract, 3rd Resp. Dis. Cont. China

10a. Odaka M, Hosoda Y, Yanagawa Y (1975) Report Series of Intractable Dis Resear. Committ. Japanese Ministry of Health and Welfare, Sarcoidosis 35-38

10b. Hosoda Y, Yanagawa Y, Odaka M et al (1973) Ibid 79-90

10c. Hosoda Y, Hiraga Y, Yanagawa Y (1973) Ibid 57-60

10d. Hayakawa N, Kurihara M (1984) Ibid. Mortality Statistics of Intractable Diseases in the World 1984, Nagoya

10e. Minowa M (1987) Ibid. Mortality Statistics of Intractable Diseases in Japan, Nagoya

10f. Urano Y, Aizawa S, Baba K et al (1984) Ibid. Statistics of Intractable Diseases from the Autopsy Data in Japan, Nagoya

11. Moriyama I (1967) In: La Sarcoidose Masson et Cie 1967, Paris pp 347-352

12. Putokonen T, Hannusela M, Mustakallio K (1966) Arch. Env. Health 12, 564-7

13. Buck A, McKusick A (1961) Amer. J Hyg 152-173, 174-188

14. Startwell PE, Edwards LB (1974) Ann R Epi 99, 250-257

15. Bresnitz EA, Stolley PD, Israel H et al (1986) Ann NY. Acad. Sci. 465, 632-642

16. Scadding JG, Mitchell DN (1985) Sarcoidosis Chapman and Hall Medical, London

17. Keller A   a) (1971) Am J. Epid. 94, 222-230
              b) (1973) Am Rev. Resp. Dis. 107, 615-620

17. Sutherland I, Mitchell DN, D'Acy Hart P (1965) Brit Med J. 2, 497-500

18. Jorgensen G, Wurm K (1964) Acta med Scand. Suppl 425, 213-5

19. Hosoda Y, Chosho M (1963) Chest Dis (J) 392-403

20. Chiba Y, Shozawa M (1950) Clinical Study of Tbc Primary Infection (J), Hoken Dojin-Sha, Tokyo

21. Shigematsu I, Hosoda Y, Odaka M et al (1964) (J) Saishin Igaku 19, 7-32

22. Hiraga M, Saitoh N, Odaka M (1987) Oral presentation at 7th Jap Soc Sarco Conf, (in print)

23. Ito Y, Toyama J, Marikawa S et al (1980) In: Sarcoidosis Alpha and Omega 121-32

24. Homma JY et al (1978) Jpn J Exp Med 48, 251-6

25. Terris M, Chaves AD (1966) Am Rev Resp Dis, 94, 50-5

26. Comstock GW, Keltz H, Sencer H (1961) Amer Rev Resp Dis Suppl 84, 130-4

27. Hosoda Y, Iwai K, Odaka M (1980) In: Sarcoidosis Alpha Omega 1980, pp 519-21

28. Hosoda Y, Hiraga Y, Odaka M et al (1976) Ann NY Acad Scien. 278, 355-67

29. Hosoda Y, Saito N, Odaka M (unpublished)

30. Eule H (1987) Personal Communication

31. Hosoda Y, Odaka M, Yamaguchi M et al (1987) Proceedings of this conference

32. Hosoda Y, Odaka M, Chiba Y (1971) Proceedings of 5th Int'l Conf Sarco, Praha, 156-159

Sarcoidosis and other granulomatous disorders
C. Grassi, G. Rizzato, E. Pozzi, editors

FAMILIAL SARCOIDOSIS:
CLINICAL, IMMUNOLOGIC, AND GENETIC FEATURES OF AN UNUSUAL VARIANT

J.L. ANDREWS, JR., T.C. CAMPBELL, R.E. ROCKLIN, M.R. GAROVOY
Lahey Clinic Foundation, Burlington; and Harvard Medical School
and Tufts University School of Medicine, Boston, Massachusetts (U.S.A.)

INTRODUCTION

Sarcoidosis is a multi-system, multi-specialty, multi-continent masquerader, which, though studied extensively, remains a perplexing puzzle.[1] Is it heredity, environment, or both that start this process of multi-organ granulomatosis? Is sarcoid one common biologic entity or many clinically similar but causally different conditions? Suspected but as yet unproved culprits include bacteria (e.g., typical and atypical mycobacteria), bacteriophages, viruses, fungi, environmental inhalants (e.g., pine pollen and beryllium), and various autoimmune disorders.[2] Studies of the patterns of heredity in sarcoidosis may identify possible genetic mechanisms in its etiology.

We describe the first reported family in which the mother, son, and daughter all have sarcoidosis. We studied both the immunologic competence and histocompatibility locus antigens (HLA) of three generations of one affected family to determine if immunologic defects were associated with familial sarcoidosis and if a common HLA haplotype was shared by affected family members. We found both.

METHODS

Migration inhibitory factor (MIF) and ^{3}H-thymidine incorporation in mononuclear cells cultured in the absence of antigen and in the presence of phytohemagglutinin (PHA), pokeweed, or Concanavalin A (ConA) mitogens and purified protein derivative (PPD), streptokinase-streptodornase (SK-SD), or Candida antigens were determined at the Brigham and Women's Hospital, Boston, Massachusetts (R.R.) by methods that have been described previously.[3] Stimulation indexes were calculated by dividing the mean counts per minute of stimulated cultures by mean counts per minute of control cultures. T cell subsets were determined by monoclonal antibody techniques by Dr. L. Cook at Lahey Clinic.

HLA typing for 20 HLA-A, 31 HLA-B, and 4 HLA-C locus specificities at the Brigham and Women's Hospital (M.G.) in 1978 used standard microlymphocytotoxicity techniques[4] with slides obtained locally and through the serum bank, National Institutes of Health (NIH), Bethesda, Maryland. Retyping, including typing for HLA-D locus, was done in 1987 at the Pulmonary Division of the NIH by the Terasaki technique using a 1984 NIH standard panel, courtesy of Dr. J. Spurzem and Dr. R. Crystal.

292

CASE REPORTS

The pedigree of the family is shown in Figure 1. All family members lived near Lawrence, Massachusetts. The mother and father are first-generation Italoamericans whose parents are from Catania, Sicily. No common occupational or environmental exposure could be identified.

Mother

This 69-year-old housewife, a bookkeeper in her husband's garage, noticed a dry cough in 1969. Her chest roentgenogram showed diffuse nodularity in the lung fields and bilateral hilar adenopathy. Intermediate strength PPD was negative. Scalene node biopsy showed noncaseating granulomas. She was treated with prednisone with symptomatic improvement and with partial clearing of the pulmonary infiltrates and hilar adenopathy. Since then she has required intermittent therapy with prednisone, 10 to 20 mg, to control her cough. Otherwise she has led an active life.

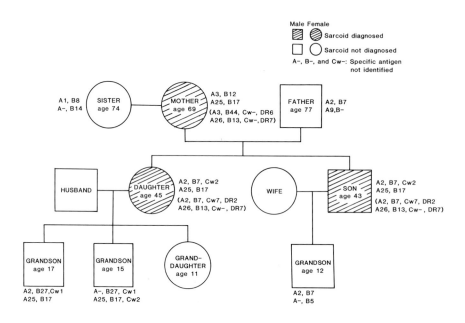

Fig. 1. Pedigree and HLA haplotypes determined in 1978 with results of 1987 studies shown in parentheses.

Daughter

This 45-year-old housewife and artist was noted to have diffuse pulmonary nodularity and an enlarged left hilar lymph node on a routine preoperative chest roentgenogram in 1975. A scalene node biopsy showed noncaseating granulomas with no acid-fast bacilli. Intermediate strength PPD gave no induration, but control skin tests for Candida and SK-SD were positive at greater than 10-mm induration. Although she had no respiratory symptoms, she was treated briefly with prednisone for pruritis, with relief. She has done well since then with no treatment.

Son

This 43-year-old trumpet player was found to have a nodule in his right lung on a routine preoperative chest roentgenogram in 1967. A repeat chest roentgenogram in 1968 showed a diffuse interstitial process in both upper lung fields and enlarged mediastinal lymph nodes. Skin tests for intermediate strength PPD, histoplasmin, and coccidioidin were negative. He underwent a right scalene lymph node biopsy, which showed noncaseating granulomas. He was treated with prednisone for six months with some improvement of the chest roentgenogram. He has remained active and stable without medication over the ensuing 20 years.

RESULTS

MIF was normal in unaffected family members and was decreased in the sarcoid subjects based on their macrophage migration inhibition of less than 20% as shown in Table I. Lymphocyte proliferation tests (Table II) reveal a slight decrease in the mother and son for some antigens as demonstrated by stimulation indices of <3. On T cell subset/monoclonal antibody studies, the daughter was normal and her mother showed increased percentages of natural killer cells, helper inducer cells, and suppressor inducer cells.

TABLE I: MIGRATION INHIBITORY FACTOR (MIF) PRODUCTION (% INHIBITION)[#]

Subject	PPD	SK-SD	Candida
Father	31	21	25
Mother*	6[†]	9[†]	12[†]
Daughter*	11[†]	8[†]	8[†]
Son*	0[†]	11[†]	-1[†]
Maternal aunt	12[†]	24	2[†]

#Greater than 20% inhibition of migration in vitro of guinea pig macrophages indicates normal MIF production by subjects' lymphocytes.
*Subject has sarcoidosis.
†Decreased MIF production.

TABLE II: LYMPHOCYTE PROLIFERATION

Subject	Unstim-ulated	Mitogens					
		PHA		Pokeweed		ConA	
Father	284±34	27,940±765	(98)#	28,447±414	(100)	16,997±2,150	(60)
Mother*	275±27	49,609±2,208	(180)	15,000±285	(55)	15,003±808	(55)
Daughter*	260±20	73,767±3,308	(284)	26,162±1,231	(101)	18,946±1,862	(73)
Son*	680±242	12,620±704	(19)	8,276±906	(12)	9,735±1,326	(14)
Maternal aunt	603±28	71,522±1,879	(119)	22,506±1,219	(37)	7,039±1,367	(12)

Subject	Unstim-ulated	Antigens					
		PPD		SK-SD		Candida	
Father	424±102	41,645±648	(98)	1,312±398	(3)	4,707±1,566	(11)
Mother*	267±40	587±149†	(2)	314±25†	(1)	2,416±287	(9)
Daughter*	355±80	1,129±394	(3)	1,792±315	(5)	1,578±283	(4)
Son*	401±154	678±179†	(1)	1,675±225	(4)	2,882±152	(7)
Maternal aunt	548±109	618±192†	(1)	2,829±244	(5)	1,019±181†	(2)

#Number in parentheses is stimulation index; >10 is a positive response for mitogens; >3 is positive response for antigens.
*Subject has sarcoidosis.
†Decreased lymphocyte response to mitogen or antigen in vitro stimulation tests.

HLA haplotypes are shown in Figure 1. The 1978 studies and the 1987 studies vary slightly as a result of changes in the NIH standard HLA panels. In both studies, the affected siblings share identical HLA genotypes. They have inherited one haplotype (A26, B13, Cw-, DR7) from their mother. In the 1978 studies two grandsons, now aged 15 and 17 years, carried the same haplotype (A25, B17) as their affected grandmother, mother, and uncle.

DISCUSSION

Familial sarcoidosis has previously been reported in over 300 families around the world. Reports on 59 sarcoid families, a review of 174 other published families by Scadding and the Research Committee of the British Thoracic and Tuberculosis Association,[5] and reviews by James[6] and Sharma et al[7] provide the following generalizations about familial sarcoidosis: Like-sex pairs predominate over unlike-sex pairs among both siblings and parent-child associations; females predominate over males and mother-child associations over father-child associations; and monozygous twins predominate over dizygous twins concordant for sarcoidosis, the latter suggesting a genetic basis for the disease.

Surveys of first-degree relatives of 62 sarcoid patients by Buck and
McKusick[8] in Baltimore found five affected families (9%). Jorgensen[9] in Germany
located 40 families by surveying 2,471 sarcoid cases (2%). Headings et al[10]
discovered 11 familial sarcoid occurrences by surveying first-degree relatives
of 80 patients in a black population in Washington, DC (14%). The 1.5% incidence of sarcoid among first-degree relatives of index cases is a 20-fold
increase over the 0.07% incidence in the black population in general. A similar
study in Ireland[11] detected sarcoidosis in at least one sibling in 11 of 114
patients (9.6%) at a sarcoid clinic. The disease prevalence among siblings was
2.4%. These studies imply that sarcoidosis is more prevalent among patients'
relatives than in the general population and that the etiology of sarcoidosis
may involve a genetic mechanism.

Although James et al[12] believed that a monogenic recessive mode of inheritance might explain the distribution of sarcoidosis in the five families they
studied, most authors hold that sarcoid inheritance must be multigenic.

While there has so far been no proof that one HLA haplotype is associated
with susceptibility to sarcoidosis in general or with familial sarcoidosis, many
have reported the association of several HLA genotypes with several clinical
subsets of sarcoidosis and with different ethnic groups. An association between
sarcoid uveitis and HLA-A1 and between sarcoid arthritis and HLA-B8 was reported
by Brewerton et al[13] and by Hedfors and Lindstrom.[14] Resolution of pulmonary
sarcoid was seen more frequently in patients with HLA-B8 by Smith et al.[15]
Ethnic HLA associations in sarcoidosis patients have been found in Germans (DR5)
by Nowack and Goebel,[16] Japanese (DRw52) by Kunikane et al,[17] South Carolina
blacks (A7, B7) by McIntyre et al,[18] and English patients (B8/Cw7/DR3), but not
West Indian blacks, by Gardner et al.[19] However, no association between a
specific HLA genotype and the development of sarcoidosis was found in 14 English
families by Turton et al[20] or in two large Swedish families by Möller et al.[21]

The findings of decreased MIF levels in all affected family members in this
study as well as decreased lymphocyte proliferation in two subjects and altered
serum T cell subsets are consistent with immunologic alterations reported in
other sarcoid subjects and cannot be linked definitely with either the cause or
effects of this family's sardoidosis.

CONCLUSION

Our family is the first reported in which a parent (mother) and members of
both sexes (son and daughter) all have proven sarcoidosis. The fact that the
affected siblings have identical HLA genotypes and share a haplotype with their
mother is suggestive but not conclusive of genetic transmission of sarcoid.

296

There is a 25% probability that this might happen by chance alone. If sarcoidosis develops in the future in the unaffected teenage grandsons who share the same HLA haplotype, the etiologic association of this haplotype with sarcoid in this family would be confirmed.

We hope that future study of more sarcoid families to the third and fourth generations and of genotypes of additional chromosomes may help to clarify further our present incomplete understanding of the role of genetic mechanisms in the etiology of sarcoidosis.

REFERENCES

1. Andrews JL Jr (1978) Lahey Clin Found Bull 27:108
2. Sharma OP, Kadakia D (1986) Semin Respir Med 8:95
3. Campbell TC, Rocklin RE, Garovoy MR, Andrews JL Jr (1981) Lahey Clin Found Bull 30:122
4. Mittal KK, Mickey MR, Singal DP, Terasaki PI (1968) Transplantation 6:913
5. Scadding JG (1973) Tubercle 54:87
6. James DG (1983) In Fanburg B (ed) Sarcoidosis and Other Granulomatous Diseases of the Lung. Marcel Dekker, New York, chap 13
7. Sharma OP, Neville E, Walker AN (1976) Ann NY Acad Sci 278:386
8. Buck AA, McKusick VA (1961) Am J Hyg 74:174
9. Jorgensen G (1965) Untersuchungen zur Genetik der Sarkoidose. Habil Schrift, Gottingen, Germany
10. Headings VE, Weston D, Young RC Jr, Hackney RL Jr (1976) Ann NY Acad Sci 278:377
11. Brennan NJ, Crean P, Long JP, Fitzgerald MX (1984) Thorax 39:14
12. James DG, Neville E, Piyasena KHG, Walker AN, Hamlyn AN (1974) Postgrad Med J 50:664
13. Brewerton DA, Cockburn C, James DCO, James DG, Neville E (1977) Clin Exp Immunol 27:227
14. Hedfors E, Lindström F (1983) Tissue Antigens 22:200
15. Smith MJ, Turton CWG, Mitchell DN, Turner-Warwick M, Morris LM, Lawler SD (1981) Thorax 36:296
16. Nowack D, Goebel KM (1987) Arch Intern Med 147:481
17. Kunikane H, Abe S, Tsuneta Y, Nakayama T, Tajima Y, Misonou J, Wakisaka A, Aizawa M, Kawakami Y (1987) Am Rev Respir Dis 135:688
18. McIntyre JA, McKee KT, Loadholt CB, Mercurio S, Lin I (1977) Transplant Proc 9(Suppl 1):173
19. Gardner J, Kennedy HG, Hamblin A, Jones E (1984) Thorax 39:19
20. Turton CWG, Turner-Warwick M, Morris L, Lawler SD (1980) In Jones Williams W, Davies BH (eds) Proceedings of VIIIth International Conference on Sarcoidosis and Other Granulomatous Diseases. Alpha Omega, Cardiff, Wales, pp 195-200
21. Möller E, Hedfors E, Wiman LG (1974) Tissue Antigens 4:299

ANTIBODIES TO TWAR- A NOVEL TYPE OF CHLAMYDIA- IN SARCOIDOSIS

Carola Grönhagen-Riska, Pekka Saikku, Henrik Riska, Bertil Fröseth &
JT Grayston
Fourth Dept. of Medicine and Dept. of Virology, University of Helsinki and
Mjölbolsta Hospital, Finland, and University of Washington, Seattle, Wash., USA

INTRODUCTION

Different chlamydial species have previously been associated with various diseases, such as
C. trachomatis, trachoma biovar, with trachoma, inclusion conjunctivitis, pneumonia of the
newborn, cervicitis and urethritis, reactive arthritis, and lymphogranuloma biovar with
Lymphogranuloma venereum (LGV) (1). The species *C. psittaci* has in mammals been found to
cause varying symptoms, e.g., arthritis, pneumonitis, conjunctivitis, carditis and
encephalomyelitis. In humans *C. psittaci* has been known to cause mainly a respiratory tract
infection with a range of mild to severe symptoms, sometimes associated with erythema
nodosum(EN), which was contracted from exposure to avian discharges and was therefore called
ornithosis/psittacosis.

Recently an apparently new species of chlamydia, TWAR (Taiwan acute respiratory), has
been identified (2,3), which causes upper and/or lower airway infections, the intensity of
which may vary from subclinical to fulminant pneumonia (4-7). It is contracted by humans
from human contact . Epidemics have been observed in Northern Europe (4,5) and endemic cases
have been reported from North America (6,7).

Chlamydiae are obligatory intracellular bacterial parasites with two nucleic acids and a
gram-negative cell wall including LPS. Infections indicate a high degree of latency, the parasites
induce their own phagocytosis through specific mechanisms associated both with the parasite and
the host cell(1). Respiratory infections would be expected to cause massive phagocytosis by
pulmonary macrophages. Phagocytosing cells are not destroyed, phagosomes do not fuse with
lysosomes, the particles multiply within the host cell and use its energy.

The most reliable and sensitive serological method for identifying anti-TWAR antibodies is
the microimmunofluorescence (micro-if) test (8,9). This test has enabled the epidemiological
studies and its use has identified two types of serologic response; slow IgG response 6-8 weeks
after often subclinical or mild disease in young persons which indicates a primary infection, and,
on the other hand, a rapidly increasing, high IgG, but a weak IgM response, associated with more
severe disease in elderly, which possibly indicates reinfection (5).

We have applied the micro-if test to detect signs of previous or on-going TWAR infection in
sarcoidosis patients.

PATIENTS

Cross-sectional pilot study. Serum samples of 29 patients with verified sarcoidosis
(mean age 47, range 18- 79 years) had been drawn in 1980-81. Twenty-three of the

patients had chronic sarcoidosis which had been diagnosed in the mid 70's or before. Nine patients were on steroid treatment, nine were considered to have inactive disease. Only one serum sample/patient was obtained.

Longitudinal follow-up study. 155 serum samples were obtained from 22 sarcoidosis patients . Most sample series were initiated in the early or mid 80's and started from the time when diagnosis was established. Patients were then followed for 7-68 (mean 32) months with a mean interval of about 5 months. Ten (45%) were men, mean age was 41 (range 21-66) years.

Control samples were 504 samples from people investigated for viral antibodies (mean age 40, range 20-50 years). 217/504 (43%) were TWAR-positive.

METHODS

TWAR IgG antibody titers were determined from frozen sera with the micro-if test, which is performed with fluorescein-conjugated goat antiserum against human IgG using purified chlamydial TWAR elementary bodies as an antigen (8,9). Activity and dissemination of sarcoidosis was determined by usual clinical examinations and tests , such as chest X-ray, pulmonary function tests, serum angiotensin-converting enzyme (ACE) activity, serum lysozyme (LZM) and immunoglobulin concentrations, dU-Ca measurements, and so on (10).

Chi-square analysis, and student's t-test and regression analysis (Statworks, Macintosh computer) were used for statistical calculations.

RESULTS

Cross-sectional pilot study. Eighteen of 29 (62%) had a positive ($\geq$ 1:32) anti-TWAR titer (range 32-1024, p< 0.05 compared with controls). Two patients with chronic sarcoidosis had clinical relapses within one year after high titers had been measured. There were no significant differences between positive and negative patients with regard to IgG concentrations, activity, chronicity or steroid requirement (33 v. 27%). Positive patients, however, were significantly older (55$\pm$12.9 versus 40$\pm$14.9, p< 0.02).

Longitudinal study. Nineteen of 22 (86%) patients had a positive TWAR titer. and the difference was highly significant compared with controls (43%, p < 0.001). Some features of the patients are presented in table 1.

In 17, the initial titer was $\geq$ 32 and 3 of these, and both patients who initially had a negative titer, had a fourfold titer increment within the first weeks or months of follow-up. Titer values remained stable in 8 and decreased in 11 patients during follow-up. All negative patients had subacute disease with stage I chest X-ray changes, which had regressed to normal without treatment within 2 years.

Mean age of the 3 negative patients was lower in this study, too. The number of positive patients with increased calcium excretion was considerably higher than has previously been reported from large patient series (11).

Positive TWAR-titers of untreated patients were correlated with IgG concentrations and with serum LZM and ACE values; r-values were -0.20 (n.s.), 0.54 (p < 0.01) and 0.50

Table 1. Some characteristics of patients included in the longitudinal study.

		TWAR-NEGATIVE	TWAR-POSITIVE		
			All	≥32-128	256-512
Patients (22)		3	19	13	6
mean age:		34.3	42.6		
Chest X-ray:	0	-	2	2	-
	I	3	5	2	3
	II	-	12	9	3
Duration at					
diagnosis:	EN	-	2	1	1
	subacute	3	14	9	5
	chronic	-	3	3	-
Chronic development:		-	6	5	1
Steroids initiated:		-	7	5	2

(p< 0.01),respectively. TWAR-titer changes did not appear as often as ACE and LZM fluctuations, especially the lower, positive titers, 1:32-1:128, seemed to remain stable for long periods of time. On the other hand, general development of titers correlated fairly well with clinically apparent fluctuations in disease dissemination and activity, table 2. Two patients presented with very high titers (1:512), both had stage II chest X-ray changes and both initially progressed, then regressed, one without, the other during steroid treatment. In both

Table 2. TWAR-titer changes compared with clinical development in untreated sarcoidosis patients.

Sarcoidosis:	progressing	stable	regressing
TWAR-titer:			
increasing	5	4	-
stable	4	7	4
decreasing	1	2	8

patients titers decreased. Steroid treatment was initiated in 7 patients, all had a positive titer (table 1), all patients reacted to treatment. However, TWAR titer changes were not equally apparent, in 2 patients immediate decrements were observed, in 2 others decrements were also recorded, but they were considerably delayed (1-2 years), in 3, titers remained stable and slightly elevated (32-64).

DISCUSSION

The pilot study indicated an increased frequency of TWAR-positivity in sarcoidosis patients. The results of this cross-sectional study of mostly chronic sarcoidosis patients were verified by the longitudinal study, in which most sera had been collected at a later date. This is interesting, since TWAR epidemics have been identified in Finland both in the late seventies, and then again in the mid 80's (4,12). These epidemies have been closely studied in military conscripts, in whom TWAR was identified as the single most usual pneumonia-causing agent (20-30%) in the years 1985-87. In the general population positive titers start appearing in school age, and at age 40, almost 50% have had a TWAR-infection. Consequently several ten thousand persons contract TWAR every year in Finland. Obviously, this frequency of infections increases the possibility of unspecifically elevated titers in sarcoidosis patients who have activated B-lymphocytes. However, no correlation between titers and IgG concentrations were observed, especially the longitudinal study indicated a considerably higher proportion of TWAR-positive sarcoidosis patients than could be expected in the general population. Positivity was more common in older patients, which was partly compatible with findings in the population in general. It may also indicate secondary TWAR infection.

Refvem et al. (13) reported positive ornithosis complement-fixing antibody titers in 16-36% of 178 sarcoidosis patients, mean 24%. The lower percentage was in patients with non-pulmonary sarcoidosis, the higher in patients with EN. Only 9% of 188 controls were positive (p < 0.001). Ornithosis-like symptoms had only been observed in some of the patients. The high number of positive controls was probably due to TWAR infections. The complement fixing antibody test is not as sensitive as the test we used and these antibodies disappear faster (usually within a year) than antibodies measured with the micro-if test.

Our results suggested a correlation between positive TWAR titers and macrophage products such as ACE and LZM. This finding was most interesting and is compatible with the pathogenesis of the infection, as chlamydiae are phagocytosed by pulmonary macrophages, but do not impede their protein synthesis (1). The number of patients studied was too small to draw any definite conclusions, but in the longitudinal study TWAR positivity seemed to correlate with various types of clinical development, chronicity was often associated with prolonged duration of slightly increased titer. Corticosteroid treatment did not usually have an immediate effect on the titers, which remained on an elevated level. All these observations may be of pathogenetic importance and may indicate an unusual response to an ordinary infection. We do not suggest that all cases of sarcoidosis are associated with a TWAR infection. Our study has not thrown any light on the immunological pecularities that induce sarcoidosis in some patients, but future epidemiological and experimental work will hopefully bring new results on the pathogenesis of this disease.

REFERENCES

1.   Schachter J (1978) N Engl J Med   298:428-435 & 490-495 & 540-549

2.   Kuo CC, Chen HH, Wang SP, et al. (1986) J Clin Microbiol 24: 1034-1037

3.   Chi EY, Kuo CC, Grayston JT (1987) J Bacteriol 169:3757-37634.

4.   Saikku P, Wang SP, Kleemola M, et al. (1985) J Infect Dis 151:832-839

5.   Grayston JT, Kuo CC, Wang SP, et al. (1986) In: Chlamydial infections. Proc. 6th Int Symp on Human   Chlamydial Infections. Ed. D Orial. Cambridge Univ Press, pp 337-340

6.   Marrie TJ, Grayston JT, Wang SP, et al. (1987) Ann Intern Med 106:507-511

7.   Grayston JT, Kuo CC, Wang SP, Altman J (1986) N Engl J Med 315:161-168

8.   Wang SP, Grayston JT (1970) Am J Ophthalmol 70:367-374

9.   Wang SP, Grayston JT (1986) In: Chlamydial infections. Proc. 6th Int Symp on Human Chlamydial Infections. Ed. D Orial. Cambridge Univ Press, pp 329-336

10.   Grönhagen-Riska C (1980) Angiotensin Converting Enzyme and Sarcoidosis (Acad Dissert ISBN 951-99272-0-4) Helsinki University

11.   Siltzbach LE, James DG, Neville E et al (1974) Am J Med 57:847-852

12.   Kleemola M, Saikku P, Visakorpi R et al (1987) J Infect Dis (in press)

13.   Refvem O, Bjornstad R, Loe K (1976) Ann NY Acad Sci 18:225-231

RETROSPECTION OF AN UNIQUE MODE TO OBTAIN COMPLETE EPIDEMIOLOGICAL DATA IN
SARCOIDOSIS

THEODOR SCHARKOFF
Department of Lung Disease, BKH Cottbus, PSF 345, 7500 Cottbus, GDR

It is a great privilege to be able to contribute to the deliberation on the
still controversial topic Epidemiology of Sarcoidosis at this International
Conference.

The main thrust of my paper will be 1) to offer you the content of our own
methodological approach and 2) to present the fundamental results obtained
under circumstances without precedent in the hitherto existing epidemiologic
inquiry in sarcoidosis.

To gain unbiased epidemiological data the author took advantage of some par-
ticularities of the public health service in the GDR (16.5 mill. inhabitants)
especially:

1. systematic unselected chest X-ray screening of the total population since
   1954,

2. compulsory registration of sarcoidosis since 1961,

3. uniform, easily accessible and well developed medical care for all citzens.

Therefore, the prerequisites to a community-related study were given. Thus,
the greatest methodological hazard resulting from the need for a resonable
representative study group has been eliminated. The really low incidence of
sarcoidosis requires a study population which is approaching the general population. The author made use of the totally ascertained sarcoidosis population
derived from the mass experiment as mentioned above in order to carry out an
analytic study (cohort analysis of incident cases (n = 1575, time: 1961 – 1975,
defined area: district of Cottbus) adjusted for several variables (27 main variables with altogether 230 subdivisions. Follow-up period: max. 25 years, min.
5 years).

The incidence is the only parameter which is suitable for reflecting the
epidemiologic situation exactly. In a disease like sarcoidosis which is curable
– mostly spontaneous – and extremely rare fatal, prevalence data are of minor
importance apart from the different usage of that term.

In the GDR the incidence established between 1970 and 1985 ranged from 8.1
to 10.2 cases pro 100,000 inhabitants without considerable variations in the
countrywide distribution. As result of the established compulsory registration,
continuity of the X-ray screening as well as the activities of specialized
medical teams in the diagnosis and the therapy of sarcoidosis the disease
remains in an epidemiological equilibrium for years (Fig. 1).

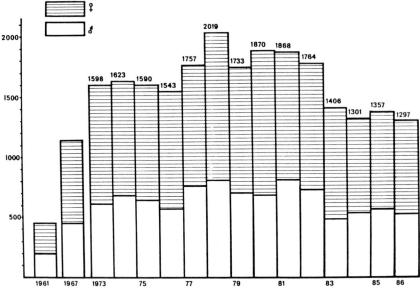

Fig. 1. Incidence of sarcoidosis in the GDR 1961 - 1985

Simultaneously with the advanced restriction of the X-ray screening the incidence curve has come to decrease in the last years (Fig. 1).

FURTHER CONCLUSIVE RESULTS
    There is a remarkable consistency in the peak age of onset (20 to 29-year
group) in both men and women (Fig. 2).
Case Fatality Rate
    death caused by sarcoidosis:
        4 cases = 0.25 % / 15 yr
    death resulting from other causes (sarcoidosis might have been partly respons-
    ible):
        45 cases = 2.85 % / 25 yr
Sex ratio:
    rough ratio male to female cases 1 : 1.54
    standardized ratio   1 : 1,46
Principal reason for the uneven sex ratio:
    Preference to females older than 30 years of age.

Residence: no significant differences between rural and urban areas.

Educational standards: emphasized predominance of the lower educational grades.

Occupation: considering the dependence of the sarcoidosis on age and sex there is no evidence for an unfavourable influence on the origin and/or the course of the disease.

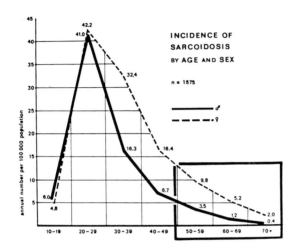

Fig. 2.   Incidence of sarcoidosis by age and sex (n = 1575)
The boxed area contains the 50-year age group and above. The group accounts for 10.2 % of the total sarcoidosis population.

DISCUSSION AND CONCLUSION

In the sixties and the seventies the sarcoidosis continued in epidemiological equilibrium in the GDR. In the last five years the decreasing incidence curve is to be traced back to the advanced restriction of the X-ray screening of the general population.

Excessive ascertainment of the asymptomatic and transient forms does not contribute to the improvement of the medical care of the diseased persons. There is no reason to suppose an increase of the disease in the last 25 years. Despite precisely collected epidemiologic data the continuous efforts to utilize both the medical as well as the socio-economic parameters with a view to pathogenesis and etiology of the disease remain without any significant results until now. The future epidemiologic research in sarcoidosis may not insist on causative aims above all.

The study presented allows reliable answers to the many unanswered questions in the epidemiology of sarcoidosis as to the influence of genetic risk factors, relationship to other diseases, overlap syndromes, socio-economic evaluation of the disease etc.

Albeit mostly disappointing yields of the epidemiological elucidation of the sarcoidosis in the past see ref. 1,2,3,4, there is really relevant progress in this respect in the eighties. Three independent European epidemiological surveys on sarcoidosis which are characterized by precise methodology and ingenious approach brought widely corresponding results see ref. 5,6,7. The author is convinced that the epidemiologic data as presented and mentioned above can be recommended as currently valid reference values for Central Europe.

REFERENCES

1. Sartwell PE (1983) Sarcoidosis and other granulomatous disorders. Pergamon Press, Paris, pp 257-260

2. Bresnitz EA, Strom BL (1983) Epidemiologr Reviews 5:124-146

3. Perdrizet S, Saltiel JC (1983) Sarcoidosis and other granulomatous disorders. Pergamon Press, Paris, pp 257-260

4. Hosoda Y, Saito S, Odaka M, Iwai K, Yanagawa H, Chiba Y, Shigematsu I (1983) Sarcoidosis and other granulomatous disorders. Pergamon Press, Paris,pp 237-244

5. Scharkoff Th (1981) Habil.-Schrift, Akademie für Ärztl. Fortbildung der DDR, Berlin

6. Hillerdal G, Nöu E, Osterman K, Schmekel B (1984) Am Rev Dis 130:29-32

7. Parkes S, Baker SB DE C, Bourdillon RE, Murray CRH, Rakshit M, Sarkies JWR, Travers JP, Williams EW (1985) Thorax 40:284-287

© 1988 Elsevier Science Publishers B.V. (Biomedical Division)
Sarcoidosis and other granulomatous disorders
C. Grassi, G. Rizzato, E. Pozzi, editors

RESULTS OF THE 1984 NATIONWIDE PREVALENCE SURVEY IN JAPAN

Y. HOSODA,[1] M. ODAKA,[2] *M. YAMAGUCHI,[3] Y. HIRAGA,[4] T. IZUMI,[5] T. TACHIBANA,[6] K. AOKI[7]

1. Radiation Effects Research Foundation, 5-2 Hijiyama Koen, Minami-ku, Hiroshima 732, (Japan), 2. JR Central Health Institute, 3. National Institute of Nutrition, 4. JR Sapporo Hospital, 5. Kyoto University, 6. Osaka Prefectural Hospital, 7. Nagoya University (* Speaker representing Japan Sarcoidosis Committee)

This report is on a study of descriptive epidemiology of sarcoidosis in Japan based on the 1984 nationwide survey combined with previous surveys.

SURVEY METHOD

As a preliminary survey, 2,921 clinical departments of hospitals with 200 beds or more were requested to report the number of sarcoidosis cases visiting their hospitals during 1984. The response rate was as high as 60%. As the secondary survey, the hospitals visited by the patients were requested to fill in the individual patient's charts comprising age, sex, residence, date of initial visit, motives of detection, symptoms, involvements, means of diagnosis, progress since the initial visit, familial sarcoidosis and type of medical insurance. Prevalence and incidence rates were estimated from the number of reported cases by Nakae's method which aimed to correct duplication, variance of residence and hospitals, and response rate by using correlation coefficients of response rate and crude prevalence rate.

RESULTS

Prevalence The respective values in the 1984 and 1972 surveys are shown below. The numbers of eligible reported cases were 1,783 and 951; crude prevalence rate per 100,000, 1.52 and 1.86 in males and 1.68 and 3.03 in females; estimated prevalence rate, 2.96 and 3.49 in males and 3.27 and 5.18 in females; (Fig. 1) histological evidence, 67.3% and 61.5%; and symptom-detected rates (other than mass X-ray), 28.5% and 45.6% in males and 50.9% and 64.8% in females, respectively. Age distribution in males formed a curve with a peak in the 20s and that in females formed a bimodal curve with peaks in the 20s and 50s, but the rate in the 40s and 50s was higher in 1984 though it was lower in 1972. In general, the patients' age seemed to have advanced. Sites involved (Fig. 2) were nearly the same in two surveys except for decrease in BHL and increase in eye lesion in 1984.

Incidence The crude rates in the 1984 and 1972 surveys were 0.90 and 1.49 per 100,000, respectively. The estimated rates have been hardly changed, being about 1.2. When the age distribution was compared among the surveys conducted in the 1960s, 1970s and 1984, the age distribution shifted to the higher age regardless of the motives of detection. The features of the increased old group were similar in all three periods.

308

In the 20s, chest lesion decreased and extrathoracic lesion, especially eye lesion, increased.

Fig. 1. Estimated prevalence   Fig. 2. Organs involved in sarcoidosis
        of sarcoidosis by age   by prevalence survey in Japan

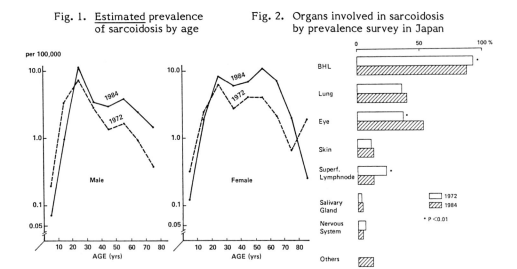

Geographical distribution   The standardized prevalence ratios (rate in a zone/rate in the entire country) were 134, 63 and 37 in 1972 in the cold, warm and very warm zones, respectively (Oxford Seasonal Climate Category), while they were 170, 51 and 57 in 1984, the difference between the warm zone and very warm zone being smaller.

SUMMARY

    In Japan, sarcoidosis prevalence increased in these 12 years. Females, old cases and cases detected by symptoms increased. Old cases also increased at first hospital visit. Old cases in incidence survey (1962-1984) showed no remarkable features, but those in the 20s had less thoracic lesions and more extrathoracic lesions.

ACKNOWLEDGMENT

    The authors wish to express their thanks to those who so willingly cooperated in this survey.

REFERENCES

1.   Report of Nationwide Survey of Intractable Diseases in 1972 (Second Report) (1973) The Intractable Diseases Research Committee, Ministry of Health and Welfare of Japan

2.   Japan Sarcoidosis Committee (1967) The Actual Condition of Sarcoidosis in Japan (Second Report)

© 1988 Elsevier Science Publishers B.V. (Biomedical Division)
Sarcoidosis and other granulomatous disorders
C. Grassi, G. Rizzato, E. Pozzi, editors

STATISTICS OF SARCOIDOSIS AUTOPSIES DURING THESE 26 YEARS IN JAPAN

KAZURO IWAI[1], TERUO TACHIBANA[2], YUTAKA HOSODA[3], YASUO MATSUI[4]

1.Research Institute of Tuberculosis,Tokyo 2.Osaka Prefectural Hospital,Osaka 3.
Radiation Effect Research Institute,Hiroshima 4.Red Cross Medical Center,Tokyo

TABLE I RATE OF SARCOIDOSIS AUTOPSY IN JAPAN, 1958-1983

	No. of total autopsy	Sarcoidosis autopsy No.	Sarcoidosis autopsy Per 100,000	
1958 - 1963	69,601	13	18.75	
1964 - 1968	99,407	22	22.11	24.44**
1969 - 1973	113,341	34	30.00	
1974 - 1978	121,574	37	30.43	35.09**
1979 - 1983	180,542	72	39.88	

** $P < 0.01$

Note: The yearly number and rate of sarcoidosis in comparison to total autopsies
is increasing significantly in Japan.

TABLE II SEX AND AGE DISTRIBUTION OF SARCOIDOSIS AUTOPSY, 1974-1983

Age	Male Total Autopsy	Male Sarcoidosis autopsy No.	Male Sarcoidosis autopsy Per 100,000	Female Total Autopsy	Female Sarcoidosis autopsy No.	Female Sarcoidosis autopsy Per 100,000
0-	17644	0	0	13670	0	0
10-	3052	0	0	1886	0	0
20-	4291	4	93.2	3251	0	0
30-	8467	7	82.7	6455	6	93.0
40-	19505	3	15.4	12179	8	65.7
50-	33580	10	29.8	19823	20	100.9
60-	44183	6	13.6	26509	19	71.7
70-	41658	5	12.0	24674	14	56.7
80-	11975	3	25.1	9326	4	42.9
Total	184355	38	20.6	117773	71	60.3

Note: Age and sex distribution of sarcoidosis showed significantly higher rate in
the females of over 40 years of age than among the males of the same age group.

310

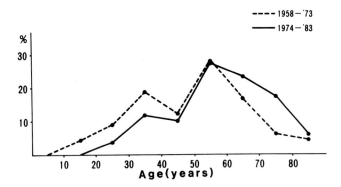

Fig. 1. Age distribution of sarcoidosis autopsy in 1958-1973 and 1974-1983
Note: Age of sarcoidosis patients shifted to higher age in recent 10 years, probably reflecting the extension of average life span of the Japanese.

TABLE III   CAUSE OF SARCOIDOSIS AUTOPSY ACCORDING TO PRESENCE OR ABSCENCE OF AN-
TEMORTEM DIAGNOSIS FOR SARCOIDOSIS, IN 1958-1973 AND IN 1974-1983

Causes of death	1958-1973 antemortem diagnosis			1974-1983 antemortem diagnosis		
	with	without	obscure	with	without	obscure
Sarcoidosis	14	32	2	29	37	0
myocardial	8	29	2	15	34	0
pulmonary	4	1	0	11	2	0
brain	2	2	0	1	1	0
others	0	0	0	2	0	0
Non-sarcoid	3	15	0	12	31	0
Unknown	0	2	1	0	0	0
Total No.	17	49	3	41	68	0
%	24.6%	71.0%	4.3%	37.6%	62.4%	0%

Note: Main cause of death was constantly myocardial sarcoidosis, and antemortem
diagnosis for sarcoidosis was made in only one third of the autopsy cases, indicating difficulties in diagnosis of cardiac sarcoidosis and few clinical sign of
the disease in some of the cases.

Rate of sarcoidosis autopsy to total autopsy,1974-1983..............36.1 per 10^5

In which, rate of sarcoidosis autopsy without antemortem diagnosis..22.2 per 10^5

Presumed prevalence rate of clinical sarcoidosis,aproximately........5.0 per 10^5

The actual number of sarcoidosis seems to be more than that of clinical cases.

SARCOIDOSIS IN NORTH INDIA : AN EMERGING CLINICAL SPECTRUM

P. BAMBERY, D. BEHERA, A. GUPTA, UPJEET KAUR, S.K. JINDAL, S. SEHGAL
S.K. MALIK AND S.D. DEODHAR
Departments of Internal Medicine, Chest Diseases, Ophthalmology, Experimental
Medicine and Immunopathology, Post Graduate Institute of Medical Education and
Research, Chandigarh-160 012 [INDIA]

INTRODUCTION

Increasing awareness has contributed substantially to the recognition of
sarcoidosis in India.[1] However, the few patients described do little justice to
our huge population, and have been indentified in large metropolitan cities where
some diagnostic facilities are available. Till 1984,[2] fewer than 100 evaluable
patients had been reported, but even in this small group some striking differences
from the Western pattern of disease were clearly discernible. Older men outnumbered
younger women, constitutional symptoms were frequently marked and ocular, bone
skin and parotid involvement were infrequent.[2]

PATIENTS AND RESULTS

Our institute serves north western India as a referral center and over the
last 7 years, we have seen 40 patients with sarcoidosis. The diagnosis was
histologically confirmed in 32 with the demonstration of granulomata in biopsy
specimens from the Kveim test site (9), liver, lungs, lymph nodes and skin (23).
Eight patients had bilateral hilar lymphadenopathy and either erythema nodosum,
or uveitis, or both.[3] There were 25 males in this group (Table 1). The mean
age at diagnosis was 47 years (range 24-68 years). Thirty nine patients had
evidence of thoracic disease but ocular involvement (16), erythema nodosum (8),
dermal plaques (2), parotid enlargement (3), fever (20) and marked constitutional
symptoms (18) were also observed. Lymphadenopathy, hepatomegaly and splenomegaly
were present in 17, 15 and 7 patients respectively. Thirty five patients were
tuberculin negative. Radiologic stages 0, I, II, and III were seen in 1, 21, 12
and 6 patients. Systemic corticosteroids were used in 24 patients while eight
received topical eye drops. The rest were treated with non steroidal anti inflammatory drugs. No patient died during the period of study but 3 had developed spirometric evidence of worsening lung function. Most of our patients had received anti
tubercular drug therapy before the diagnosis of sarcoidosis was considered and
confirmed.

DISCUSSION

The pattern of disease observed by us confirms the male domination reported
but differs from earlier Indian descriptions in the prevalence of ocular, dermal

and parotid involvement. Our patients were similar to those described by Prof. D. Geraint James.[4] A comparison of the incidence of various organ system involvement by saroidosis worldwide[5], reveals marked variation. While observer bias may contribute to this, ethnic, racial and genetic factors also play a part. We feel that the differences observed between our patients and those described by Dr. Samir Gupta,[2] may well reflect this diversity in India. The spectrum of sarcoidosis in India is now emerging, and with improving standards of health care, we feel, many more patients will be described soon.

TABLE I

SARCOIDOSIS : CLINICAL AND LABORATORY MANIFESTATIONS : REST OF THE WORLD & INDIA %

COUNTRY CITY	UK		USA		ITA	FRA	JAP	YOGO	INDIA	
	LON	EDN	NY	LA	NAP	PAR	TOK	N.SAD	CAL	CH
TOTAL PATIENTS	818	502	311	150	624	350	282	285	90	40
FEMALES	61	64	68	67	53	45	47	60	35	37
40 YRS	74	72	71	69	77	72	74	37	44	25
THORACIC	88	95	92	93	99	94	87	90	62	97
OCULAR	27	6	7	10	0.4	9	22	4	8	40
E.NODOSUM	34	33	11	9	4	7	4	11	2	20
C.N.S.	9	3	4	2	0	4	4	2	11	13
PAROTID	6	5	8	6	0	6	5	3	0	8
HEPATOMEGALY	12	x	x	x	x	x	x	x	42	37
SPLENOMEGALY	10	6	18	15	0	9	5	3	27	17
LYMPHADENOPATHY	27	33	37	31	0.3	23	23	12	19	42
RADIOLOGIC STAGE										
0		4	8	7	1	6	5	10	1	2
I	65	52	43	25	64	38	51	57	38	53
II	22	29	35	35	28	49	30	21	29	30
III	13	15	14	33	7	7	6	11	32	15
KVEIM +	84	64	92	72	56	77	54	81	89	45
MANTOUX -	70	58	63	85	70	80	62	43	69	88

REFERENCES

1. James DG, Jones Williams W. (1985) Sarcodosis and other granulomatous disorders, WB Saunders Co. Philadelphia.

2. Gupta SK, Mitra K, Roy M, Dutta SK. (1985) Ind.J.Chest.Dis.All.Sci. 27: 55-63.

3. Winterbauer RH, Belic N, Moores KK. (1973) Ann.Intern.Med. 78: 65-71.

4. James DG. (1983) J.Roy.Coll.Phys.Lond. 17: 196-204.

5. James DG, Neville E, Siltzbach LE. et al. (1976) Ann.N.Y.Acad.Sci. 278: 321-334.

SARCOIDOSIS DEATHS - THE HOWARD UNIVERSITY HOSPITAL EXPERIENCE 1975 - 1987

ROBERT L. HACKNEY JR., ROSCOE C. YOUNG JR., OCTAVIUS D. POLK JR., EARL M. ARMSTRONG

Department of Medicine, Pulmonary Division, Howard University Hospital, 2041 Georgia Avenue, N.W., Washington, D.C.

INTRODUCTION

In the past respiratory failure complicated by tuberculous or non-tuberculous lung infections was the most common cause of death in sarcoidosis patients (1-4). We studied the records of our 28 biopsy proven sarcoidosis patients who died between 1975 and 1987 to determine if such patients now die of the same problems.

THE GROUP STUDIED

There were 19 women and 9 men whose mean age was 44 years. The mean duration of sarcoidosis before death was 11 years. All the patients were black. Chest x-ray films were classified as follows: Stage I - Bilateral hilar lymphadenopathy (BHL) alone; Stage II - BHL with diffuse pulmonary lesions (DPL); Stage III - DPL without BHL and Stage IV - Stage III with cysts. Patients were considered to have Chronic respiratory failure if the PaO_2 was less than 55mmHg (at an FIO_2 of 20.79%) at least 6 months.

RESULTS

In addition to the 19 patients with chronic respiratory failure 6 others had Stage IV chest x-ray film patterns (See Table I).

TABLE I

THE CAUSES OF DEATH OF 28 HOWARD UNIVERSITY HOSPITAL SARCOIDOSIS PATIENTS 1975 - 1987

Causes of Death	No. Patients (%)
I. Chronic Respiratory Failure	19 (68)
A. Simple with or without Cor Pulmonale	7 (25)
B. With superimposed Acute Respiratory Failure	8 (29)
C. With Malignancy	4 (14)
II. Cardiac Sarcoidosis	6 (21)
III. Steroid Therapy Related	3 (11)

The total of such x-ray patterns was 25 or 89% of the entire group.

DEATHS DUE TO ACUTE RESPIRATORY FAILURE SUPERIMPOSED ON CHRONIC RESPIRATORY FAILURE

Three (3) patients with pulmonary embolism (See Table I) were wheelchair confined because of severe hypoxemia which required them to use continuous oxygen. Both patients who died from pulmonary hemorrhage had fungus balls in upper lobe cysts.

DEATHS DUE TO MALIGNANCY AND CHRONIC RESPIRATORY FAILURE

These were the oldest patients in the group and have had Sarcoidosis longer than any of the others. Primary Cancer sites were: 1 patient-bilateral breast and bladder, 1 each-breast, pharynx and stomach respectively. Sarcoidosis was present at least 5 years before the initial diagnosis of Cancer was made in all of the patients.

CARDIAC SARCOIDOSIS PATIENTS

Four (4) patients died from ventricular arrhythmias one (1) of whom had extensive neurosarcoidosis and another had testicular lesions and lupus pernio. Death was due to acute respiratory failure with acute cor pulmonale in another patient and due to intractable congestive heart failure in a final one.

STEROID THERAPY RELATED

Gram negative sepsis accounted for the death of 1 patient and peritonitis due to multiple ruptures of colonic diverticuli in another. The last patient discontinued his prednisone and died from acute adrenocortical insufficiency.

SUMMARY

Chronic respiratory failure caused the deaths of 68% (19 of 28) of our patients most of whom had superimposed acute respiratory failure or Cancer. cardiac sarcoidosis accounted for 6 and steroid therapy another 3 of the deaths. These causes of death differ considerably from those previously reported.

REFERENCES
1. Sones M, Irael HL (1960) Course and Prognosis of Sarcoidosis. Amer J. Med 29:84-93
2. Mayock RL, Bertrand P, Morris CE, Scott JH (1963) Manifestations of Sarcoidosis. Analysis of 145 Patients with a Review of Nine Series Selected from the Literature. Amer J Med 35:67-89
3. Reisner D (1967) Observations of the Course and Prognosis of Sarcoidosis. Amer Rev Respir Dis 96:361-380
4. Huang CT, Heuric AE, Sutton AL, Lyons HA (1981) Mortality in Sarcoidosis. A Changing Pattern of the Causes of Death. Eur J Respir Dis 62:231-238

SMOKING DOES NOT AFFECT PREVALENCE OR SHORT TERM FUNCTIONAL OUTCOME OF SARCOIDOSIS IN IRELAND

KEVIN WARD, MUIRIS X. FITZGERALD

Dept. of Medicine, University College Dublin, St. Vincent's Hospital, Elm Park, Dublin 4, Ireland

INTRODUCTION

Cigarette (cigs.) smoking is associated with a no. of respiratory disorders (1). However smokers maybe at a decreased risk of developing extrinsic allergic alveolitis or ulcerative colitis (2). Compared to non-smokers it has been suggested both that smokers are less likely (3) and equally likely (4) to develop sarcoidosis.

MATERIAL AND METHODS

Details of smoking habits, at the time of diagnosis, of pts. at our Sarcoid Clinic were obtained by personal interview or by chart review. Data was available on 335 pts.; 177 men (mean 31 yrs) and 158 women (mean 32 yrs). Regular smokers were those who smoked >5 cigs./day for >6 months. Patients who stopped regular smoking within 6 months of diagnosis were classed as regular smokers. The control group were interviewees from the annual survey by the Health Education Bureau (HEB) and Irish Marketing Surveys Ltd. into the smoking habits of 1000 members of the adult population. Follow-up (mean 49 months, minimum 12 months) of pulmonary function tests is reported for 208 pts.

RESULTS

One hundred and twenty three sarcoid pts. (37%) were regular smokers at their time of diagnosis. This was approx. the same as the 10 year average for smoking in the general population (37.5%). Forty one sarcoid pts. (12%) were ex smokers.

TABLE 1

No. regular smokers; sarcoids and controls, different age ranges

Age Range (years)	Sarcoids: regular smokers	Controls: regular smokers
18 - 24	35 of 78 pts. (44%)	37%
25 - 34	58 of 146 pts. (40%)	41%
35 - 44	16 of 60 pts. (27%)	38%
45 - 54	5 of 19 pts. (41%)	41%

No significant differences

316

There was no difference between the prevalence of smoking between the male (37%) and female (36%) pts. and the male (42%) and female (33%) controls. Smokers comprised 36% of those presenting with erythema nodosum (n=88) and 35% of pts. with significant eye problems (n=89) ; 37% of 217 pts. without eye problems were smokers.

TABLE 2

No. regular smokers; sarcoids and controls, different years of diagnosis

Year of diagnosis	New sarcoids Smokers (%)	Nonsmokers	Control Smokers (%)
1978	7 (35%)	13	39%
1979	7 (27%)	19	36%
1980	16 (53%)	14	36%
1981	12 (36%)	21	35%
1982	10 (45%)	12	35%
1983	10 (29%)	25	32%
1984	15 (37%)	26	32%
1985	5 (24%)	16	32%
1986	10 (34%)	19	31%

No significant differences

TABLE 3

Sarcoid smokers and non-smokers; initial and latest pulmonary function tests

Pulmonary Function Test	Sarcoid smokers n = 75 (mean % predicted +- SD)		Sarcoid non smokers n = 108	
	1st	Last	1st	Last
FVC	89 (16)	94 (17)	90 (19)	95 (18)
FEV1	90 (21)	93 (21)	86 (19)	89 (22)
DLCO	88 (20)	95 (17)	85 (19)	91 (20)

No significant differences

SUMMARY

There was no difference in smoking habits between the sarcoid pts. and the control population. Our findings are in keeping with other negative studies (4). This survey of the smoking habits of Irish sarcoid pts. finds no evidence that smoking protects against the development of sarcoidosis or ameliorates its pulmonary consequences.

REFERENCES

1. Smoking and health: a report of the surgeon general. Washington, DC.; U.S. Government Printing Office, 1979. (DHEW publication no. (PHS)79-50066).

2. Jick H, Walker AM. Cigarette smoking and ulcerative colitis. N Engl J Med 1983; 308:261-3.

3. Douglas JG, Middleton WG, Gaddie J et al. Sarcoidosis: a disorder commoner in non-smokers? Thorax 1986; 41:787-91.

4. Bresnitz EA, Stolley PD, Israel HL, Soper K. Possible risk factors for sarcoidosis. Ann NY Acad Sci 1986; 465:632-642.

SARCOIDOSIS IN BARCELONA: SPRING CLUSTER OF LÖFGREN SYNDROME

F. Badrinas (*), J. Morera (***), J. Mañá (*), E. Fité (**), J. Valverde (*), R. Vidal (**) and
J. Ruiz-Manzano (***)
Hospital de Bellvitge (*), Hospital Vall d´Hebró (**) and Hospital `` Germans Trias i Pujol´´(***).
BARCELONA. SPAIN.

INTRODUCTION

The sarcoidosis incidence rate in Barcelona is 1.2 per 100.000 (1), and subacute forms with erythema nodosum (Löfgren syndrome) are very frequent (44% in our series of 423 patients).

AIM OF THE STUDY

The purpose of the study is demonstrate the seasonal variations of Löfgren syndrome at onset (2-5).

MATERIALS AND METHODS

During the 15-years period, 1971 through 1986, from a series of 423 patients with confirmed sarcoidosis, 186 having Löfgren syndrome were studied. 166 were female (89%) and 20 were male (11%).
Mean age: 39 years (range: 14 to 67 years). Race: caucasian.
The statistical analysis is a goodness of fit test using the Chi-square method the null hypotesis is that the date follow a uniform distribution

RESULTS

Among 186 patients having Löfgren syndrome, 91 (49%) were diagnosed during the spring months of April, May and June. Significant statistical differences were found between spring and other seasons (p < 0.0001)

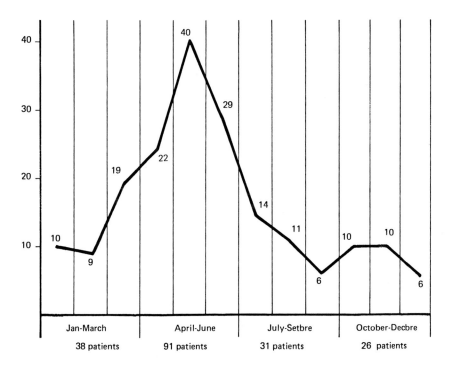

	Jan-March	April-June	July-Setbre	October-Decbre
	38 patients	91 patients	31 patients	26 patients

318

CONCLUSION

This findings strongly suggest the intervention of hypothetical enviromental factor in the etiology of this disorder.

REFERENCES

1. Morera Prat J., Aranda Torres A. and Badrinas Vancells F. Sarcoidosis in Spain. In: IX International Conference on Sarcoidosis and Other Granulomatous Disorders. J. Chretien, J. Marsac and J.C. Saltier (eds) Pergamon Press, Paris, 1983; pp 625.
2. Hosoda Y., Hiraga Y., Odaka M., et al. A cooperative study of sarcoidosis in Asia and Africa: analytic epidemiology. Ann N Y Acad Sci, 1976; 278: 355-367.
3. Putkonen T., Hannuksela M., and Mustakallio K.K. Cold season prevalence of the clinical onset of sarcoidosis. Archs environ Hlth, 1966; 12: 564-568
4. Poukkula A., Huhti E., Lilja M. and Saloheimo M. Incidence and clinical picture of sarcoidosis in a circumscribed geographical area. Br J Dis Chest, 1986; 80: 138-147.
5. Henke C.E., Henke G., Elveback L.R., Beard C.M.Ballard D.J. and Kurland L.T. The epidemiology of sarcoidcsis in Rochester, Minnesota: a population-based study of incidence and survival, Am J Epidemiol 1986; 123: 840-845

© 1988 Elsevier Science Publishers B.V. (Biomedical Division)
Sarcoidosis and other granulomatous disorders
C. Grassi, G. Rizzato, E. Pozzi, editors

SARCOIDOSIS AND TUBERCULOSIS OF LYMPH NODES :
AN EPIDEMIOLOGICAL STUDY OF 25 YEARS

K. GOURGOULIANIS, A. STEFIS, S. GOUGOULAKIS, F. SCOTTI,
TSAKRAKLIDES. V.
1. Athens Hospital of Thoracic Diseases
2. Pathology Department of Social Security Institute
3. Diagnostic Therapeutic Center "HYGEIA"

The incidence of sarcoidosis and tuberculosis of lymph nodes
can not be determined accurately because the diagnostic methods
particularly for sarcoidosis are not absolutely defined. The
purpose of this study was the evaluation of the epidemiological
characteristics of the above diseases in Greece the last twenty
five years.

MATERIAL AND METHODS

We reviewed 4711 lymph nodes biopsies performed during the
years 1961- 1985 from the files of the Pathology Department of
Social Security Institute. The diagnosis of sarcoidosis was made
in 158 patients (3%) and the diagnosis of tuberculosis in 582
patients (12%). The diagnosis was based on patients files and on
the histological examination of the material from two
pathologists.

RESULTS

The percentage of sarcoidosis was much higher during the late
years (1981-1985), 46 patients, than during the early years
(1961-1965), 8 patients. The percentage of tuberculosis was
higher during the early years (1961-1965), 129 patients, than
during the late years (1981-1985), 69 patients (Table I). The
incidence of sarcoidosis was higher in the elderly than in the
other age groups. The number of women with sarcoidosis of lymph
nodes (112) was higher than the number of the man (46), an
average of 7 women to 3 men. The mean age for women was 56 and
the mean age for men was 41 years old (p<.01). The mean age for
patients with sarcoidosis was 54 and the mean age for patients
with tuberculosis was 44 years old (p<.01) (Table II).

DISCUSSION

The biopsy of lymph nodes is one of the most frequent
diagnostic method of sarcoidosis; 40% of the diagnosis of
sarcoidosis was based on it (Siltzbach, 1974). The data indicate
that the tuberculosis of lymph nodes is 4 times more frequent
than sarcoidosis of lymph nodes. The same ratio in Algeria was
40:1 (Benjaoui, 1986). The sarcoidosis attacks the women more
frequently than tuberculosis, two times more often than men. In
the years 1981-1985 the two diseases have the same distribution
in Greece. Consequently the tuberculous lymphadenitis is
decreasing giving its place to sarcoidosis, a new health problem
with an increasing incidence in the Greek population.

REFERENCES

1. Benzaoui Z.,Berrabah Y.,Lelloy S. Sarcoidosis in Western Algeria. An epidemiological study. Sarcoidosis 1986; 3:171.

2. Siltzbach LE.,James GD., Turiaf J.,Battesti JP.,Sharma OF., Hosoda Y.,Mikami R., Odaka M., (1974). Course and prognosis of sarcoidosis around the world. Am J Med 57(6):847.

TABLE I

	SARCOIDOSIS	TUBERCULOSIS	
1961-65	8	129	(6%)
1966-70	23	161	(14%)
1971-75	39	127	(31%)
1976-80	42	96	(44%)
1981-85	46	69	(67%)
	158	582	(27%)

Distribution of sarcoidosis and tuberculosis of lymph nodes per five years

TABLE II

	SARCOIDOSIS	TUBERCULOSIS
WOMEN	56.4 (SD 13.1)	46 (SD 16.6)
	t-test 6.26 (p<.001)	
MEN	48.6 (SD 14.7)	41 (SD 17.7)
	t-test 3.1 (.01>p>.001)	
MEAN AGE	54	44

Age at diagnosis

© 1988 Elsevier Science Publishers B.V. (Biomedical Division)
Sarcoidosis and other granulomatous disorders
C. Grassi, G. Rizzato, E. Pozzi, editors

OCULAR SARCOIDOSIS IN THE NETHERLANDS

A.Rothova[1,3], C.Alberts[2], A.Kijlstra[3], E.Glasius[3], A.C.Breebaart[1]

1) Academic Medical Centre, Dept. of Ophthalmology, 2) Academic Medical Centre, Dept. of Pulmonology, 3) Netherlands Ophthalmic Research Institute, Amsterdam, The Netherlands

INTRODUCTION

Ocular involvement in sarcoidosis remains controversial. It has been reported in 25-65% of the patients, depending on geographical factors, population sample, extent of ophthalmologic examination and follow-up. The aim of our study was to determine the frequency and extent of ocular involvement and to identify a clinical profile of patients at risk to develop ocular disease.

MATERIALS AND METHODS

We studied two groups of sarcoidosis patients using a computer analysis of more than 25 variables per patient, including the results of ophthalmologic and general examinations as well as the laboratory and radiological findings.

Group 1 consisted of 163 patients with clinical diagnosis sarcoidosis consulting the sarcoidosis clinic in Amsterdam between 1979 and 1986. Group 2 included 75 consecutive patients with biopsy proven sarcoidosis from group 1, who presented at the sarcoidosis clinic between 1983 and 1986. Our study included 66 black patients (41%) in group 1 and 35 black patients (47%) in group 2.

RESULTS

Ocular involvement was present in 71 patients (44%) of group 1 and 41 patients (55%) of group 2. Half of those with eye manifestation were black. Uveitis was the most common ocular manifestation of sarcoidosis (63% in both groups, see table 1). Legal blindness (vision <0.1) was always due to (posterior and pan) uveitis complications. No difference was observed in the frequency of uveitis when the patients were subdivided according to sex, age, race and chronicity of sarcoidosis. General clinical symptoms of sarcoidosis patients with uveitis did not significantly differ from the symptoms of sarcoidosis patients without uveitis.

The uveitis patients (n=26, group 2) were classified according to the localisation of uveitis in an anterior or posterior/panuveitis group (table 2). Female patients suffered more frequently from ocular sarcoidosis than male patients ($p<0.001$ group 1; $p<0.02$ group 2). In black patients anterior uveitis was more frequent ($p<0.005$ group 1 and 2), whereas in white patients posterior and panuveitis was more common. The complication rate was significantly higher in the posterior and panuveitis group (p<0.005). Chronic posterior uveitis associated with ocular complications was most frequently observed in white female patients (p<0.001 group 1 and 2).

CONCLUSIONS

Based on this study we conclude that chronic posterior uveitis associated with serious ocular complications occurred most frequently in white female sar-coidosis patients. Since ocular involvement was present in half of sarcoidosis patients, we conclude that ophthalmologic examination is necessary in order to recognise this disease and prevent its complications or visual handicap.

TABLE 1

OCULAR FINDINGS IN SARCOIDOSIS

	ocular involvement in clinical sarcoidosis (group 1)		ocular involvement in biopsy proven sarcoidosis (group 2)	
	n	%	n	%
conjunctival involvement	29	40	17	41
lacrimal gland involvement	23	32	15	36
uveitis	45	63	26	63
anterior uveitis	19	27	12	29
posterior and panuveitis	26	37	14	34
visual acuity $\leqslant$0.1	6	8	3	7
no. of patients	71		41	

TABLE 2

CHARACTERISTICS OF UVEITIS PATIENTS IN BIOPSY PROVEN SARCOIDOSIS

	total uveitis	anterior uveitis	posterior and panuveitis
no. of patients	26	12	14
age at the onset (y)	35	30*	42*
sex ratio (male to female)	1:2,3	1:1,4	1:3,6
race ratio (white to black)	1:1	1:3*	2,5:1*
acute to chronic uveitis ratio	1:1,8	2:1*	1:13*
ocular complications	16	3[+]	13[+]
visual acuity $\leqslant$0.1	3	0	3

* p<0.05

[+] p<0.005

FINAL RESULTS OF 15-YEARS FOLLOW UP STUDY OF 168 SARCOID PATIENTS

B. DJURIĆ, N. ŽAFRAN, DJ. POVAŽAN

Institute of Lung Diseases and Tuberculosis, 21204 Sremska Kamenica,
Yugoslavia

The aim of this study is to estabilish the course and outcome of sarcoidosis over a longer period of time after the diagnosis was made. Therefore,
we studied the course of sarcoidosis of 168 patients who had this disease
diagnosed approximately 15 years ago (cases covered the time span from 14 to
22 years).

When the diagnosis was made the average age of the patients was 42 years,
with patients between the ages of 20 and 70.60% of the patients were females and 40% were males. We had 102 patients (61%) with stage I of intratho
racic sarcoidosis (enlarged hilar lymph nodes), 40 patients (24%) with stage II (enlarged hilar lymph nodes + granulomatous lung lesions or only granulomatous lung lesions), and 26 patients (15%) with stage III (diffuse fibrotic lesions).

Extrathoracic sarcoid lesions were discovered in liver in 50% of the cases,
in eyes in 20%, in bones in 15, in skin in 4%, in periferal lymph nodes in
13% and in parotid gland in 2%.

68% of the patients had symptoms and they manifested as: cough in 65% of
the cases, weakness in 40%, dyspnoea in 33%, sweating in 28% and arthralgia
in 18%. Erythema nodosum was present in 16% of the patients. 32% of all sarcoid patients were without any symptoms.

Tuberculin test was negative in 46% of our patients.

Pulmonary function tests have shown decrease of vital capacity in 34.3%
of patients with stage I, in 82% of patients with stage II and all the patients with stage III.

Total endobronchial resistance was increased in 16.4% of the patients.

84% of cases were treated with corticosteroids.

The analysis of the 15 years follow-up study of the described patients
have shown following results:

Total regression of pulmonary lesions was established in 87.2% of the cases with stage I. Enlarged lymph nodes still persisted in 7.8%. 4.9% of the
cases had progression towards pulmonary fibrosis. Among 40 patients who had
stage II, 15 years ago, now 30 of them (75%) have normal chest X-ray. 7.5%
evolved towards pulmonary fibrosis, but in 7 patients (17.5%) chest X ray

was unchanged. Over the period of 15 years there have not been noticed any improvements on chest X-ray of patients with stage III.

18.3% of our patients had relapses. 86% of the relapses occurred in the first three years after the diagnosis of sarcoidosis was made. 11% of relapses occurred in the period from 3 to 6 years and 3% of relapses occurred in the period from 6 to 9 years after the sarcoidosis was diagnosed. The average age of patients with relapses (49.5 years) was higher than average age of the whole group (42 years).

In the period of observation 27 persons (15.1%) died. 70.3% of all fatalities were patients with diffuse pulmonary fibrosis. In 14 cases (51.8%) the cause of death was pulmonary insufficiency. Cerebrovascular insult was a cause of death in 14.8% of the cases. In 26% of fatalities the cause of death could not be determined because the data were not available to us.

The results of the pulmonary function tests in the majority of cases have shown improvement except in patients with stage III.

Analysing the symptoms of sarcoid patients we have found that now arthralgia is present in 23.1% of cases, even a little more than it was in the beginning of the disease (18%).

Evaluating the results of radiological regression, pulmonary function test and the existance of symptoms, 15 years after sarcoidosis was diagnosed, 72% of patients had normal results and were without any symptoms. 28% of the patients had abnormalities on chest X ray, disturbance in pulmonary function or had symptoms.

A CONTINUATION OF THE WORLDWIDE STUDY ON SARCOIDOSIS

B. DJURIĆ (YU), A.G.KHOMENKO (SU), M.MAYER (CSR)
G. RIZZATO (I), O. SCHWEIGER (H), R.CHRIST (GDR)
N. SEČEN (YU)

INTRODUCTION

Results of retrospective study of 3676 patients with sarcoidosis were reported in 1976 in New York, on the Seventh International Conference on Sarcoidsis and Other Granulomatous Disorders. In that study the next features were
investigated: sex, race, intrathoracic and extrathoracic localisation, positive Kveim-Siltzbach and negative tuberculin test, systemic corticosteroid therapy and mortality due to sarcoidosis. The purpose of this study is to continue former investigation on the sarcoidosis features in some European countries (Italy, Soviet Union, Czechoslovakia, Hungary, German Democratic Republic
and Yugoslavia).

MATERIAL, METHODS AND RESULTS

Out of examined patients with sarcoidosis, 333 patients were from Italy,
55 from Soviet Union, 277 from Czechoslovakia, 16 from Hungary, 512 from
GDR and 285 from Yugoslavia.

Except from Hungarian patients (small statistical model) in whom sarcoidosis was predominatly in males, in all other countries the greater frequency
of sarcoidosis was diagnosed in felmales, in 860 patients (58.18%). 994 patients (63.87%) were younger than 40 years. There were 1378 (93.23%) patinents
with intrathoracic sarcoidosis.

Ocular involvement was found in 43 patients (2.90%); all patients were
from Yugoslavia. Erythema nodósum occurred in 270 patients (18.26%).The
most freguent was in patients from Czechoslovakia - 67 cases 24% , the least frequent was in patients from Yugoslavia - 31 cases (11%). Other skin
lesions were in 71 patients (4.80%).

Parotid gland enlargement was seen in 34 patients (2.30%). Nervous-system
involvement occurred in 13 patients (0.87%). Bone involvement occurred
in 36 patients (2.43%), mostly in the group of patients from Yugoslavia. Bone cystes were not registrated in patients from Itraly, Hungary and GDR.

Lymphadenopathy and splenomegaly were simulataneously registrated in 58 patients (3.92%). Lymphadenopathy was found in 445 patients (30.10%) and splenomegaly in 18 patients (1.21%) . Hepatomegaly was observed in 59 patients
(3.99%).

Heart changes occurred in 65 patients (4.39%).

Lacrimal gland involvement was found in 4 patients (0.27%). They were from Czechoslovakia and GDR. Kidney involvement was registrated in 5 patients (0.33%). Four patients were from Czechoslovakia and one patient was from Hungary.

Changes in upper respiratory tract were observed only in one patient from Czechoslovakia.

861 patients (58.25%) were treated with systemic corticosteroids. None of the patients from Italy used corticosteroids, while 92% of the patients from Yugoslavia were treated with this kind of therapy.

Kveim-Siltzbach test was positive in 283 patients (72%). The most frequent positive Kveim-Siltzbach test was in patients from Yugoslavia (81%).

Negative tuberculin test was registrated in 654 patients (63%).

Hyperglobulinemia occurred in 12.1% of the patients and hypercalcemia in 3.11%.

CONCLUSION

The group of 1193 sarcoid patients from Italy, Soviet Union, Czechoslovakia, Hungary, German Democratic Republic and Yugoslavia, were analyzed in the same principle as the group of 3676 patients whose results of examination were shown on the Seventh International Meeting on Sarcoidosis and Granulomatous Disorders which now comprises total 4869 patients.

Sarcoidosis was found to be the same or rather similar disease in all analyzed countries. However, males were found to be predominant in the Hungarian sarcoid group and ocular involvement was mostly found in the Yugoslav group. Parotid gland enlargement as well as nervous system changes were frequently found in Yugoslav and Czechoslovak group. Heart changes were most often diagnosed in the examined group from Czechoslovakia. Kidney involvement was more frequently diagnosed in Hungary than in other countries.

Corticotherapy was applied in almost all patients from Yugoslavia,but in other countries it was applied in a less percentage, but it was not applied to any patient from Italy.

Kveim-Siltzbach test was positive 40-85% on the average 72%,i.e. sarcoid patients reacted in a similar way in all countries. Tuberculin test was the least positive in the Yugoslav group of patients and the most positive in the Czechoslovak group.

Correspodence: Prof. dr B. Djurić, Institute of Lung Diseases, 212o4 Sremska Kamenica, Yugoslavia

SARCOIDOSIS AND CANCER: A PROSPECTIVE STUDY

FRODE K RØMER
Department of Medicine, Silkeborg Central Hospital,
DK-8600 Silkeborg (Denmark)

INTRODUCTION

The occurrence of cancer in sarcoidosis patients has been described in occasional cases and in a few small series. In one register study (from Denmark) an increased occurrence of malignant lymphomas and lung cancer was found, based upon the Danish Sarcoidosis Register and compared with the general population risk.

However, these results were seriously challenged in a later revision of the series (Rømer 1978), leaving no evidence of an increased incidence of cancer in those series.

Thus, it remains unsolved whether the frequency of malignant diseases in sarcoidosis is higher than in the general population.

The present study is designed to evaluate the long term risk of cancer development in a well-defined Danish series of sarcoidosis patients.

MATERIAL AND METHODS

The total number of patients is 578, mean age 31 years, all whites. All patients had the diagnosis of sarcoidosis in the years 1960-1981. All but seven had pulmonary sarcoidosis (type I 57%, type II 36%, type III 6%), erythema nodosum was present in 19% and other extrathoracic manifestations in 28%.

By cooperation with the Danish national population register (which covers the whole population) and the Danish Cancer Register (to which notification is compulsory for physicians and medical institutions) all relevant data are computerized. When this procedure is finished it will be possible to obtain the following results; 1) mortality, time and causes of death, 2) number, time and nature of malignant diseases, 3) association between these and the clinical and demographical features of the sarcoidosis patients, 4) comparison with the expected mortality and cancer morbidity in the general population.

RESULTS

The input of data on computer is not yet finished. But a preliminary, although incomplete screening in 1982, unveiled only 6 cases of malignancies following sarcoidosis in 526 patients, followed for 1-20 years. This figure was not higher than expected.

CONCLUSION

It is still open for debate whether cancer occurs more frequently than expected in patients with sarcoidosis. We hope that this prospective study may throw light on this problem. The final results are planned to be available at 1987-88, covering 6-27 years of observation. Regular reevaluations are planned.

EPIDEMIOLOGY OF SARCOIDOSIS. OUTLOOK.

M. FREITAS E COSTA
Clínica de Doenças Pulmonares - Faculdade de Medicina de Lisboa.
Av. Prof. Egas Moniz, 1699 Lisboa Codex (Portugal)

The edpidemiological workup of any pathologic entity carry multiple problems, exemplified by sampling, evaluation and interpretation of data.

As sarcoidosis is concerned, the epidemiologic studies are even more difficult and complex. This is based on its unknown etiology, multisystemic and plurifaced characteristics, inconstant symptomatic exuberance and expression resulting in a several speciality analysis, designately in the field of the pneumologist, dermatologist, ophtalmologist and neurologist.

Nevertheless, some important work on epidemiology of sarcoidosis has come out, mostly exemplified by the studies of Geraint James and Jones-Williams, which somehow clarify aspects of such a fascinating nosologic entity.

As I was charged to perform an Outlook of the Epidemiology of Sarcoidosis for the XI World Congress, in Milan, it seemed appropriate to develop a short inquiry about some elements of epidemiologic importance. So far, this short inquiry was elaborated and mailed to 220 Pneumologists or Pneumologic Centers throughout the World (Europe - 100; North America - 30; Latin America - 30; Africa - 20; Asia - 20; Middle East - 10 and Australia - 10), requesting information about new cases of sarcoidosis diagnosed in 1985 and 1986. The number of patients, age, sex, race, clinical setting, stage, smoking habits, tuberculin skin test, SACE and Kweim test were required.

Of 220 inquiries mailed, only 46 positive and satisfactory responses were received (20.9%), but it must be stressed that the inquiry was frequently divulgated by inquired colleagues, as it was the cases of Belgium, Italy and Sweden, resulting in a whole of 76 contributors (Table I).

So, it was possible to obtain data about 2636 new cases of Sarcoidosis (Europe - 2242; North America - 237; Asia - 122 and Middle East - 35) proceeding from 24 countries, from which at least one response was received (Table II), (A and B).

EPIDEMIOLOGY – SARCOIDOSIS

COUNTRY	CONTRIBUTORS
AUSTRIA	H. KLECH
BELGIUM	BOGAERTS, D. BRUART, L. CALLENS, M. DEMETS, P. DESCHEPPER, R. DEVOPELAIRE, J. P. DIERCKX, C. GILLARD, HUYBRECHS, HENNEGHIEN, F. LENAERTS, MAIRESSE, J. P. MOLLE, R. PANNIER, J. PRIGNOT, RENACLE, Y. J. ROBIENCE, VAN RINHERGHEN, P. VERHAGE, VERSIJP, A. VERSTRAETEN and J. M. VERSTRAETEN
BULGARIA	P. DOBREV and STOYAN IVANOV
CANADA	G. M. DAVIES
CHINA	WANG ZENGLI
CZECOSLOVAKYA	Z. VOSLÁŘOVÁ, V. VOTAVA and KŘIVINKA
FINNLAND	EERO TALA
FRANCE	J. MIGUERES and MAX PERRIN-FAYOLLE
GERMANY	DIERKESMANN and HUZLY
IRELAND	M. X. FITZGERALD
ISRAEL	I. BRUDERMAN and HTOPILSKY
ITALY	L. ALLEGRA, F. BAUJI, A. BLASI, L. CARRATU, A. CIPRIANI, C. GRASSI, D. OLIVIERI, G. PESCETTI, E. POZZI, G. RIZZATO and G. SEMENZATO
JAPAN	Y. HIRAGA, Y. HOSODA and T. IZUMI.
KOREA(S)	DONG-SOON KIM
NORWAY	A. GULSVIG, S. HUMERFELT and V. KAUG
POLAND	JAN ZIELINSKI
PORTUGAL	A. R. ALMEIDA, R. ÁVILA, J. M. ABREU BARRETO, A. MARTINS COELHO, M. YGLÉSIAS DE OLIVEIRA and M. FREITAS E COSTA
ROMANIA	V. MANGIULEA
SPAIN	A. XAUBET-MIR and A. AGUSTI VIDAL
SWEDEN	I. BRADVIK and B. G. SIMONSSON, BOMAN, J. SJÖGREN, T. WEGNER
SWITZERTALND	PH. LEUENBERGER
THAILAND	SOMCHAI BOVORNKITTI
UNITED KINGDOM	D. C. FLENLEY and 11 col.
USA	H. ISRAEL, J. A. RANKIN, H. REYNOLDS and Om P. SHARMA
TOTAL **24 Countries**	**70 Contributors**

TABLE I

It is clear the handicap to withdraw conclusions from these data, specially relating to the incidence of Sarcoidosis throughout the World.

However, relating to Europe, with 2242 cases, it is my opinion that some items should be stressed.

So, the number of cases disclosed in Czechoslovakia is remarkable, owing to the fact that only the total of new cases are reported (618).

Also the number of new sarcoidosis cases reported by Sweden (301) and refered to an wide area of the country, leads us to admit its high incidency rate.

The high number of Belgium contributors (22 and 141 patients) must express a fairly good outlook of this country situation. The same may be accepted for Italy, with 386 new cases in 1985-86.

In what Portugal is concerned, with 97 new cases in a population which includes approximately $2_{/3}$ of the whole country, the prevalence should be approximately 0.7 per 100.00, a relatively low prevalence. However it is worth to remeber that 20 years ago, the prevalence estimate by T.G. Villar was 0.2 per 100.000 inhabitants.

Other data merit some remarks. It has been described that sarcoidosis affects predominantly patients less than 40 years old and females, which our inquiry confirms in its whole ($<$ 40 years - 58.6%; females - 60%).

Nevertheless I state that, in some countries, this is not the rule as in Czechoslovakia, where 52.5% of patients are older than 40, or in Norway, Ireland and Poland which yield a predomine of males, respectively of 75%, 57% and 54%.

Other aspects are also interesting. So, for the clinical setting, the average of patients with ophtalmological abnormalities is 7.2%, but in Portugal this rate is of 15.6%, in the United States of America of 19.9% and in Japan of 44.8%. Also the dermatological involvement displays a noticiable variation. The whole rate being 20.6%, in Poland it is of 2.6% only, as far as in the United Kingdom it goes to 31.7%, in Portugal to 32.9% and in Ireland to 40%.

Other important differences may be retrieved in our data, but those refered above are elucidative of the impossibility to set standards for several aspects of Sarcoidosis.

Some other clues deserve a special remark. The low incidence of smoking habits among patients must be stressed, once more (16.7%).

Curious enough, is the performance of tuberculin skin test in 71.6% of patients, 16.8% of whom were positive, and of SACE in only

COUNTRY	N.° PATIENTS	AGE		SEX		RACE			SMO-KERS	CLINICAL PRESENTATION					
		<40	>40	♂	♀	CAUC	AF	AS		RX	DERM	OST	RESP	OPH	NEUR
AUSTRIA	70	51	19	28	42	69	1	0	11	64	15	3	36	1	7
BELGIUM	141	7b	63	65	76	130	11	0	31	74	24	11	59	6	4
BULGARIA	105	56	49	34	71	105	0	0	13	102	7	11	80	7	5
CANADA	21	16	5	12	9	14	7	0	3	21	5	5	15	2	0
CHINA	1	1	0	1	0	0	0	1	1	1	0	0	1	0	0
CZECOSLOVAKIA	618	294	324	205	413	618	0	0	108	61	134	68	422	10	5
FINLAND	19	6	13	8	11	19	0	0	3	1J	3	5	11	2	0
FRANCE	56	37	19	24	32	55	1	0	13	15	9	11	5	4	4
GERMANY (GFR)	54	28	26	21	33	54	0	0	16	54	9	6	19	0	2
IRELAND	70	53	17	40	30	70	0	0	19	6	28	2	18	7	2
ISRAEL	35	13	22	14	21	35	0	0	10	33	6	9	19	4	1
ITALY	386	217	169	155	231	386	0	0	78	286	106	69	175	18	5
JAPAN	105	66	39	45	60	0	0	105	30	73	7	1	4	47	1
KOREA(S)	12	5	7	2	10	0	0	12	0	9	6	0	6	2	0
NORWAY	33	25	8	25	8	33	0	0	22	33	8	11	21	2	1
POLAND	117	78	39	64	53	117	0	0	?	117	3	6	40	3	1
PORTUGAL	97	62	35	39	58	92	4	1	20	29	32	23	51	15	6
ROMANIA	60	45	15	21	39	60	0	0	18	52	9	20	21	1	0
SPAIN	19	9	10	9	10	19	0	0	7	3	7	2	8	0	0
SWEDEN	301	199	102	110	191	298	3	0	?	89	41	88	96	14	5
SWITZERL	36	27	9	20	16	36	0	0	12	36	0	0	25	0	0
THAILAND	4	3	1	2	2	0	0	4	1	4	0	0	2	0	0
U.K.	60	34	26	29	31	60	0	0	24	11	19	2	24	1	3
USA	216	144	72	81	135	84	131	1	?	142	51	20	112	43	18
TOTAL	2636	1547	1089	1054	1582	2354	158	124	440	1325	529	373	1270	189	72
		58,6%	41,4%	40%	60%	89,3%	6%	4,7%	16,7%	50,3%	20,1%	14,2%	48,2%	7,2%	2,7%

TABLE II - A

COUNTRY	N.º PATIENTS	SMOKERS	STAGE				TUBERCULIN		SACE		KWEIM	
			0	I	II	III	+	-	>	N	+	-
AUSTRIA	70	11	6	39	16	9	7	63	51	19	—	—
BELGIUM	141	31	6	65	47	23	14	80	38	44	—	—
BULGARIA	105	13	3	46	54	2	13	92	30	5	—	—
CANADA	21	3	0	12	6	3	—	—	18	0	—	—
CHINA	1	1	0	1	0	0	0	1	1	0	1	0
CZECOSLOVAKIA	618	108	18	436	113	31	171	402	3	2	33	14
FINLAND	19	3	2	5	12	0	5	13	5	13	1	1
FRANCE	56	13	2	26	24	4	13	15	31	18	—	—
GERMANY (GFR)	54	16	0	19	30	5	4	25	14	18	—	—
IRELAND	70	19	3	22	34	11	—	—	39	31	—	—
ISRAEL	35	10	0	19	10	6	9	26	—	—	24	1
ITALY	386	78	39	156	116	75	43	179	235	102	20	8
JAPAN	105	30	10	72	18	5	41	61	58	46	—	—
KOREA(S)	12	0	2	6	4	0	1	7	3	2	3	—
NORWAY	33	22	0	9	18	6	4	29	8	8	—	—
POLAND	117	?	0	41	50	26	25	59	—	—	—	—
PORTUGAL	97	20	2	32	43	20	16	70	45	30	—	—
ROMANIA	60	18	7	31	14	8	3	42	10	3	—	—
SPAIN	19	7	1	9	2	7	0	17	—	—	—	—
SWEDEN	301	?	45	109	129	8	57	139	70	28	106	16
SWITZERL	36	12	0	14	12	10	—	—	18	12	—	—
THAILAND	4	1	0	3	1	0	1	3	2	2	1	—
U.K.	60	24	4	27	16	13	4	23	19	7	20	5
USA	216	?	18	70	86	42	12	91	98	114	3	1
TOTAL	2 636	440 16,7%	168 6,4%	1 269 48,1%	755 28,6%	313 11,9%	448 16,8%	1 447 54,8% 71,6%	796 30,2%	504 19,1% 49,3%	212 8,9%	46 1,7% 9,7%

TABLE II - B

49.3%, of cases (19.1% of whom with normal values).

The lack of disponibility of a reliable Kweim-Siltzbach test is expressed by the fact that only in 9.7% of patients reported the mentioned test had been performed. Although in Sweden the test was performed in 40.5% of cases.

It may be infered so far, from the short analyses on our abreviated inquiry that many aspects of the study of sarcoidosis go unrevealed or blurred. This justifies the large value of every work which may contribute for its knowledge, as the useful papers and posters here in the topic "Epidemiology" of the XI World Congress on Sarcoidosis and Other Granulomatosis, some aspects of which should be stressed and commented, begining with the prevalence and evolution of Sarcoidosis: some differences were stated, perhaps no more than apparent, as in the case of German Democratic Republic, where the disease is obligatorily declared (Scharkoff).

It may be concluded that this prevalence is changeable and that, in some countries or places, sarcoidosis may be rare (Bambery et al; Abbas et al; Amoli and Masjeti).

Racial factors may still justify these differences, as well the reported discrepances for sex and age incidences.

Just as Hosoda pointed out in his State of the Art, climatic conditions may also be the reason for differences retrieved. Also organs involvement in sarcoidosis remains controversial as it occurs, for instance, in ocular involvement (Rothova et al).

The mortality rate is surely difficult to evaluate, owing to the fact that Sarcoidosis is a chronic and multisystemic disease with different analytic criteria. On some statistics, respiratory insufficiency is pointed as the main cause of death (Djuric et al; Hackney et al), while others ellect the cardiovascular system as the main responsable (Iway et al).

Other important oppinion states that the frequency of Sarcoidosis is increasing, which should not be attributed only to better diagnostic techniques. As I already mentioned, from my personal experience, the increase of incidence of Sarcoidosis seems a fact also in Portugal. In contrast, some countries, as German Democratic Republic do not report this increase.

Although the pathogenesis of sarcoidosis remains a mistery, this Congress greatly contributed for a better recognition of the problem, which suggests a diversity of causes for the disease or, at least, which may intervene in its pathogenetic pathways (Rocklin et al; Gröhagen-Riska et al; Ward and FitzGerald; Badrinas et al; Ablashi et al; Andrews et al).

Anyway, and should be drawn any statements from the short inquiry hereby reported and analysing the important knowledge obtained from the presented works, I should conclude that a long way has to be walked on the Study of the Epidemiology of Sarcoidosis.

In order to obtain important and worthwhile progress, it is fundamental :

1 - A multidisciplinary participation and contribution in order to know the true prevalence of Sarcoidosis;

2 - To standardize diagnostic and clinical evaluation criteria for Sarcoidosis;

3 - To obtain and organize data which be valuable to better understanding and classification of sarcoidosis pathogenesis.

REFERENCES

1. ABBAS M., AYADY S., DJEBBAR A., MADACHE M., NAFIR F.Z., BELAID F. - "Epidemiological Study of Sarcoidosis" (1987) - XI World Congress on Sarcoidosis and Other Granulomatous Disorders, Milan.

2. ABLASHI D., SALAHUDDIN Z., IMAM P., BIBERFELD P., DALGHLIESH A., EKLUND A., HANNGREN A., GALLO R. - "Serological Association of a New Herpes Virus (HBLV) with Sarcoidosis" (1987) - XI World Congress on Sarcoidosis and Other Granulomatous Disorders, Milan.

3. AMOLI K., MASJEDI M.R. - "Some Aspects os Sarcoidosis in Iran" (1987) - XI World Congress on Sarcoidosis and Other Granulomatous Disorders, Milan.

4. ANDREWS J.L., CAMPBELL C., ROCKLIN R., GREINEDER D. - "Familial Sarcoidosis: Clinical, Immunological and Genetic Features of an Unusual Variant" (1987) - XI World Congress on Sarcoidosis and Other Granulomatous Disorders, Milan.

5. BADRINAS F., MORERA J., MAÑÁ J., FITÉ E., SISÓ C., VIDAL R., RUIZ-MANZANO J. - "Sarcoidosis in Barcelona" (1987) - XI World Congress on Sarcoidosis and Other Granulomatous Disorders, Milan.

6. BADRINAS F., MORERA J., MAÑÁ J., FITÉ E., VALVERDE J., VIDAL R., RUIZ-MANZANO J. - "Sarcoidosis in Barcelona: Spring Cluster of Lofgren Syndrome" (1987) - XI World Congress on Sarcoidosis and Other Granulomatous Disorders, Milan.

7. BAMBERY P., BEHRA D., GUPTA A., UPJEET KAUR, JINDAL S.K., SEHGAL S., MALIK S.K., DEODHAR S.D. - "Sarcoidosis in North India: an

Emerging Clinical Spectrum" (1987 - XI World Congress on Sarcoidosis and Other Granulomatous Disorders, Milan.

8. HENDRIK M., BEUMER M. - "Historical Development of Sarcoidosis"
(1987) - XI World Congress on Sarcoidosis and Other Granulomatous Disorders, Milan.

9. BROTZU G., FALCHI S., LANTINI V., MONTISCI R. - "Twenty Cases of
Mediastinal and Pulmonary Sarcoidosis in Sardinian" (1987) - XI
World Congress on Sarcoidosis and Other Granulomatous Disorders,
Milan.

10. CASTRIGNANO L., CREMONCINI M., GRANATA S. - "Serum Angiotensin
Converting Enzyme (SACE) Levels in smokers and Non Smokers. Pre-
liminary Data" (1987) - XI World Congress on Sarcoidosis and
Other Granulomatous Disorders, Milan.

11. DJURIC B., KHOMENKO A.G., MAYER M., LOGLISCI T., SCHWEIGER O.,
CHRIST R., SECEN N. - "A Continuation of the Worldwide Study
on Sarcoidosis" (1987) - XI World Congress on Sarcoidosis and
Other Granulomatous Disorders, Milan.

12. DJURIC B., ZAFRAN N., POVAZAN Dj. - "Late results of 15-Year
Long Follow-Up of 168 Sarcoid Patients" (1987) - XI World Congress on Sarcoidosis and Other Granulomatous Disorders, Milan.

13. GOURGOULIANIS K., STEFIS L., GOUGOULAKIS S., SCOTTI F.,
TSAKRAKLIDES V. - "Sarcoidosis and Tuberculosis of Lymph Nodes:
A Epidemiological Study of 25 Years" (1987) - XI World Congress
on Sarcoidosis and Other Granulomatous Disorders, Milan.

14. GRÖNHAGEN-RISKA C., SAIKKU P., RISKA H., FRÖSETH B. - "Chlamy-
dia Psittaci (TWAR) Antibodies in Sarcoidosis Patients" (1987)-
XI World Congress on Sarcoidosis and Other Granulomatous
Disorders, Milan.

15. HACKNEY RL Jr., YOUNG RC Jr., POLK OD Jr. - "Sarcoidosis Deaths
- 1977-1986: An Analysis of the Experience at Howard University
Hospital" (1987) - XI World Congress on Sarcoidosis and Other
Granulomatous Disorders, Milan.

16. HOSODA Y., ODAKA M., YAMAGUCHI M., HIRAGA Y., IZUMI T.,
TACHIBANA T., AOKI K. - "Results of the 1984 Nation-Wide Prevalence Survey in Japan" (1987) - XI World Congress on Sarcoidosis and Other Granulomatous Disorders, Milan.

17. HOSODA Y. - "Epidemiology". State of the Art (1987) - XI World
Congress on Sarcoidosis and Other Granulomatous Disorders, Milan.

18. IWAI K., TACHIBANA T., HOSOSDA Y., MATSUI Y. - "Statistics of
Sarcoidosis Autopsies During these 25 Years in Japan" (1987) -

XI World Congress on Sarcoidosis and Other Granulomatous
Disorders, Milan.
19. JAMES D.G., WILLIAMS W.J. - "Sarcoidosis and Other Granulomatous
Disordes" - (1985) - London, W.B. Sounders Company.
20. MAFFRE J. Ph., MASSON CH., CAST Ch. St., HADETT M., OURY M.,
TUCHAIS E. - "Lofgren Syndrome (LS) : Epidemiologic and Clinical
Data About 40 Cases" (1987) - XI World Congress on Sarcoidosis
and Other Granulomatous Disorders, Milan.
21. PRANDI E., AZZOLINI L., CAPPELI O., TORALDO M.D., RICHELDI L.,
FONTANA A., PELLEGRINO M., VELLUTI G. - "An Epidemiologic Study
on 226 Patients Affected with Sarcoidosis and Submitted to
Alveolar Lavage" (1987) - XI World Congress on Sarcoidosis and
Other Granulomatous Disorders, Milan.
22. ROMER F.K. - "Sarcoidosis and Cancer: a Prospective Study" (1987)
- XI World Congress on Sarcoidosis and Other Granulomatous
Disorders, Milan.
23. ROTHOVA A., ALBERTS C., KIJLSTRA A., BREEBAART A.C. - "Ocular
Sarcoidosis in the Netherlands" (1987) - XI World Congress on
Sarcoidosis and Other Granulomatous Disorders, Milan.
24. NABIL S. SAMARA - "Sarcoidosis in Jordan" (1987) - XI World Congress on Sarcoidosis and Other Granulomatous Disorders, Milan.
25. SCHARKOFF Th. - " Retrospective of an Unique Mode to Obtain
Complete Epidemiological Data in Sarcoidosis" (1987) - XI World
Congress on Sarcoidosis and Other Granulomatous Disorders,Milan.
26. WARD S., FITZGERALD M.X. - "Smoking Does Not Affect Prevalence
or Short Term Functional Outcome of Sarcoidosis in Ireland"
(1987) - XI World Congress on Sarcoidosis and Other Granulomatous Disorders, Milan.

FUNCTIONAL IMPAIRMENT

FUNCTIONAL IMPAIRMENT IN SARCOIDOSIS* - STATE OF THE ART

Om P. Sharma, M.D.**
Professor of Medicine
University of Southern California
School of Medicine
2025 Zonal Avenue
Los Angeles, CA 90033

*Part of the study was performed during the author's stay in Chest Disease Institute, Kyoto, JAPAN, as a Japanese Society for the Promotion of Science Research Fellow.

With no other disease did pulmonary physiologists have so much fun as with sarcoidosis. More is yet to come, because so much remains unexplained. I will restrict my remarks to the following three aspects of the functional impairment in sarcoidosis:

    I. AIRWAY OBSTRUCTION

    II. DIFFUSING CAPACITY: EFFECT OF POSTURAL CHANGE

    III. RESPIRATORY MUSCLE DYSFUNCTION

I. AIRWAY OBSTRUCTION

A. Does Sarcoidosis Produce Airway Obstruction?

Extensive physiological studies, with a few exceptions, emphasized functional changes typical of a "restrictive impairment," i.e., reduction in static pulmonary volumes, impaired diffusing capacity (transfer factor) and reduced pulmonary compliance.[1,2] Little emphasis was placed on airway involvement. It was rather odd, because as long as 30 years ago, Longcope and Frieman demonstrated the common occurrence of bronchial or peribronchial granulomas in the disease.[3]

Holmgren and Svanborg found that four of the 11 patients with hilar adenopathy and no pulmonary infiltration (Stage I) had significantly reduced maximal mid-expiratory flow rates (MMF); three of the four patients also had increased airway resistance obtained from timed pressure volume loops (Fig. 1). These observations were echoed in another study of 18 patients with Stage I sarcoidosis; five (27%) had increased airway resistance (Fig. 2). Levinson et al measured static and dynamic pulmonary volumes, diffusing capacity, static transpulmonary pressures, closing volumes, and frequency dependent dynamic compliance in 18 sarcoidosis patients. The airway function was abnormal in every patient by at least one of these tests, and nearly always in multiple tests.[5] Miller pointed out that the airway obstruction is common in sarcoidosis.[6] Recently, we studied 123 consecutive Black patients with sarcoidosis; 78 (63%) patients had airway obstruction. The diffusing capacity was impaired in 49 (60%) of 76 patients. Thus, airway obstruction is a common feature of sarcoidosis; its incidence, however, varies considerably.

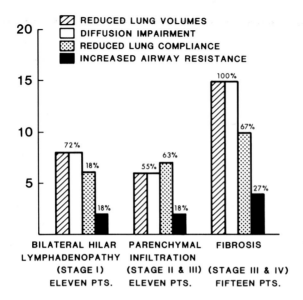

Fig. 1.: LUNG FUNCTIONS IN SARCOIDOSIS
(Adapted from Savanborg, N., Acta Med Scandinav Vol. 180 (Supp. 366)

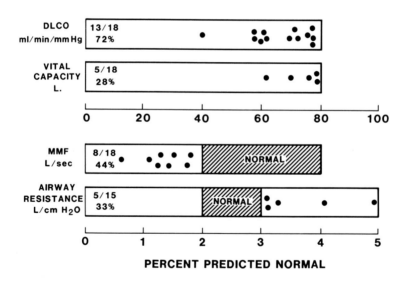

Fig. 2.: LUNG FUNCTIONS IN 18 PATIENTS WITH BILATERAL HILAR LYMPHADENOPATHY
(Stage I)

B. WHAT IS THE SITE OF AIRWAY OBSTRUCTION?

One reason why airway obstruction did not attract enough attention might
have been related to lung compliance. Reduced lung compliance tends to
increase maximum expiratory flow rates, thereby obscuring the flow impairment produced by airway narrowing. Macklem tells us that there are three
airway function tests which are relatively independent of lung elasticity:
1) The upstream resistance, as measured from the maximum flow static
recoil curve; 2) the effect of helium on maximum expiratory flow at 50%;
and 3) the effect of helium on pulmonary resistance.[7]

Kaneko et al studied 21 patients with sarocidosis; all but one had
decreased total lung capacity; and 17 showed reduced vital capacity. They
compared the instantaneous forced expiratory flow rate after 50 per cent
of the FVC had been exhaled (FEF 50%) with the predicted value for FEF 50%
calculated, using the patients' forced vital capacity (FVC). In nine of 21
patients, the FEF 50% was greater than the loss of volume, suggesting the
airway's obstruction. Further analysis revealed that the low conductance
of the upstream segment at 50 per cent of the FVC, in addition to the
decreased FEF 50%, implying that the flow impairments were due to peripheral
airways' narrowing.[8] Levinson et al contend that diminished ratios of the
forced expiratory volume in one second over the forced vital capacity
(FEV_{10}/FVC) and ratios of the closing volume over the vital capacity (CV/VC)
were indicators of the small airway dysfunction.

The airway obstruction in sarcoidosis is common, and it can involve
either the central or the peripheral, or both, airways.

C. WHAT CAUSES AIRWAY OBSTRUCTION IN SARCOIDOSIS?

The following factors, acting either alone or in combination, may produce airway narrowing in sarcoidosis.

i. Structural Changes

Longcope and Freiman pointed out that granulomas may compress the airways and cause obstruction.[3] Endobrochial protuberances of 2-3mm in diameter are frequently seen during bronchoscopy; gross mucosal abnormalities,
however, are uncommon. In one of the patients described by Levinson et al,
microscopic examination revealed a small airway surrounded by granulomatous
inflammation.[5] Main, segmental and subsegmental bronchi may all be involved.[9] (Fig. 3.)

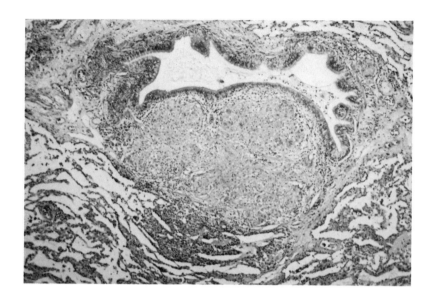

Fig. 3. A lung biopsy specimen showing sarcoidosis granulomas in the wall of a bronchiole, causing airway obstruction.

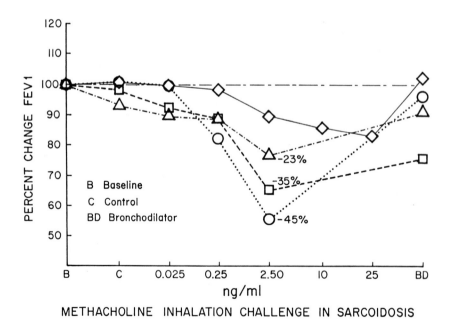

METHACHOLINE INHALATION CHALLENGE IN SARCOIDOSIS

Fig. 4. Four patients with acute sarcoidosis showing FEV1^{o} recuctions in response to methacholine inhalation.

ii. CHEMICAL MEDIATORS OF BRONCHOSPASM

Hyperexcitability of the bronchial tree was demonstrated by Bechtel et al.[10] Ten of their 20 patients with sarcoidosis exhibited a positive methacholine response. This state of bronchial hyperresponsiveness is present even in early (Stage I) sarcoidosis.[11] When challenged with methacholine, 18 (69%) of our 26 patients showed a 20 per cent or greater fall in FEV_1 (Fig. 4). The mechanism of this bronchial hyperactivity is not clear. Flint et al found that the number of bronchoalveolar lavage mast cells in sarcoidosis patients was much higher than the controls. Moreover, anti-IgE induced histamine release from the bronchoalveolar lavage cells was also markedly exaggerated.[12,13] How these observations may relate to either the bronchial hyperactivity or clinical airway obstruction is unclear.

iii. ROLE OF COMPLEMENT AND COMPLEMENT-SPLIT PRODUCTS

This exciting part of the story starts with the knowledge that C_{4a}, and C_{5a} (anaphylotoxins), degradation products of C_3, C_4, and C_5, increase vascular permeability and produce smooth muscle spasm. Previously, studies from our clinic had shown that alveolar macrophages from patients with sarcoidosis produce 1,25 dihydroxy vitamin D_3.[14] Using culture supernates from eight sarcoidosis patients, Glovsky, in our laboratory, has measured C_{3a}, C_{4a}, and C_{5a} by using radioimmunoassay kits (Upjohn Diagnostics, Kalamazoo, Michigan) and C_3 and C_4 by radial diffusion using immunoplates (Behring Diagnostics, La Jolla, California). C_3 levels in the patients were higher than in controls ($p < .05$). C_4 levels, although high, were not statistically significant (Fig. 5). Measurements of C_{3a} and C_{4a} showed much variability. Whether the C_{3a} and C_{4a} found in the culture supernates are cleaved *in vitro* from C_3 and C_4 remains to be determined. Thus, it appears that the activated macrophage not only can synthesize C_3 and C_4, but also can cleave the protein to C_{3a} and C_{4a} which, in turn, induces airway narrowing. (Table I.) Although, studies have demonstrated complement activity in the bronchoalveolar lavage fluid and the presence of arachidonic and metabolities in sarcoid alveolar macrophages, fuller studies are needed to establish the role of anaphylotoxins in sarcoidosis.[15,16] It appears that the activated macrophage, a prominent constituent of the noncaseating granuloma, contributes toward the production not only of angiotensin converting enzyme and 1,25-$(OH)_2$-D, but also of anaphylotoxins.

TABLE I. Production of C_3, C_4, C_{3a}, and C_{4a} by Supernates from Cultured Alveolar Macrophages from Patients with Sarcoidosis and other nonsarcoidal Pulmonary Diseases.**

Patient Number	C_3 (µg)	C_4 (ng)	C_{3a} (ng)*	C_{4a} (ng)*
1.	2.97	190	178	30
2.	.78	150	79	30
3.	.94	640	135	30
4.	.34	120	275	36
5.	.60	898	57	30
6.	.60	188	91	30
7.	.78	90	55	30
8.	2.70	1,169	334	44
9.	2.32	768	260	52
10.	1.96	673	273	67
11.	1.56	452	173	30
12.	13.04	2,703	1,111	934
13.	9.59	2,920	590	294
14.	1.50	90	49	30

*10% fetal calf serum = < 50 ng/ml - C_{3a} and C_{4a}.

**0.5-1.0 x 10^6 Alveolar Macrophages per well. Values as expressed are either µg/ml (C_3') or ng/ml.

Patients Nos. 1-6 are non-sarcoidosis supernates.
Patients Nos. 7-14 are sarcoidosis supernates.

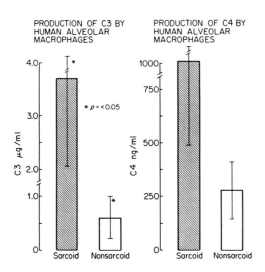

Fig. 5.: PRODUCTION OF C_3 AND C_4 BY ALVEOLAR MACROPHAGES IN PATIENTS WITH SARCOIDOSIS AND NONSARCOIDAL PULMONARY DISEASES

II. DIFFUSING CAPACITY: EFFECT OF POSTURAL CHANGE

In normal subjects, single breath diffusing capacity for carbon monoxide increases in the supine, as compared to the sitting, position. This
normal change is regarded as being due either to distension or to recruitment of the pulmonary capillary bed.[17,18] In pulmonary sarcoidosis, the
loss of diffusing capacity for carbon monoxide remains the common and perhaps the earliest physiological abnormality. It is conceivable that occurence of granulomatous angitis may affect the distensibility of the pulmonary capillaries. In order to test the hypothesis that a fixed pulmonary
capillary bed might exist in sarcoidosis, we measured the coefficient of
diffusion (KCO) in 20 patients with sarcoidosis, and 10 normal controls.
The normal group increased the KCO by 12.8%, ($p < 0.05$), in supine position.
In the sarcoidosis group, however, no significant change of KCO occurred in
supine position, suggesting that vascular involvement in sarcoidosis may
play an important role. (Figs. 6, 7.)

III. RESPIRATORY MUSCLE DYSFUNCTION

Although skeletal muscle is commonly affected in sarcoidosis, the
incidence of respiratory muscle involvement is not known. Routine biopsies
of these muscles are not performed, and respiratory muscle functions are
not regularly included in the evaluation of lung functions. Discrepancies
between subjective, radiologic and physiologic assessment of sarcoidosis
raises the spectre of respiratory muscle involvement. Athos et al reported patients with sarcoidosis who had normal lung volumes and diffusing
capacity, but had significantly abnormal exercise tolerance tests.
Dimarco et al observed that some patients with sarcoidosis had reduced PI
Max, suggesting decreased pressure generating ability.[19]

We studied maximum expiratory pressure (PE Max) and maximum inspiratory pressure in 33 paitents with biopsy-proven sarcoidosis, and 38 normal
volunteers. Result was considered abnormal if it was 2SD of predicted
mean. Effort was good in all patients. Three patients complained of
chest pain during testing. Of the 38 control subjects, 35 were normal,
one had abnormal PE Max, one had abnormal PI Max, and one had abnormal
PE Max and PI Max. Of the 46 patients, 16 showed significant muscle dysfunction (Table II) ($p < 0.005$ by M^2 test). Further evaluation of respiratory muscle in sarcoidosis patients is indicated.

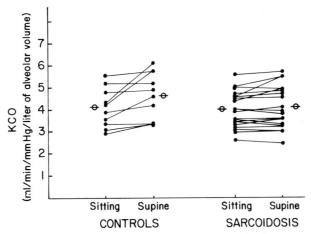

Fig. 6.: EFFECT OF POSTURE ON THE COEFFICIENT OF DIFFUSION (Kco) IN SARCOIDOSIS

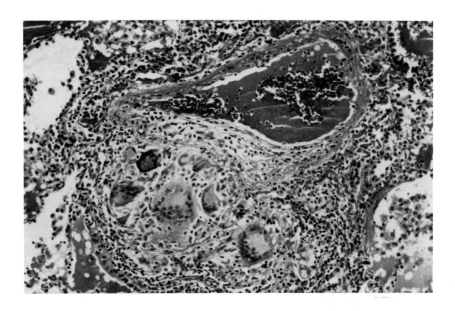

Fig. 7. Sarcoid granulomata involving a pulmonary vessel (HE x150).

TABLE II: Respiratory Muscle Dysfunction in Sarcoidosis.

	PATIENTS		CONTROLS	
NUMBER	46		38	
	NO	%	NO	%
NORMAL	18	39	35	92
PE Max <2SD	11	23	1	2.6
PI Max <2SD	1	2	1	2.6
BOTH PE Max and PI Max	16	35	1	2.6
TOTAL	46	100	38	100

REFERENCES

1. Svanborg N (1961) Acta Medica Scandinav (Supplement 366):170

2. Young RCC, Carr TG, Shelton M et al (1967) Am Rev Respir Dis 95:224-38

3. Longcope WT, Freiman DG (1952) Medicine 31:1

4. Sharma OP, Colp C, Williams MH Jr (1966) Arch Intern Med 17:436-40

5. Levinson RS, Metzger LF, Stanley NN et al (1977) Am J Med 62:51-59

6. Miller A, Teirstein AS, Jackler I et al (1974) Am Rev Resp Dis 109:179-189

7. Macklem PT (1981) In: Chretien, Marsac, Santiel (eds) Sarcoidosis and other granulomatous diseases. Pergamon Press, Paris, pp 310-311

8. Kaneko K, Sharma OP (1977) Bull Eur Physiopathol Respir 13:231-240

9. Honey M, Jepson E (1957) Thorax 12:18-22

10. Bechtel JLT, Starr T III, Dantzker DR et al (1981) Am Rev Respir Dis 124:759-761

11. Manresa PF, Romero CP, Rodriguez SB (1986) Ann NY Acad Sci 465:523-9

12. Flint KC, Leung KB, Hudspith BN et al (1986) Thorax 41:94-99

13. Rankin JA, Kaliner M, Reynolds HY (1987) J Allergy Clin Immunol 79:371-377

14. Adams JS, Sharma OP, Mercedes A et al (1983) J Clin Invest 72:1856-60

15. Lambre CR, LeMaho S, di Bella G et al (1986) Am Rev Respir Dis 134:238-242

16. Bachwich PR, Lynch JP III, Kunkel SL (1987) Clin Immunol Immunopathol 42:27-37

17. Hyland RH, Krastins IRB, Aspin N (1978) Amer Rev Resp Dis 117:1045-53

18. Bates DV, Pearce JF, (1956) J Physiol 132:232-242

19. Dimarco AF, Kelsen SG, Cherniack MJ, Gothe B (1983) Am Rev Respir Dis 127: 425-430

THE SPECTRUM OF AIRWAYS OBSTRUCTION IN SARCOIDOSIS

ALBERT MILLER, M.D., ALVIN S. TEIRSTEIN, M.D., MARK PILIPSKI, B.A., LEE K. BROWN, M.D.
Pulmonary Laboratory, Box 1232, The Mount Sinai Medical Center, New York,
New York 10029 USA

INTRODUCTION

In evaluating pulmonary function (pf) in the more than 5,000 patients who have been registered at the Sarcoidosis Clinic of The Mount Sinai Hospital in New York, we have had a unique opportunity to observe the many physiologic manifestations of this disease. That many of these involve obstruction to various sites in the airway is not sufficiently appreciated.

In this paper, we review the observations we have made on airway function in sarcoidosis (sarc). In addition, we analyzed spirometric tests performed on 351 recent patients to provide an indication of the frequency of airways obstruction (AO) detectable on the forced expiratory effort.

MATERIALS AND METHODS

351 sarc patients who performed acceptable [1] tests in 1982 – 1984 were placed into mutually exclusive spirometric categories using the following criteria: Normal (NL): Nl. FVC, FEV_1/FVC AND MMF; Suggestive Restrictive (Sugg Rest): As above but FEV_1/FVC $\geq$ 0.90 (age $\leq$ 39) or 0.86 (age $\geq$ 40); Restrictive (Rest): FVC < 95% lower confidence interval (CI) but > 54% predicted, FEV_1/FVC nl ($\geq$ 0.65 age $\geq$ 60, 0.70 age 30-59, 0.75 age < 30); Severe Restrictive (Sev Rest): As above but FVC $\leq$ 54% pred; Obstructive (Obs): FVC nl, FEV_1/FVC below limits defined above; Severe obstructive (Sev Obs): FVC nl, FEV_1/FVC < 0.55 age < 30, < 0.50 age $\geq$ 30; Small Airways Dysfunction (SAD): FVC nl, FEV_1/FVC neither ↓ nor ↑ , MMF < 95% CI; Combined, primarily restrictive (Comb Rest): Both FVC and FEV_1/FVC ↓ ; ↓ in FVC $\geq$ ↓ FEV_1/FVC; Combined, primarily obstructive (Comb Obs): ↓ in FEV_1/FVC > ↓ in FVC.

Smoking categories were: Nonsmokers (NS) smoked less than one cigaret a day, had smoked $\leq$ 10 cigarets a day for $\leq$ 6 months or smoked only cigars and pipes. Current smokers (SM) exceeded these limits and did not discontinue smoking > 2 years previously. Ex-smokers (XS) exceeded these limits and discontinued smoking > 2 years previously.

THE SPECTRUM OF AIRWAYS OBSTRUCTION IN SARCOIDOSIS

I. Bronchial hyperreactivity (HR)

HR to methacholine was reported in half (10 of 20) the sarc patients studied (13 were in stages II and III). [2] We have tested 31 patients in all stages, 16 of whom (52%) showed HR; several responders had normal baseline pulmonary function. Two other investigators variously reported 1/3

(13 of 39 [3] and 1 of 14 [4] to have HR but found that the sarc patients as a whole did not differ from normals in the median provocative concentration; 10 of the 14 patients in the second study were stage I. HR is probably more likely when bronchial inflammation is greater (stages II - III vs. I) or airway caliber is diminished.

II. Small Airways Dysfunction (SAD)

Changes of SAD were reported in 16 of 18 consecutive patients with restrictive impairment: $\uparrow$ upstream Raw, $\spadesuit$ closing volume, $\downarrow$ MMF/VC, $\uparrow$ frequency dependence of compliance; [5] 6 had $\downarrow$ FEV$_1$/VC suggestive of overt AO. We have previously reported SAD ($\downarrow$ flow - volume ratios at low lung volume without $\downarrow$ FEV$_1$/FVC) in 6 of 25 stage I and 2 of 19 stage II patients. [6] Greek investigators noted findings of SAD in a variable proportion of nonsmokers in stages I - II, ranging from 17% with $\downarrow$ FEF$_{25-75\%}$/VC to 37% with $\uparrow$ CV/VC to 45% with frequency dependence of compliance and 62% with $\uparrow$ upstream Raw [7].

III   Overt Airways Obstruction (AO)

While AO (defined most simply as $\downarrow$ FEV$_1$/FVC) is not typical of stages I and II, we reported FEV$_1$/FVC values $\leq$ 0.74 in 9/46 patients (20%) in these stages [6]. In a later investigation of consecutive new patients, [8] FEV$_1$/FVC $\leq$ 0.74 was noted in 26% (9/34) patients in these stages; 5 of the 9 were NS. Of the 18 in stage 1, FEV$_1$/FVC was reduced in 4 (22%).

A useful radiographic predictor of AO was evidence of fibrosis (bullae, microcysts and/or retraction of hila, mediastinum or diaphragm: BMR). When patients in stages II and III were separated into those with (20) and those without (14) BMR, FEV$_1$/FVC was $\downarrow$ in 4 in the latter (29%) and 10 of the former (50%)[8]. These observations confirmed our report in 1974 [9] that 11 of 16 patients with BMR (69%) had $\downarrow$ FEV$_1$/FVC. Of these 11 patients with AO, 9 had $\downarrow$ VC and 8 $\downarrow$ FRC, indicating that theirs was a true combined restrictive - obstructive impairment. This ventilatory disorder may be said to be characteristic of BMR in sarc. In our 1980 series, combined impairment was present in 7 of the 10 obstructive patients with BMR compared with only 2 of the 8 obstructive patients without BMR [8]. This disorder seldom responds to bronchodilators.

Our review of 351 recent patients relates the prevalence of $\downarrow$ FEV$_1$/FVC (as defined in Methods) to smoking history: This was present in 14% of NS, 26.5% of SM and 34.5% of XS, for an overall prevalence of 20%.

IV. Bullae

Air spaces (often called bullae or cysts) are common in chronic pulmonary sarc. We have reported [10] 2 unusual patients with progressively enlarging giant bullae who could be characterized as a "vanishing lung syndrome".

Both had severe AO. One of these was followed through a typical evolution of sarc, the other was thought to have bullous emphysema and found to have sarc only when tissue at bullectomy showed characteristic granulomas. Two other cases of "vanishing lungs" which developed in the course of sarc have been reported [11,12].

V. Stenosis of one or multiple large bronchi

This has been reported in sarc at least since 1941 [13]. In the first reported wide use of bronchoscopy in the diagnosis of sarc (many years before the advent of the fiberoptic bronchoscope), Friedman et al from this hospital noted stenosis of lobar or segmental bronchi in 8 of 35 patients [14]. Many patients with isolated atelectasis have been thought to have bronchial neoplasms while those with multiple stenoses resulting in AO have been thought to have "COPD". Stenosis of a main bronchus may result in a biphasic expiratory flow-volume (F-V) curve. Stenosis of both main bronchi is described below.

VI. Upper Airways Obstruction (UAO)

Sarc has long been known to involve the nose, sinuses, nasopharynx, larynx and trachea. Stridor is a common symptom. A laryngeal aperture as small as 2mm has been reported [15]. Variable extrathoracic UAO has been suggested by inspiratory and expiratory F-V curves [16]. We have recently reported (17) 2 patients with characteristic fixed UAO due to sarc. They were unusual in that the obstruction resided in both main bronchi, almost the entire lengths of which were stenotic. Peak flows were 1.37L and 1.38L/sec respectively, consistent with an orifice <4mm in diameter. One patient had florid sarc, the other had no other stigmata and was proven to have the disease on the basis of a positive Kveim test and conjunctival biopsy.

SUMMARY

We have reviewed our previous and recent experience with pf in sarc, as well as that of other investigators, to present a spectrum of obstruction from the distal small airways through the segmental, lobar and main bronchi into the upper respiratory tract. We have presented commonly encountered pf patterns (bronchial HR, SAD, AO) often not considered in this disease as well as unusual cases of "vanishing lungs" and fixed UAO from bilateral bronchial stenosis.

354

REFERENCES

1. Ferris BG. (Principal Investigator). (1978) Epidemiology standardization project. Am Rev Respir Dis 118, Part 2.

2. Bechtel JJ, Starr T III, Dantzker DR, Bower JS. (1981) Am Rev Respir Dis 124:759-761.

3. Konietzko N, Kraft J. (1982) Am Rev Respir Dis 126:943.

4. Olafsson M, Simonsson BG, Hansson SB. (1985) Thorax 40:51-53.

5. Levinson RS, Metzger LF, Stanley N, Kelsen SG, Altose MD, Cherniack NS, Brody JS. (1977) Amer J Med 62:51-59.

6. Miller A, Chuang M, Teirstein AS, Siltzbach LE. (1976) Ann NY Acad Sci 278:292-300.

7. Argyropoulou PK, Patakas DA, Louridas GE. (1984) Resp 46:17-25.

8. Miller A, Einstein K, Thornton J, Teirstein AS, Siltzbach LE. (1980) In: Eighth International Conference on Sarcoidosis and other Granulomatous Diseases. WJ Williams and BH Davies (eds.). Alpha Omega Publishing Ltd., Cardiff, pp. 331-336.

9. Miller A, Teirstein AS, Jackler I, Chuang M, Siltzbach LE. (1974) Am Rev Respir Dis 109:179-189.

10. Miller A. (1981) Brit J Dis Chest 75:209-214.

11. Harden KA, Barthakur, A. (1959) Dis Chest 35:607.

12. Zimmerman I, Mann N. (1949) Ann Intern Med 31:153.

13. Benedict EH, Castleman B. (1941) NEJM 224:186-189.

14. Friedman OH, Blaugrund SM, Siltzbach LE. (1963) JAMA 183:120-124.

15. Di Benedetto, Lefrak S. (1970) Am Rev Respir Dis 102:801-807.

16. Bower JS, Belen JE, Web JG, Dantzker DR. (1980) Am Rev Respir Dis 122:325-332.

17. Miller A, Brown LK, Teirstein AS. (1985) Chest 88:244-248.

© 1988 Elsevier Science Publishers B.V. (Biomedical Division)
Sarcoidosis and other granulomatous disorders
C. Grassi, G. Rizzato, E. Pozzi, editors

BRONCHIAL HYPERREACTIVITY IN SARCOIDOSIS

KIYOSHI SHIMA, SINOBU TAKENAKA,
KOICHRO FUKUDA, KOJI TERAMOTO.

Internal medicine Dept., Kumamoto Municipal Hospital, 1-1-60,
Kumamoto city, Kumamoto.
(Japan)

INTRODUCTION

There are several reports that the airway obstruction[1,2] occurred and
the changes in bronchial walls were observed by flexible fiberoptic bronchoscopy in sarcoidosis patients. Therefore, it would be
thought that increased airway hyperreactivity would occurred in
sarcoidosis patients. So, we have investigated in the bronchial
hyperreactivity in sarcoidosis patients using Astograph.

MATERIALS AND METHODS

Forty patients with sarcoidosis (SA) : mean age of 48 years (range
18-72) male 10 female 30, 7 patients with chronic bronchitis (CB)
mean age of 51 years (range 38-64) male 4 female 3 and 35 patients
of bronchial asthma (BA) : mean age of 41 (range 21-56) male 18
female 17 were studied. All 40 of sarcoidosis patients were diagnosed by the histology of scalene nodes biopsy and transbronchial
lung biopsy. Sarcoidosis patients who had the corticosteroid
treatment within six months, smorking habit and atopic history
were excluded.

Bronchial hyperreactivity (BHR) was examined by using ASTOGRAPH
(model TCK-6100H, chest co. JAPAN) deviced by prof. Takishima,
which is the direct graphical recorder of the cumulative dose-
response curves of the airway reactivity to the methacholine
broncho-provocation : 25, 12.5, 6.25, 3.125, 1.563, 0.781, 0.39,
0.195, 0.098, 0.049 mg/dl in concentration.

This curve is expressed as respiratory resistance by osscilation.

Dmin (dose minimum) is a amount of inhaleted methacholine when
respiratory resistance in curve began to increase and express the
sensitivity of bronchial airways.

C min (concentration minimum), also express the sensitivity of
bronchial airways.

Sd is a ratio of the increasing respiratory resistance to inhaleted methacholine dosis when the respiratory resistance began to

increase, and expresses the reactivity of bronchial airways.

PGF, PGE, histamine, C-AMP, C-GMP, TxB2, ACE in peripheral venous blood (PVB) and broncho-alveolar lavage fluid (BALF) were measured by BML co. Tokyo, JAPAN. within one month when ASTOGAF was performed. Spirometry was performed with ST460 spirometer. (Fukuda co. Japan)

Gallium scintigrams was performed by the administration of two mci ^{67}Ga before 72 hours.

Statistical analysis of the data was performed using the t test.

RESULTS

As presented in table 1,

Twenty-six of sarcoidosis patients (65.0%), 6 of 7 CB patients (85.7%) and 35 of 35 BA patients (100%) showed BHR. The levels of Cmin were 5.23 in SA patients, 4.76 in CB patients and 1.25 in BA patients. The levels of Sd were 0.56 in SA patients, 1.18 in CB patients and 2.04 in BA patients. Therefore the intensity of BHR in SA patients was much more weaker than the BHR in CB and BA patients.

Table 1 Bronchial hyperreactivity in respiratory disease

	Sarcoidosis	Chronic bronchitis	Bronchial asthma
n	26/40 (65.0%)	6/7 (85.7%)	35/35 (100%)
Rrs cont	4.62±1.21	4.17±1.20	5.21±1.65
Cmin	5.23±6.74	4.76±4.65	1.25±2.29
Dmin	7.61±9.87	7.18±7.07	1.76±3.29
Sd	0.56±0.88	1.18±2.24	2.04±2.24

Table 2 Case distribution

	BHR +	BHR −
No. cases	26	14
Sex	M5 F21	M5 F9
y.o. Aver.	47.5+15.3	50.1±16.1
	(18~72)	(21~68)
Stage		
I	6	5
II	17	6
III	1	2
0	2	1

As presented in table 2, SA patients showing BHR were 26 cases, male 5 : female 21, 47.5 in mean age and stage I:6, II:17, III:1, 0:2. SA patients without BHR were 14 cases, male 5 : female 9, 50.1 in mean age and stage I:5, II:6, III:2, 0:1.

There were no difference between BHR(+) and BHR(−) in the lung function test %VC, FEV1.0% and % DLco (table 3).

As presented in table 4, among the patients showing the change in bronchial wall, the cases of positive BHR were 10 patients (66.7%) and the negative were 5 patients.

Table 3 Lungfunction

	n	B H R +	n	B H R −
% V C	24	94.78+13.28	1 1	95.23±14.15
F E V₁ %	24	82.28+8.57	1 1	82.26±9.56
% DL co	18	78.27+14.81	8	82.81±15.42

Table 4 Changes in bronchial wall

changes	B H R +	−
+	1 0(66.7%)	5
−	1 3(61.9%)	8
T o t a l	2 3(63.9%)	1 3

As presented in table 5, among the patients showing higher than 21.3 I.U. in S-ACE levels, the cases of positive BHR were 16 patients (59.3%) and the negative 11 patients.

Table 5 S − A C E

ACE levels	B H R +	−
21.3>	16 (59.3%)	11
21.3<	10 (76.9%)	3
T o t a l	26 (65.0%)	14

Table 6 G a − S c i n

Ga (+)	B H R +	−
+	12 (57.1%)	9
−	13 (72.2%)	5
T o t a l	25 (64.1%)	14

As presented in table6, among the patients showing the accumulation of Ga scintigrams, the cases of positive BHR were 12 patients. (57.1%) and the negative were 9 patients.

As presented in table 7, among the patients showing 0 to 20 % in the number of lymphocytes of BALF, the positive BHR groups were 7 patients (70%) and the negative were 3 patients. Among the patients showing 21 to 40 % and more than 40%, the positive BHR were 7 patient (53.8%) and 9 patients (64.3%).

Table 7 Lymphocytes in BALF

BALF Ly (%)	BHR +	−
0 − 20	7 (70%)	3
21 − 40	7 (53.8%)	6
41 <	9 (64.3%)	5
Total	23 (62.2%)	15

Table 8 Several factors in peripheral venous blood

		BHR +		−
	n		n	
Histamine	19	5.64±3.37	13	7.64±3.80
PGF	20	391.55±208.71	13	351.23±199.35
PGE	19	98.32±56.24	13	93.77±96.28
c−AMP	20	17.06±3.20	13	15.51±4.10
c−GMP	20	5.25±2.11	13	5.60±2.14
TxB₂	7	58.71±21.09	5	40.00±9.75
ACE	26	18.72±6.64	14	19.15±6.77
OKT4/8	17	1.78±0.87	10	1.53±0.55
IgE	26	228.92±333.76	14	129.57±151.29
Eosinophil	26	139.7±132.7	14	99.2±92.3

As presented in table 8, histamine levels in PVB were 5.64ng/ml in BHR positive group, 7.64 in BHR negative group, Thromboxan B2 levels were 58.71ng/ml in BHR(+), 40.00 in BHR(−). IgE levels were 228.92IU/ml in BHR(+), 129.57 in BHR(−) and Eosinophil cells were 139.7 in BHR(+), 99.2 in BHR(−).

The slight difference of these levels between BHR(+) and BHR(−) was found, but not statistically significant. No difference of the levels of PGF, PGE, C−AMP, C−GMP, S−ACE and OKT4/8, ratio between BHR(+) and BHR(−) was found.

As presented in table 9, histamine levels in BALF were 4.10 in BHR(+) 2.60 in BHR(−). OKT4.8 rations in BALF were statistically higher, 4.86 in BHR(+) than 1.51 in BHR(−) (P< 0.05),The levels of PGF, C−AMP, C−GMP, S−ACE and the percentage of lymphocytes in BALF were not statistically different.

Table 9 Several factors in bronchoalveolar lavage fluid

		BHR +		−
	n		n	
Histamine	9	4.10±3.35	6	2.60±1.61
PGF	9	101.33±148.31	6	111.00±157.62
c−AMP	9	1.70±0.58	6	2.14±1.20
c−GMP	8	0.41±0.26	5	0.32±0.11
ACE	15	1.31±1.27	12	1.19±0.92
OKT4/8	11	4.86±4.91	8	1.51±1.03
Ly (%)	23	34.22±17.66	14	32.00±15.21

DISCUSSION.

Using the technique of flexible fiberoptic Bronchoscopy, the changes in sarcoid brochial wall was revealed in sarcoidosis patients, and also lymphocytes alveolitis, namely inflammation of lower airways was observed. It is considered that these bronchial inflammatory changes will occure BHR in sarcoid bronchial airways.

Bechtel et al[5] report the increase airway reactivity in 10 of 20 sarcoidosis patients. We have also experienced the BHR in 26 of 40 sarcoidosis patients, but its intensity of reactivity and sensitivity to the methacholine is more weaker than those of CB and BA. But molafssen et al[6] report that measuring by recording the FEV1.0 after increasing doses of methacholine, BHR was not found in sarcoidosis patients except three with asthma. Also, monietzko et al[7] do not find the BHR in 39 sarcoidosis patients and report that there was any difference in subgroups of patients of ACE, lysozyme or atopy. These different reports might due to different staging and activity in sarcoidosis.

Our method to examine the BHR in sarcoidosis patients is different from these investigaters. Using the same increasing dosis of methacholine, but the respiratory resistance curve by oscillation was used to measure the BHR in sarcoid bronchial airways. We also exermined the BHR using the FEV1.0 changing rate and abtained the results that BHR was observed in 2 of 20 sarcoidosis patients. From this results, our method may be more sensitive to detect the BHR in sarcoidosis than usual method using the FEV1.0 changing rate.

The mechanism why the BHR observes in BA, CB and farmer's lung now is not known in details. As the results of our measuring several mediators and othors in PVB and BALF, low histamine levels, low Thromboxan B2, high IgE and eosinophile in PVB and high histamine, high OKT4.8 ratio in BALF even if these data was not statistically significant except OKT4/8 ratio. It is possible that cause of BHR in sarcoid bronchial airways will be associated with high histamine and high OKT4/8 tatio in BALF, namely sarcoid activity, for reasons these factors in BALF will be more reflected on the bronchial airways than those in PVB.

SUMMARY

Bronchial reactivity was examined in 40 sarcoidosis patients, 7 chronic bronchitis patients and 35 bronchial asthma patients

using the respiratory resistance curve by oscillation after in
halating methacholine. Twenty-six of 40 sarcoidosis patients was
more lower hyperreactive to methacholine than 6 of 7 chronic
bronchitis patients and 35 bronchial asthma patients.

Histamine levels and OKT4,8 ratio in BALF was higher in hyperreactive sarcoidosis patients than in non-reactive.

REFERENCES
1. Olsson T, Bjornstad-Petterson H, stjernberg NL. Bronchostenosis
   due to sarcoidosis.
    Chest 75:663, 1979.
2. Miller A, Terstien AS, Jackler I, chang M. Siltzbach LE. Airway
   function in chonic pulmonary sarcoidosis. Am. Rev. Respir. Dis.
   109:179, 1974.
3. Friedman OH, Blaugrund SM, Siltzbach G.E. Biopsy of bronchial
   wall as an aid in diagnosis of sarcoidosis.
   JAMA 183:120, 1963.
4. Takishima, T., Hida W., Sasaki, H., Suzuki, S., Sasaki, T.
   : Directwriting recorder of the dose-response curves of the
   airway to methacholine. Chest, 80:600, 1981.
5. Bechtel J.J. Aerway hypersensitivity patients with sarcoidosis.
   Am. Rev. Respir. Dis. 124:759, 1981.
6. Molafsson BG, et al: Bronchial reactivity in patients with
   recent pulmonary sarcoidosis. Thorax 40:51, 1985.
7. Monietzko N. et al : Airway huperreactivity in patients with
   sarcoidosis. Am. Rev. Respir, Dis. 126:943, 1982.

© 1988 Elsevier Science Publishers B.V. (Biomedical Division)
Sarcoidosis and other granulomatous disorders
C. Grassi, G. Rizzato, E. Pozzi, editors

THE EFFECT OF CORTICOSTEROID THERAPY ON THE BREATHING PATTERN
IN INTERSTITIAL LUNG DISEASE (ILD).

P.M. RENZI, G.D. RENZI,
St. Luc and Notre-Dame Hospitals, Montreal, Québec, Canada.

INTRODUCTION

The breathing pattern in ILD is generally characterized by increased ventilation per minute with smaller tidal volumes and higher
frequencies. This pattern of breathing results from the modification of the inspiratory neuromuscular output (P.1) and the timing
of the breathing cycle. The output and timing vary primarily as a
function of the magnitude of the lung elastance, the higher is the
elastic load, the greater will be the static neuromuscular output
and shorter will be the duration of the inspiratory time (1-2).

Other factors such as inflammatory, will also alter the breathing
pattern in ILD. These consist primarily of chemical mediators.

The object of this study was to evaluate the effect of corticosteroids on the neuromuscular drive and breathing pattern in ILD.

TABLE 1. EXPERIMENTAL PROTOCOL:

1. Lung volumes, spirometry and arterial blood gases.

2. Static pressure volume charactaristics of the lungs.

3. Volume and time components of the respiratory cycle.
    Tidal volume (VT), frequency in breaths per min.
    Inspiratory (TI) expiratory (TE), total time (TTOT) sec.

4. Ventilatory drive parameters.
    Mean inspiratory flow (VT/TI). Mouth occlusion pressure
    (P.1) cmH$_2$0.
    Inspiratory time over total time (TI/TTOT).

TABLE 2. PATIENT POPULATION:

1. **Group S:** 11 patients with ILD (mean TLC 73% of pred.) and
    tests performed prior and after 6 months of prednisone.

2. **Group C:** 6 patients with ILD (mean TLC 72% of pred.) served
    as controls, received no treatment and were tested at 6
    months intervals.

3. **Group N:** 25 normal subjects (mean FVC 101% of pred.) matched
    for age, weight, height and sex, were compared to the other
    2 groups.

TABLE 3. ANTHROPOMETRIC CHARACTERISTICS AND INITIAL LUNG FUNCTION
VALUES IN 11 ILD PATIENTS RECEIVING CORTICOSTEROIDS (S) AND 6
CONTROL ILD PATIENTS (C).

	STEROIDS		CONTROLS	
	(MEAN	± SD)	(MEAN	± SD)
Age (years)	39.8	17.2	39.7	13.3
Height (m)	1.6	0.11	1.65	0.13
Weight (kg)	68.7	6.6	60.3	13.9
TLC (pred)	73.9	16.4	72.	14.7
FVC (% pred)	72.9	15.2	56.5	14.7
FEV_1/FVC (%)	77.9	9.7	75.6	5.9
LUNG ELASTANCE (cm H_2O/L)	11.3	4.7	13.8	6.6
PaO2 (mmHg)	75.9	10.5	65.7	9.2
PaCO2 (mmHg)	40.3	6.1	41.	2.6

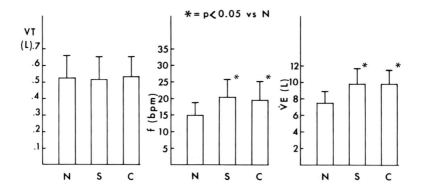

Fig. 1. Compares the initial tidal volume, frequency breaths/min.&
minute ventilation in the 3 groups. N equals normals, S equals ILD
before steroids and C equals ILD control group. The bars indicate
1 SD. The * indicates P <0.05 vs N. As noted, there is no difference in the 3 groups for tidal volume. Frequency is higher in
the ILD groups when compared to normals. Ventilation is also
greater in ILD groups than in normals.

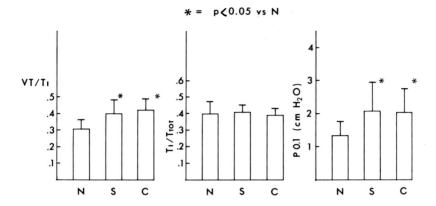

Fig. 2. shows the initial drive parameters in the 3 groups, N vs
S vs C. The * indicates p <0.05 vs N. VT/TI is greater in the ILD
groups before treatment than the normals. TI/TTOT is similar in
the 3 groups. P0.1 is significantly increased in the ILD groups
indicating increased neuro-muscular drive.

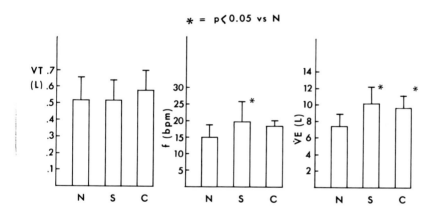

Fig. 3. now compares the final ventilatory parameters in the 3
groups, N vs S vs C. The * indicates p <0.05 vs N. There is no
difference for tidal volume. Frequency in breaths per min. remains
increased in the S group after steroid therapy, but the control
group is not statistically different from the normals. Minute
ventilation remains increased in the ILD group after steroids
as well as in the ILD group control.

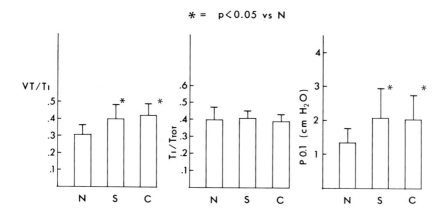

*= p<0.05 vs N

Fig. 4 now shows the final drive parameters in the 3 groups. The * indicates p <0.05 vs N. VT/TI remains increased in the ILD group after steroids as well as the ILD control group. TI/TTOT remains unchanged in the 3 groups. PO.1 is still increased in the ILD group (S) as well as the ILD control group (C).

In order to evaluate factors besides elastance that influence the pattern of breathing, we plotted ventilatory parameters as a function of total elastance in 33 normal subjects breathing with inspiratory elastic loads.

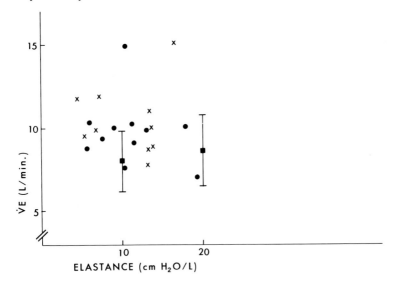

Fig. 5. compares elastance (cm H_2O/L) on the horizontal axis vs ventilation (VE L/min.) on the vertical axis. The full squares indicate normal subjects with inspiratory elastic loads. The bars indicate 1 SD. The full circles represent ILD patients before steroids,

and the X, ILD patients after steroids. Please note that several
subjects have increased ventilation above that predicted by
elastance and this persists in the ILD group after steroids.

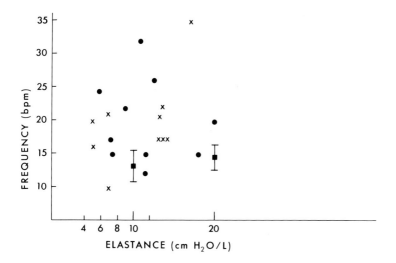

Fig. 6 relates elastance (cm H_2O/L) on the horizontal axis vs
frequency (bpm) on the vertical axis. The full squares indicate
normal subjects with inspiratory elastic loads. The bars indicate
1 SD. The full circles show ILD patients before steroids and the
X's, ILD patients after steroids. Please note that most of the
subjects breathe more rapidly than that predicted by elastance and
even after steroid therapy, the increased frequency persists.

CONCLUSIONS

1. The abnormal breathing pattern and increased neuromuscular
    drive in ILD are not corrected by corticosteroids.
2. The persistence in increased neuromuscular drive and ventila-
    tion is greater than that predicted by elastance alone.

Hypothesis: These modifications may be due to a) a persistent
inflammatory response in spite of steroids or b) reflexes generated
by lung fibrosis.

REFERENCES

1. Renzi G, Milic-Emili J, Grassino A. (1982) The pattern of
    breathing in diffuse lung fibrosis. In: Bull europ Physiopath
    resp 18:461-472

2. Renzi G, Milic-Emili J, Grassino A (1986) Breathing pattern in
    Sarcoidosis and Idiopathic Pulmonary Fibrosis. In: Ann NY
    acad sci 465:482-490

© 1988 Elsevier Science Publishers B.V (Biomedical Division)
Sarcoidosis and other granulomatous disorders
C. Grassi, G. Rizzato, E. Pozzi, editors

RESPIRATORY CLEARANCE OF 99Tc-DTPA AND GRANULOMA SURFACE AREA IN RAT LUNG
GRANULOMATOSIS INDUCED BY COMPLETE FREUND ADJUVANT.

M. MORDELET-DAMBRINE, G. STANISLAS-LEGUERN, D. HENZEL, L. BARRITAULT, J.
CHRETIEN, G. HUCHON.

Unité INSERM 214, Hôpital Laennec,75340 Paris Cedex 07 and Unité INSERM 13,
Hôpital Claude Bernard, 75944 Paris Cedex 19, France.

INTRODUCTION

Epithelial permeability may be assessed by the respiratory clearance of 99m
technetium radiolabeled diethylene triamine pentaacetate (RC-DTPA). RC-DTPA
might be increased in pulmonary sarcoidosis. To investigate that phenomenon, we
carried out a study in rats in which we induced lung granulomatosis by the
injections of Complete Freund Adjuvant (CFA). RC-DTPA measurements and
morphometric examinations were performed.

MATERIALS AND METHODS

Experimental conditions. Two groups of 25 rats were studied: control and CFA
groups, this animals received two intravenous injections of saline solution or
CFA, 48 hours apart. RC-DTPA was measured before and 28, 42, 56, 70, 112 days
after the second injection in each animal. After the second measurement of
RC-DTPA, the animals were killed.

Respiratory clearance. We determined RC-DTPA in rats as described by Minty and
Royston. RC-DTPA is the negative slope of the regression line through the values
of corrected pulmonary radioactivity and is expressed in %/min.

Morphometric study. After bleeding the animal, the whole left lung was fixed
and cut in 5 μm slices and stained with hematoxylin and eosin. One lung slice
was randomized in each animal for determining of section surface area,
granuloma, bronchiole, and vessel surface areas on 100 random fields. Surface
areas were measured with a videocamera. Data were expressed as the ratio of
granuloma surface area over the respiratory surface tissue area without

368

bronchioles and vessels (Gr/RT%)

RESULTS

Time	RC-DTPA (%/min)			Gr/RT(%)
	Control	CFA	p	
Before	0.4 (0.1)	0.4 (0.1)		0
After				
28 days	0.4 (0.1)	0.9 (0.2)	<0.01	1.6 (0.4)
42 days	0.8 (0.1)	1.7 (0.3)	<0.001	2.6 (1.0)
56 days	0.4 (0.1)	0.7 (0.1)	<0.01	2.2 (1.1)
70 days	0.5 (0.1)	0.9 (0.2)	<0.05	2.5 (0.5)
112 days	0.4 (0.1)	1.2 (0.4)	<0.001	1.7 (0.5)

Granuloma were present in all pulmonary sections of lung rat of the CFA group, mainly in peribronchovascular and subpleural tissues. The central part of granuloma contained macrophages and epithelioid like cells; lymphocytes remained at the periphery of granuloma; collagen was seen in the larger granulomas and these granulomas were more numerous after 42 days.

SUMMARY

1 - CFA injections induced pulmonary granulomas.

2 - Granuloma surface areas increased up to the 42th day and they remained high until the 112th day.

3 - RC-DTPA increased from 42 to 112 days.

CONCLUSION

The presence of lung granulomas is associated with an increased clearance of 99mTc-DTPA.

SARCOIDOSIS, BRONCHIAL REACTIVITY AND BAL

A. COLLODORO, A. FERRARA, P. ROTTOLI, L. ROTTOLI, A. STURMAN, M.G. PIERONI, M. REFINI, N. CHILARIS, A. PERRELLA AND S. BIANCO

Istituto Tisiologia e Malattie Apparato Respiratoriom, Universita' di Siena, Italy

Bronchial hyperreactivity has been recently observed in patients with pulmonary sarcoidosis (PS). The aim of the present study was to confirm these findings and to assess to what extent BAL can modify bronchial reactivity in sarcoidosis.

METHODS

We studied 25 patients with PS; 9 men and 16 women, mean age of 48.4 years (range 26-66), 6 were smokers. The standard spirometry revealed 16 normal, 7 restrictive, 1 obstructive and 1 mixed pattern. Mean VC, FEV1 and TLC as percentage of predicted were, respectively: 86.8 ± 16.6, 87.8 ± 15.4 and 91.08 ± 15.2 Nine patients were in Stage I, 13 were in Stage II, and 3 were in Stage III. Mean SACE was 56.8 ± 17.9 UI/min ml. Fourteen patients had respiratory symptoms (cough and/or dispnoea). Six patients had steroid therapy. The patients were challenged with doubling doses of methacoine, from 10 to 20.000 mcg, by means of a "Mefar" dosimeter. A positive response was defined as a $\geq 20\%$ decline in FEV1 during the test. In 15 patients the challenge was repeated 24 hrs after the BAL. It was performed with an Olympus Fiberoptic Bronchoscope, following local anesthesia, by infusing eight-ten 30 ml aliquots of sterile saline solution in subsegmental bronchus of middle lobe or lingula and gently aspirating.

RESULTS

A moderate degree of hyperreactivity, methacholine PD 20 mcg 3515 ± 3513 (M $\pm$ SD), was observed in 16 patients (64%), whereas 9 (36%) were normal. No significant difference was found in pulmonary functional test, stage and SACE of the two groups. In the patients undergoing the BAL, 9 (60%) showed a moderate degree of hyperreactiviy, metacholine PD 20 mcg 4250 ± 3586, whereas 6 (40%) were normal. No change in bronchial reactivity was observed after BAL: PD 20 before BAL 4250 ± 3586 mcg vs PD 20 4802 ± 4497 after BAL. No correlation was found between airway responsiveness and examined parameters: SACE, stage, lung function, BAL (% recovery; total cells; % lymphocytes; T4/T8 ratio). Only a slight, non statistically significant decrease of the baseline lung volumes was found in the responders group (VC 84.3 ± 19.5; FEV1 84.6 ± 17.6; vs 89.2 ± 9.2; 93.5 ± 8.9) and a slight increase in lymphocytes number of BAL (38.5 ± 16.7 vs 22.18 ± 13.2) in the same group. The patients with bronchial hyperreactivity also showed more evidence of cough and/or dispnoea.

DISCUSSION

The aim of the study was to confirm the presence of the bronchial hyperr-eactivity in patients with PS, and to assess the changes of such a hyperreactivity after BAL. Whereas some AA. (1, 2, 3) found bronchial hyperreactivity in patients

370

with PS in different stages, others (4, 5) exclude it as being a "true hyperreactivity" and refer to it as depending on a lung volume decrease which is sometimes present in these patients. Our data showed the presence of the moderate degree of hyperreactivity in patients with PS. No other significant difference was found either in the lung volumes of the responder and non responder groups or in any other considered parameters. The presence of increased lymphocytes in the BAL of the responder group was noticeable, even if not statistically significant. This finding confirms the presence of a lymphocytic alveolitis, which could determine the mediators release (6), with related epithelial damage and subsequent increase of epithelial permeability and the uncovering of nerve endings. Further data based on larger studies are necessary to confirm this finding. The second part of the study (BAL- hyperreactivity) clearly showed that BAL does not alter airway responsiveness in patients with PS (Table 1). A similar study was recently carried out in asthmatic patients which demonstrated no change of hyperreactivity after BAL in these more responsive subjects (8). This is further confirmation of the safety of this technique.

TABLE 1

Effect of BAL on methacholine airway responsiveness in patients with pulmonary sarcoidosis.

Patients No	Average age	Sex	Stage	Baseline FEV1 (% pred)	Methacholine PD 20 (mcg) pre-BAL	post-BAL
1	50	m	I	96	10.700	14.000
2	54	f	III	69	5.000	5.500
3	43	f	II	59	2.500	600
4	58	f	I	100	10.000	500
5	50	f	I	55	1.100	1.280
6	52	f	II	86	1.000	10.000
7	29	f	II	74	750	340
8	65	m	III	86	5.000	5.000
9	43	f	I	119	2.200	6.000
mean	49.3			82.6	4.250	4.802
± SD	10.2			20.6	3.586	4.497

REFERENCES

1. Bechtel JJ et al. Am Rev Resp Dis 1981;124:759.
2. Amaral-Marques R et al. Abstracts, 5th Eur Conf Sarcoidosis, Vienna, 27-30 August 1986, p 166.
3. Olafsson M et al. Thorax 1985;40:51.
4. Konietzko N, Kraft J. Am Rev Resp Dis 1982;126:943.
5. Konietzko N, Faupel-Bauer B. Abstracts, 5th Eur Conf Sarcoidosis, Vienna, 27-30 August 1986, p 124.
6. Clancy L et al. Europ J Resp Dis 1986,69(suppl 147):199.
7. Laitinen AL et al. Europ J Resp Dis 1983,64(suppl 131):267.
8. Kirby et al. Am Rev Resp Dis 1987;135:554.

© 1988 Elsevier Science Publishers B.V. (Biomedical Division)
Sarcoidosis and other granulomatous disorders
C. Grassi, G. Rizzato, E. Pozzi, editors

371

IMPAIRED AIRWAY FUNCTION IN SARCOIDOSIS STAGE II

WOLFGANG PETERMANN, JÜRGEN BARTH, PETER ENTZIAN,
STEFAN HOPPE-SEYLER

Dept. of Internal Medicine, University of Kiel, 2300 Kiel 1,
Schittenhelmstrasse 12, Fed. Rep. of Germany

Depending on activity and stage of the disease, changes of the
lavage cell count and T-cell subsets in sarcoidosis are well known
[1-4]. Among other functional disturbances, particularly diffusing
disorders, small airway disease in sarcoidosis are described [5-7].
We have investigated relationships between lung lavage cell counts
and lung function tests.

Functional and radiological evaluations and bronchoalveolar lavages were performed in 17 patients (12 male, 5 female, aged 18-52
years) with histologically proven sarcoidosis before and after 6
month of steroid treatment. The therapy was required because of
either an involvement of extrapulmonary organs (e.g. eyes, skin)
or a progression of the pulmonary sarcoidosis. All patients had
sarcoidotic pulmonary infiltrates with and without hilar adenopathy. Following treatment we saw in 14 out of 17 patients a complete normalization of the chest radiograph and in 3 patients a
diminution of the reticular pattern of the lung. Total lung capacity, vital capacity, residual volume, airway resistance, forced
vital capacity in 1 s related to VC, expiratory peak flow, and arterial oxygen tension have been normal before and after therapy.

On the contrary, we saw significant differences between the results before and after treatment concerning the maximal expiratory
flow at 25, 50 and 75% of FVC (MEF_{25}, MEF_{50}, MEF_{75}), maximal mid-
expiratory flow between 25 and 75% of FVC (FEF_{25-75}) and the single breath diffusing capacity of the lung for CO (DLCO)(table 1).

Table 1:
Physiological tests before and after treatment (median/SD, U-test)

	MEF_{25}	MEF_{50}	MEF_{75}	FEF_{25-75}	DLCO
		% predicted			
before	88/ 8	69/ 6	56/ 6	62/ 7	67/ 5
after	106/ 8	83/11	88/ 8	93/ 8	101/ 5
p	<0.01	<0.01	<0.001	<0.001	<0.001

Regarding to BAL the medians of total cell count and percentage of lymphocytes did not differ considerably before and after therapy. On the other hand, the percentage of T-helper cells decreased significantly whereas the percentage of T-suppressor-cells showed a marked increase by means of steroid treatment. Accordingly, the T_H/T_s-ratio decreases highly significant (table 2).

Table 2:
Cells in BAL-fluid before and after treatment (median/SD, U-test)

	total cells (x 10^6)	lympho (%)	T_H-cells	T_s-cells	T_H/T_s
			(% of lymphocytes)		
before	30.2/12.0	29/ 7	73/ 7	12/ 5	6.4/1.8
after	16.4/11.1	17/ 6	59/ 6	17/ 3	3.4/0.8
p	ns	ns	<0.01	<0.01	<0.001

There were strong correlations between FEF_{25-75} and DLCO (r=+ 0.83) and between T_H/T_s-ratio and both DLCO (r=-0.79) and FEF_{25-75} (r=-0.81). We conclude, that in active sarcoidosis (determined by BAL) small airway disease is not uncommon besides the well known disorder of diffusing capacity.

REFERENCES

1. Ceuppens JNL, Laquet ML, Marien G, Demedts M, van den Eckhout A, Stevens, E (1984) Alveolar T-cell subsets in pulmonary sarcoidosis. Am Rev Respir Dis 129:563-568

2. Chretien J, Venet A, Danel D, Israel-Biet D, Sandron D, Arnoux A (1985) Bronchoalveolar lavage in sarcoidosis. Respiration 48:222-230

3. Keogh BA, Hunninghake GW, Line BR, Crystal RG (1983) The alveolitis of sarcoidosis. Am Rev Respir Dis 128:256-265

4. Rossi GA, Sacco O, Cosulich E, Risso A, Balbi B, Ravazzoni C (1986) Helper T-lymphocytes in pulmonary sarcoidosis. Am Rev Respir Dis 133:1086-1090

5. Le Merre C, Rousset G, Prefaut CH (1986) Sous-estimation de l' obstruction bronchique dans la sarcoidose. Respiration 50:88-96

6. Renzi GD, Renzi PM, Lopez-Majano V, Dutton RE (1981) Airway function in sarcoidosis: effect of short-term steroid therapy. Respiration 42:98-104

7. Scano G, Monechi GC, Stendardi L, Lo Conte C, van Meerhaege A, Sergysels R (1986) Functional evaluation in stage I pulmonary sarcoidosis. Respiration 49:195-203

© 1988 Elsevier Science Publishers B.V. (Biomedical Division)
Sarcoidosis and other granulomatous disorders
C. Grassi, G. Rizzato, E. Pozzi, editors

373

VENTILATION-PERFUSION RELATIONSHIPS IN PULMONARY SARCOIDOSIS

A. ZWIJNENBURG[*], C. ALBERTS", C.M. ROOS", H.M. JANSEN", H.R. MARCUSE[*]
[*] The Netherlands Cancer Institute, Dept. of Nuclear Medicine.
" Academic Medical Centre, Dept. of Pulmonary Medicine. Amsterdam, The
Netherlands.

INTRODUCTION

Disturbed gas exchange in pulmonary sarcoidosis may be the result of
a reduced diffusing capacity of the alveolar-capillary membrane or of
an uneven distribution of ventilation-perfusion. The diffusing capacity
for carbon monoxide (DLCO) is an estimate of the diffusing capacity of
the alveolar-capillary membrane, but may also be influenced by ventilation-
perfusion inequality.

The present study investigates the presence of ventilation-perfusion
inequality in patients with pulmonary sarcoidosis using quantitative
analysis of ventilation-perfusion single photon emission computed
tomography (SPECT).

PATIENTS AND METHODS

We studied 14 patients (mean age 45 yrs.) One patient had radiographic
stage II and 13 patients had radiographic stage III pulmonary sarcoidosis.
In all patients the diagnosis was confirmed by tissue biopsy.

Pulmonary function tests included spirometry, body plethysmography,
DLCO (single breath) and blood gas analysis at rest.

SPECT was performed using a dual head rotating gamma camera system.
Kr-81m gas was used as a ventilation tracer and Tc-99m microspheres as a
perfusion tracer. For each camera head 30 images of Kr-81m and Tc-99m
activity were acquired simultaneously over 180 degrees. From the resulting
images transaxial slices were reconstructed and in each slice the lung
contour was detected. Within the lung contour $\dot{V}/\dot{Q}$ was calculated in 6.3
cubic mm pixels. Histograms were made of the distribution of ventilation and
perfusion over $\dot{V}/\dot{Q}$. As a measure of ventilation perfusion inequality the
log standard deviation (lnSD) of these distributions was calculated as
well as the percentage of ventilation with $\dot{V}/\dot{Q} \geqslant 10$ and the percentage
of perfusion with $\dot{V}/\dot{Q} \leqslant 0.1$.

RESULTS

Table I summarizes the results. In all patients considerable defects in
ventilation and perfusion were found. Despite this, 6 patients had normal
$\dot{V}/\dot{Q}$ distributions. Only one of these 6 patients had a decreased DLCO.

In 8 patients abnormal distributions of $\dot{V}/\dot{Q}$ ratios were found. Six of these patients also had a decrease in DLCO. Only one patient showed a decrease in pO2 at rest.

TABLE I.

No. of pts	DLCO/VA	pO$_2$	* ln SD (V/Q)	# %V/Q $\geqslant$ 10
			SPECT	
5	N	N	N	N
1	↓	N	N	N
2	N	N	N	↑
4	↓	N	N	↑
1	↓	N	↑	↑
1	↓	↓	↑	↑

N=normal, * N $\leqslant$ 0.4, # N $\leqslant$ 10%

DISCUSSION

The normal $\dot{V}/\dot{Q}$ distribution which was found in 6 patients means that the defects were completely matched, leaving the rest of the lung unaffected. These defects are functionally non-existent and therefore have no influence on gas exchange other than decreasing lung volume.
This was reflected by a normal pO2 in these 6 patients and a normal DLCO in 5 of them. One patient had a decreased DLCO which was attributed to a reduced diffusing capacity of the alveolar-capillary membrane. In 6 of the patients with abnormal $\dot{V}/\dot{Q}$ distributions a decrease in DLCO was found and 1 of these patients had a hypoxaemia at rest. These effects may partly be a result of ventilation-perfusion inequality in these patients.

It was concluded that ventilation-perfusion SPECT can give valuable information about the pathophysiology of gas exchange in pulmonary sarcoidosis, in addition to the classical pulmonary function tests.

Multiple inert gas elimination technique in interstitial lung disease: analysis of ventilation-perfusion relationships.

R. Prediletto, B. Formichi, G. Viegi, E. Fornai, E. Begliomini, A. Santolicandro, C. Giuntini.

C.N.R. Institute of Clinical Physiology and 2nd Medical Clinic of the University of Pisa, Italy.

Introduction

There are still few studies on the mechanisms underlying arterial hypoxemia in interstitial lung disease. From these studies arterial hypoxemia was suggested to be a result of various mechanisms: the thickening of alveolar interstitium which reduces the diffusing capacity for oxygen (1, 2); the reduction of alveolar capillary bed (3); the alteration of alveolar capillary membranes in a non uniform manner, thus causing a ventilation-perfusion mismatching (4); the low mixed venous oxygen tension due to low values of cardiac output and the shortened time available for diffusion of oxygen across the alveolar-capillary membrane due to pulmonary vascular involvement present in advanced interstitial lung disease (5, 6).
Our present study was therefore performed with the aim to analyse the probable causes of hypoxemia in patient with interstitial lung disease by the assessment of ventilation-perfusion relationships from multiple inert gas technique (4). This method is a useful approach for the evaluation of pulmonary gas exchange and, in particular, for the analysis of the relationships between the distribution of ventilation ($\dot{V}$) and perfusion ($\dot{Q}$) in respect to their $\dot{V}/\dot{Q}$ ratio.
In this brief paper the preliminary results on three patients have been reported.

Material and Methods

Three patients (2 men and 1 woman aged 54 to 64 years) with a diagnosis of interstitial lung disease were submitted to the study. The diagnosis of interstitial lung disease was based on clinical findings, radiographic evidence of interstitial damage (presence of nodular pattern with infiltration and fibrosis, more evident in two patients) and on functional data. At the time of the investigation none of patients was being treated with corticosteroid or bronchodilator drugs. Two patients had never smoked and one was ex-smoker.
Patients were investigated through: chest radiograph, perfusion lung scan, lung function tests with a Hewlett-Packard computerized system in order to determine static lung volumes (% RV) and flow volume curves indexes (% FEV1), single breath carbon monoxide diffusing capacity (%DLCOSB), alveolar to arterial oxygen and arterial to alveolar carbon dioxide gradients (A-aDO2, a-ADCO2) with a computerized breath by breath technique by using a respiratory mass spectrometer and finally multiple inert gas elimination technique to assess the $\dot{V}/\dot{Q}$ match and to calculate the arterial oxygen tension that could develop from the $\dot{V}/\dot{Q}$ match and to compare it with the PaO2 measured.

This work was supported with the funds from CNR (National Research Council) Cardio-Respiratory Group.

Results

The patients showed reduction of static lung volumes (e.g. RV 52, 41 and 79%), a decreased %FEV1 (e.g. 67, 92, 52%), a marked level of hypoxemia (e.g. PaO2 57, 68, 53 mmHg), a normal values of mixed venous oxygen tension (e.g. PvO2 34, 35 and 33 mmHg), a marked increase of A-aDO2 (e.g. 71, 50 and 72 mmHg), and of a-ADCO2 (e.g. 14, 11, 13 mmHg). Moreover, they showed a decrease of %DLCOSB (e.g. 52, 68 and 22%).

The distribution of $\dot{V}$ and $\dot{Q}$ by multiple inert gas technique showed the presence of $\dot{V}/\dot{Q}$ inhomogeneity, slightly in one patient and markedly in the others. The main fraction of $\dot{Q}$ was located in regions with $\dot{V}/\dot{Q}$ ratio of .1, .6 and .6, whereas the mean fraction of $\dot{V}$ was located in regions with $\dot{V}/\dot{Q}$ ratio of 2.8, .9 and 1.6. The venous shunt (i.e. the compartment with $\dot{V}/\dot{Q}$ of zero) was 2, 4 and 0% of cardiac output. Regions of low $\dot{V}/\dot{Q}$ ratios (.1) were observed in those patients with more $\dot{V}/\dot{Q}$ inhomogeneity. Alveolar dead space ventilation (i.e. the compartment with $\dot{V}/\dot{Q}$=infinity) was 44, 30 and 43%. PaO2 calculated from the $\dot{V}/\dot{Q}$ distribution (e.g. 60, 64 and 59) did not differ significantly from that measured in two patients.

Discussion

These preliminary results, that need to be confirmed in a larger sample of patients, showed that the calculated PaO2 was not very different from that measured in two patients, thus suggesting a diffusion limitation to gas exchange in patient with interstitial lung disease (2). The observed hypoxemia could be explained by the presence of regions with low $\dot{V}/\dot{Q}$ units and by the wide dispersion of $\dot{V}/\dot{Q}$ ratios, more evident in two patients.
In conclusion, different mechanisms (reduction of oxygen diffusion capacity across the alveolar capillary membrane, $\dot{V}/\dot{Q}$ inhomogeneity, perfusion of poorly ventilated regions) could explain the impairment of pulmonary gas exchange in interstitial lung disease and these hypotheses are in agreement with the results obtained in literature (2, 5, 6).

Bibliography

1) Finley T., Swenson E. W., Comroe J. H.jr: The cause of arterial hypoxemia at rest in patients with alveolar capillar block syndrome. J. Clin. Invest. 1962, 41: 618-622.
2) Wilhelmsson Y.J., Hornblad Y;, Hedenstierna G.: Ventilation-perfusion relationships in interstial lung disease. Eur. J. Respir. Dis. 1986, 68: 39-49.
3) Hamer J.: Cause of low arterial saturation in pulmonary fibrosis. Thorax 1964, 19: 507-514.
4) Wagner P.D., Saltzman H.A., West J.B.: Measurement of continuous distribution of ventilation-perfusion ratios: theory. J. Appl. Physiol. 1974, 36: 588-599.
5) Wagner P.D., Dantzker D.R., Dueck R. et al.: Distribution of ventilation-perfusion ratios in patients with interstitial lung disease. Chest 1976, 69 (suppl.): 256-257.
6) Wagner P.D.: Multiple inert gas techniques: results in normal subjects and in patients. Prog. Resp. Res. 1981, Vol. 16: 245-249.

RADIOLOGICAL PULMONARY CHANGES IN SARCOIDOSIS : A MODIFICATION OF INTERNATIONAL STAGING SYSTEM

SAMIR K GUPTA, SURENDRA K SHARMA
Sarcoidosis Unit, The Calcutta Medical Research Institute and Institute for Respiratory Diseases, Calcutta.

INTRODUCTION

Standard international radiological staging system in sarcoidosis[1] (Stages 0-3) was found to be inadequate when radiological assessment was undertaken in 715 Xray plates of chest, during a period of 14 years (1972-1986) in Calcutta, India. Hence, a modified system was devised to see if it could help in more accurate assessment, especially with respect to prognosis and further progress.

MATERIAL AND METHODS

All the cases were thoroughly investigated[2] before a diagnosis of sarcoidosis was made. Histological confirmation was obtained from more than one tissue[3]. All radiological pictures taken during 1972-86 were analysed by 3 independent observers, all with adequate radiological training. Majority verdict was accepted in cases of divided opinion. A total of 715 X-ray plates were analysed and these included postero-anterior, lateral, and tomographs. Various changes during treatment, remission and relapses were analysed in details. During analysis, it became apparent that some of the radiographs could not be accurately classified under the existing Staging system[1], hence Stages IA, IIB and IIIA and IV were added. Further explanation is provided in the Table 1 itself.

RESULTS

These changes are expressed in Table 1. Further modification of the international staging system is shown in the left hand columns of the table. It appeared to project a little more accurately the radiological changes occuring during treatment and was seen to be better related to prognosis and course (as detailed in the table).

TABLE - 1
ROENTGENOGRAPHIC STAGING OF SARCOIDOSIS

International		Modified
Stage 0	normal CXR	Stage 0 Same
Stage I	hilar lymphadenopathy (HL) No pulmonary change	Stage I hilar lymphadenopathy A-unilateral (UHL) 45% in this series B-bilateral (BHL) 55% 77% (both A & B) may progress

International		Modified	

Stage II	HL with mottling and/or fibrosis	Stage II	UHL/BHL
			A-mottling (73%)
			  may clear initially
			B-fibrosis (27%)
			  rarely disappears

Stage III	only mottling and/or fibrosis (NO HL)	Stage III	A-only mottling (16%)
			  may clear initially
			B-Streaky fibrosis (84%)
			  usually persistent

		Stage IV	pleural effusion, miliary lesions, bullae, cyst, cavity, solitary nodules (sarcoidoma) temporary paralysis of hemidiaphragm etc.

DISCUSSION

HL or hilar lymphadenopathy (Stage 1) is regarded as an early development and it undergoes resolution in about 90% within 2 years in Western countries[4]. Though unilateral HL (Stage 1A) is uncommon in the West, it was fairly common and was seen in nearly half the cases.[2,5] Nearly 77% progressed to bilateral HL (Stage IB) or/and then direct to Stages II or III.

In Stage II, prognosis was better when the lesions were associated with mottled opacities (Stage IIA, 73%) - these cleared initially with treatment. Streaky opacities (Stage IIB, 27%) showed poor resolution during treatment and often progressed to Stage III disease.

In Stage III, mottled opacities (Stage IIIA), seen in 16%, were rare but had better prognosis with initial clearing in nearly one third of cases, whereas streaky opacities suggesting fibrosis, seen in 84% (Stage IIIB), nearly always persisted.

Stage IV[1,6] included a large group of unclassified radiological pictures including solid tumour - like shadows ('sarcoidoma'), bullae, cyst or cavity, mycetoma, consolidation, pleural effusion (6% of our cases), reversible SVC obstruction (2 cases) and temporary hemidiaphragmatic palsy (3 cases), probably due to associated periglandular mediastinitis[8] etc. In many cases the lesion ultimately cleared but cysts or bullae persisted.

It is concluded that the modified staging system can classify the radiological changes better and more accurately during treatment than the existing system. Mottled opacities (Stages IIA and IIIA) have better prognostic value than the streaky opacities (Stages IIB or IIIB)[9]. Stage IV is an added necessity as many radiological pictures cannot be classified satisfactorily under the present system.

REFERENCES

1. De Remee RA. The roentgenographic staging of sarcoidosis. History and contemporary perspectives. Chest 83 : 128-133, 1983.

2. Gupta Samir K, Mitra K, Chatterjee S, Chakravarty S. Sarcoidosis in India. Br J Dis Chest 79 : 275 - 283, 1985.

3. Gupta Samir K, Mitra K, Chatterjee S et al. Multiple biopsies in the diagnosis of sarcoidosis. Indian J Chest Dis & All Sci. 26 : 65-75, 1984.

4. James DG, Jones Williams W. Sarcoidosis and other granulomatous disorders. WB Saunders, London, p 222, 1985.

5. Gupta Samir K, Chatterjee S, Sharma SK. Radiological presentation of sarcoidosis in India. Indian J Radiol. 37 : 319-323, 1983.

6. Sharma OP. Sarcoidosis. A Clinical approach. CC Thomas, Springfield, Illinois. p 30, 1975.

7. Gupta Samir K, Mitra K. Superior vena caval obstruction in sarcoidosis. Lung India 5 : 86-87, 1987.

8. Gupta Samir K. Essentials of Medical Syndromes. Oxford & IBH, Delhi, p 647-648, 1986.

9. Gupta Samir K, Dutta Subir, Mitra K, Roy M. Effect of treatment of sarcoidosis in India. In : Proceedings of the 11th International conference on sarcoidosis, Milan, in press.

© 1988 Elsevier Science Publishers B.V. (Biomedical Division)
Sarcoidosis and other granulomatous disorders
C. Grassi, G. Rizzato, E. Pozzi, editors

COMPARISON OF NEW CSF, NEUROPHYSIOLOGICAL AND NEURORADIOLOGICAL STUDIES IN
NEUROSARCOIDOSIS

VIRPI OKSANEN [*]

The Minerva Foundation Institute for Medical Research, P.O. Box 819, SF-00101
Helsinki and Department of Neurology, Helsinki University Hospital (Finland)

INTRODUCTION

Neurological involvement occurs in 5% of sarcoidosis patients and can be
the presenting sign of sarcoidosis (1,2). Clinical diagnosis is often difficult
and routine laboratory parameters are nonspecific; thus new methods for both
diagnosis and follow-up are needed.

The present study assessed the value of the following examinations in
neurosarcoidosis: measurements of cerebrospinal fluid (CSF) angiotensin
converting enzyme (ACE), lysozyme (LZM), and beta-2-microglobulin (B2m), brain
computed tomography (CT), visual evoked potentials (VEPs), and brainstem
auditory evoked potentials (BAEPs).

PATIENTS AND METHODS

Twenty neurosarcoidosis patients (14 women, 6 men) were examined. Their
mean age was 45 years (range 24-69 years). Neurological symptom was the
presenting sign of sarcoidosis in 10 of them. The main neurological lesion was
localized to the cranial nerves in 7 patients and to the central nervous system
(CNS) in 13 patients (11 cerebral, 2 spinal).

CSF-ACE was measured by a sensitive inhibitor binding assay (3,4), -LZM by
a modified RIA method (5) and -B2m by a commercial RIA kit (Pharmacia, Sweden).
CT scans were performed with the EMI CT 1010 head scanner or Siemens Somatom 2
body scanner. In VEPs and BAEPs only delayed latencies or absent responses were
recorded as abnormal.

RESULTS

Table I shows the number of abnormal findings. CSF-ACE was elevated in all
7 patients with cranial nerve lesions, -LZM and -B2m in 6 of them. At least one
of the parameters was elevated in all neurosarcoidosis patients. CSF-LZM and
-B2m correlated significantly, but CSF-ACE did not correlate to -LZM or -B2m.

CT was normal in all 7 patients with cranial nerve and in 5 with CNS
lesions. Abnormalities were white matter low density lesions (4 patients),
ventricular enlargement (3 patients), mass lesions (2 patients), old
infarction, cerebral atrophy and plexus chorioideus enhancement.

Milan prize winner for authors under 35 years.

382

VEP was abnormal in 8 patients without visual symptoms and BAEP in 6 patients without auditory symptoms.

Table I.

NUMBER OF ABNORMAL CSF, CT, VEP AND BAEP FINDINGS

	Cranial nerve lesions (7 patients)	CNS lesions (13 patients)
CSF-ACE	7/7	8/13
-LZM	6/7	8/11
-B2m	6/7	6/11
VEP	2/7	8/13
BAEP	3/7	5/13
CT	0/7	8/13

CONCLUSIONS

For a complete evaluation of a patient with suspected neurosarcoidosis, combination of diagnostic methods is needed. CSF studies were useful in cerebral lesions but especially in cranial nerve lesions where CT usually fails to detect abnormalities. CT can reveal unexpected cerebral lesions and should be performed to all neurosarcoidosis patients. VEP and BAEP are noninvasive, sensitive and easily repeatable, and may also reveal subclinical lesions.

REFERENCES

1. Stern BJ et al. (1985) Arch Neurol 42: 909-917.
2. Oksanen V (1986) Neurosarcoidosis: a clinical, laboratory and neuroradiological study. Thesis, University of Helsinki.
3. Fyhrquist F et al. (1984) Clin Chem 30: 696-700.
4. Oksanen V et al. (1985) Neurology (NY) 35: 1220-1223.
5. Oksanen V et al. (1986) J Neurol Sci 73: 79-87.

RETROPERITONEAL INVOLVEMENT IN SARCOIDOSIS

LUCIA CASTRIGNANO[1], GIORGIO FASOLINI[2], MARCO NOZZA[2], ARRIGO SCHIEPPATI[2]
1: Sarcoidosis Clinic, E.O. Niguarda, Milan, Italy; 2: Ospedali Riuniti,Bergamo, Italy.

INTRODUCTION

Retroperitoneal lymphnodes involvement in pulmonary sarcoidosis was described by a few Authors (1, 2, 3,) by lymphography.

We report 4 cases of sarcoid patients with a retroperitoneal lymphnodes enlargement detected by abdominal computerized tomography (CT).

CASES REPORT

A 29 years old man with a history of longstanding histologically proven pulmonary sarcoidosis was admitted to hospital because of acute onset obstructive jaundice (total bilirubin 7.7mg%) and urinary tract obstruction (creatinine 6.6 mg%; blood urea nitrogen 2.08mg%). Abdominal ultrasonographic examination (Fig.1 Panels A and B) and computerized tomography scan showed lymphnodes compression on liver hylum and on both renal pyelocalyceal system; he underwent dialysis for 12 days while high dose steroid therapy was given for 2 months with early relief of obstruction.After 1.3 and 13 months of this therapy retroperitoneal lymphnodes were strongly decreased (Fig.1 Panels C and D)and sarcoidosis was silent with normal bilirubinemia, blood urea nitrogen and daily urinary volume.

After seeing this patient, we submitted 12 consecutive patients with st. I or II histologically proven sarcoidosis to abdominal CT scan: in 2 of them increased retroperitoneal lymphnodes could be shown.In one of these patients, admitted to hospital because of chest pain, erythema nodosum and exertional dyspnoea, we observed a symptom-free right hydronephrosis due to lymphnodes compression.A steroid therapy was given with a good improvement.In the other, many retroperitoneal lymphnodes were discovered without compression.

A further(non consecutive)patient with longstanding pulmonary sarcoidosis was admitted to hospital because of fever,hepatomegaly and wide splenomegaly. Abdominal CT scan showed many periaortic and retrocaval lymphnodes and lymphography showed lymphnodes grouping with structural rearrangement.

384

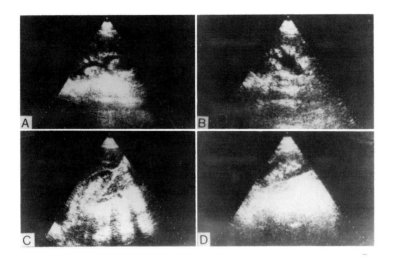

Fig. 1. Panels A and B: bilateral hydronephrosis (right kidney panel A,left B).
Panels C and D: no hydronephrosis after steroid therapy (right kidney panel C,
left D).

DISCUSSION

In our study we submitted 14 patients with longstanding pulmonary sarcoidosis
to abdominal CT scan. All scans but 4 were normal. In 2 on these 4 pts, scans
showed hydronephrosis.In one of these 2 pts we observed right symptom free hydronephrosis while in the other we discovered a clinical acute renal insufficiency
due to bilateral hydronephrosis. In the others two pts abdominal CT scan showed
retroperitoneal lymphnodes involvement without compression. We conclude that a
retroperitoneal involvement in sarcoidosis is more frequent than previously
suspected; the physician should maintain a high index of suspicion towards
its complications.

ACKNOWLEDGEMENTS

We thank Prof. G. Rizzato for permitting the presentation of his patients in
this study and for his helpful suggestions.

REFERENCES

1. Akisada M. et al: Radiology 93, 1273, 1969
2. Traianos G. et al: Hellen ARMED Forces Med. Rev. 6, 671, 1972
3. Thibaud G. et al: Ann. Med. Nancy. 12, 1125, 1973

© 1988 Elsevier Science Publishers B.V. (Biomedical Division)
Sarcoidosis and other granulomatous disorders
C. Grassi, G. Rizzato, E. Pozzi, editors

CONCLUSIVE SUMMARIZING REMARKS AND OUTLOOK

PROFESSOR H. HERZOG, BASEL (SWITZERLAND)

If one compares the actual tendencies of research in functional impairment
of patients with sarcoidosis with those of the last twenty years one can
observe a clear change of interest amongst the actual investigators. While
in the last two decades, the sixties and the seventies, the targets were
largely impairment of volumes, diffusion capacity and compliance of the lung,
the interest of research workers in Sarcoidosis is now concentrating clearly
on airway function.

This is probably due to the availability of several tests for bronchial
clearance es well as to the progress in Asthma research which has resulted
in the concept of bronchial hyperreactivitiy and of airway inflammation as
basis of asthmatic obstruction.

Results like those from Marshall and Karlish (Fig. 1) concerning the behaviour
of vital capacity, lung compliance and D_{CO} along the radiological stages of
pulmonary Sarcoidosis are now classical knowledge. The same is true for blood
gas tensions measured in the different stages of Sarcoidosis as shown on
figure 2 with results from Svanborg.

On the other hand, the teams of Levinson and of Cherniack in Philadelphie, of
Stanley in England and of Brody in Boston have been among the first to draw
the attention on the influence of sarcoidosis on airway function and breathing
mechanics. In a famous article in the American Journal of Medicine in 1977,
they showed a strong increase of transpulmonary pressure, a decrease of FEV_1 in
% of FVC, an increase of closing volume (Fig. 3) and a distinct tendency of
dynamic compliance to decrease with increasing breathing frequency as a sign
of airways obstruction (Fig. 4). Finally, the same research teams were able to
demonstrate in patients with sarcoidosis, non-smokers and smokers that the
ratio of maximal expiratory flow to static transpulmonary pressure was smaller
than normal in all but two patients (Fig. 5). This ratio however indicate an
abnormally high upstream resistance i.e. the resistance of the small bronchi
down to the equal pressure point. Sarcoidosis may influence airway function in
two ways: on the one hand, granulomas may compress or intrude upon the lumen
of large and small airways. On the other hand, granulomas formed in the pulmonary interstitium may modify the supporting structures around terminal
and respiratory bronchioles leading to airway collapse.

Finally, early in the sixties, Svanberg compared diffusing capacity with
pulmonary vascular resistance in the different stages of sarcoidosis. Looking
at figure 6 it becomes quite clear that, since decreasing D_{CO} is invariably

FIG. 1.

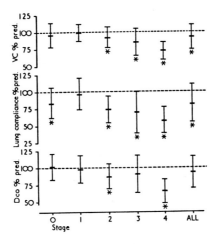

FIG. 1.   Vital capacity, lung compliance (percent of normal predicted from
the patient's expected functional residual capacity), and diffusing capacity
(predicted from the equation of Williams et al. (1961) in the different stages
of sarcoidosis. Mean values and one coefficient of variation. * indicates that
the mean is significantly different from normal. (2)

FIG. 2.

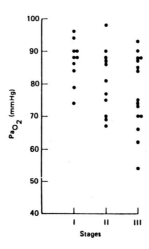

FIG. 2.   Arterial PO_2 in patients with sarcoidosis in stage I (hilar
adenopathy without abnormality of the x-ray film of the chest), stage II
(pulmonary infiltrates), and stage III (pulmonary fibrosis). (3)

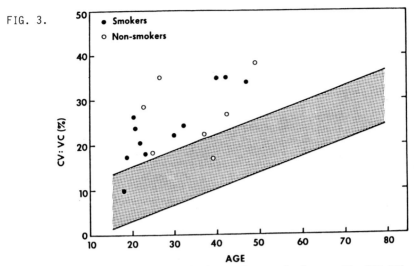

FIG. 3. The relationship of closing volume: vital capacity (CV:VC) ratios to age in patients with sarcoidosis. The shaded area represents the normal range. (1)

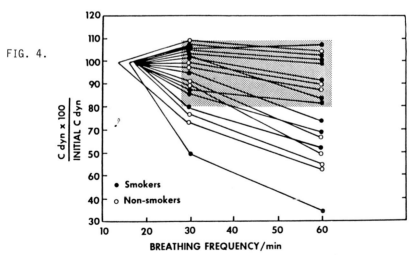

FIG. 4. The relationship of dynamic compliance (C dyn) to breathing frequency in patients with sarcoidosis. The shaded area represents the normal range. (1)

FIG. 5.

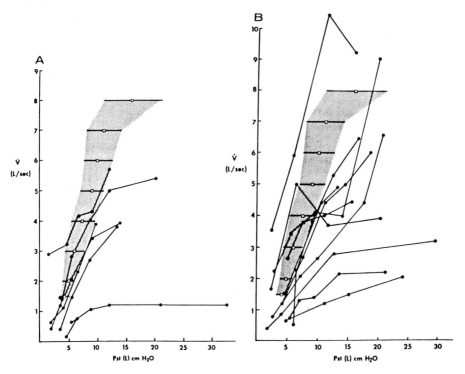

FIG. 5.   A, the relationship of maximal flow to transpulmonary pressures in nonsmoking patients with sarcoidosis. B, the relationship of maximal flow to transpulmonary pressures in smoking patients with sarcoidosis. The shaded area represents the normal range. (1)

FIG. 6.

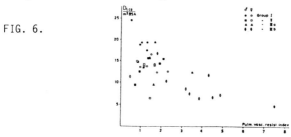

FIG. 6.   Pulmonary diffusing capacity for carbon monoxide ml STPD/min/Hg per sq. m. body surface area, D_{LCO}/m^2 BSA, during exercise in sitting position (ordinate) in relation to pulmonary vascular resistance index,

$$\frac{\overline{P}_{PA} - \overline{P}_{PCV}}{\dot{Q}/m^2 BSA}$$, during exercise in supine position (abscissa). (4)

coupled with increasing vascular resistance, arterial hypoxia in more advanced stages or sarcoidosis is largely due to capillary destruction and not
so much to ventilation / perfusion mismatch.

So far with history of sarcoidotic impairment of the functions of the respiratory tract. Let us now have a look at the presentations and posters of the
session we just have assisted to.

AEROSOL CLEARANCES STUDIES

After the excellent introductory lecture by Sharma, presenting the actual
state of the art on functional impairment of respiratory organs in sarcoidosis, there were two papers on airway epithelium clearance of micronic
acrosolized Technetium 99m-DTPA (Rc-DTPA) from the group around Chrétien in
Paris. On the one hand, as long as respiratory clearance remains normal the
course of Sarcoidosis is favourable. When however lung function declines,
Rc-DTPA increases and constitutes an indication for steroid therapy. On the
other hand, the same team uses the respiratory clearance (RC) of 99m Tc-DTPA
in rats for the control of the influences of sarcoidotic granulomas in the
respiratory tract. Rc-DTPA increases when granulomas induced by Freund's
adjuvant are present, because there is no aerosol transport. Following injection of complete Freund's adjuvant, RC is always increased. Thus aerosol
clearance can be a very useful tool for the control of granuloma density
within the lungs.

BRONCHIAL HYPERREACTIVITY

Bronchial hyperreactivity in sarcoidosis was discussed in two papers. The
Japanese Group around Shima states that the alterations of bronchial walls, well
known from fiberoptic investigations, are generally combined with increased
resposiveness of the airways demonstrated by methacholine challenge as well as
by provocation test with histamin. Bronchial hyperreactivity was observed in
65% of patients with sarcoidosis while the same authors found that 86% of
patients with chronic bronchitis and of course 100% of asthmatics were hyper-
responsive. The team thinks that bronchial hyperreactivity in sarcoidosis is
correlated to the changes of the bronchial wall as well as to the histamin
receptor activity of its structures and depends finally on the activity of the
sarcoidosis lesions.

The Siena group around Bianco was wondering if and in what extent bronchoalveolar lavage (BAL) modifies bronchial responsiveness measured by metha-
choline-challenge. The autors observed a rather marked decrease of airway
reactivity after BAL which is so far unrelated to SACE, to the precentage of

lymphocytes in BAL, to the stage of the disease and to the lung function values.

AIRWAYS OBSTRUCTION

Airways obstruction in sarcoidosis was discussed by three groups of authors.
The New York team around Miller and Teirstein attribuates bronchial narrowing
to several causes: bronchial hyperreactivity, small airways obstruction, pulmonary bullae, bronchial stenoses by COPD, and upper airways obstruction. The
group from Kiel around Petermann, concludes, that airways dysfunction in sarcoidosis is localized particularly in the small airways. This may decrease by
increasing the $\dot{V}$ / $\dot{Q}$-mismatch, the value of the CO-diffusing capacity in addition to anatomical destruction of blood capillaries. In a poster of Sharma,
Los Angeles, finally the importance of airway obstruction is evaluated. He
found a bronchial narrowing in 63% of patients with sarcoidosis. When challenged with methacholine 60% of 26 patients showed a 20% or greater fall in FEV_1.
In macrophage culture supernates of patients with sarcoidosis he found besides
chemical mediators including chemotactic peptides, increased levels of C3, C4,
C5 and the anaphylatoxines C3a and C4a. He concludes that the relative role of
macrophage-produced mediators in bronchial hyperreactivity of sarcoidosis is
still to be established.

VENTILATION / PERFUSION RELATIONSHIPS

Ventilation / Perfusion relationship has been examined by three groups of
workers. The Amsterdam team with Zwijnenburg has combined for this purpose two
techniques which are both equally precise but technically and intellectually
sophisticated, namely the multiple inert gas infusion technique developed by
Wagner and West and the single photon emission computed tomography (SPECT) by
which regional pulmonary functions is visualized and gives a three dimensional
mapping of activity distribution. By introduction of Krypton 81 m-gas as a
ventilation tracer and of Technetium 99 m-microspheres as a perfusion tracer
the Amsterdam group was able to develop a technique for the quantitative analysis of simultaneous ventilation / perfusion SPECT studies. This method can
yield values for ventilation and perfusion as well as $\dot{V}$ / $\dot{Q}$-ratios for pulmonary regions as small as 6,3 cubic millimeters. Furthermore the technique
is able to deliver continuous distribution control of regional ventilation /
perfusion ratios. In a group of 10 patients in pumonary sarcoidosis stages III
to IV with still normal blood gases or slight hypoxemia at rest, it was possible to confirm or to rule out regional ventilation / perfusion inequality
as cause for disturbed gas exchange and to confirm in some cases a capillary
perfusion defect as basis for decreased diffusion capacity. However this

elegant technique is certainly highly professional and not feasible by everyone.

Multiple inert gas technique was also applied by the Pisa team around Prediletto for the investigation of the possible mechanisms of hypoxemia in interstitial lung disease. The conclusion from the results in three patients with advanced disease was, that the hypoxemia could mainly be explained by mechanisms like $\dot{V}$ / $\dot{Q}$-inhomogeneity, regions with low $\dot{V}$ / $\dot{Q}$-units or impaired diffusion.

Finally the group of Bologna around Falcone used Ventilation / Perfusion scintigraphy for the study of airway involvement in 12 patients with sarcoidosis in stage I, mainly II and some in stage III. The authors combined the evaluation of the Gallium - 67 scan with the Technetium 99 m Perfusion-Scan and Technetium 99 m Ventilation-Scan. This team did not find any correlation between the scanning results and the stage or the duration of the disease. However, the technique seams usefull in the evaluation of airway involvement in the follow-up of pulmonary sarcoidosis.

SPIROMETRIC METHODS COMBINED TO NUCLEAR PROCEDURES

The conventional methods of spirometry, exercise test and blood gas analysis have however not disappeared but are still applied in sarcoidosis in combination with the modern nuclear procedures.

CONTROL OF EFFECTS OF STEROID-TREATMENT

Another Pisa team around Palla and Giuntini studied young subjects with pulmonary sarcoidosis stage I to II who had normal spirometry and ACE-values but mildly abnormal D_{CO}- and Gallium-Scan values as well as sarcoidotic lesions on the x-ray. The team found linear correlations of x-ray-score with 67 Gallium-line-index as well as with FVC, FEV1, D_{CO} and ACE. After 6 months of high (25mg) or low (5mg) prednisone treatment, most of the considered parameters showed average improvement in the high as well as the low prednisone group which tended to remain stable in the subsequent 6 months.

MECHANISMS OF DYSPNEA

The group around Lo Cicero in Milano tried to explain the mechanisms of dyspnea in patients with pulmonary sarcoidosis who were normoxemic at rest but showed hypoxemia in exercise. The degree of pulmonary involvement was evaluated by methods such as Gallium-scan, transbronchial lung biopsy and CO-Diffusion test in steady state. - The team observed that the exercise-desaturation test agreed with the Gallium 67-results in a high percentage of the cases.

LUNG TRANSFER - FACTOR

Lung transfer-Factor and K_{CO} in sarcoidotic subjects were investigated by
Sergi and his group in Milano. They found that for patients with normal total
lung capacity, transfer factor- and K_{CO}-values were equally discriminant. But
in patients with restrictive disease, the values of K_{CO} expressed in percentage
of the predicted values at TLC, is erroneous and theoretical values at sub-
maximal VA should be used.

RESPIRATORY MUSCLE DYSFUNCTION

The investigation by Mir, Laroche and Green in London on respiratory muscle
dysfunction in sarcoidosis led to the conclusion that phrenic nerve- and dia-
phragma muscle function remained intact in patients with pulmonary sarcoidosis
and that eventual defects in the motricity of respiration were rather caused
by spinal lesions at the phrenic nerve roots.

BAL - FINDINGS AND FUNCTIONAL IMPAIRMENT

The team around Rust and Meier-Sydow in Frankfurt investigated the correlation
of bronchial lavagefluid findings with the functional impairment in patients
with sarcoidosis. The conclusion was, that only the neutrophil count in BAL can
be used as parameter for the extent of the functional impairment in Sarcoidosis
patients. As the neutrophil count is normal in early stages of the desase,
this parameter can indicate progression to pulmonary fibrosis.

BREATHING PATTERNS

Finally, Renzi, Milic-Emily and their group in Montreal were interested in
the effect of steroid therapy on the breathing pattern in patients with
interstial lung disease. Ventilation, flow rates and breathing frequency
were controlled. It was concluded that corticosteroid therapy did not correct
the abnormal breathing pattern nor the increased neuromuscular drive in interstitial lung disease. If inflammatory mediators are suppressed by steroids,
the resulting fibrosis perpetuates reflex mechanisms responsible for maintaining the altered breathing pattern.

OUTLOOK

The techniques for functional evaluation of lungs in sarcoidosis are certainly at a degree of perfection, wich is hard to push much higher anymore.
Where however, the field is still wide open, is the combination with
immunological and biochemical methods. The moving front is certainly on this
side. But it has always been a wise attitude, to control biological methods

by procedures stemming from classical mathematics and physics. In this sense, a multiplicity of methods is now completing the mosaic of functional parameters, which is already now more able than before to evaluate the sarcoidotic patients condition, thus permitting to determine the starting point for steroid therapy or to describe a better screening of new and better treatments for Sarcoidosis we need so urgently.

REFERENCES

1. Levinson, R.S., Metzger, L.F., Stanley, N.N., Kelsen, S.G., Altose, M.D., Cherniack N.S., Brody, I.S.: Airway function in sarcoidosis Am J. Med. 62, 51 (1977)

2. Marshall, R., Karlish, A.J.: Lung function in sarcoidosis. Thorax 26,402 (1971)

3. Williams jr., M.H.: Pulmonary function in: sarcoidosis and other granulomatous discason of the lung, Fanburg B.L. ed., Marcel Dekker, New York, Basel P.77, 1983

4. Svanborg, N.: Cardiopulmonary function in sarcoidosis; general discussion. Acta Med. Scand. 170, Suppl. 366, 119 (1961)

CLINICAL ASPECTS OF PULMONARY SARCOIDOSIS

SARCOIDOSIS : CLINICAL ASPECTS. STATE OF THE ART

SAMIR K GUPTA
Chief, Sarcoidosis Unit, Respiratory Diseases Dept., The Calcutta Medical Research Institute and Institute for Respiratory Diseases, Calcutta.

Sarcoidosis is a syndrome-complex (still inadequately defined), which affects several systems, all of which show monotonously uniform[1], regular, non-caseating granulomas in all of the affected tissues. The definition accepted at the 7th International Conference on sarcoidosis at New York, 1975, is in fact a shortened clinical description of the syndrome, as seen clinically in the West; all the 134 words were adjusted in 14 sentences[2]. However, sarcoidosis in different races and geographical regions presents quite a few interesting variations,[3] which will be the subject matter of this paper.

PREVALENCE

No doubt sarcoidosis is a world wide phenomenon. The prevalence has been noted to be inversely related to the intensity of infection of tuberculosis and leprosy in the community.[3] The available data for either prevalence or incidence (i.e. the annual attack rate) is not adequate for many developing countries like India where a few cases are reported due to a variety of reasons like prevalence of tuberculosis, absence of 'sarcoid-conscious' physicians, absence of MMR surveys etc. Even in developed countries, many asymptomatic cases are never reported in life time. Hence, autopsy figures may be upto 640 per 100,000 population, as shown by Hagerstrand and Linell.[4] In USA, the prevalence varies from one state to other (from 11-71, per 100,000 population)[5]. Arctic regions seem to be free from this syndrome. In European countries, the figure varies from 0.04 (Spain) to 64 (in Sweden)[3]. In some countries like Japan the figure has risen from 3 to nearly 12 over a period of 18 years[6].

RACE

In many countries having multiracial societies, the different races show a varying predilection. In USA[5] and South Africa[7], the black population is nearly 10-12 times more prone than the local whites. American Red Indians and American Chinese, Australian aborigines and Maoris in New Zealand are rarely affected.

In London, the prevalence rate varies from 27 (in local-born English) to 213 (in young immigrant Irish women[3]). In Calcutta, India, a small sect of Marwaris (constituting only 2% of population) accounts for nearly 33% of the known cases in the city of Calcutta. It may be that being wealthy, they only could afford the high cost of investigation and could go round doctors in

India and abroad before a diagnosis was made.

AGE

In the West, sarcoidosis affects the young age group (3rd and 4th decades)[3]. However, all ages between 3 months[8] to eighty years[9] have been reported to be affected. In India, patients are usually above 40 years of age,[10] partly because of the delay in diagnosis. Such elderly subjects are affected in Jamaica, Finland and some other countries.

SEX

Sharma,[11] after a review of available data, has concluded that black women are twice as prone as their men, while amongst the whites both sexes show equal propensity. Males predominate in India[10] (5:3) and in Israel (3:1), Singapore (7:5), Malayasia (8:5), Jamaica etc.[12]

FAMILIAL INCIDENCE

Nearly 200 patients have been described till 1983[3]; James and his co-workers reported 31 of these cases[13]. Monozygotic twins are more affected than the dizygotic twins. Brother-sister relationship is the commonest, followed by mother-child combination. Djurić et al[14] have reported sarcoidosis in a pair of monozygotic twins, living 35 miles apart but developing the disease at the same time. We have 2 brothers (one living and developing the disease in Canada, the other in India) and a father-daughter combination-the latter being distinctly uncommon[3]. Husband-wife combination has been reported in a few.[3,15]

CLINICAL PRESENTATION

This depends on a variety of factors namely duration of illness, the site and extent of the tissue involvement, the degree of activity of the disease etc. Racial factors and geographical location may influence the pattern of the disease. It can conveniently be grouped into acute, subacute and chronic types.[16]

Acute. (meaning sudden and often asymptomatic[16]) onset of sarcoidosis is fairly frequent in the Americas, Europe and Japan. Acute sarcoidosis, in its true sense, is uncommon in West except in Sweden, immigrant Irish women in London, Puerto Ricans in New York and Martinique women in Paris,[3] where often a combination erythema nodosum (EN), bilateral hilar lymphadenopathy (BHL) with arthralgia and eye manifestations is seen mostly in young females during pregnancy and lactation. This combination, the so called Löfgren syndrome,[17,18] is seen in less than 5% of cases in India.[19] It is uncommon also in USA, Japan and most of the tropical countries. Other uncommon acute presentation may involve any system, as detailed later.

Subacute. all these cases usually present with a history of symptoms having duration less than two years.[16] These patients predominate in India (nearly 60% of our series in Calcutta) - they often have periodic fever, ranging between 99°F - 101°F but are not acutely ill. Unlike in West, history spans for several years and diagnosis is missed owing to a variety of reasons, enumerated earlier and elsewhere.[10,19]

Chronic. all these cases have a history of more than two years.[16] They have a slow progressive course and may come up with chronic respiratory insufficiency, disfiguring cutaneous lesions, eye problems etc. Many cases in India and other tropical countries and the black population in USA and South Africa may develop this form of disease, either at the time of diagnosis or later.

Most of the symptomatic cases appear to the physician either   i) due to non-specific constitutional symptoms or ii) due to symptoms related to specific organ involvement.

Nearly one third of Sharma's cases at Los Angeles appeared with non-specific constitutional symptoms.[11] Nearly all our cases in India had constitutional symptoms as low grade fever, anorexia, malaise, fatigue, myalgia, arthralgia[19] etc.

Most of these cases come to the chest physicians with a varying complaints of cough, dyspnoea, wheezing, pain in chest, haemoptysis or heaviness in chest due to pleural effusion. Lung was involved in 87% in World-wide series,[20] 88% in James series,[3] more than 90% cases[11] at Los Angeles and in 98% in our own series at eastern India.[19] Many cases with marked changes in chest Xray may be asymptomtic. While paucity of symptoms may be striking when compared to the radiological changes, signs in chest are even more disproportionate, when compared to the Xray changes. This has been termed as 'clinico-radiological dissociation' by us[21] and has been confirmed by other workers.[22] Rarely symptoms occur due to a variety of complications as superior vena caval obstruction,[23] cor pulmonale, segmental collapse and pneumonia, acute respiratory failure due to pulmonary fibrosis (causing 11 of 14 deaths in our series[21]) etc. Cyst and bullae formation, cavitation etc. may be present without accompanying symptoms. Three cases of temporary left hemidiaphragmatic palsy had been noted in our series with BHL, possibly due to associated periglandular mediastinitis.[24]

Fairly large number of sarcoidosis cases appear to a general physician with pyrexia of unknown origin, anorexia, malaise, nausea, weight loss, fatigue, arthralgia with or without myalgia, hepato-splenomegaly, lymphadenopathy etc. Though uncommon in West, a low grade fever is often present in our subjects in India.[21] These patients, as a rule, are little inconvenienced with fever of 100°F. (patients can do often their daily office work or even play games), in contrast with tuberculosis patients, who may be bedridden with 99°F. Fatigue and weight loss is not so profound as seen in tuberculosis. Enlargement of lymph nodes (28% world series,[20] 39% in James' series[3] and 19% in India[21]) is usually painless. Several earlier series from USA, including many black people, have reported high incidence of lymphadenopathy (69% to 100%[25,26]). It is difficult to conjecture why some of these earlier series had such high incidence of lymph node enlargement. Most of these are cervical nodes and are firm, without matting and may at times enlarge to fairly large size (upto 2-6 cms in diameter). Abscess or sinus formation is rare. Hepatosplenomegaly is extremely common in some countries and is seen in nearly 70% of cases in India[27] while in the West, it is not so common (10% in James' series[3]).

Many a sarcoidosis patient comes to the department of dermatology as cutaneous manifestations[3,28] are fairly common (nearly 25% of most of the series). Erythema nodosum occurs as an acute entity and may appear as an integral part of Löfgren syndrome[17,18] and has been stressed earlier. Lupus pernio is quite characteristic of a chronic disease, associated with lung fibrosis, chronic uveitis and bone changes.[29] Cutaneous plaques, either psoriasiform or angiolupoid, with telangiectatic vessels, are not uncommon, when lymphadenopthy and splenomegaly may be associated. Maculo-papular eruptions, scars and subcutaneous nodule are also seen in sarcoidosis. Some cases may develop severe pruritus. Alopecia, keloid-like lesions and mucosal patches are also described.[30]

Some cases are referred from the rheumatology department with arthritis or arthralgia. Arthalgia is usually monoarticular in India,[10] polyarticular in the Puerto Ricans in New York[11] and affects usually the larger joints-this symptom is often transient and may not be divulged and is often available only on leading questioning.[19,21] Rarely the picture may mimic rheumtic or rheumatoid illness. Löfgren syndrome,[17,18] already discussed, is usually associated with a good prognosis.[30,31] Bone cysts, associated with chronic skin lesions,[28,32] are often painless while painful dactylitis is rare. Persistent chronic arthritis and deformity are rare except in blacks in USA[11,31] and South Africa.[7] Some cases may resemble having rheumatoid disease very closely.[11,30] Asymptomatic granulomatous muscle involvement seems frequent (50-80%) in the West[34] but rare in India.[35] Other forms of muscle involvement are palpable muscle nodules, polymyositis-like features, chronic myopathy or isolated sarcoid myopathy.[11]

In the recent world-wide survey,[20] the incidence of eye involvement was fairly common in London (27%) and Tokyo (32%). It is rather infrequent (8%) in India,[10,36] Thailand,[37] Taiwan[38] and neighbouring countries. Repeated conjunctival biopsies have failed to elicit a single case of conjunctival involvement in India.[35,36] There may be features of uveitis (acute, subacute or chronic) uveo-parotitis, retinal vasculitis, choroidoretinitis, glaucoma, early cataract, optic neuritis, keratic precipitate, visual loss etc. Fundoscopy may reveal, in addition, snow-ball clumps in vitreous, mutton-fat appearance in fundus, papilloedema etc.[39] Several ophthalmological syndromes are associated with sarcoidosis as Sicca, Sjögren, Löfgren, Mikuliiz, Heerfordt[18,40] etc. Most of the earlier reported large series show ocular involvement in nearly 20-27% of cases,[41-44] while the incidence has become less[20] now, probably due to a large number of case-detection by MMR (often early and asymptomatic).

Radiologists may refer most of these cases as some forms of radiological abnormalities in sarcoidosis are quite common. In Western countries and Japan, where MMR surveys are frequently undertaken, bilateral adenopathy are referred for clinical assessment as patients are often asymptomatic. Other pulmonary abnormalities, which can give rise to various symptoms, are mottlings, miliary shadows, honey - comb appearance, patchy consolidation, solitary shadows (so called 'sarcoidoma'), cysts or bullae, cavitation, pleural effusion, widening of mediastinal shadow (with clinical features of superior vena caval obstruction[23]), temporary hemi-diaphragmatic paralysis (seen in 3 of our patients temporarily[24]), pleural effusion etc. Other bones may show radiolucent, either permeative or destructive, lesions. Joints may show effusion, thining of periarticular bones[3,11] etc. Clinical features depend on the underlying pathology.

Neurologists are likely to see a few of these cases. In some earlier series the incidence was high[44,45] (16-29%) but the world-wide review[20] had shown a much lower figures (1-4% mostly). Clinically four groups are discernible[11]: i) cranial nerve involvement; ii) peripheral nerve affection; iii) CNS lesions (including brain, meninges and spinal cord) and iv) psychiatric problems. Facial palsy is recorded in nearly half the cases,[46] most of these are unilateral (65%). Other cranial nerves as optic, glossopharyngeal, vagus etc. are occasionally affected. Facial nerve may at times be involved with swelling of the ipsilateral parotid gland.[46,47] Papilloedema is uncommon but it affects more women than men[3]; optic paiplla may be affected at times.[47] Hypothalamic involvement is rare but has been reported by Turkington and MacIndoe[48] in 11 cases and Caro et al[49] in 5 cases. Some of these patients had profound hyperprolactinaemia.[50] Other forms of CNS involvement are recorded as obstructive hydrocephalus, hemiparesis, mental confusion, epileptiform convulsion etc. Focal granulomas may occur at any part but most commonly basal region of the brain is involved. Peripheral neuropathy may involve both motor and sensory or either of them separately.[46] There may be associated cranial nerve palsy also. Psychiatric manifestation may need admission of the patient to a mental hospital; agitation, hallucination, memory loss, irritability, lethargy, paranoia, apathy, confusional state etc. have been recorded.[51] Cerebrospinal fluid may at times show remarkable pleocytosis and raised protein level.[51]

Several recognised syndromes (as Fröhlich, Diencephalic, Pineal etc.[18]) may be noticed. We have recorded an incidence of 11% neurosarcoidosis in the all-India series.[21] It is rather uncommon in eastern India[27] (5%) and in countries in South-East Asia.[37,38]

Clinically recognisable cardiac lesions occur more in subjects over 40 years and in elderly women in Japan.[20] Suggestive clinical features may be seen only in 5% cases while in autopsy cardiac involvement is seen in 20% cases.[52,53] Symptoms like pain in chest, sudden loss of consciousness, tachycardia, palpitation, oedema feet etc. may be associated with arrhythmia, conduction defects like right or left bundle branch block, complete heart block with Stokes - Adams attacks, cardiomyopathy, pulmonary hypertension, congestive cardiac failure, valvular lesions, myocardial infarction, pericardial involvement[3,11] etc. In eastern India, cardiac lesions were detected in 11% cases[54] following ECG, 2-mode echo-cardiography, tread-mill test etc., most of whom had few clinical symptoms. Sudden death due to probable cardiac involvement has been recorded and may occur in 15% of the cases with sarcoidosis, affecting heart.[53]

Involvement of kidneys may often be asymptomatic and may be due to granulomatous involvement of renal tissue. Sarcoid nephritis with clinical features of uraemia has been described.[55] Hypercalcaemia, by itself or by causing nephrocalcinosis, can cause renal damage.[3,30]

Gastroenterologists may find sarcoidosis cases while investigating hepato-splenomegaly, hepatic granulomas, intrahepatic cholestasis, Crohn's disease like features or Whipple syndrome[18]-like illness, portal hypertension etc.[3] Asymptomatic affection of pancreas has been proven by autopsy[56,57]. Adult form of diabetes mellitus has been noticed in 12% patients in our series : the incidence is nearly 4 times higher than in the general population. Peritoneal involvement has been described by several authors, causing ascites.[58]

Only a few cases are seen by ENT Surgeons when the mucosa of the nose, larynx or pharynx is involved. Symptoms were noticed in only 6% of the London series of James.[3] Nasal obstruction, crusting, discharge, hoarseness, stridor, nasal intonation of voice etc. are complained of.[59]

Immunological and biochemical disturbances are usually present without symptoms or signs except lymphadenopathy. Most of these cases suffer little from pyogenic infections. Disturbances of calcium metabolism have been referred to earlier.

Sarcoidosis is only a rare paediatric problem (4% in world series : 6% in our own[60]). School surveys by MMR have revealed asymptomatic cases in Japan[61] and Hungary[62]. Black children get a more severe symptomatic disease in USA, while children below 4 years may develop rash, arthritis and uveitis with little chest complaints.[3] Peripheral lymphadenopathy, hepatosplenomegaly are usually commoner than in adults. Severe eye involvement and erythema nodosum were uncommon in Japan but were seen in USA. Like adults in India,[19,21] the children with sarcoidosis may show signs of relapse.[64]

Pregnancy may prove a boon to young females with sarcoidosis, when some show distinct clinical improvement.[65]

CLINICAL COURSE

How does the clinical course run ? It differs again in different countries. Typically an American black (often a female) will have more respiratory symptoms with fever, loss of weight, skin and eye lesions. She will tend to run a more severe disease with an indolent course with more probability of developing a chronic disease with complications. In comparison, the American white will have a much milder disease with a chance of spontaneous resolution within a period of 2 years.[3,30]

European whites have similar features as American whites with a fair chance of resolution, even if no treatment is given to a majority with a Stage I radiological disease, a substantial number in Stage II and in some in Stage III.[3,11,30]

South African blacks[7,66] have more arthritis, bone cysts and skin lesions with nail dystrophy than the local whites or mixed races.

Patients in the Indian subcontinent get subacute episodes with fever, arthralgia, cough, dyspnoea with high sedimentation rate, hypergammaglobulinaemia, hypercalciuria and high SACE[19,21]

ACKNOWLEDGEMENT

I am indebted to many colleagues in India and abroad, especially Drs.Om Sharma, Los Angeles, D.Geraint James, London, S.Bovornkitti, Bangkok, Y.Hosoda & Y.Nittu, Japan, for helping me in collecting data.

REFERENCES

1. Drury RAB. Problems in histological interpretation in sarcoidosis. Postgrad Med J. 46 : 478, 1970.

2. Proceedings of the 7th International Conference on Sarcoidosis and other Granulomatous Disorders, Siltzbach LE. (ed.), Ann NY Acad Sci. 278 : p 1, 1976.

3. James DG., Jones Williams W. Sarcoidosis and other Granulomatous Disorders London, WB Saunders, 1985.

4. Hegerstrand I, Linell F. The prevalence of sarcoidosis in the autopsy material of a Swedish town. Acta Med Scand. 1976 (suppl.425) : 103, 1964.

5. Israel HL. Influence of race and geographic origin on incidence of sarcoidosis in the United States. In : Levinsky L and Macholda F. (eds.) Proceedings of the 5th International Conference on Sarcoidosis, Prague, Karlova University p 235, 1971.

404

6. Hosoda Y, Iwai K, Odaka M. Recent Epidemiological features of sarcoidosis in Japan : Proceedings of the 6th International Conference on Sarcoidosis, Iwai K, Hosoda Y. (eds.),Tokyo, Univ Tokyo Press p 519, 1980.

7. Benatar S. Sarcoidosis in South Africa. In : Proceedings of the 8th International Conference on Sarcoidosis. Jones Williams W, Davies BH (eds.), Cardiff, Alpha and Omega Press p 508, 1980.

8. Naumann O. Contribution to knowledge of Schaumann's benign lymphogranulomatosis : Besnier - Boeck - Schaumann's disease. Z Kinderheilk. 60 : 1, 1938.

9. Leitner SJ. Diagnosis, etiology and therapy of epitheloid cell granulomatosis, Besnier-Boeck-Schaumann's disease. Neue Med Welt. 1 : 1044, 1950.

10. Gupta Samir K, Mitra K, Roy M, Dutta SK. Sarcoidosis in India. Indian J Chest Dis All Sci. 27 : 55, 1985.

11. Sharma OP. Sarcoidosis : A Clinical Approach. Springfield, Illinois, CC Thomas, 1975.

12. Hosoda Y, Koguda T, Yamamoto M, Hongo O, Mochizumi H. et al. A cooperative study of sarcoidosis in Asia and Africa; descriptive epidemiology. Ann NY Acad Sci. 278 : 347, 1976.

13. James DG. Genetics and familial sarcoidosis. In : Sarcoidosis and Other Granulomatous Disease of the Lung. B.L. Fanburg (ed.), New York, Marcel ekker Inc. p 135, 1983.

14. Djurić O , Burković' D, Dostanić' D. Sarcoidosis in twins. Sarcoidosis 3 : 172, 1986.

15. British Thoracic and Tuberculosis Association. Familial association in sarcoidosis. Tubercle 54 : 87, 1973.

16. James DG. Clinical concept of sarcoidosis. Am Rev Resp Dis. 84 : 14, 1961.

17. Löfgren S. Primary pulmonary sarcoidosis. Acta Med Scand. 145 : 424, 1953.

18. Gupta Samir K. Essentials of Medical Syndromes. New Delhi, Oxford and IBH, 1986.

19. Gupta Samir K, Chatterjee S, Roy M. Clinical profile of sarcoidosis in India. Lung India 1 : 5, 1982.

20. James DG, Neville E, Siltzbach LE, et al. A worldwide review of sarcoidosis. Ann NY Acad Sci. 278 : 321, 1976.

21. Gupta Samir K, Mitra K, Chatterjee S and Chakraborty SC. Sarcoidosis in India. Br J Dis Chest 79 : 275, 1985.

22. Loudon RG, Boughman RP. Crackles in sarcoidosis and in fibrosing alveolitis. Sarcoidosis 3 : 164, 1986.

23. Gordonson J, Trachenberg S, Sargent EN. Superior vena cava obstruction due to sarcoidosis. Chest 63 : 292, 1973.

24. Gupta Samir K. The syndrome of spontaneous laryngeal palsy in pulmonary tuberculosis. Br J Laryngol Otol. 74 : 106, 1960.

25. Riley EA. Boeck's sarcoid : a review based upon a clinical study of 52 cases. Am Rev Tuberc. 62 : 231, 1950.

26. Israel HL, Sones M. Sarcoidosis : Clinical observations on 160 cases. Arch Int Med. 102 : 766, 1958.

27. Gupta Samir K. Sarcoidosis in India. The past, present and the future (Merck Oration) Lung India. In press.

28. James DG, Thomson AD. Dermatological aspects of sarcoidosis. Q J Med. 28 : 109, 1959.

29. James DG. Lupus pernio. In : Proceedings of the 9th International Conference on Sarcoidosis and other Granulomatous Diseases. Chretien J, Marsac J, Saltiel JC (eds.), Paris, Pergamon Press. p 465, 1983.

30. Scadding JG, Mitchell, DN. Sarcoidosis, 2nd ed., London, Chapman and Hall, 1985.

31. Siltzbach LE, Derberstein JL. Arthritis in Sarcoidosis. Clin Orthop. 57 : 31, 1968.

32. James DG. Sarcoidosis of the skin. In : Dermatology in General Medicine. 3rd ed., Fitzpatrick TC (ed.), New York, McGraw Hill, 1984.

33. Spilberg I, Siltzbach LE, McEwen C. The arthritis of sarcoidosis. Arthritis Rheum. 12 : 126, 1969.

34. Lebacq E, Ryelle M. Les manifestations articulares de la sarcoidose. Rev Rheum. 11 : 611, 1966.

35. Gupta Samir K, Mitra K, Chatterjee S, Banerjee D, Roy M. Multiple biopsies in the diagnosis of sarcoidosis. Indian J Chest Dis All Sci. 26 : 65, 1984.

36. Das A, Chatterjee S, Bagchi S, Gupta Samir K. Ocular involvement in sarcoidosis. Indian J Ophthalmol. 34 : 195, 1984.

37. Bovornkitti S. Sarcoidosis in Thailand. In : Proceedings of the 6th International Conference of Sarcoidosis. Iwai K, Hosoda Y. (eds.), Tokyo, Tokyo University Press. p 311, 1974.

38. Yang SP, Wu MC. Sarcoidosis in Taiwan. In : Proceedings of the 6th International Conference of Sarcoidosis. Iwai K, Hosoda Y. (eds.), Tokyo, Tokyo University Press p 309, 1974.

39. James DG. Anderson R, Langley D, Ainslie D. Ocular sarcoidosis. Br J Ophthalmol. 48 : 461, 1964.

40. James DG. Multi-system ocular syndromes. J R Coll Physicians London, 9 : 63, 1974.

41. James DG, Sharma OP. Extrathoracic sarcoidosis. Proc R Soc Med. 60 : 692, 1967.

42. Longcope WT, Freiman DG. A study of sarcoidosis. Medicine 31 : 1, 1952.

43. Siltzbach LE. Sarcoidosis : Clinical features and management. Med Clin North Am., 51 : 483, 1967.

44. Mayock RL, Bertrand P, Morrison CE, Scott JH. Manifestation of sarcoidosis : analysis of 145 patients with a review of nine series selected from the literature. Am J Med. 35 : 67, 1963.

45. Gendel BR, Young JM, Greiner DJ. Sarcoidosis. Review with 24 additional cases. Am J Med. 12 : 205, 1952.

46. Colover J. Sarcoidosis with involvement of the nervous system. Brain 71 : 451, 1948.

47. Blain JG, Riley MD, Logothetis J. Optic nerve manifestations of sarcoidosis. Arch Neurol. 13 : 307, 1965.

48. Turkington RW, MacIndoe JH. Hyperprolactinaemia in sarcoidosis. Ann Int Med. 76 : 545, 1972.

49. Caro JF, Glennon JA, Israel HL. Neuroendocrine studies in sarcoidosis. In : Proceedings of the 8th International Conference on Sarcoidosis. Jones Williams W, Davies BH (eds.), Cardiff. Alpha and Omega Press p 587, 1980.

50. Malarkey WB, Kataria YP. Sarcoidosis and hyperprolactinaemia. Ann Int Med. 81 : 116, 1974.

51. Hook O. Sarcoidosis with involvement of the nervous system. Arch Neurol Psychiat. 71, 554, 1951.

52. Roberts WC, McAllister HA, Ferrous VJ. Sarcoidosis of the heart. Am J Med. 62; 86, 1977.

53. Fleming HA, Bailey SM. Sarcoid heart disease. J R Coll Physicians, London. 15 : 245, 1981.

54. Gupta Samir K. Sarcoidosis in eastern India : A critical analysis. J Assoc Phys India, in press.

55. Tiwari SC, Kaushal R, Singh MK, Dhingra K. Granulomatous sarcoid nephritis : review with report of a new case. J Assoc Phys India 34 : 209, 1986.

56. Ryrie DR. Sarcoidosis with obstructive jaundice. Proc R Soc Med. 47 : 879, 1954.

57. Ekelund C. Schaumann's disease and its relation to pancreatic disturbance. Nord Med. 30 : 817, 1946.

58. Wong M, Rosen SW. Ascites in sarcoidosis due to peritoneal involvement. Ann Int Med. 57 : 277, 1962.

59. James DG, Barter S, Jash D, MacKinon DM, Carstairs LS. Sarcoidosis of the upper respiratory tract. J Laryngol Otol. 96 : 711, 1982.

60. Gupta Samir K, Mitra K. Sarcoidosis in children. Indian Pediatrics. in press.

61. Nittu Y, Horikawa M, Suetake T, Hasegawa S, Kubota H, Komatsu S. Intra-thoracic sarcoidosis in children. In : Proceedings of the 6th International Conference on Sarcoidosis. Iwai K, Hosoda Y. (eds.·), Tokyo, Univ Tokyo Press, p 507, 1974.

62. Loos T. Sarcoidosis in children. In : Proceedings of the 3rd European Conference on Sarcoidosis. Djurić B (ed.), Yugoslavia, Novi Sad, New Faculty, p 335, 1982.

63. Heatherington S. Sarcoidosis in young children. Am J Dis Children 136 : 13, 1982.

64. Gupta Samir K Mitra K. Paediatric sarcoidosis in India. J Assoc Phys India, in press.

65. Agha FP, Yade A, Amendola MA, Cooper RF. Effects of pregnancy on sarcoidosis. Surg Gynecol Obstet. 155 : 817, 1982.

66. Morrison JGL. Sarcoidosis in the Bantu. Br J Dermatol. 90 : 649, 1974.

ELEVATED SERUM LEVELS OF SOLUBLE INTERLEUKIN-2 RECEPTOR IS CHARACTERISTIC OF BUT NOT SPECIFIC FOR ACTIVE PULMONARY SARCOIDOSIS

E. CLINTON LAWRENCE, VENESSA A. HOLLAND, MARK B. BERGER, KAREN P. BROUSSEAU, RICHARD J. WALLACE, JR., LAWRENCE E. MALLETTE, CAROLE E. KURMAN, DAVID L. NELSON

The Rockwell-Keough Pulmonary Immunology Laboratory and the General Clinical Research Center of The Methodist Hospital, and the Veterans Administration Hospital, and the Department of Medicine, Baylor College of Medicine, Houston, Texas 77030; the Metabolism Branch, National Cancer Institute, National Institutes of Health, Bethesda, Maryland 20892; and The University of Texas Health Science Center, Tyler, Texas 75910.

INTRODUCTION

Lymphocyte activation is the end-product of a complex series of cellular and lymphokine-mediated events. Effector T-cell responses are characterized by the release of interleukin-2 (IL-2) by activated T-cells (1) and the subsequent binding of IL-2 to its specific cell-surface receptor (IL-2R) (2). Recent studies have demonstrated the release of a soluble form of IL-2R in vitro by activated T-lymphocytes (3), and elevated serum levels of soluble IL-2R have been reported in certain lymphoreticular malignancies (4).

Sarcoidosis is characterized by activation of T-lymphocytes, including the release of IL-2 (5-6). We have previously reported that levels of soluble IL-2R in sera and bronchoalveolar lavage fluids are elevated in active pulmonary sarcoidosis (7). The purpose of the present study was to extend our knowledge of soluble IL-2R in serum in sarcoidosis and other disease states.

MATERIAL AND METHODS

Study Population

The patient population consisted of 25 patients with active untreated sarcoidosis, 7 patients with inactive sarcoidosis, 15 patients with active idiopathic pulmonary fibrosis (IPF), 8 patients with active pulmonary tuberculosis and 26 patients with primary hyperparathyroidism and hypercalcemia.

Assay for Soluble Interleukin-2 Receptor

The enzyme-linked immunosorbent assay (ELISA) for soluble IL-2R was performed as described (3). Alternate rows of the inner 60 wells of Immulon-1 flat-bottomed 96-well microtiter plates (Dynatech Laboratories, Alexandria, Va.) were coated with 150 µl of the monoclonal anti-IL-2R antibody, anti-Tac (kindly provided by Dr. Thomas A. Waldmann, Bethesda, Md.), at a concentration of 1 µg/ml in carbonate buffer or buffer alone. The plates were incubated overnight at room temperature, washed, and 100 µl of an appropriate dilution of fluorescein-isothiocyanate (FITC)-modified 7G7/B6 in PBS contain Tween - 20 and 1% FCS (PBS/Tween/FCS) was added to all wells. After another 2 hour incubation at room temperature, the plates were again washed and 100 µl of an appropriate dilution of alkaline phosphatase-conjugated rabbit anti-FITC in PBS/Tween/FCS was added to each well. The plates were incubated at room temperature for an additional hour, and then washed prior to the addition of 100 µl of p-nitrophenyl phosphate substrate at a concentration of 1 mg/ml (Sigma Chemical Co., St. Louis, Mo.) to each well. The absorbance values at 405 nM in the wells were determined using the Titertek ELISA reader (Flow Laboratories, Rockwell, Md.). The absorbance of control wells was subtracted from that of experimental wells and this value was compared to a standard curve generated from a known standard source of IL-2R (3) to convert absorbance values to concentrations of IL-2R expressed as U/ml.

Statistical Analysis

The data were analyzed using the computing capacities of the CLINFO data analysis system. Values for soluble IL-2R were first converted to $\log_{10}$ as previous studies have shown release of soluble IL-2R to be a geometric function (8). Data for soluble IL-2R levels in sera of normals vs patients were compared using Student's t-test for groups with equal variances.

RESULTS

Sera from patients with active sarcoidosis and parenchymal lung disease (radiographic Stages II or III) had geometric mean values for soluble IL-2R of 1975 units/ml compared to 640 units/ml for normal controls ($p < 0.001$, Student's t-test). By contrast, soluble IL-2R were lower (989 units/ml, $p < 0.05$ compared to normals) in patients with active sarcoidosis but no radiographic evidence for parenchymal disease (Stages 0 or I). Soluble IL-2R levels were not elevated in patients with inactive sarcoidosis. Three of the 4 sarcoidosis patients with the highest levels of soluble IL-2R also manifested hypercalcemia. While levels of soluble IL-2R were elevated for the group of patients with IPF (1171 units/ml, $p < 0.05$ compared to normals), the striking elevations of soluble IL-2R noted in active sarcoidosis were not seen and there was greater overlap with normal values, suggesting that marked serum elevations of soluble IL-2R are more indicative of active pulmonary sarcoidosis than IPF. To further define the specificity of elevation of soluble IL-2R in serum for sarcoidosis, a comparison was made between normals and patients with active pulmonary tuberculosis (Table 1). As expected, the mean level of soluble IL-2R

was also elevated in patients with tuberculosis, indicating that soluble IL-2R
levels may be elevated in other granulomatous diseases. By contrast, serum
levels of soluble IL-2R were not elevated in patients with hypercalcemia
related to primary hyperparathyroidism. Thus, the marked elevations of soluble
IL-2R seen in patients with sarcoidosis and hypercalcemia likely reflects
greater granulomatous inflammation.

TABLE 1

SOLUBLE IL-2R LEVELS IN SERUM IN TUBERCULOSIS AND PRIMARY HYPERPARATHYROIDISM

	Norm	Tb	*1^{0}HP
n	52	8	26
mean	637	2396	480
(SEM)	(108)	(1.42)	(1.14)
p value		<.05	NS

* 1^{0}HP = primary hyperparathyroidism

DISCUSSION

Previously, we have reported increased levels of soluble IL-2R in sera and
bronchoalveolar lavage fluids of patients with active sarcoidosis (7). We also
noted a fall in levels of soluble IL-2R in sera after 6 weeks of corticosteroid
treatment associated with clinical improvement (7). These findings suggested
that serial measurements of soluble IL-2R in sera might be clinically useful in
the management of sarcoidosis.

The present study has extended our previous observations regarding soluble
IL-2R by comparing serum levels from normals to those from patients with active
sarcoidosis, with or without radiographically apparent parenchymal disease,
patients with inactive sarcoidosis, and patients with active IPF. Although
mild elevations of soluble IL-2R were noted in the group of IPF patients and
patients with active sarcoidosis who lacked obvious parenchymal involvement
radiographically, the greatest elevations of soluble IL-2R occurred in those
patients with active sarcoidosis and pulmonary infiltrates. The only patient
classified as having active sarcoidosis without pulmonary infiltrates who
exhibited increases in soluble IL-2R had hypercalcemia and evidence of
parenchymal lung involvement on transbronchial lung biopsy. Three of the four
sarcoidosis patients with the greatest elevations of soluble IL-2R (including
the 1 patient classified as not having parenchymal disease) also had
hypercalcemia. However, serum levels of soluble IL-2R were not elevated in

patients with hypercalcemia related to primary hyperparathyroidism, suggesting that the marked elevations of soluble IL-2R seen in patients with sarcoidosis and hypercalcemia was related to greater granulomatous inflammation.

Any systemic disease process associated with activation of the T-cell system might be associated with serum elevations of soluble IL-2R, as has been described for certain lymphoreticular malignancies (4). Patients with active pulmonary tuberculosis also had elevated levels of soluble IL-2R in serum. Thus, elevated serum levels of soluble IL-2R is characteristic of active pulmonary sarcoidosis and may be a useful marker to follow (9). However, elevations of soluble IL-2R in serum is not specific for sarcoidosis.

ACKNOWLEDGEMENTS

Supported in part by Research Grants from The National Institutes of Health (HL-29542) The McKelvey Fund, and The Veteran's Administration.

Computational assistance was provided by the CLINFO project, funded by the Division of Research Resources of the NIH under grant number RR-00350.

REFERENCES

1. Smith KA (1980) T-cell growth factor. Immunol Rev 51:337-357.

2. Leonard WJ, Depper JM, Robb RJ, Waldmann TA, Greene WC (1983) Characterization of the human receptor for T cell growth factor. Proc Natl Acad Sci 80:6957-6961.

3. Rubin LA, Kurman CC, Fritz ME, et al (1985) Soluble interleukin-2 receptor are released from activated human lymphoid cells in vitro. J Immunol 135:3171-3177.

4. Greene WC, Leonard WJ, Depper JM, Nelson DL, Waldmann TA (1986) The human interleukin-2 receptor: Normal and abnormal expression in T cells and in leukemias induced by the human T-lymphotropic retroviruses. Ann Int Med 105:560-572.

5. Hunninghake GW, Bedell GN, Zavala DC, Monick M, Brady M (1983) Role of interleukin-2 release by lung T-cells in active pulmonary sarcoidosis. Am Rev Respir Dis 128:634-638.

6. Pinkston P, Bitterman PB, Crystal RG (1983) Spontaneous release of interleukin-2 by lung lymphocytes in active pulmonary sarcoidosis. N Eng J Med 308:793-800.

7. Lawrence EC, Brousseau KP, Kurman CC, Nelson DL (1986) Soluble interleukin-2 receptors are present in serum and bronchoalveolar lavage fluids in active sarcoidosis. Clin Research 34:579A.

8. Nelson DL, Rubin LA, Kurman CC, Fritz ME, Boutin B (1986) An analysis of the cellular requirement of the production of soluble interleukin-2 receptors in vitro. J Clin Immunol 6:114-120.

SARCOIDOSIS AND TRACE METALS AS INVESTIGATED BY NEUTRON ACTIVATION ANALYSIS

R. PIETRA[1], J. EDEL[1], E. SABBIONI[1] and G. RIZZATO[2]

1   CEC Joint Research Centre, 21020 Ispra (Varese) Italy

2   Ospedale Niguarda Ca' Granda, Divisione Medica Vergani, Milano, Italy

INTRODUCTION

Trace metals have played a recognized role in clinical medicine for many years.

Although clinical recognition is limited to a few elements (Fe, I, Cu, Mn, Zn) it may be expected that other metals are associated with clinical diseases. Areas where trace metals may be implicated etiologically are atherosclerosis, cardiomyopathy, muscular distrophy, cancer and diseases of the central nervous system (1). Clinical interest in trace metals is also expanding in the field of pulmonary diseases. Subjects affected by some forms of lung fibrosis had obviously abnormal levels of metals in the pulmonary tissue as well as in other tissues and body fluids (2). However, it is not known whether trace metals might be directly or indirectly involved in the etiology of granulomatous lung disorders, including sarcoidosis. The great experimental difficulties in measuring accurately minute quantities of trace metals in tissues and body fluids, particularly during the lifetime of the patients, is still a major factor responsible for this situation.

In order to investigate possible relationships between sarcoidosis and trace elements, research strated using neutron activation analysis (NAA), a very sensitive and reliable multielement analytical technique which greatly facilitates the acquirement of fundamental data on trace metal content in human tissues including lung biopsies and bronchoalveolar lavage (3). This paper shows preliminary rcoults related to three sarcoidosis patients and two subjects with suspected sarcoidosis.

MATERIALS AND METHODS

Samples analyzed were collected from subjects admitted to the Niguarda Hospital, Milan. They were : (i) lung biopsy of two sarcoidosis subjects (F.R. and L.D.) and two patients (P.M. and P.A.) exposed to hard metals (Co, Cr, Ta, W), who had interstitial fibrosis initially confused with sarcoidosis owing to high serum ACE level (ii) BALs of a sarcoidosis subject (Z.C.) and of the two hard

TABLE I

TRACE METAL LEVELS OF THE LUNG BIOPSY OF TWO SARCOIDOSIS SUBJECTS (F.R. AND L.D.) AND TWO PATIENTS WITH SUSPECTED SARCOIDOSIS (HARD METAL WORKERS, P.M. AND P.A.)

Element	Metal content(ng g^{-1} wt.w.)				
	F.R.	L.D.	P.M.	P.A.	Controls
Cd	1000	< 500	–	–	145
Co	< 100	110	2440	830	55
Cr	< 500	201	3050	12000	327
Cs	80	30	–	–	19
Cu	760	975	–	–	1600
Mo	–	630	–	–	70
Rb	15000	12500	–	–	4920
Ta	< 18	< 22	32500	29000	10
Zn	1250	10000	–	–	11100
W	< 5	1.7	107000	52000	1.5

TABLE II

TRACE METAL LEVELS OF BALs OF A SARCOIDOSIS SUBJECT (Z.C.) AND OF THE PATIENTS WITH SUSPECTED SARCOIDOSIS (HARD METAL WORKERS, P.M. AND P.A.)

Element	Metal content (ng g^{-1} wt.w.)			
	Z.C.	P.M.	P.A.	Controls
As	7.5	–	–	0.9
Co	2.1	1.2	2.1	0.6
Cs	4.4	0.3	–	0.4
Cu	50	–	–	250
Mo	150	65	–	8.9
Rb	160	40	–	60
Ta	< 1.5	1010	0.9	0.25
Zn	470	800	–	695
W	2.1	60	24.5	1.5

metal workers P.M. and P.A.

Controls were subjects analyzed in the context of a research programme on
trace metals in the human lung (4). The NAA procedures used have been described elsewhere (5). Briefly, samples were irradiated in the Triga Mark II reactor of the Pavia University or in the HFR reactor, Petten, the Netherlands, at
a thermal neutron flux ranging from 5×10^{12} to 2×10^{14} neutrons $cm^{-2} sec^{-1}$. Standards used were multielement National Bureau of Standards SRM 1571 Orchard
Leaves, SRM 1577 Bovine Liver and synthetic standards. Irradiated samples were
directly counted and/or submitted to radiochemical separations in order to eliminate the background radiation of interfering radioisotopes such as ^{24}Na, ^{32}P,
^{82}Br. The counting of the radioisotopes was carried out by γ-ray spectrometry using a Ge(Li) detector connected with a 4096 multichannel analyser
(Elscint, FRG).

RESULTS

Table I gives the concentrations of ten elements, expressed as ng g^{-1} of wet
tissue, of the lung biopsy of the two subjects affected by sarcoidosis (F.R.
and L.D.). Six of them (Cd, Cs, Cu, Mo, Rb, Zn) show variations considered significant in comparison to the controls. No definitive conclusions can be drawn
for Co, Cr, Ta and W although the results seem to suggest that no variation occurs. A similar conclusion is also for fifteen other elements tested (Ag, Au,
Ce, Eu, Ga, Hg, Ir, La, Sb, Sc, Sn, Th, U, Yb, values not reported).

Table I shows also the concentrations of Co, Cr, Ta and W in the lung biopsy
of the two hard metal workers. The obviously high levels of these elements suggest the hard metal origin of the fibrosis (case of false sarcoidosis).

Table II shows the concentration of metals in the BALs of sarcoidosis patient
(Z.C.) and of the hard metal workers. Six elements (As, Cs, Cu, Mo, Rb, Zn) in
the BAL of the sarcoidosis subject show variations in comparison to the normal
values. Co, Ta and W were without appreciable variations, similarly to fourteen
other elements tested (As, Cd, Ce, Fe, Ga, Hf, Hg, La, Sb, Sc, Sn, Tb, Th, Yb,
values not reported).

CONCLUSIONS

To the best of our knowledge this is the first attempt to study the relationship between trace metals and sarcoidosis. Despite the very limited number of
subjects analyzed the following indications can be drawn : (i) Cs, Rb and Mo
show higher levels in the lung and BAL of sarcoidosis patients while Cu levels
seem to be lowered. These findings, if confirmed, would be of particular importance due to the biochemical role that these elements play in humans. Molybdenum is a constituent of flavin-dependent enzymes and reduces copper retention
in the presence of inorganic sulphate (6). Rubidium most resemble potassium
and these two elements have a great degree of metabolic interchangeability (7)
(ii) the use of NAA is particularly suited as an analytical tool in the medical
diagnosis. Determination of Co, Ta and W in the lung and BAL is sometimes decisive to identify false sarcoidosis (8). In the sarcoidosis subjects the levels
of these elements seem to change in comparison to controls. Their detection is
important in the diagnosis of hard metal fibrosis, a lung disease showing an
X-ray of the chest which can be easily confused with that of sarcoidosis subjects.

RECOMMENDATIONS FOR FUTURE RESEARCH

(i) determination of trace metal levels in sarcoid tissues at different stages
(granulomata formation and fibrosis), in order to establish relationships
between trace metal concentrations and clinical and physical examinations. Particular attention should be paid to elements such as Cs, Rb, Cu, Mo taking into
account a great number of patients. Studies on autoptic tissues of sarcoidosis
subjects are strongly recommended.

(ii) analysis of specimens as possible indicators of trace metal changes in
sarcoidosis patients. They would include blood, urine, hair, nails, saliva.
High priority would be given to the determinatin of trace metal levels in the
BAL, including its different cell population.

(iii) specific studies on single elements for which variation in sarcoid tissues would be observed. They would include investigations on intracellular
distribution and interaction with biochemical components. In this context the
use of radiotracers with very high specific radioactivity was proved to be
particularly suitable (9).

ACKNOWLEDGEMENTS

We are greatly indebted to JRC–Petten,Mr. J.P. Konrad, HFR Division and Mr. L. Ubertalli, JRC–Ispra for their technical assistance in the neutron irradiations.

REFERENCES

1. Friberg L, Nordberg G, Vouk V (1980) In: L. Friberg et al.(eds) Introduction, Elsevier, North Holland Biomedical Press 1979

2. Sulotto F, Romano C, Berra A, Botta GC, Rubino GF, Sabbioni E, Pietra R Amer. J. Ind. Med. (1986) 9:567–575

3. Sabbioni E, Pietra R, Rizzato G (1983) Proc. 6° Convegno di Igiene Industriale, Università Cattolica, 5–7 Dicembre 1983, Roma, Tipar Press, Roma, pp. 210–224

4. Vanoeteren C, Cornelis R, Sabbioni E (1986) Report EUR 10440, CEC Luxembourg

5. Sabbioni E, Pietra R, Gaglione P, Vocaturo G, Colombo F, Zanoni M, Rodi F (1982) Sci. Total Environ. 26:19–32

6. Friberg L, Boston P, Nordberg G, Piscator M, Robert KH (1975) Molybdenum– a Toxicological Appraisal, Report US EPA, Washington DC (under contract No 68–02–1210)

7. Meltzer HL, Lieberman KW (1971) Experientia 27:672–676

8. Rizzato G, Lo Cicero S, Barberis M, Torre M, Pietra R, Sabbioni E (1986) Chest 89:101–106

9. Edel J, Pietra R, Sabbioni E, Rizzato G, Speziali M (1986) Acta Pharmacol. Toxicol. 59:52–55.

© 1988 Elsevier Science Publishers B.V. (Biomedical Division)
Sarcoidosis and other granulomatous disorders
C. Grassi, G. Rizzato, E. Pozzi, editors

THE COURSE AND MANAGEMENT OF 53 PATIENTS WITH HEMOPTYSIS IN SARCOIDOSIS

CJ JOHNS, SA SCHONFELD, PP SCOTT

Respiratory Division, Johns Hopkins Hospital, Baltimore, MD 21205 USA

Hemoptysis is observed in patients with sarcoidosis most frequently in association with advanced fibrocystic changes in the lungs. Mycetomas are frequently identified in these patients.[1] In a few patients, endobronchial disease may result in bleeding and occasionally localized cystic changes may develop relatively early. Other causes of bleeding must always be excluded, especially tuberculosis.

MATERIAL AND METHODS

Both inpatient and Sarcoid Clinic outpatient records of The Johns Hopkins Hospital from 1960-1987 were reviewed. Approximately 4% of the sarcoidosis patients admitted did have some hemoptysis. Computerized diagnostic codes were utilized.

RESULTS

Studies identified 53 patients with hemoptysis felt to be related to sarcoidosis, with no other cause identified. The group included 51 black and two white patients. Forty were female and 13 male. In 41 patients, the bleeding was recurrent but occurred only once in 8 patients. Fibrocystic disease was observed radiographically in 39 of 48 patients.

Mycetomas.

Mycetomas were identified radiograpically in 28 patients, and strongly suspected in four others, for a total of 32 patients. This group is analyzed in detail. Sarcoidosis was diagnosed 3-33 years previously, with a mean follow-up of 15.5 years. The first hemoptysis occurred 9.3 (0.7-22) years prior to last visit, and the mycetoma was known for a mean of 8 (1-18) years. Two patients with mycetomas had some early blood streaking of sputum, and then no hemoptysis for 16 and 18 years respectively. Aspergillus fumigatus was cultured from 19 patients. The degree of hemoptysis is presented in Table 1, for the total group and for those patients with a mycetoma.

418

TABLE I

DEGREE OF HEMOPTYSIS IN SARCOIDOSIS PATIENTS

| | No. of Patients | |
Hemoptysis	Mycetoma Present	Total No.
Minor < 150ml/24hrs	13	31
Major 150-600ml/24hrs	6	9
Massive > 600ml/24hrs	13	13
Total	32	53

Table II presents the outcome of the patients with mycetomas, with the numbers of those living and known dead. One patient with massive hemoptysis was lost to follow-up after four months. The mean period of survival was 9.0 (0.7-22) years for 31 patients. Twenty living patients survive for 9.5 years after the initial hemoptysis, with 4.5 years for the four patients with fatal hemoptysis and 7.0 years for the 7 patients dying with pulmonary insufficiency. The latest study reveals a mean forced vital capacity of 56.6% of predicted for the 20 living patients, 44.2% for the 4 patients who died with hemorrhage and 39.6% for the seven who died with pulmonary insufficiency.

TABLE II

HEMOPTYSIS: OUTCOME OF 32 MYCETOMA PATIENTS

| | No. of Patients | | | | |
| Hemoptysis | Living | Uncertain | Dead | | Total |
			Hem	Resp	
Massive	5	1	4	3	13
Major	5		0	1	6
Minor	10	—	—	3	13
Total	20	1	4	7	32

Hem = Fatal Hemoptysis   Resp = Respiratory Failure

Massive Hemoptysis.

This was observed in 13 patients and occurred from 1 month to 15 years after the first hemoptysis, with a mean interval of 7.3 years. The time interval between the first hemoptysis and the first massive hemoptysis ranged from a few hours or days in two patients, and up to 12 (mean 4) years. In one patient a major hemoptysis of 240 ml occurred 1 month prior to his fatal massive hemorrage. In two patients the fatal hemorrhage was the first massive hemoptysis and one had a fatal hemorrhage one year after a prior massive hemoptysis. Seven of these patients died, but only four from fatal hemorrhage.

These occurred 2,3,5,and 8 years after the first hemoptysis. Three others died
of pulmonary insufficiency three to ten years later.

Elective Therapeutic Embolization.

  Six patients with massive bleeding had elective therapeutic embolization
(embolotherapy) of bronchial arteries or collateral transpleural vessels.
Bronchoscopy was performed as the bleeding subsided to determine the site of
bleeding. Preliminary arteriography was used to define the anatomy of the
bronchial arteries and collateral supply, including intercostal vessels. None
of the patients were actually bleeding at the time of embolization. Embolic
agents usually were surgical gelatin (Gelfoam) or polyvinyl alcohol (Ivalon) or
microfibrillar collagen (Avitene). Bronchial arteries were sometimes found to
be enlarged. The details of these patients are presented in Table III.

TABLE III

ELECTIVE THERAPEUTIC EMBOLIZATION

Age/Race/ Sex	Years of Sarcoidosis	% Predicted Forced Vital Capacity	Follow-up Years	Outcome
27 BF	3	47	0.5	Streaking only
27 BF	8	36	1	Fatal Hemorrhage
29 BF	7	59	5	Minor - Lost
47 BF	17	78	7	Streaking
57 BM	33	?	0.3	Minor - Lost
64 BF	18	57	1.7	Minor

(B - Black   F - Female   M - Male)

  The first patient had eight hospital admissions over a 3 month period,
because of recurrent hemoptysis, requiring antibiotics and transfusion with 29
units of blood. She had four arteriographic procedures and two elective
embolizations. For the last five months she has had only occasional minimal
blood streaking of her sputum and no further hospitalization. She continues on
rotating antibiotics with tetracycline, ampicillin, erythromycin and
trimethoprim-sulfamethoxazole (Bactrim). Another 27 year old black female had
recurrent serious hemoptyses for 5 years. She had only minor bleeding for a
year following embolization, but then had a massive fatal hemorrhage. The mean
period of survival after the embolotherapy is 2.6 years.

Medical Management.

  Continued low dose maintenance corticosteroids with 5-15 mg of prednisone
daily have been used in almost every patient to control the sarcoid granulomas.

420

No invasive fungal disease has been observed, even in autopsy material, and
the mycetomas appear to be saprophytic. No anti-fungal agents were used.

Because of bilateral diffuse restrictive disease and frequent bilateral
mycetomas, no patients were treated surgically. In such patients surgery is
hazardous and complications frequent.[3,4,5]

Chronic purulent sputum is a characteristic of most patients where a mycetoma
is identified. Bacterial studies reveal both gram positive and gram negative
organisms. Broad spectrum antibiotics are standardly utilized. In many ways,
these patients resemble the clinical picture of bronchiectasis. Chest physical
therapy and postural drainage are also helpful. Cough suppressants are used
during bleeding.

SUMMARY

Thirty-two of 53 patients with hemoptysis and sarcoidosis were found to have
mycetomas present, often bilaterally. A prolonged course is frequent with the
mean period of survival 9.0 years after the first hemoptysis. Massive bleeding
of more than 600ml/24 hours occurred in 13, with 4 fatal hemorrhages. Six of
these patients had embolotherapy, with diminished bleeding for 4 months to
seven (mean 2.6) years. One died from hemorrhage at one year. Seven patients
died with pulmonary insufficiency and cor pulmonale.

No invasive fungal disease was observed and anti-fungal agents were not used.
Low dose corticosteroid treatment is utilized. Bacterial infection plays a
prominent role and the judicious use of antibiotics seems beneficial as these
patients resemble those with bronchiectasis. Surgery is not recommended
because of bilateral restrictive disease. Long term conservative medical
management can ameliorate the hemoptysis and is recommended in fibrocystic
sarcoidosis.

REFERENCES

1. Kaplan J, Johns, CJ (1979) Mycetomas in pulmonary sarcoidosis. Johns
    Hopkins Med J 145:157-161

2. Remy J, Arnaud A, Fardou H et al (1977) Treatment of hemoptysis by
    embolization of bronchial arteries. Radiology 122:33-37

3. Faulkner SL, Vernon R, Brown PP, Fisher RD, Bender HW, Jr. (1978)
    Hemoptysis and pulmonary aspergilloma: operative versus non-operative
    treatment. Ann Thorac Surg 25:389-392

4. Israel HL, Lenchner GS, Atkinson GW (1982) Sarcoidosis and aspergilloma:
    the role of surgery. Chest 82:430-432

5. Johns CJ (1982) Management of hemoptysis with pulmonary fungus balls.
    Editorial in Chest 82:400-401

FACTORS WHICH ADVERSELY AFFECT THE COURSE OF SARCOIDOSIS: An Analysis of 111
Autopsied Cases of Sarcoidosis

Om P. Sharma, M.D., E. Klatt, M.D., Sarcoidosis Clinic and Department of Pathology, Los Angeles County-University of Southern California School of Medicine,
1200 North State Street, Los Angeles, California 90033

Recently, we analyzed clinical records of 111 patients who were found to have
sarcoidosis at autopsy. The diagnosis of sarcoidosis was on the basis of noncaseating granulomas, either in the lung or in two or more tissue systems associated
with negative smears and cultures for bacteria (acid-fast and non-acid-fast) and
fungi. All microscopic sections showing granulomas were studied under polarizing
light for birifringent foreign body particles.

Most surprising was the realization that in 75 (68%) of 111 cases, multisystem sarcoidosis was discovered for the first time at autopsy. The disease in
these individuals had remained silent, benign, and asymptomatic; the death occurred of causes unrelated to sarcoidosis (Table I). The remaining 36 (32%) patients
were known to suffer from sarcoidosis. These patients had advanced multisystem
disease which pursued a relentless course, and finally succumbed to complications
of sarcoidosis (Table II).

Of 36 patients who were known to suffer from sarcoidosis before their deaths,
83% were Black. Black patients developed sarcoidosis earlier and died before 40
years of age. Black women suffered more than either Black men or White men and
women. White patients with sarcoidosis lived a full life and died much later, of
causes not related to sarcoidosis. Initial chest X-ray appearance and the number
of organs involved by the disease had an impact on the prognosis (Figs. 1 and 2).

TABLE II: CAUSE OF DEATH IN 36 AUTOPSIED
CASES OF KNOWN SARCOIDOSIS

Cause of Death	Number of Patients
Corpulmonale	12
Myocardial Sarcoidosis	6
Respiratory Failure	4
Renal Failure	2
Amyloid/Sarcoidosis	2
Infection*	2
Diabetes (Acute MI)	2
Cerebrovascular Accident*	2
Neurosarcoidosis	1
Carcinoma*	1
GI Bleeding	1
SBE*	1
	36

*Not directly related to Sarcoidosis

TABLE I: CAUSE OF DEATH IN 75 CASES WHERE SARCOIDOSIS WAS DIAGNOSED AT AUTOPSY
(SILENT)

Cause of Death	Number of Patients
Cerebrovascular Accident	17
Gastrointestinal Bleeding	9
(Alcoholism and complications)	
Myocardial Infarction	7
Pulmonary Emboli	2
Respiratory Failure	5
Dissecting Aneurysm	4(1*)
Renal Failure	4(1*)
Congestive Heart Failure (ASHD)	3(1*)
Diabetes Mellitus (and complications)	3
Rheumatoid Arthritis	2
Carcinoma of Colon	2
Lymphoma	2
Carcinoma (Pancreas & Liver, Cervix)	2
Amyloidosis	1*
Guillian-Barre' Syndrome	1*
Carcinoma of Esophagus	1
Auto Accident	1
Miscellaneous	9
	75

*Related to Sarcoidosis

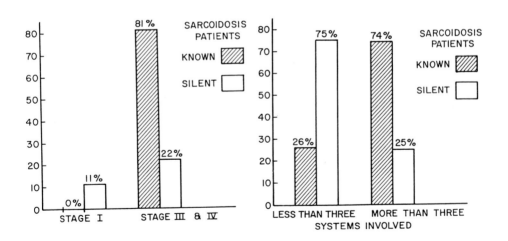

SMOKING CAUSES AN ALTERATION OF BALF CELL FINDINGS IN PATIENTS WITH BHL
SARCOIDOSIS BUT NO EVIDENCE COULD BE FOUND THAT SMOKING AFFECTS THE NATURAL
COURSE OF BHL SARCOIDOSIS

TAKATERU IZUMI, SONOKO NAGAI, MASANORI KITAICHI, SHUNSAKU OSHIMA
Chest Disease Research Institute, Kyoto University, Sakyo-ku,
Kyoto 606 (Japan)

INTRODUCTION

Sarcoidosis is a systemic disease with a characteristic manifestation of epithelioid cell granuloma formation. Examination of the cells in bronchoalveolar
lavage fluids (BALF) of patients with this disease has shown formation of lung
lesions due to cellular immune responses associated with an increase, accumulation, and activation of macrophages and T lymphocytes.[1] The effects of smoking
on the body, especially the lungs, have long been known, but in addition to its
effects as nonspecific stimulation, smoking was recently shown to have immunological effects as well.[2] This suggests that smoking affects the pathogenesis
and course of sarcoidosis, an allergic lung disease.

Under this assumption, we examined differences in BALF cell findings and
spontaneous disappearance of bilateral hilar lymphadenopathy (BHL) shadows
observed in chest x-rays between non-smoking (NS) and smoking (S) sarcoidosis
patients.

I. DIFFERENCES IN BALF CELL FINDINGS BETWEEN NON-SMOKERS AND SMOKERS

MATERIALS AND METHODS

Patient and control populations. Fourteen NS (8 males and 6 females) and 17 S
(14 males and 3 females) sarcoidosis patients were included in this study.
These patients were 1) within 6 months of detection of BHL (stage I in 12 NS and
all S patients and stage II in 2 NS patients) by general health screening, at
which they were asymptomatic, 2) diagnosed on the basis of biopsy findings (7 NS
and 6 S patients) or high serum ACE levels (>43 U/ml), 3) without extrathoracic
lesions, and 4) not treated with corticosteroids. The controls were sex- and
age-matched healthy individuals with no complaints, no abnormalities in chest
x-rays, and normal pulmonary function (%VC>80%, FEV$_1$%>70%). Cigarettes/day in
patients with sarcoidosis was 23.8 ± 11.3 (Mean $\pm$ SD) and those in healthy
controls was 17.9 ± 8.1. Patients and healthy individuals with occupational or
environmental exposure to dust were excluded from this study.

Brochoalveolar lavage. BAL was performed by infusing and recovering 50 ml
saline 6 times for a total of 300 ml.

TABLE 1

EFFECTS OF CIGARETTE SMOKING ON BALF CELL FINDINGS IN HEALTHY AND SARCOIDOSIS PATIENTS

	Healthy controls		Sarcoidosis	
	NS	S	NS	S
No. (M, F)	14 (8, 6)	17 (14, 3)	14 (8, 6)	17 (14, 3)
Ages	28.0 ± 6.6*	28.1 ± 6.4	31.1 ± 12.1	26.4 ± 6.4
Recovery of fluids (%)	73.7 ± 6.8	71.9 ± 5.9	76.8 ± 6.8	71.6 ± 10.6
Recovered cells ($\times10^5$/ml)	0.53 ± 0.22	2.45 ± 2.11	1.26 ± 0.78	1.67 ± 1.03
Macrophages (%)	83.8 ± 10.9	95.7 ± 33.5	67.3 ± 19.8	81.7 ± 16.4
($\times10^3$/ml)	43.8 ± 21.1	237.2 ± 206.0	75.6 ± 42.4	138.9 ± 94.5
Lymphocytes (%)	15.3 ± 10.6	3.9 ± 3.2	32.1 ± 20.0	17.9 ± 16.1
($\times10^3$/ml)	8.6 ± 5.7	7.0 ± 5.2	49.3 ± 50.0	27.4 ± 33.1
Neutrophils (%)	0.7 ± 0.6	0.3 ± 0.4	0.4 ± 0.4	0.3 ± 0.4
($\times10^3$/ml)	0.3 ± 0.3	0.8 ± 1.9	0.5 ± 0.7	0.3 ± 0.4
OKT4$^+$/OKT8$^+$	2.38 ± 0.80	0.83 ± 0.33	4.21 ± 1.90	3.88 ± 2.61

Significance brackets:

Recovered cells: Healthy NS vs S $P<0.005$; Healthy S vs Sarcoidosis NS $P<0.005$**

Macrophages (%): Healthy NS vs S $P<0.001$; Sarcoidosis NS vs S $P<0.05$; Healthy vs Sarcoidosis (NS) $P<0.02$; Healthy S vs Sarcoidosis S $P<0.005$

Macrophages ($\times10^3$/ml): Healthy NS vs S $P<0.005$; Sarcoidosis NS vs S $P<0.05$; across groups $P\ 0.05$

Lymphocytes (%): Healthy NS vs S $P<0.001$; Sarcoidosis NS vs S $P<0.05$; Healthy vs Sarcoidosis $P<0.02$

Lymphocytes ($\times10^3$/ml): Healthy vs Sarcoidosis (NS) $P<0.01$; across groups $P<0.02$

Neutrophils (%): Healthy NS vs S $P<0.02$

OKT4$^+$/OKT8$^+$: Healthy NS vs S $P<0.001$; across groups $P<0.005$; $P<0.001$

* Mean ± SD
** Significant differences between two groups

Evaluation of cells recovered by bronchoalveolar lavage. The cells recovered were washed and the number of cells per volume of the BALF recovered was cal- culated. Cell populations in 500 cells were counted in centrifuged specimens after May-Grünwald-Giemsa staining. T cell subsets were identified using OKT3 (pan T), OKT4 (helper/inducer), and OKT8 (cytotoxic/suppressor) mouse monoclonal antibodies (Ortho Pharmaceutical, Raritan, N.J.) and the percent of positive cells was measured by using a flow cytometry, Ortho Spectrum III.

The statistical significance of the differences among the groups was examined by Student's t-test.

RESULTS

The results are shown in Table 1. In healthy controls, the number of re- covered cells was greater and the percentage and number of macrophages were significantly higher, but the percentages of lymphocytes and neutrophils and the OKT4$^+$/OKT8$^+$ ratio were significantly lower in S as compared with NS. In sarcoidosis patients, on the other hand, the percentage of macrophages was higher but the percentage of lymphocytes lower in S as compared with NS, but no significant difference in recovered cells or in the OKT4$^+$/OKT8$^+$ ratio was observed.

II. EFFECTS OF SMOKING ON SPONTANEOUS DISAPPEARANCE OF BILATERAL HILAR LYMPHO- ADENOPATHY SHADOWS IN SARCOIDOSIS PATIENTS

MATERIALS AND METHODS

Subjects. The subjects were 47 NS (13 males and 34 females, mean age ± SD 23.6 ± 7.6 years) and 35 S (34 males and 1 female, 25.3 ± 5.7 years) who were found by chest x-rays in general health screening to have BHL sarcoidosis without any symptoms and without extrathoracic lesions. They were followed up for at least 5 years, during which time they continued to smoke without inter- ruption. Cigarettes/day in smoking patients was 20.0 ± 3.2. Among NS, histo- logical diagnosis was made in 13, lesions were determined by chest x-ray to be stage I in 44 and stage II in 3. In S, histological diagnosis was made in 24, and the lesions were stage I in 30 and stage II in 5. The NS consisted of more females and the S of more males (P<0.005), and more S were histologically diagnosed than NS (P<0.005).

Evaluation. Spontaneous disappearance of BHL was compared in chest x-rays between the S and NS 6 months, and 1, 2, 3, 4, and 5 years after detection.

RESULTS

The results are shown in Table 2. Disappearance of BHL was not different between the two groups at any time of evaluation, and no findings suggestive of the effects of smoking on the course of BHL were obtained.

TABLE 2
EFFECTS OF CIGARETTE SMOKING ON THE DISAPPEARANCE RATE OF BHL SHADOWS IN SARCOIDOSIS

| Groups | No | \multicolumn{6}{c}{Shadows not disappeared (%)} | | | | | |
		1/2	1	2	3	4	5 years
NS	47	40 (85)	23 (49)	14 (30)	6 (13)	6 (13)	4 (9)
S	35	27 (77)	16 (46)	9 (26)	4 (11)	3 (9)	2 (6)

III. DISCUSSION

Effects of smoking on sarcoidosis patients were studied in those showing BHL without extrathoracic lesions, whose disease was detected by general health screening. These patients were selected to eliminate effects of the diversity of lesions observed in sarcoidosis patients.

A significantly greater number of cells were recovered from the BALF of non-smoking patients than from those of non-smoking healthy controls, but such a difference was not observed in S; the number of cells was smaller in smoking patients than in the smoking controls. This reduction in the number of cells recovered from lavage fluid in smoking sarcoidosis patients may be considered to be due to limitations in collection of lung cells caused by formation of granulomatous lesions, rather than a real reduction in lung cells. Previous reports[3-6] indicated that the percentage of lymphocytes is reduced in S compared to NS in the BALF obtained from sarcoidosis patients. Our results were in agreement with these reports. Both the percentage and number were greater in sarcoidosis patients than in the healthy controls regardless of the smoking habit, but S showed 3.9 times increase in the mean number of lymphocytes as compared with 5.7 times increase in NS. Considering that the number of lymphocytes was similar between S and NS in healthy controls, there may be some inhibition against expansion of lymphocytes in smoking sarcoidosis patients. In healthy controls, the $OKT4^+/OKT8^+$ ratio was significantly smaller in S than NS, but no significant difference was observed in sarcoidosis patients, in agreement with previous report.[7] These findings suggest that smoking has no inhibitory effects on selective expansion of $OKT4^+$ cells. From these observations, smoking is considered to affect BALF cell findings in sarcoidosis patients as well as in healthy controls, but the effects in patients are not as distinct as in healthy individuals. Part of the effect of smoking, therefore, appears to be eliminated by the appearance of sarcoid granuloma lesions.

Comparison of chest x-rays between non-smoking and smoking sarcoidosis patients during a 5-year period showed no difference in spontaneous disappearance of BHL, and there was no evidence that smoking affects the prognosis of BHL sarcoidosis. This result is considered to be the first report on the effect of smoking on the prognosis of sarcoidosis, and there appears to be little possibility that smoking exerts adverse effects on BHL sarcoidosis. However, this may not apply to patients with pulmonary involvements. Further studies are needed in such patients as well as on the relationship between the amount of smoking and its effects.

SUMMARY

Effects of smoking on BALF cell findings and changes in chest x-rays were evaluated in patients with BHL sarcoidosis without extrathoracic lesions, which was detected by general health screening.

1. Smoking affected BALF cell findings in sarcoidosis patients as well as in healthy controls, but its effects in patients were not as distinct as in controls.

2. Smoking did not influence spontaneous disappearance of BHL in chest x-rays.

However, these findings obtained in patients with asymptomatic BHL sarcoidosis may not apply to patients with distinct pulmonary involvements or those with symptomatic sarcoidosis.

REFERENCES

1. Hunninghake GW, Gadek GE, Kawanami O, Ferrans VJ, Crystal RG (1979) Amer J Pathol 97:149-206

2. Hersey P, Prendengast D, Edwards A (1983) Med J Aust 2:425-429

3. Arnoux A, Mansac J, Stanislas-Leguerin G, Huchon G, Chretien J (1982) Path Res Pract 175:62-79

4. Rossman MD, Dauber JH, Cardillo ME, Daniele RP (1982) Am Rev Respir Dis 125:366-369

5. Radermecker M, Gustin M, Saint-Remy P (1984) Eur J Respir Dis 65:189-195

6. Leuenberger Ph, Vonmoos S, Vejdovsky R (1985) Eur J Respir Dis Suppl 139:72-75

7. Lawrence EC, Fox TB, Teague RB, Bloom K, Wilson RK (1986) Ann NY Acad Sci 465:657-664

VALUE OF BRONCHOALVEOLAR LAVAGE LYMPHOCYTE SUBPOPULATIONS FOR THE DIAGNOSIS OF SARCOIDOSIS

U. COSTABEL, A. ZAISS, D.J. WAGNER, R. BAUR, K.H. RÜHLE, H. MATTHYS

Abteilung Pneumologie, Med.Univ.Klinik, D-7800 Freiburg, FRG

INTRODUCTION

Pulmonary sarcoidosis is characterized by a lymphocytosis with an increase in the T4/T8 ratio and a decrease in the % of $Leu7^+$ natural killer cells in broncho-alveolar lavage (BAL) fluid, dependent on the stage of activity (1-4). The lymphocytosis is a nonspecific finding present in various granulomatous and other interstitial lung disorders. The T4/T8 ratio might be more specific since some important diseases, e.g. hypersensitivity pneumonitis, have decreased ratios. Except for one preliminary report, studies about the sensitivity and the specificity of BAL parameters for sarcoidosis are lacking, however (5).

The aim of our study therefore was to assess the diagnostic value of different BAL variables for sarcoidosis in comparison with other lung diseases.

MATERIAL AND METHODS

Study groups

All untreated patients with biopsy proven sarcoidosis (n=126) were unselective-ly evaluated at the time of diagnosis when they entered our department (Table I). Their mean age was 39 $\pm$ 13 years. 34 of them presented with chest radiographic stage 1, 69 with stage 2, and 23 with stage 3.

48 patients with a clinical picture consistent with sarcoidosis but with unpro-ven histology, were excluded from the study.

There remained 363 patients who were definitely diagnosed to have no sarcoido-sis (Table I).

TABLE I	SARCOIDOSIS (biopsy proven, untreated)	126
STUDY GROUPS	NON-SARCOIDOSIS	363
	Hypersensitivity Pneumonitis	32
	Silicosis	29
	Asbestosis	12
	Tuberculosis	8
	Histiocytosis X	8
	Diffuse Fibrosing Alveolitis	31
	Malignancies	25
	Other Conditions	218
	TOTAL	489

BAL

The BAL was performed with 5 x 20 ml physiologic saline. In addition to total and differential cell counts, lymphocyte subpopulations were determined by surface marker analysis with an immunoperoxidase slide assay using a battery of mono-clonal antibodies (6).

Statistics

The statistical analysis was performed with the following BAL parameters: lymphocytes expressed as % of total cells; ratio of T4+ helper/inducer cells to T8+ suppressor/cytotoxic cells; and Leu7+ natural killer cells expressed as % of lymphocytes. Mean values ± SD were calculated, and the groups compared with the Student's t-test. The sensitivity and specificity for sarcoidosis of different values of the parameters were stepwise calculated with four fold tables. In addition, a discriminant analysis was performed.

RESULTS AND DISCUSSION

Shown in table II are the mean values of the BAL data from the sarcoidosis and the non-sarcoidosis group. The differences are significant (P< 0.001, all comparisons).

Shown in table III are sensitivity and specificity rates for sarcoidosis of selected values of % lymphocytes. The upper limit of normals in our laboratory is 13% lymphocytes in BAL fluid (6). Taking this as cut off point, the sensitivity is high. 90 % of all sarcoidosis patients are equal

TABLE II

VARIABLES IN BAL FLUID

mean ± SD	Sarcoidosis	Non-Sarcoidosis
Lymphocytes (%)	41 ± 21	23 ± 24
T4/T8 (ratio)	5.1 ± 4.3	1.6 ± 1.4
Leu7 (% of ly)	6 ± 5	13 ± 11

TABLE III

VALUE OF BAL % LYMPHOCYTES FOR THE DIAGNOSIS OF SARCOIDOSIS

Lymphocytes %	Sensitiv. %	Specific. %	Chi-square
13	89.7	50.6	62.7
17	85.7	58.0	71.1
32	64.3	72.2	52.6
40	54.0	75.9	37.9

to or beyond this limit. But the finding is non-specific, since 50 % of the non-sarcoidosis patients also show an increase in BAL % lymphocytes above normals. The best cut off point for lymphocytes is at 17% (maximum chi-square value), but the specificity remains low.

Shown in table IV are the sensitivity and specificity rates for different T4/T8 ratios. The best cut off point is at a ratio of 3.5 and higher (maximum chi-square value). This ratio corresponds to the upper limit of normals in our laboratory (6). The sensitivity is low: only 53% of all sarcoidosis patients have increased T4/T8 ratios. But the finding has a high specificity of 93%. If a higher cut off ratio of 5.0 is chosen, the specificity rises to 98% at the expense of a fall in sensitivity to 47%. At a ratio of ≥ 10.0, a specificity rate of 100% is achieved, but this extreme increase in the T4/T8 ratio is seen in only 11% of sarcoidosis patients.

Shown in table V are the results of a discriminant analysis which took into account the 3 variables. The number of patients in each group is smaller, because Leu7 was not determined in all cases. The stepwise analysis shows that the T4/T8 ratio is the best single discriminating variable followed by the % lymphocytes. An improvement in sensitivity is observed when the 2 variables % ly and T4/T8 are combined. The best discrimination is obtained by the combination of the 3 variables % ly, T4/T8, and Leu7 (sensitivity 71%, specificity 89%, accuracy 84%).

In the non-sarcoidosis group, an elevated T4/T8 ratio ≥ 3.5

TABLE IV

VALUE OF BAL T4/T8 RATIOS FOR THE DIAGNOSIS OF SARCOIDOSIS*

T4/T8 ratio	sensitiv. %	specific. %	Chi-square
1.0	93.7	41.3	52.3
2.0	78.6	72.2	99.7
3.5	53.2	92.8	128.6
5.0	47.3	97.5	111.8
7.5	22.2	98.6	64.6
10.0	11.1	100.0	41.5

* Four fold table

TABLE V

DISCRIMINANT ANALYSIS*

Variable	Sensitiv.	Specific.	chi-squ.
Ly ≥ 17%	85.7	58.0	38.0
T4/T8 ≥ 3.5	57.4	91.2	104.2
Leu7 < 10%	80.2	50.0	27.9
Ly + T4/T8	62.4	90.5	116.3
Ly+T4/8+Leu7	71.3	88.7	136.1

* Sarcoidosis n = 101
Non-Sarcoidosis n = 284

was found in 22 patients; these were 7/12 with asbestosis, 5/12 with pulmonary fibrosis associated with collagen vascular diseases, 3/7 with drug induced pneumonitis (bleomycin, busulfan, cyclophosphamide), 2/19 with idiopathic pulmonary fibrosis, 1/32 with hypersensitivity pneumonitis, 1/25 with malignancies, 1/8 with histiocytosis X, 1 with chronic pneumonia, 1 with acute bronchitis.

Berylliosis and some collagen vascular diseases like Crohn's disease, primary biliary cirrhosis, and Sjögren's syndrome, are known to be disorders which may have increased BAL T4/T8 ratios (7,8). We recently described elevated T4/T8 ratios in patients with asbestosis and in subjects after asbestos exposure (9). When we exclude such disorders by history, by detection of asbestos bodies in the BAL fluid, or by knowing the underlying collagen vascular disease, then a T4/T8 ratio greater than 3.5 is of high diagnostic value for sarcoidosis.

We conclude that in these cases (T4/T8 ≥ 3.5) the diagnosis of sarcoidosis can be made by the determination of BAL lymphocyte subpopulations. This may avoid the need for more invasive biopsy procedures.

SUMMARY

The sensitivity and specificity of different BAL variables (% lymphocytes, T4/T8 ratio, % Leu7$^+$ cells) were assessed for sarcoidosis (n = 126) in comparison with other lung diseases (n = 363). Elevated % lymphocytes ($\leqslant$13%) was a sensitive (90%) though non-specific (51%) finding. Elevated T4/T8 ratio ($\leqslant$3.5) had a low sensitivity (53%) but a high specificity (93%). A discriminant analysis combining the three BAL variables yielded a sensitivity of 71%, a specificity of 89%, and an accuracy of 84%. We conclude that the determination of multiple BAL variables, including the T4/T8 ratio, may be of diagnostic help in sarcoidosis.

ACKNOLEDGEMENT

This study was supported in part by grant Co 118/2-2 from the Deutsche Forschungsgemeinschaft.

REFERENCES

1. Hunninghake GW, Crystal RG (1981) N Engl J Med 305: 429-434

2. Costabel U, Bross KJ, Matthys H (1983) Klin Wochenschr 61:349-356

3. Rossi GA, Sacco A, Cosulich E, Damiani G, Corte G, Bargellesi A, Ravazzoni C (1984) Thorax 39:143-149

4. Semenzato G, Agostini C, Pezzutto A, Gasparotto G, Cipriani A, Chilosi M, Pizzolo G (1984) J Clin Lab Immunol 13:25-28

5. Selland M, Winterbauer RH, Springmeyer SC, Noges J, Dreis DF, Pardee NE (1986) Chest 89:519S

6. Costabel U, Bross KJ, Matthys H (1985) Bull Eur Physiopathol Respir 21:381-387

7. Rossman MD, Greenberg J, Kern J, et al (1986) Am Rev Respir Dis 133:A195

8. Wallaert B, Bart F, Grosbois JM, Ramon Ph, Tonnel AB, Voisin C (1987) In: Paramelle B, Brambilla C, Pin I, Blanc-Jouvan F (eds) Compte Rendu du Congrès de Pneumologie de Langue Francaise. Grenoble, June 11-13, 1987, pp 169-178

9. Costabel U, Bross KJ, Huck E, Guzman J, Matthys H (1987) Chest 91:110-112

EARLY NEUTROPHIL ALVEOLITIS IN LOFGREN SYNDROME.

J. Ph. MAFFRE*, E. TUCHAIS*,M.F. CHRETIEN**, M. OURY*

*Service de Pneumologie C.H.R. 490033 ANGERS CEDEX,**Laboratoire de cytologie,
C.H.R 49033 ANGERS CEDEX, FRANCE.

INTRODUCTION

Lofgren Syndrome (LS) is considered as an acute onset of sarcoidosis (1). Its
prognosis is almost always favourable in caucasian (2). Few data are available
about lung cell populations at early phase of sarcoidosis. We therefore studied a
group of eighteen LS who underwent a Broncho-alveolar lavage (BAL) between eight
and one hundred days after beginning of erythema nodosum (EN)

PATIENTS AND METHODS

18 patients with LS (LS group) defined by the association of EN, bilateral
hilar lymphadenopathy (BHL) were studied. All were caucasian, female (mean age
$34,8 \pm 14,8$ years, one smoker). We considered that clinical and radiological
features where enough for diagnosis of LS (3). However sarcoidosis was histologically proven in 11 cases. All patients had complete examination for other etiologies (e,g, various infectious agents, drugs). Evolution and/or elevation of serum
angiotensin converting enzyme (SACE) confirmed diagnosis all cases. Patients were
followed up for at least one year. Spirography was performed in all patients at
time of diagnosis and during evolution.

This LS group was compared to a group of 9 recently diagnosed stage I sarcoidosis (ST I group), matched for age ($30,1 \pm 8,6$ yrs) including 6 males and 3 females, (one smoker). None ot these patients were treated at time of BAL. BAL was
performed in all patients at time ranging from 8 to 100 days after onset of EN.
First aliquot was eliminated to lessen bronchial contamination. Numeration was
performed using a grid cytometer (Lemaur 0,4 mm) and differential cell count was
made after cyto-centrifugation (700 rpmn) and coloration with May Grunwald Giemsa.
Student t test was used to compare different groups.

RESULTS

Endoscopic examination did not show evidence of bacterial infection in tracheo-
bronchial tree. Data are presented in table 1. One Patient had 6 % eosinophil in
her BAL fluid. As expected, evolution showed complete resolution of both clinical,
roentgenographic and biological (SACE) manifestations in less than one year. No
increase of PMN count in peripheral blood was seen although inflammatory changes
were noted.

Alveolitis	LS Group (mean ± SD)	ST I Group (mean ± SD)	Significance
Total cell Yield (x 10 /ml)	352 ± 211	441 ± 247	NS
Lymphocytes (%)	47,6 ± 16,3	48, 9 ± 16,2	NS
Neutrophils (%)	4,16 ± 3,7	1,66 ± 1,5	p<0,05

Table : 1 LS patients BAL fluid compared with St I group.

Fig. 1 shows that elevated PMN count in BAL fluid is mostly seen between15 and 20 days after onset of EN (PMN = 6,0% ± 3,9 before 25 dys, VS 1,87% ± 1,8 at/or after 25 dys, p<0,005)

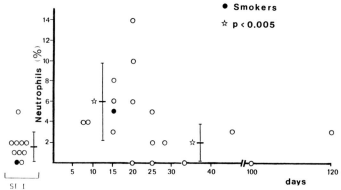

Fig 1 : Percentage of PMN in BAL of lofgren syndrome patients as a function of time. Compared with recently diagnosed Stage I sarcoidosis.

DISCUSSION

To our knowledge, we demonstrate for the first time that PMN can be seen at early phase of EN. The fact that LS is an acute onset of sarcoid alveolitis is supported by a low proportion of elevated SACE titers at diagnosis although secondary rise of SACE is seen in almost all cases. PMN alveolitis in LS appears to be slight and transient. Our data are consistent with other studies (4) where LS alvolitis after 3 weeks did not show high percentage of PMN. However an other study (5) did not mention PMN alveolitis in BAL from more recent LS (Less than 1 month).

It is now currently admitted that PMN in BAL fluid is related to fibrotic process (6). Clinical and functionnal evolution of our patients are not consistent with this fact. Early and transient PMN alveolitis has been shown in other interstitial diseases during experimental conditions.In hypersensitivity pneumonitis

(HP) Fournier et al (7) showed a transient but intense PMN alveolitis wich resolved in few days after antigen challenge, then followed by mononuclear cell infiltration. By analogy, one can evoke an immune complex (IC) mechanism in early phase of sarcoidosis with EN. This hypothesis is supported by the fact that IC have been seen in sarcoidosis especially with EN (8). Relevance of IC in different stages of sarcoidosis remains to be elucidated. In experimental Antigen Antibody challenge in guinea-pig, Robbins et al (9) pointed out that alveolar macrophage released neutrophil chemotactic factor (NCF) . This release is mediated by cell surface C5. Interestingly in human HP, NCF detected in patients blood is attributed to C5a (10). Comparison of lung cell comportments in HP and sarcoidosis is a classical way of investigation of the unknown triggering mechanism of the latter (11). Our results could bring additional clue in this way. Indeed, PMN are seen in HP in experimental conditions or rarely in acute antigen exposition. Then one can imagine, that LS could result from an intense antigen exposure wich initiates alveolitis.

Further, dispersion in percentage of PMN at 2 or 3 weeks and relative low intensity of PMN alveolitis (compared to experimental conditions in HP) could be explained by differences in (i) doses or specificity of antigen and/or (ii) mesestimation ot the time elapsed since the real beginning ot the disease. (EN is often preceded by arthralgia and fever).

CONCLUSION

Thus early and transient neutrophil alveolitis can be seen in LS. Analogy with other clinical and experimental features lead to think that PMN may not be solely relevant for a fibrotic evolution. The role of immune complexes and complement probably represents interesting ways ot investigations. The neutrophil may be involved in early inflammatory response to an immunological challenge. However the inititing agent remains to be founded.

Acknowledgements : we wish to thank Mrs A. ROSIERE for technical assistance and Mrs DEFAYE M. tor valuable secretarial assistance.

REFERENCES

1 - SILTZBACH L.E, JAMES D.G., NEUVILLE E, et al. Course and prognosis of sarcoidosis around the world (1974) Am. J. Med. 57 : 847-52.

2 - TURIAF J, BATTESTI J.P, DOURNOVO P. L'érythème noueux de la sarcoïdose (1976) Now Press Med 5 : 2603-5.

3 - LEVINSKY L, SVANDOVA E, MUNZONA J et al
    Incidence of lofgren's syndrome in Czechoslovakia in 1979.

CHRETIEN J. MARSAC J, SALTIEL JC (Eds) : Sarcoidosis and other granulomatous disorders IX th international conference Paris 1981 Pergamon Press.

4 - VALEYRE D,SAUMON G, GEORGES R et al : The relationship between disease duration and non invasive pulmonary explorations in sardoidosis with etythema nodosum
(1984) Am. Rev. Respir. Dis, 129 : 938-43.

5 - WARD K, O'CONNOR C, VAN BREDA A et al : Erythema nodosum confounds the
pronostic value of broncho-alveolar lavage T lymphocyte helper : suppressor ratio
in sarcoidosis (Abstract)(1987)Am Rev. Respir. Dis. 135, n°4 supplement, A 28

6 - ROTH C, HUDRON G.J. ARNOUX A et al : Bronchoalveolar cells in advanced
pulmonary sarcoidosis. (1981) Am. Rev. Respir. Dis 124 : 9 - 12

7 - FOURNIER E, TONNEL A. B., GOSSET Ph et al : Early neutrophil alveolitis
after antigen inhalation in hypersensivity pneumonitis (1985) Chest 88 : 563-6

8 - GUPTA R.C., KUEPPERS F, DE REMEE R.A et al : Pulmonary and extrapulmonary
sarcoidosis in relation to circulating immune complexes (1977) Am. Rev. Respir.
Dis. 116 : 261-6.

9 - ROBBINS R.A, RUSS W. D, THOMAS K. R et al : Complement component C5 is
required for release of alveolar macrophage derived neutrophil chemotactic
activity (1987) Am Rev. Respir. Dis. 135 : 659-64

10 - TONNEL A. B, FOURNIER E, MALLART A et al : Apport du lavage broncho-
alvéolaire à la physiopathologie des pneumopathies d'hypersensibilité (1985)
Immunologie médicale 11 : 47-50.

11 - THOMAS PD, HUNNINHAKE G. W : Currents concepts of the pathogenosis of
sarcoidosis (1987) Am. Rev. Respir. Dis 135 : 747-60.

© 1988 Elsevier Science Publishers B.V. (Biomedical Division)
Sarcoidosis and other granulomatous disorders
C. Grassi, G. Rizzato, E. Pozzi, editors

ANALYSIS OF UNUSUAL THORACIC MANIFESTATIONS OF SARCOIDOSIS: A REVIEW OF RADIOGRAPHIC FEATURES

S. David Rockoff, M.D. and Prashant Rohatgi, M.D.

George Washington University Medical Center, 901 23rd Street, N.W., Washington, D.C. 20037, U.S.A.

INTRODUCTION

Atypical thoracic sarcoidosis is often confusing and may lead to erroneous diagnoses. We present an analysis of the unusual manifestations of thoracic sarcoidosis for the guidance of physicians dealing with patients with possible sarcoidosis.

MATERIAL AND METHODS

A review of our clinical material as well as a comprehensive review of the literature led to the development of a clinically useful analysis of the unusual thoracic manifestations of sarcoidosis. We present the relative frequency with which the unusual manifestations occur. Pertinent references can be found in our prior publications.[1,2]

RESULTS

Bony Lesions

Involvement of bone is usually in the chronic phase of the disease and is generally associated with cutaneous, pulmonary and other systemic manifestations. The overall frequency of bony lesions is 3% (range, 1%-13%) with involvement of bones other than the hands and feet being very rare. We have found five sarcoid lesions involving the ribs, 13 of the thoracic vertebrae and 2 of the sternum. Thoracic vertebral lesions are usually multiple and generally associated with other bony lesions and most often there is collapse of the involved vertebral body. The radiographic appearance of the involved bones is not typical and may be seen as infiltrative or as punched-out lesions.

Pleural lesions

Pleural effusions in sarcoidosis, originally thought to be rare, have been shown to occur in 2.4% in 3,146 cases. They are usually asymptomatic, may be unilateral or bilateral, and may be seen any time during the course of the illness. They may be of any size, rarely even massive. In the fluid there is usually a predominance of lymphocytes. Additionally, two cases of chylothorax and 12 cases of pleural thickening ascribed to sarcoidosis have been described.

A radiographic sign not commonly appreciated is development of apical pleural thickening in patients with fibrocystic sarcoidosis due to colonization of the cysts with the Aspergillus organism. (Figure 1). Six such cases have been reported and we have seen 5 others. The apical cap may precede the appearance of the fungus ball by several years.

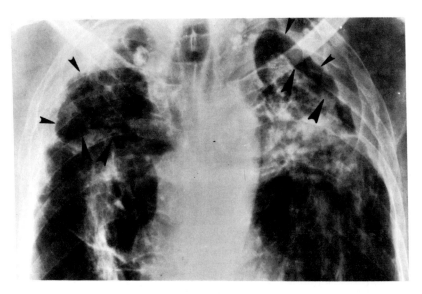

Fig. 1 Bilateral apical caps (small arrowheads) as a sign of Aspergillus colonization of pulmonary cysts in fibrocystic sarcoidosis and fungus balls within the apical cysts (large arrowheads).

Mediastinal Lesions

Paratracheal and hilar adenopathy occur in 80-90% of patients with thoracic sarcoidosis. However, isolated mediastinal adenopathy, with little or no lung involvement, is uncommon and may lead to erroneous diagnoses. Predominant middle mediastinal adenopathy (i.e paratracheal, subcarinal, aortico-pulmonary and retroazygos) has been reported 18 times. Anterior mediastinal adenopathy occurs rarely, either alone or in combination with other lymph node enlargement. Predominant posterior mediastinal adenopathy has been reported 11 times and has a preferred location in the lower paravertebral position. Tracheal lesions have been reported to affect 1% to 3% of patients.

Hilar Lesions

Unilateral hilar adenopathy, especially when it occurs in the absence of radiographically visible lung lesions, presents a confusing picture and is said to occur in 1% to 7% of cases. Hilar adenopathy of sarcoidosis rarely causes bronchial compression. Egg-shell calcifications of hilar lymph nodes occurs rarely in sarcoidosis with 14 cases reported. Calcification of hilar and/or mediastinal lymph nodes may occur in 3% to 20% of such patients, acknowledging that it is difficult determine exact etiology without pathology.

Unusual Pulmonary Lesions

Sarcoid lesions of the lungs rarely can appear as <u>solitary pulmonary nodules</u>. This was reported once in a series of 887 resected nodules and we have found a total of five such cases. <u>Unilateral reticulonodular</u> and <u>unilateral "alveolar"</u> lesions are occasionally encountered, with 12 unilateral interstitial and 2 unilateral "alveolar" lesions documented.

A troublesome lesion in pulmonary sarcoidosis is <u>the true primary pulmonary cavitary lesion</u>. The walls of such lesions are formed by noncaseating granulomas with little fibrosis and are believed to be due to ischemic necrosis. There are only six proven cases in the literature and we have seen four others. Such lesions are usually thick walled but may be thin walled (Figure 2).

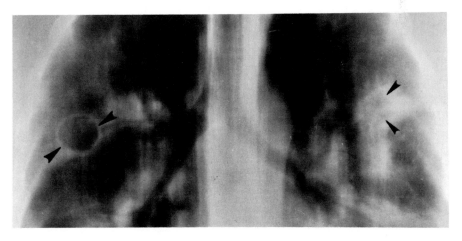

Fig. 2. Frontal tomogram of chest with thick walled sarcoid cavity in the left lung and thin walled sarcoid cavity of the right lung (arrowheads).

The <u>endobronchial lesions of sarcoidosis</u> can be visualized broncho scopically as well as by bronchography (Figure 3). These can cause hemoptysis or bronchial obstruction. Chronic bronchial obstruction due to endobronchial lesions may lead to acute or chronic inflammation of the involved lobe or segment with bronchiectasis often being present in the involved lobe.

Cardiovascular Lesions

<u>Cardiomegaly</u> occurs in 5% of patients. Rarer lesions include <u>pulmonary hypertension</u> in the absence of severe diffuse lung disease, presumably due to

440

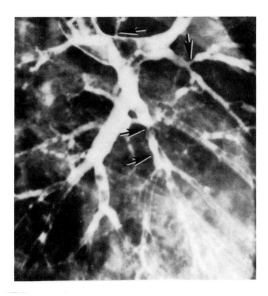

Fig. 3 Bronchogram of left lung showing endobronchial sarcoid granulomas (arrows).

involvement of the peripheral pulmonary vasculature. Vascular obstructions due to sarcoidosis include 10 cases of superior vena caval obstruction, four cases of innominate or left brachiocephalic vein obstruction, and 11 cases of pulmonary artery obstruction.

SUMMARY

Although thoracic sarcoidosis is a common disease and its usual radiographic manifestations are well recognized, there are a number of unusual and potentially confusing radiographic manifestations which may mimic other disease entities and cause diagnostic confusion. Our presentation tabulates and analyzes the unusual manifestations of thoracic sarcoidosis so that clinicians may be alerted to their occurrence and consider sarcoidosis in the differential diagnosis when they are encountered.

1. Rockoff SD, Rohatgi P. Unusual manifestations of thoracic sarcoidosis. Am J Roentgenol 1985;144:513-528.
2. Rockoff SD. Atypical sarcoidosis: The thoracic mimic. Contemp Diagnos Radiol 1986;9:1-6.

© 1988 Elsevier Science Publishers B.V. (Biomedical Division)
Sarcoidosis and other granulomatous disorders
C. Grassi, G. Rizzato, E. Pozzi, editors

PULMONARY SARCOIDOSIS IN THE ELDERLY : INCIDENCE AND ROENTGENOGRAPHIC,PHYSIOLO= GIC,BRONCHOALVEOLAR LAVAGE,AND SCINTIGRAPHIC CHARACTERISTICS.

CLAUDIO MARIA SANGUINETTI,BRUNO BALBI,FAUSTA VASSALLO,CARLO ALBERA,
STEFANO GASPARINI,PAOLO GHIO,GIOVANNI ARTURO ROSSI.
Pulmonary Divisions,Ancona,Turin,and Genoa Hospitals,Italy.

INTRODUCTION

Sarcoidosis is a multisystem granulomatous disorder of unknown origin,often asymptomatic and most commonly affecting young adults.Nevertheless,cases in the late middle age,mainly in women,have been described (1).

It has been reported that the age of patients at the onset of the disease seems to affect the prognosis,a younger age being associated with a more favourable course (2),but other Authors (3) found no relationship between age of subjects and clinical presentation or prognosis of sarcoidosis.

Only occasional and partial reports have dealt with the hallmarks of sarcoi= dosis in the elderly.

Thus,the aim of the present study is to seek for clinical,radiographic,physio= logic,and laboratory characteristics of sarcoidosis in older subjects.

MATERIAL AND METHODS

Reported here are the records of 37 subjects older than 60 years at diagnosis, belonging to a group of 303 patients with biopsy proven pulmonary sarcoidosis, who came under observation between 1980 and 1986 in three pulmonary divisions of northern and middle Italy.

They were 30 females and 7 males,mean age 66 yrs(range 60-78) and none was current smoker.

Of each of the 37 patients,chest roentgenograms,respiratory function data, bronchoalveolar lavage (BAL) findings,and Gallium 67 (^{67}Ga) lung scans were re- examined.

Chest roentgenograms were typed using the following classification:stage I, bilateral hilar adenopathy;stage II,diffuse interstitial lung disease with hilar adenopathy;stage III,diffuse parenchymal changes only.

Vital capacity(VC),total lung capacity(TLC),forced expiratory volume in one second (FEV$_1$) and diffusing lung capacity for carbon monoxide (DLCO;single breath method,corrected for alveolar volume and haemoglobin) were measured with Pulmorex Fenyves & Gut(Basel,Switzerland) and with Spirotest 3 Jaeger(Wurzburg Main,West Germany).Bronchoalveolar lavage was performed with Olympus BF-B3 using a total of 100 ml of sterile saline solution in aliquots of 20 ml.Total and dif= ferential cell counts and lymphocyte subsets characterization were performed as previously described (4,5).Gallium scans were obtained with a rectilinear scan= ner(Dyna Camera 4C,Picker Corp.,Highland Heights,Oh,USA),48 hours after IV in= jection of 50 μCi/kg of ^{67}Ga citrate.Gallium index was computed according to Line et al (6).

RESULTS

In our study the peak incidence of sarcoidosis was in the age group 30-39,but 37 out of 303 patients (12.2 %) were 60 yrs old or more at diagnosis.

The female/male ratio in these 37 subjects was significantly increased (4.3:1) compared to younger patients(1.4:1)(p < 0.01,x^2 test),with a twfold mean(+SEM) duration of the disease(12+2 months) compared to subjects aged under 60(6+1 mon= ths;p < 0.02,unpaired t-test).Most patients were symptomatic at diagnosis.

In patients over 60 yrs rx stage I was present in 4 subjects,stage II in 19, and stage III in 14,while in those aged under 60 rx stages I and II were preva= lent (p < 0.01;x^2 test).

VC was on the average 75.4 + 3.5(SEM) % pred;TLC 84.0 + 3.0 % pred;FEV$_1$ 76.4 + 4.4 % pred;% FEV$_1$/VC 90.9 + 3.0 % pred;DLCO 72.0 + 4.0 % pred.These values are all significantly reduced compared to those found in younger patients(p< 0.02, unpaired t-test).

Bronchoalveolar lavage analysis showed:increase in total cell count,in % lym= phocytes,neutrophils and eosinophils,and decrease in % macrophages compared to normal values (table 1).Lymphocyte subpopulations typing demonstrated increase in T cells and in helper/suppressor (H/S) ratio (table 1).In addition,29 pa= tients (78%) had increased percentages of lung T lymphocytes with H/S ratio greater than 3:1.

Gallium 67 scans were performed in 23 patients and resulted positive in 74 % of them.

Table 1

BAL FINDINGS IN 37 PATIENTS WITH SARCOIDOSIS AGED 60 YRS OR MORE AT DIAGNOSIS
(Mean values $\pm$ SEM)

Parameter		Sarcoidosis Patients	Normal values
Total no. of cells (x 10^6)		17.8 $\pm$ 3.1	10.3 $\pm$ 2.2
Macrophages	(%)	53.3 $\pm$ 4.8 *	93.0 $\pm$ 4.0
Lymphocytes	(%)	36.0 $\pm$ 4.4 *	7.0 $\pm$ 1.0
Neutrophils	(%)	5.9 $\pm$ 1.8 **	0.5 $\pm$ 0.5
Eosinophils	(%)	4.7 $\pm$ 1.8 **	0.5 $\pm$ 0.5
T cells	(%)	80.6 $\pm$ 3.5	73.0 $\pm$ 4.0
B cells	(%)	5.3 $\pm$ 1.1	8.0 $\pm$ 3.0
H/S ratio		4.1 $\pm$ 0.3 *	1.8 $\pm$ 0.2

* $p < 0.01$ and ** $p < 0.05$ vs normal value.

DISCUSSION

An extensive survey carried on sarcoidosis patients showed a marked prevalence for the ages 20 to 40 (7).In subjects older than 60 yrs the incidence is repor= ted to vary from 5 % to 8.5 % ,but our study clearly demonstrates that this incidence may be higher (12.2 %).

According to other Authors (1,8,9) we found that usual predilection of sarcoi= dosis for females is markedly increased in the elderly.The reason why this oc= curs remains obscure,but one might suppose that constitutional,hormonic,and other sex-linked factors are able to enhance those pathogenic mechanisms which lead to disease.Thus,this prevalence in females should be taken into account in the attempt to ascertain the etiology of sarcoidosis (10).

Most patients in our study were symptomatic at diagnosis.This finding is in accordance with that of Hillerdal et al (9),whose older patients were mainly identified because of symptoms.On the contrary,Scharkoff et al (11) observed that sarcoidosis in older than 50 yrs was characterized by asymptomatic or sym= ptom-poor course.It does not seem odd that patients with impaired,even though not conspicuously,lung function,as the ours are,may be more frequently diagnosed for the presence of respiratory symptoms.Probably,sarcoidosis in elder patients started several years before the diagnosis and it elapsed quite asymptomatic for a long time,until it is discovered because of respiratory symptoms.This beha= viour might also explain why we found a prevalence in rx stage III and an increase in BAL neutrophils and eosinophils.In fact,we previously demonstrated a significant progression with time from rx stage I to III (12).In addition,Roth et al (13) showed an increased percentage of neutrophils in BAL fluid from pa= tients with advanced sarcoidosis.

These findings agree with the presence of more fibrotic lesions in older sar= coidosis patients.Nevertheless,the activity of pulmonary alveolitis is still well evident in these subjects,as witnessed by the increase in T-helper lympho= cytes of BAL and the high incidence of positive gallium scans.

On the ground of our results we conclude that sarcoidosis is not rare in the elderly and it can maintain high intensity alveolitis.Thus,this diagnosis should be taken into account especially in old women presenting with diffuse intersti= tial lung disease.

REFERENCES

1. British Thoracic and Tuberc.Assoc. (1969) Tubercle 50:211-248

2. Rømer FK (1984) Acta Med Scand 213 (suppl 690): 1-93

3. Teirstein AS,Lesser M (1983) In:Fanburg BL (ed) Sarcoidosis and other Gra= nulomatous Diseases of the Lung.Marcel Dekker,New York,pp 101-134

4. Rossi GA,Sacco O,Cosulich E,Damiani G,Corte G,Bargellesi A,Ravazzoni C (1984) Thorax 39:143-149

5. Sanguinetti CM,Giulioni S,Bartocci C,Montroni M (1985) Riv Pat Clin Tuberc Pneumol 56:165-184

6. Line BR,Fulmer JD,Reynolds HY,Roberts WC,Jones AE,Harris EK,Crystal RG (1978) Am Rev Respir Dis 118:355-365

7. James DG,Neville E,Siltzbach LE,Turiaf J,Battesti JP,Sharma OP,Hosoda Y et al (1976) Ann N Y Acad Sci 278:321-334

8. Yanagawa H,Hosoda Y,Odaka M,Mikami R,Hashimoto T,Shigematsu I (1979) In: Sarcoidosis,University Tokyo Press,pp 355-377

9. Hillerdal G,Nou E,Osterman K,Schmekel B (1984) Am Rev Respir Dis 130:29-32

10. Israel HL,Sones M (1958) Arch Intern Med 102:766-776

11. Scharkoff H,Scharkoff Th (1983) Prax Clin Pneumol 37:546-548

12. Sanguinetti CM,Montroni M,Balbi B,Prete M,Gasparini S,Rossi GA (1987) Sarcoidosis 4:18-24

13. Roth C,Huchon GJ,Arnoux A,Stanislas-Leguern G,Marsac JH,Chretien J (1981) Am Rev Respir Dis 124:9-12

© 1988 Elsevier Science Publishers B.V. (Biomedical Division)
Sarcoidosis and other granulomatous disorders
C. Grassi, G. Rizzato, E. Pozzi, editors

CT VERSUS RADIOGRAPHY IN SARCOIDOSIS

LEE SIDER, M.D.
EDWARD S. HORTON JR. M.D.
Department of Radiology, Northwestern University Medical School,
Superior Street and Fairbanks Court, Chicago, Illinois

INTRODUCTION

Computed tomography (CT) is the major diagnostic imaging tool in the evaluation of the mediastinum and hili. One of CT's great advantages over the chest radiograph is in allowing detection of small lymph nodes regardless of their mediastinal location. This has led to a detection of adenopathy in sarcoidosis in previously unsuspected or unusual locations. We recently reviewed the CTs of 25 patients with proven sarcoidosis to help reassign the frequency of involvement of the different mediastinal lymph node groups as compared to previous reports using only the chest radiograph.

MATERIAL AND METHODS

The CTs of 25 patients were reviewed retrospectively. All scans were obtained on a GE 8800 or 9800 at 1 cm intervals. Nodes greater than 1.5 cm in the hili or mediastinum were considered enlarged for the purpose of this study.

RESULTS

Lymphadenopathy was consistently found in right paratracheal and pretracheal groups (25/25). Hilar adenopathy was present in 23 patients. Less frequently present was AP window (22/25), subcarinal (16/25), anterior mediastinal (12/25), and posterior mediastinal adenopathy (6/25). Supraclavicular (4/25) and axillary (2/25) adenopathy was considerably less often observed.

Lymph node groups were also categorized according to the combination of involvement. Beyond the consistent involvement of pretracheal, paratracheal, and hilar nodes, we found no statistically significant difference in the combination of areas which were involved. There was a fairly even distribution of combinations in patients with generalized mediastinal adenopathy (Table 1).

TABLE I

	Cases	% of Total	Peripheral Adenopathy	Splenomegaly	Pleural Effusion
P + R + H	2	8%	-	-	-
P + R + AP	1	4%	-	-	-
P + R + AP + H	2	8%	2	-	-
P + R + H + AM	1	4%	1	-	-
P + R + H + AP + AM	3	12%	1	1	1
P + R + AP + SC + H	5	20%	-	-	1
P + R + AP + SC	1	4%	2	-	-
P + R + AP + SC + H + AM	6	24%	-	1	-
P + R + AP + SC + H + PM	2	8%	-	-	-
P + R + AP + SC + H + AM + PM	2	8%	-	-	-

P = pretracheal, R = right paratracheal, AP = AP window, H = hilar, SC = subcarinal, AM = anterior mediastinal, PM = posterior mediastinal

DISCUSSION

Sarcoidosis appears to be a generalized process involving various mediastinal and hilar nodal groups. While certain groups are more consistently involved, apparently any mediastinal group may demonstrate adenopathy. CT does not appear to give further assistance over radiography in distinguishing sarcoidosis from a neoplastic process with multicompartmental mediastinal and hilar involvement.

ADVERSE EFFECT OF CHRONIC TONSILLITIS ON REGRESSION OF BILATERAL
HILAR LYMPHADENOPATHY IN SARCOIDOSIS

TOGO IKEDA, HIROSHI KOTOH, KENTAROU WATANABE, NOBUAKI SHIGEMATSU
Research Institute for Diseases of the Chest, Faculty of Medicine,
Kyusyu University, Fukuoka (Japan)

INTRODUCTION

Bilateral hilar lymphadenopathy (BHL) on chest x-p regress
spontaneously in most cases of sarcoidosis on long-term base.
However, there are considerable cases whose regression of BHL
delay. We have experienced frequent association of chronic
tonsillitis, sinuitis, and dental caries in these patients. We
hypothesized the presence of focal infection may affect adversely
on natural regression of sarcoidosis. We recommended tonsillectomy eagerly even in cases relative indication for tonsillitis
itself. We analyzed the effect of tonsillectomy on regression
of BHL.

MATERIAL AND METHODS

We experienced 217 cases of intrathoracic sarcoidosis during
the years 1970 through 1986. Among them, 74 cases were carefully
examined by rhinolaryngologist. The presence of chronic tonsillitis was observed in 55 cases (74%). Adrenocorticosteroids
were administered in 30 cases. Serial change of BHL was reviewed
in the rest of 25 cases.

RESULTS

Tonsillectomy was performed in 13 cases. In these 13 cases
(4 males, 9 females, mean age 35.4 ± 12.5), BHL regressed in 10,
unchanged in 2, and enlarged in 1 during the mean follow-up period
of 4 years. On the other hand, in 12 cases without tonsillectomy
(5 males, 7 females, mean age 41.8 ± 14.7), BHL regressed in 4,
unchanged in 6, and enlarged in 2 during the mean follow-up period
of 3 years. In the present series of 25 cases, new lesion (heart,
lung, or skin) appeared during the follow-up period in one case
after tonsillectomy and in four cases without tonsillectomy.
Decrease of serum angiotensin-converting enzyme often followed
tonsillectomy. Overall morbidity of 25 cases were fairly good.
Pulmonary function deterioration observed in one case who received

tonsillectomy. He showed BHL enlargement and increase in pulmonary infiltrates. Cardiac arrhythmia appeared in two cases without tonsillectomy. Arrhythmia persisted in one case after tonsillectomy and steroid administration.

TABLE EFFECT OF TONSILLECTOMY ON SERIAL CHANGE OF BHL IN SARCOIDOSIS PATIENTS WITH CHRONIC TONSILLITIS

Tonsillectomy	BHL on chest x-p		
	regressed	unchanged	enlarged
+	55F 49F 45F 37F 29F 29F 24M 23F 20M 16F	46F 44M	43M,L
	10/13(77%)	3/13(23%)	
−	54F,S 54F 31F 31F	60F,H 56F 56F 50F 37M 23M	31M,H 18M
	4/12(33%)	8/12(67%)	

Number indicate age, M: male, F: female.
Letters after comma indicate new lesion appearing during the follow-up period. L: lung, S: skin, H: cardiac arrhythmia.

DISCUSSION

The presence of focal infection other than tonsil may affect the result. We focused on tonsil for the sake of simplicity of analysis and clarity of the effect of operation. Even though the above problem, the effect of tonsillectomy deserve notice. The presence of chronic tonsillitis may affect giving an antigenic agent or unknown irritant and interfere with natural regression of disease activity of sarcoidosis.

SUMMARY

In 25 cases of sarcoidosis with chronic tonsillitis, the effect of tonsillectomy was analyzed. BHL regressed in 10 of 13 (77%) after tonsillectomy and in 4 of 12 (33%) without tonsillectomy. The presence of chronic tonsillitis adversely related to the regression of BHL in sarcoidosis.

© 1988 Elsevier Science Publishers B.V. (Biomedical Division)
Sarcoidosis and other granulomatous disorders
C. Grassi, G. Rizzato, E. Pozzi, editors

HIGH RESOLUTION COMPUTED TOMOGRAPHY IN SARCOIDOSIS

G. STANISLAS-LEGUERN   , J. FRIJA , P. MOREL , A. HIRSCH , M. LAVAL-JEANTET ,

J. CHRETIEN .

1 - Clinique de Pneumophtisiologie, Hôpital Laennec, 2 - Services de
Pneumologie, de Radiologie Centrale et de Dermatologie, Hôpital Saint-Louis, 1
avenue Claude Vellefaux 75010 Paris, France.

INTRODUCTION

The objective of this work was to study the sensitivity of high resolution
chest computed tomography (HRCT) in detecting parenchymal abnormalities in
sarcoidosis.

MATERIEL - METHODS

Thirty-one patients (14 men, 17 women, mean age, 36 ± 10.5 yrs) with proven
sarcoidosis underwent postero-anterior chest radiography (CR) and HRCT. Based on
the CR results, the patients were divided into four groups: group 0, normal CR
(n=4); group I : bilateral hilar lymphadenopathy (BHL) (n=14); group II, BHL
with parenchymal abnormalities (n=8); group III, parenchymal abnormalities
without BHL (n=5). For the HRCT studies, one mm slices were performed, every 10
mm, from apex to diaphragm during apnea after deep inspiration. Each lung was
divided into 3 zones by 2 horizontal lines (total zones n=186). Six categories
of parenchymal abnormalities were assessed: small nodules (SN, < 10mm 0), large
nodules (LN >10mm 0), honeycomb (HC), Kerley lines (K), ground glass (GG) and
pleural involvement (Pl). A CR and HRCT ccore was calculated by giving points
for each involved zone as follows: 1 = scarce SN, HC, K, GG (< half a zone), Pl;
2 = SN without confluence, GG (> half a zone); 3 = SN with confluence; 4 = LN (<
half a zone); 5 = LN (> half a zone).

RESULTS

Ten out of the 14 patients of group I had parenchymal abnormalities. Five of
the patients in group III had lymphadenopathies that were seen with HRCT.

56/186 zones were implicated by CR vs 94/186 by HRCT. The main results are shown in tables I and II.

TABLE I

Means and standard error of the mean of radiological scores in CR and HRCT in each group and in all 3 groups I, II and III.

| | GROUPS | | | | |
SCORE	I	II	III	II+III	I+II+III
CR	0	11.9±3.5	11.6±4.0	11.7±2.5	5.7±1.7
HRCT	3.7±1.2	16.7±3.3	20.8±4.4	18.8±2.6	10.7±2.0
P	<0.01	NS	NS	<0.01	<0.001

TABLE II

Frequency of the six parenchymal abnormalities in groups I, II and III (n=27)

| | COMPUTED TOMOGRAPHY | | | | | |
| CHEST RADIOGRAPHY | Absence | Presence | Absence | Presence | Absence | Presence |
	SN		LN		GG	
Absence	90	32	134	11	111	51
Presence	12	28	11	6	0	0
	K		HC		Pl	
Absence	138	22	144	6	149	7
Presence	0	2	12	0	0	6

The percentage of false negative with CR is 53% (32/60) for SN, 100% for GG and HC, 92% (22/24) for K and 50% (7/13) for Pl.

CONCLUSION

The results of this study show that small nodules and ground glass are the most frequent abnormalities in sarcoidosis. SN are detected by both CR(71%) and HRCT (64%). GG is only observed with HRCT (53% vs 0% with CR). Kerley lines are better detected by HRCT (25% versus 3.5% CR zones). We conclude that HRCT is more sensitive than CR to detect parenchymal abnormalities and to better analyse the basic parenchymal abnormalities seen in sarcoidosis.

© 1988 Elsevier Science Publishers B.V. (Biomedical Division)
Sarcoidosis and other granulomatous disorders
C. Grassi, G. Rizzato, E. Pozzi, editors

TRANSBRONCHIAL LUNG BIOPSY IN THE DIAGNOSIS OF SARCOIDOSIS

A. CIPRIANI, G. DI VITTORIO, G. FESTI, A. TOMMASINI
University of Padua, Italy, Pneumology Dept.

The diagnosis of Sarcoidosis is essentially based on:
- suggestive clinical and radiological findings,
- no evidence of fungi or bacteria in biopsies, sputum or any other body fluid,
- histological evidence of non-caseating granuloma, necessary to confirm the clinical radiological hypothesis.

Superficial, enlarged lymph nodes, skin lesions, conjuntival nodules should be considered first as possible sites of biopsy, because they can be easily done on an outpatient basis.

Other procedures, including scalene lymph node biopsy, mediastinoscopy, liver biopsy, open lung biopsy require admission in a surgical ward, general anesthesia, and greater risk of complications.

The lung is affected in 88-90% of cases so transbronchial lung biopsy (TLB) with fiberoptic bronchoscope is widely used. Because of its high diagnostic yield (70-90%), TLB is currently the best way to obtain a lung parenchima specimen.

TLB requires local anesthesia only. It is routinely preceded by bronchoalveolar lavage (BAL), and may be performed under fluoroscopy to prevent pneumothorax.

Contraindications are: severe pulmonary hypertension, hemorragic disorders, severe pulmonary insufficiency. Complications are limited to pneumothorax and hemoptysis.

Diagnostic yield is correlated to number of biopsies and radiological stage. In our experience four biopsies are necessary. The preferred sites are either the superior or inferior lobes; depending on radiological findings or Gallium 67 uptake.

Between January 1984 and September 1986, 104 new patients (54 males, 48 females, age range 18-70 yrs) with clinical and radiological picture suggestive of sarcoidosis were admitted to our Pneumology Division and underwent TLB without fluoroscopy. For each patient at least 4-5 biopsies were taken, preferably on right upper lobe or in the area radiologically most affected. Histological diagnosis was made in 85 patients (82%).

Percentage of positive biopsies was related to radiological stage: 50% (2/4) at 0 stage, 72% (34/47) at first stage, 90% (37/41) at second stage, and reached 100% (12/12) at third stage. Reported complications were three cases of mild, spontaneously re-solving pneumothorax and one case of hemoptysis (more than 50 ml).

Because TLB results in high diagnostic yield, is well tolerated by patients, has limited and minor complications, and may be repeated frequently, it is the first choice procedure in the diagnosis of sarcoidosis; long before more invasive mediastinoscopy or open lung biopsy.

CLINICAL FINDINGS AND BRONCHOSCOPIC ABNORMALITIES IN SARCOIDOSIS

C. MELISSINOS, M. VESLEMES, D. BOUROS, D. ZARIFIS, M. ZAHARIADIS AND
J. JORDANOGLOU
From Athens University, Pulmonary Department, Athens, Greece

INTRODUCTION

Sarcoidosis affects the bronchi commonly, as indicated by histologic, bronchoscopic and airway function data. Attempts to correlate such data with symptoms
and signs from the Respiratory System are complicated mainly by the inclusion of
smokers in most series with sarcoidosis and the difficulties in objective evaluation of macroscopic bronchoscopic findings.

In this study clinical findings in non smokers with sarcoidosis are correlated
to bronchoscopic findings reported by two bronchoscopists with special interest
and endoscopic experience for the disease.

MATERIAL AND METHODS

We present here twenty seven patients with the final diagnosis of sarcoidosis
consecutively examined in our bronchoscopy Lab. All patients were non smokers
without other cardiovascular or pulmonary disease, and with no history indicating
atopy. On admission a complete History and Physical examination was performed in
all patients by the same investigator, according to the protocol.

A second physician examined blindly all patients and only findings confirmed by
both examiners are reported here. Routine Pulmonary function tests and Chest films
were available prior to Bronchoscopy.

Fiberoptic bronchoscopy was performed transnasaly under local anesthesia
Bronchoscopic findings were recorded separately by two experienced bronchoscopists and the ones confirmed by both, are reported.

RESULTS

Our findings are summarized in Table I and II.

TABLE I
BRONCHIAL MUCOSAL ABNORMALITIES

None	10	(37%)
Diffuse	11	(41%)
Local	3	(11%)
Diffuse and local	3	(11%)
Any abnormality	17	(63%)

TABLE II
CLINICAL FINDINGS

Dyspnea	14	(52%)
Cough	11	(41%)
Crepit. rales	4	(15%)
Wheezes	2	(7%)

Bronchoscopic Findings. A wide main carina was observed in 3 patients.

Mucosal abnormalities reported as of more than of slight degree (i.e. moderate or severe) were found in 17 patients.

The bronchoscopic abnormalities were diffuse in 11 patients, local in 3 and diffuse and local in 3.

Clinical Findings. Dyspnea was reported by 14 patients (52%), and was equally frequent among patients with normal and abnormal mucosa (50% and 53%).

Cough was present in 10 of the 17 patients with positive bronchoscopy and in only one of the patients with normal mucosa.

Auscultatory findings were detected in 6 patients (22%), 4 had crepitant rales and 2 wheezes.

5 of the 6 patients with auscultatory findings had also an abnormal broncho-scopy.

SUMMARY

Sarcoidosis (27 pts) – ⊖ : with dyspnea
 Ø : FEV$_1$/FVC

We conclude that in Sarcoidosis most patients with cough and additional chest sounds are expected to have an abnormal bronchoscopy. Our data suggest that cough in Sarcoidosis originates mainly from bronchial mucosal abnormalities. Along these lines the similarities between the fiberoptic bronchoscope range of visible bronchial tree and the distribution of cough receptors in the bronchial wall is of interest.

Further studies are needed though, in order to establish the time sequence and findings in sarcoidosis.

RECENT PULMONARY SARCOIDOSIS MIMICKING IDIOPATHIC PULMONARY FIBROSIS.

FREDERIC BART (1), CHRISTIAN DELERIVE (2), VINCENT MASSART (1)
(1) Département de Pneumologie, (2) Laboratoire d'Anatomie et Cytologie
Pathologique, Hôpital A. Calmette, Lille. FRANCE.

Pulmonary fibrosis may arise during the chronic stage of pulmonary
sarcoidosis, after several years of evolution (1). We described 3 cases
of acute and recent pulmonary sarcoidosis mimicking idiopathic pulmonary
fibrosis at initial presentation. Two men (smokers) and one woman (non
smoker), with mean age of 37 ± 10 years, were free of previous pulmonary
disease. In the three cases, onset of symptoms was abrupt with severe
dyspnea, fatigue and weight loss. Physical examination revealed crackles
in lung fields. All patients had normal chest X ray before admission but
at this time, pulmonary infiltrates (with hilar adenopathy in 2 cases).

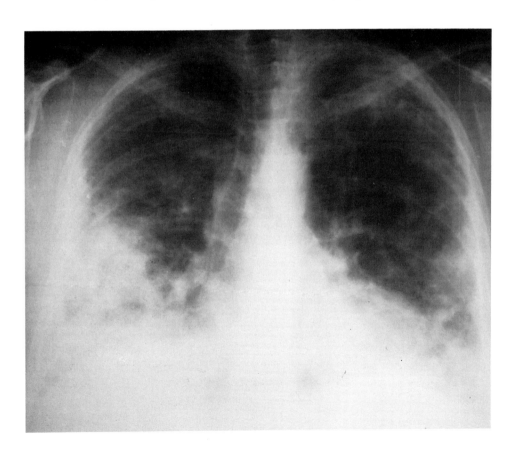

Research for bacterial, viral, mycotic or parasitic infection was negative. All patients were free of medication and they had no exposition to gaz, mineral or organic compounds known to be associated with interstitial lung disease.

P.P.D. skin tests (10 T.U. and 50 T.U.) were negatives. Serum angiotensin converting enzyme levels were high : 62 ± 5 U/l (normal value < 35 U/l). Gallium 67 lung scanning revealed an increase uptake. Bronchoalveolar lavage and pulmonary function tests (table I) were performed. Open lung biopsies and histologic examination showed the same lesions in three cases : multiple coalescent sarcoid granulomas with important surrounding collagen fibrosis and disorganization of normal lung architecture. High dose corticosteroid treatment was prescribed in each case with intermittent bolus (30 mg/kg) in two. The first patient showed progressive remission after 2 years. The second patient was stable after 3 years of corticosteroid and the third one was also stable with steroids but significantly improve clinically, radiographically and functionally after 4 months of cyclophosphamide. In our three patients, clinical symptoms and signs, radiographic patterns, severe functional impairment and high percentage of neutrophils in bronchoalveolar lavage were more suggestive of idiopathic pulmonary fibrosis. However diagnosis of pulmonary sarcoidosis was confirmed on open lung biopsies. Our data suggest that acute and recent pulmonary sarcoidosis may mimick idiopathic pulmonary fibrosis.

Patients	1	2	3
BRONCHOALVEOLAR LAVAGE			
Total cell count (10^4/ml)	30.4	27.6	3.5
Macrophages (%)	74	82	66
Lymphocytes (%)	10	4	22
Neutrophils (%)	15	13	12
Eosinophils (%)	1	1	0
CD4/CD8	ND	6.3	2.6
PULMONARY FUNCTION TESTS			
TLC (% predicted)	73	45	58
FEV_1 (% predicted)	88	44	60
FVC (% predicted)	80	48	58
DLCO (% predicted)	59	50	79
PO_2 (mmHg)	64	59	67

Table I

REFERENCE

(1) Scadding JG (1967). Sarcoidosis. Eyne and Spottiswoode, London

© 1988 Elsevier Science Publishers B.V. (Biomedical Division)
Sarcoidosis and other granulomatous disorders
C. Grassi, G. Rizzato, E. Pozzi, editors

LYMPHOCYTE KARYOTYPES IN PULMONARY SARCOIDOSIS

Y. PACHECO*, C. CHARRIN**, G. COZON**, F. GORMAND*, M. PERRIN-FAYOLLE*,
D. GERMAIN**

* Service du Pr PERRIN-FAYOLLE - Centre Hospitalier Lyon-Sud -
   69310 Pierre-Bénite - France

** Service central d'hématologie - Hopital Edouard Herriot -
   69374 Lyon Cedex 08 - France

INTRODUCTION

In spite of an extensive search for specific infectious agents and immunological reactions, the etiology of sarcoidosis remains unknown. The occurence of sarcoidosis in members of the same family has suggested that genetic factors might involved (1) but no firm relationship has been demonstrated. Various manifestations of sarcoidosis may be associated with specific antigens of major histocompatibility loci (2-3). Veien and col. (4) showed with chromosome analysis of blood lymphocytes a significantly greater number of hypomodal cells among patients with sarcoidosis disease. Recently chromosomal aneuploidy has been described in sarcoid granuloma cells (5).

We report in the following study the results of blood lymphocytes chromosomal analysis in 30 sarcoidosis patients.

MATERIAL AND METHODS

Thirty patients (15 women and 15 men) with clinical evidence of sarcoidosis as well as histological verification of this diagnosis participated in the study. Seven patients received steroids at the time of Karyotype analysis and five have received Azathioprin (150 mg/day).

Blood lymphocytes karyotypes were analyzed with RHG method according to the technic of DUTRILLAUX and COUTURIER (6).

RESULTS

Among the sarcoidosis patients : 28 had normal karyotype but two had abnormalities of their blood lymphocyte karyotypes. The karyotype of the first patient (non treated) showed initially high percentage of non specifically broken chromosomes but it became normal after two months of steroid therapy.

The second patient, who was treated with Azathioprine (AZ), one year ago during six months presented an apparently balanced TRANSLOCATION 46 XX, t (11;11) (P 12-p 14) in blood T lymphocytes (picture 1) but not in skin fibroblast culture (picture 2). This translocation persisted after two months of steroid therapy but was not found after six months and disease improvement.

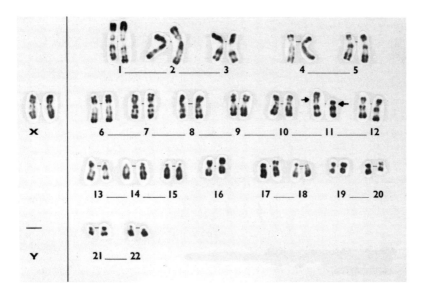

Picture 1. Blood T Lymphocytes.

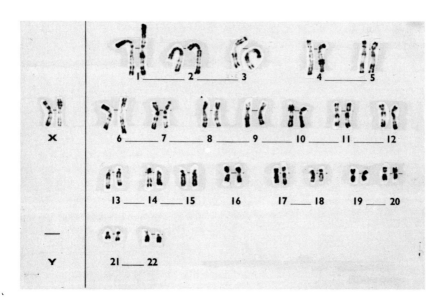

Picture 2. Skin Fibroblasts.

COMMENTS

Various hypotheses can be discussed to explain this chromosomal translocation : a direct toxic effect of AZ or genomic abnormality depending upon sarcoidosis disease and possibly revealed by AZ.

In four other patients who presented with pulmonary sarcoidosis and were treated with AZ, blood lymphocytes karyotype were normal, nervertheless this observation indicates that AZ must be used carefully in sarcoidosis.

The second hypothesis needs further chromosomal examination on alveolar T lymphocyte and genotype studies in order to be clarified.

It is important to note that this translocation interested a region of the short arm of chromosome 11 where Harvey Ras I and parathormone genes have been located and we hypothesize this possible mechanism of sarcoidosis disease.

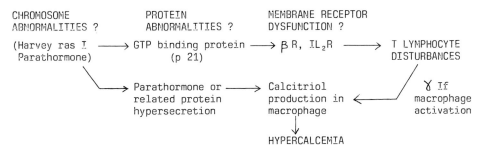

REFERENCES

1. Prendiville J, Robinson A, Young M (1982) Ir J. Medical Sci. 151:258-60

2. Guyatt GH, Bensen WG, Stolman LP, Fagnilli L, Singal DP (1982) Can. Med. Assoc. J 127:1005-1006

3. Smith MJ, Turton CW, Mitchell DN, Turner Warwick M, Morris LM, Lawler SD (1981) Thorax 36:296-298

4. Veien NK, Wulf HC (1980) Arch Dermatol Res 168:9-13

5. Okabe T, Suzuki A, Ishikawa H, Watanabe I, Takaku F (1986) Am Rev Respir Dis 134:300-304

6. Prieur M., Dutrillaux B, Lejeune J (1973) Ann Genet 16:39-46

461

CLINICAL RISK ASSESSMENT IN SARCOIDOSIS. OUTLOOK

HEINRICH KLECH   M.D.,F.C.C.P.
2nd Med.Dep.Wilhelminenspital,Montleartstraße 37, 1171 Vienna (Austria)

SUMMARY

   Although 80 percent of patients with sarcoidosis experience a favourable prognosis and a resolution of the disease within 2 years the remaining 20% need to
be consistently observed and possibly treated. In this attempt the adequate
assessment of the patients individual risk to develop complications in involved
target organs is the main challenge for the clinician. The current review focuses
on the clinical value of established and newly developed investigational tools in
order to predcit the development of lung fibrosis in patients with pulmonary
sarcoidosis.

   Although chest radiography and volumetric lung function tests remain to be used
routinely in follow up of patients with sarcoidosis they are less sensitive to
predict lung fibrosis. However, DLCO and oxygen saturation studies are reasonably
predictive. Serum Angiotensin converting enzyme and Lysozyme are of same value
when serially assessed. Among the newer biochemical tests the serial follow up of
Prokollagen III peptide, hyaluronate, - Interferon, Fibronectin or soluble
Interleukin-2 receptors may attain particular importance as soon as conclusive
data from more prospective longitudinal studies are available. 67 Gallium is a
well established tool. however, its use is restricted because of its costs and
radiation load. Assessment of epithelial permeability by use of 99m Tc-DTPA
appears to be sensitive measurement of lung epithelial integrity when distorted
by chronic inflammatory processes. However, as with CT densitometry and Nuclear
Magnetic Resonance imaging of the lung these means for time being are still in
an too early developmental stage in order to draw conclusions for clinical purposes.

   Studies on bronchoalveolar lavage (BAL) in the past extended largely our knowledge and understanding of pathophysiologic processes in pulmonary sarcoidosis.
However, BAL apart from some exceptions still has to be regarded as investigational and experimental tool, although it is widely used by clinicians. Evaluation
of T-cell subsets in sarcoidosis seems more valuable than mere lymphocyte counts.
Studies on macrophage activation and on non cellular components of BAL fluid may
give more consistent information , as soon as todays basic problems of standardisation and reproducibility of BAL data are satisfactorily resolved.

   In conclusion, since the major attributing factors which lead to pulmonary fibrosis are not fully understood, the clinician still has to rely largely on clinical experience.However, new investigative tools are increasingly helpful.

INTRODUCTION

Sarcoidosis is a multisystem granulomatous disorder which in most cases has a good prognosis. About 60% of patients experience a spontaneous resolution of the granulomatous process even without any therapy (1). However, the severity of the disease and the likelihood of a non favourable prognosis increases the number of involved organs (1). The most frequent severe complications which are seen in patients with multisystem sarcoidosis are listed in Table 1.

TABLE 1

FEATURE	POSSIBLE ORGAN IMPAIRMENT	RISK ASSESSMENT
HYPERCALCIURIA	renal failure	Ca-metabolism
OCULAR INVOLVEMENT	loss of sight	Fluorescin angiography
CNS INVOLVEMENT	neuritis, palsies hydrocephalus	CT scan, NMR
CARDIAC INVOLVEMENT	arrhythmia, cardiac insufficiency sudden death	ECG, 201-Thallium scanning, myocardial biopsy
PULMONARY INVOLVEMENT	lung fibrosis respiratory insufficiency	lung function tests, X-ray, biochemical markers of activity BAL, radioisotopes

Hypercalciemia is seen in 11% of patients worldwide, but showing a large variation within various racial groups (2). Hypercalciuria is greatly associated with chronic persistent multisystem sarcoidosis (3).

Pathophysiologically the disturbance of the calcium metabolism is due to an overactivity of calcitriol (1,2-dihydroxychole-calciferol) which is a metabolite of Vitamin D3, intestinal calcium absorption (4) resulting in hypercalcemia and hypercalciuria. Chronic hypercalcemia leads to calcinosis of the kidneys and further to renal failure.

Examination of Ca^{++} levels is a routine procedure in sarcoidosis. Corticosteroid treatment given in time usually normalizes the Ca^{++} metabolism.

Granulomatous involvement of the ocular system is reported in about 25% in patients with sarcoidosis (3). Several features like uveitis, granulomatous retinitis etc. may lead to sight impairment and in severe cases to progressive loss of sight. Therefore close examination of the eyes is a routine procedure in patients with sarcoidosis. Fluorescin angiography of the retinal arteries gives early clues of posterior ocular uveitis involvement (5).

Central nervous system involvement is reported in about 5% of patients (3) which clinically may result in neuritis, palsies etc. The use of CT scans and NMR (nuclear magnetic resonance) improved markedly our diagnostic possibilities (6).

Cardiac involvement comprises the emergence of granulomas in the myocardium causing cardiac insufficiency or when appearing in the endocardium causing arrhythmia. The diagnosis is difficult and proper clinical assessment apart from ECG and holter monitoring are expensive (Thallium-201 scanning) or invasive (His-bundle excitation, myocardial biopsy) (7). Cardiac involvement usually is under-reported. Sudden death due to myocardial sarcoidosis is more common in younger adults as previously suggested.

RISK ASSESSMENT FOR PULMONARY FIBROSIS

Involvement of the pulmonary system is the most frequent feature in sarcoidosis. Only 8 percent of patients present and continue to have a normal chest radiograph (3). However, in these cases lung function tests, particularly gas transfer may be abnormal and transbronchial biopsies may show granuloma. Some of these patients will meet the criteria of active lung involvement using the new investigative techniques, such as bronchoalveolar lavage (BAL) and Gallium scanning.

However, patients with type-0 or type-1 sarcoidosis in about 80% will experience a spontaneous resolution within a 2-year period. Of the remaining 20%, in about the half there is progression of stage II with persistent or progressive pulmonary infiltrates, and the other half will be left with persistent bilateral lymphadenopathy, usually associated with skin lesions (8).

The longer the pulmonary infiltrates persist, the more likely it is that fibrosis will develop. Overall 5 to 10% of all patients with intrathoracic sarcoidosis will end up with some degree of pulmonary fibrosis (8). It is the clinicians task to recognize any development of lung fibrosis in time. Ideally they should identify patients at risk by careful monitoring the course of the disease.

Following a critical review is given to what extent the clinicianis capable to meet this challenge and secondly which armamentarium he has available today.

CONVENTIONAL TECHNIQUES:

I. CHEST RADIOGRAPHY

Recording of symptoms and close observations of changes by serial X-rays and lung function tests are traditionally the classical means which has been used for many years. However, the value of chest radiography in this context is limited because of various reasons:

1) Although the classical staging of pulmonary sarcoidosis due to historic reasons is based on mere radiographic features, it does not necessarily reflect the real pathomorphological distribution of grnauloma within the lung. Chest radiography showing bilateral hilar lymphadenopathy suggesting stage I sarcoidosis does not exclude interstitial or endobronchial granuloma formation which could be substantiated by transbronchial lung biopsy (9, 10, 11) or intrapulmonary uptake of ^{67}Gallium (10, 12). Additionally in these cases significant changes in the pulmonary distribution of alveolar cells obtained by bronchoalveolar lavage (BAL) or changes of lung epithelial permeability (LEP) can be noted (13, 14). Thus, intrapulmonary sarcoid lesions can only be visible on the chest radiograph, when a certain degree of granulomatous accumulation in the lung tissue is exceeded.

2) Diagnosis of lung fibrosis cannot primarily depend on chest radiographic findings. In case of radiologic deterioration the chest radiograph cannot reliably distinguish between granuloma and fibrosis unless additional information is available.

   In conclusion serial chest radiographs remain to be routinely used in patients with pulmonary sarcoidosis because of its low costs and overall availability, however, its limitation to distinguish between granulomatous lesions or lung fibrosis at least in subtle cases is obvious.

II. LUNG FUNCTION TESTS

Respiratory symptoms like dyspnoe, cough and chest pain generally are neither strongly correlated to lung function abnormalities nor to radiographic changes in pulmonary sarcoidosis except in patients with advanced irreversible fibrosis (11, 15). Most of the respiratory symptoms (dyspnoe and cough) are due to 1) bronchial changes like endobronchial granuloma formation (sarcoid bronchitis), 2) mucosal swelling and 3) increased nonspecific airway reactivity. The latter could be recently substantiated by increased numbers of mastcells and histamine, obtained from BAL fluids of patients with sarcoidosis (13).

TABLE 2

PROGNOSTIC VALUE OF LUNG FUNCTION TESTS

	SIGNIFICANCE	POSSIBLE INTERFERENCE
VITAL CAPACITY	moderate, sensitive unspecific	exclude bronchial airflow obstruction
FEV$_1$	unspecific	
DLCO	sensitive, specific	exclude bronchial airflow obstruction
ARTERIAL OXYGEN SATURATION AT REST	sensitive, unspecific	exclude bronchial airflow obstruction
ARTERIAL OXYGEN SATURATION ON EXERCISE	sensitive, specific	

Consistent dyspnoe at exertion usually in connection with decreased DLCO and restrictive lung function tests, however, is characteristic for irreversible lung fibrosis but will be noted only in advanced cases. This may correlate to diminishing of airflow and increased airway resistance when measurements of small airway function are included (16). However, these changes can be found in any radiographic stage of the diseases and are not necessarily correlated to changes in spirometric lung volumes (12, 17). In stages II and III the consistent major abnormality is a reduction in gas transfer (DLCO) which correlated well with granuloma density and the extent of interstitial cellular infiltration in lung biopsies (11). A simple blood gas analysis (e.g. arterial oxygen saturation on exercise) basically can yield similar results (18).

In conclusion, although there is a trend to worsening pulmonary function with increasing radiographic stage, there may be considerable disparity between the chest radiograph and the results of the lung function tests. Breathlessness correlates better with the results of pulmonary function data (in particular when measuring airflow obstruction) rather than with the radiographic extent of pulmonary infiltration. However, airflow limitation is common in all stages in sarcoidosis and therefore has no prognostic significance. Spirometric measurements of lung volumes (VC, TLC, etc.) remain to be helpful to document a restrictive pattern of pulmonary function impairment in patients with established lung fibrosis but are of limited value during short term follow ups to signal a prognostic risk (17). DLCO and arterial oxygen saturation on exercise seems to be the most reliable prognostic indicator for the early development of lung fibrosis. However, in case of concomitant airflow limitation - which is common in those patients - obtained DLCO values may be incorrect (18, 19).

III. EXTRAPULMONARY SIGNS OF PROGRESSION

Sicne sarcoidosis is a multisystem granulomatous disorder, extrapulmonary manifestations are frequent and in many cases helpful to give prognostic clues for the further course of the disease. As an example erythema nodosum together with bihilar adenopathy usually has a very favourable prognosis whereas chronic skin lesions, bone cysts or hypercalcemia are associated with a chronic course of the disease likely to develop irreversible pulmonary fibrosis. A prognostic index of various features of sarcoidosis is given in Table 3.

TABLE 3   Probability (%) for resolution of intrathoracic sarcoid lesions in presence of various features of sarcoidosis.Adapted from (3).

FEATURE	PROBABILITY (%) FOR CHEST RESOLUTION
Acute arthritis	69%
Erythema nodosum	64%
Parotid	49%
Peripheral adenopathy	46%
Spleen	39%
CNS	39%
Heart	33%
Lupus pernio	29%
Upper respiratory tract	21%
Bone	19%
Nephrocalcinosis	11%

NEW TECHNIQUES:

I. BIOCHEMICAL MARKERS

1. Serum Angiotensin Converting Enzyme

Angiotensin converting enzyme (ACE) since over 10 years is routinely used in the management of patients with sarcoidosis. ACE can be expected elevated in about 60% of patients with sarcoidosis (20). Although due to its low specificity ACE is of limited use for the diagnosis of sarcoidosis, it is helpful in follow up and monitoring the disease. It is positive also in patients with extrathoracic sarcoidosis and probably reflects the granuloma mass of the body. ACE behaves differently according to the radiographic stage: In stage 0 ACE levels are raised in 27% of patients, in stage I in 56%, stage II in 72% and in stage III 56% of patients show elevated levels of ACE (20). However, highest levels usually are seen in stage II rather than in patients with stage III (21). This phenomenon probably can be best explained by the enhanced granulomatous mass usually observed in stage II disease compared to stage III. Indeed, in patients with stage III sarcoidosis with advanced lung fibrosis the ACE levels may be lower because the natural producers of ACE which are the capillary endothelial cells of the lung are rarified. In these cases of advanced pulmonary sarcoidosis any significant rise of ACE during follow up studies is of prognostic importance and may signal deterioration sometimes more reliable than serial chest radiographs. S-ACE in most series in patients with a chronic disease show a positive correlation to hypocalcemia (22) which is known to be associated with an unfavourable prognosis (Table 3).

ACE has been successfully determined in BAL fluid and proposed by some investigators as a marker of sarcoid activity of the lung superior to mere Serum-ACE levels (23, 24). However, S-ACE levels from practical reasons are far easier to examine. ACE tends to be positively correlated to 67 Gallium activity (25), because both tests probably measure a quite similar phenomenon (accumulation of epitheloid cells and granulomas). ACE levels are affected by steroid therapy as well as the 67 Ga uptake. Therefore both ACE and 67 Ga scans should be performed one week after the steroid has been discontinued (25,26). In contrast, during serial long term follow up measurements after cessation of steroid therapy ACE rises more quickly to elevated levels than the 67 Gallium scan will turn positive (12, 27).

In conclusion ACE reflects closely the activity and the mass of granulomas in the body. This is of particular interest and importance in chronic cases, because any prolongation of the granulomatous process in the lung tissue is known to increase the risk for development of irreversible lung fibrosis (28). As a rule, the longer granulomatous lesions are present in the lung in a particular patient the more attention should be paid to elevated S-ACE levels. Thus, S-ACE despite its limited value for the initial diagnosis of sarcoidosis it remains to be a valuable, non invasive and inexpensive tool in follow up of patients with sarcoidosis.

2. Lysozyme

Lysozym is a low moluecular weight kationic enzyme that can be detected in epitheloid cells and in the macrophages of the sarcoid granuloma. In patients with sarcoidosis elevated Lysozym-levels follow quite closely to those of ACE reflecting the mass of the epitheloid cell granuloma (29, 30, 31) and its prognostic significance is similar to ACE (26).

3. Newer biochemical markers of sarcoid activity

Apart from serum assays of ACE and Lysozym several other biochemical markers have been investigated and suggested for clinical use in patients with sarcoidosis (Table 4).

TABLE 4   Biochemical serum markers of sarcoid activity

MARKER	SUGGESTED SOURCE
ACE	epitheloid cells, granulomas
LYSOZYM	macrophages, granulomas
BETA-2-MICROGLOBULIN (30)	activated lymphocytes
THERMOLYSIN-LIKE	unknown
SERUM METALLENDOPEPTIDASE (32)	
TRANSCOBALAMIN II (30)	
GAMMA INTERFERON (33)	activated T-lymphocytes, granulomas
NEOPTERIN (33)	macrophages
SOLUBLE INTERLEUKIN-2-RECEPTORS (35)	activated T-lymphocytes
PROKOLLAGEN-III-PEPTIDE (37,38, 39, 41, 43)	activated fibroblasts

As with ACE some of them reflect the activity and load of the body granuloma mass, and in most instances correlate to ACE despite the source of the molecule is sometimes different. This is true for Thermolysin like Serum Metalloendopeptidase (32) and beta-2-microglobulin (30). However, these markers do not appear to show advantages to simple ACE serum assays, and no long term serial follow up data are available so far. Maintenance of enhanced T-helper lymphocyte activity within the lung tissue (T-helper alveolitis) leads to granuloma formation. Prolonged per- sistance of intrapulmonary granuloma is suggested to be primarily responsible for development of lung fibrosis in patients with sarcoidosis (28). (Fig.1).

PATHO-IMMUNOLOGY OF PULMONARY SARCOIDOSIS

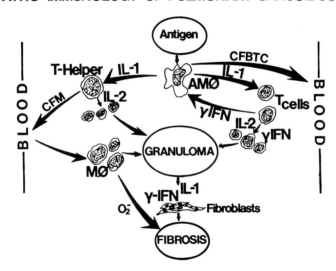

Gamma-Interferon is produced by activated T-lymphocytes and is the most likely factor to stimulate alveolar macrophages to secrete neopterin. In a recent study we could show that patients with advanced and progressive pulmonary sarcoidosis (type II and III) showed higher levels of gamma-Interferon than patients with type-I sarcoidosis or normal controls. Serum gamma-Interferon levels were positi- vely correlated to elevated levels of neopterin, to ACE and a 67 Gallium score (33).

In pulmonary sarcoidosis Interleukin-2 is produced by activated T-lymphocytes (34) and is responsible for intrapulmonary T-cell replication which anteceded pulmonary granuloma formation (Fig.1). Determination of serum levels of soluble Interleukin-2 Receptors in patients with sarcoidosis had been recently demonstrated by Lawrence et al (35). Highest levels were found in patients with parenchymal lung sarcoidosis and some correlation could be seen with ACE, 67 Ga scanning and hypercalcemia.

Intrapulmonary recruitment of fibroblasts is suggested to be primarily responsible for development of lung fibrosis. Increase of procollagen III peptid (PCP) concentrations is suggested to reflect the number of activated fibroblasts which are stimulated to produce collagen (36). Increased concentrations of PCP had been successfully demonstrated in sera of patients with idiopathic pulmonary fibrosis and with sarcoidosis (37, 38) as well as in BAL fluid of patients with sarcoidosis and farmer's lung (39, 40). In our series of patients highest levels of PCP were found in patients with idiopathic pulmonary fibrosis and in patients with active intrapulmonary sarcoidosis (type II and III) rather than in patients with type-I sarcoidosis. Serum levels of PCP correlated significantly to levels of serum ACE but not with lysozyme or gamma-Interferon (41, 42). BAL levels of PCP in sarcoidosis were positively correlated to the number of BAL T-helper cells (43). Corticosteroid therapy drastically lowers PCP levels.

Thus, determination of PCP in serum seems to be an excellent means to assess fibroblast activity. However, more serial data are warranted to confirm these observations.

II. ROLE OF RADIOISOTOPES

1. 67 Gallium scanning

Today we are looking back at about 10 year experience with 67 Ga scanning in patients with sarcoidosis. A recent overview is given by Klech et al (12). Despite some controversion about the real clinical value and cost-benefit-risk-factors of 67 Gallium, the use and indication of 67 Ga as a supplement to chest radiography and other markers of activity in sarcoidosis today has been reasonably established. It is selectively indicated
   a) For assessment of extent, location and inflammatory activity of sarcoid lesions
   b) For follow up progression or response to treatment
   c) To detect disseminated interstitial disease that escapes visualization by chest radiography.
As previously outlined serial chest radiography is less sensitive than

67 Gallium to document deterioration of lung lesions (10, 27). 67 Ga may be of particular value in patients with chronic sarcoidosis and having fibrotic lesions over years. Reappearance of granuloma in the lung parenchyma sometimes can be better documented by 67 Ga scanning rather than chest radiography and lung function tests (17, 27). Chest radiography obviously cannot discriminate between granuloma and fibrosis. Similarily volumetric lung funtion tests are basically not helpful to detect an early deterioration (12).

Numerous studies tried to determine the predictive value of 67 Ga scanning for assessment of progression of the intrapulmonary granulomatous process in conjunction with other markers of activity (44, 45, 46, 47). Line et al (44) suggested to use 67 Gallium scanning together with an increased percentage (> 28%) of BAL lymphocytes (high intensity alveolitis) as an index of bad prognosis showing a close correlation of both tests. Although their findings had been confirmed by some other groups (45, 48) there are subsequent studies which came to other conclusions (46, 47, 49, 50, 51).

Todays knowledge suggests that a persistence of an increased ratio of BAL T-helper/suppressor cell do better correlate to clinical deterioration rather than mere BAL lymphocyte counts (52). An increase of mast cells in BAL cell counts - which has been reported to be linked to a progressive evolution of the lung granuloma towards lung fibrosis - has been predominantly observed in patients with positive 67 Ga lung scans (13).

In conclusion despite obvious controversies about the value of 67 Gallium scanning in conjunction with other markers of disease activity (which are basically due to different modes of evaluations in various studies or to the fact that any described marker measures different features of sarcoidosis) 67 Gallium provides useful information about the extent and persistence of the granulomatous process within the lung (12). 67 Ga is more sensitive thatn chest radiography and when used selectively - is of reasonable value for follow up and for therapeutical decisions in pulmonary sarcoidosis within the framework of other markers of activity.

2. Measurement of lung epithelial permeability with 99m Tc-DTPA

Under normal conditions the epithelium is impermeable to fluid and protein,but injury due to various causes may result in abnormal transepithelial transport or leakage of water and solutes from the vascular space into the alveolar space. Inhalation of 99Tc-Diethylenetriaminepenta-aceticacid (99Tc-TDPA) is used as a small solute tracer (molecular weight 492 daltons) for measurement of lung epithelial permeability (53). Aerosol radioactivity then will be measured over the lungs. Recently we proposed the measurement of 99mTc-DTPA in the urine as a more simple means which gives same results as thoracic imaging (54). Increased clearance rates were reported in various interstitial lung diseases like systemic sclerosis, idiopathic pulmonary fibrosis (55), hypersensitivity pneumonitis (53) and in sarcoidosis (14, 55, 56,57a,b,58).Because of the incompleteness of available data so far it is difficult to compare LEP to other present available means for sarcoid activity. However, some findings can be elicited already:

a) Patients with stage 0 or stage I sarcoidosis have normal LEP whereas patients with pulmonary lesions demonstrated increased LEP (56). However, in our study (58) we could show pathologic permeability in stage I disease as well, but this was, however, less pronounced than in stage II/III patients.

b) No significant correlation could be found to BAL lymphocytes or markers of macrophage activation.

c) LEP appears to correlate better to 67 Gallium activity and to the inflammatory course of the disease.

d) Smoking markedly increases permeability (59).

e) Corticosteroid therapy improves pathologic permeability in sarcoidosis.

In conclusion LEP measurement is suggested to reflect the integrity of the pulmonary epithelium. Although LEP only is able to measure the amount of leakage between the alveolar space and the plasma volume, it seems very likely that it reflects any inflammatory alveolar-interstitial processes as well. Thus, increased 99mTc-DTPA clearance may be a valuable indicator to assess inflammatory processes in the lung interstitium. Establishing the potential role of LEP measurements in the non invasive evaluation of management of sarcoidosis will depend on well designed long term prospective studies in treated and untreated patients.

III. NEW IMAGING TECHNIQUES

1. Lung density studies

The density of the lung parenchyma can be measured with a computed tomography technique of the thorax by use of special lung masks which match the pulmonary tissue. Increase of pulmonary density in sarcoidosis is correlated to impairment of lung function tests (60). CT densitometry appears to be more sensitive than plain chest radiography. However, more comparative data to ACE , 67 Gallium scanning and BAL are badly needed. It remains questionable that CT densitometry provides more sensitive information than other means unless the results of prospective clinical trials will be made available.

2. Proton Magnetic Resonance Imaging (MRI)

Recently the hypothesis was tested whether MRI can differentiate the exudative

phase of interstitial lung diseases (alveolitis) from the relative acellular fibrotic phase (61). Although MRI in some cases followed clinical improvements by
successful treatment the value of MRI to predict the clinical course is regarded
to be limited.The issue of availability, costs and some unresolved technical problems (61) have to be mentioned anyway; the need of well designed prospective
clinical trials with MRI is obvious.

IV. BRONCHOALVEOLAR LAVAGE: A RELIABLE TOOL FOR ASSESSMENT OF RISK IN PULMONARY SARCOIDOSIS ?

Bronchoalveolar lavage (BAL) today is widely used in several aspects of pulmonary diseases (62, 63, 64). In particular its application in pulmonary sarcoidosis led to a new pathophysiologic understanding and growing interest in this
disease. BAL has taught us much about new immunological aspects of sarcoidosis
(Fig.1) and it helped us understand the compartmentalization of the disease process (65, 66, 67).

In the few studies which have correlated BAL cells with cells isolated from
lung biopsy tissue the percentages of lymphocytes, macrophages and inflammatory
cells have corresponded well (64, 68) .   An immunohistological analysis of BAL
cells and transbronchial biopsy tissue using a battery of monoclonal antiserums
against macrophages and various lymphocytes, found good qualitative concordance
(69).This and the large amount of immunologic data about alveolar cells in health
and disease explain why pulmonary scientists are so exited about BAL. But what is
the benefit of BAL for the pulmonary physician who observes and treats patients
with sarcoidosis

> - for diagnostic purposes and
> - what is the prognostic value and how helpful is BAL for follow
>   up examination ?

Actually numerous centers wordlwide today perform BAL routinely in their patients with sarcoidosis. In a recent international survey we found a remarkable
concordance how various investigators are handling some of the technical aspects
of BAL, however, there was a considerable disparity how to express and interprete
the results – since common ranges of normal values are not firmly defined –
at what time BAL should be performed and are there clinical consequences on
basis of obtained results (71). At the time of survey in 1985/1986 69% of re-
sponding centers would have regarded a high lymphocyte alveolitis (28% lymphocytes – high intensity alveolitis) as one of an important indicator to start
steroid treatment (71). In the meantime the overall opinion might have changed.

How predictive are BAL lymphocyte counts in sarcoidosis ?

In 1981 Line et al (44) presented the concept of the high intensity alveolitis (BAL lymphocytes > 28%) in pulmonary sarcoidosis, which together with a positive 67 Gallium scan were suggested to signal an unfavourable prognosis with impairment of lung function within the 6 months. Their data were basically supported by Keogh et al in 1983 (71) and some other authors as well suggesting that with active untreated alveolitis lung function will decrease. Since then their data were subject to some criticism (72).One might speculate that their data were generated from a comparatively small number of patients followed for the most part only a short while in the overall course of their sarcoidosis. Because spontaneous remission can occur, a longer follow up may be needed to address the natural history of the disease. In fact several other studies that have correlated results of BAL with response to therapy in the meantime could show that it might be too restrictive to rely only on 1 BAL count (47, 73, 74, 75).

In conclusion a mere lymphocytic count is not sufficient to predict the outcome at the first examination and consequently, to decide whether or not to treat sequential BAL are needed. BAL is particularly useful at the 12 months of follow up and is of predictive value only at this time (76). Diagnostically elevated BAL lymphocytes are only of limited value for the initial diagnosis of sarcoidosis since other pulmonary diseases as well may show elevated BAL lymphocytes, like hypersensitivity pneumonitis (63, 64, 77) systemic sclerosis (78),rheumatoid arthritis (74) and even in assymptomatic farmers (80). However, such finding as a screening procedure in interstitial lung disease may redirect or confirm a diagnosis (81, 82).

Are T-lymphocyte subsets predictive ?

Increased T-lymphocyte with a consistent increased ratio of helper(T4)/suppressor cells (T8) are regarded as an important diagnostic feature in particular for discrimination to hypersensitivity pneumonitis (63,77).Moreover, Costabel et al (52) could demonstrate that sarcoid patients with a high helper/suppressor ratio will experience a less favourable course of their disease. Their results are confirmed by Ceuppens et al (74) who could demonstrate that in patients undergoing successful steroid treatment the initial high ratio went down accordingly to the clinical course. Baughman et al (47) could show a reverse relationship of impaired vital capacity to the BAL T_4/T_8 ratio. Thus, a high T_4/T_8 ratio is more predictive for progressive disease than mere lymphocyte counts.

Are other BAL cells apart from lymphocytes predictive ?

Predominance of BAL-PMN neutrophils with or without eosinophils are the characteristics of patients with Cryptogenic fibrosing alveolitis (83, 84).

However, the role of those cells in BAL fluid of patients with sarcoidosis is still unclear. Roth et al (85) reported enhanced BAL-PMN granulocyte and eosinophil counts in patients with advanced pulmonary fibrosis. Intringuingly on the other hand enhanced BAL-PMN neutrophils had been recently reported in patients with Löfgren syndrome as well (86). However, Löfgren syndrome is known to be associated with an excellent prognosis.

Increase of mast cells in BAL has been reported in patients with sarcoidosis by Bjermer et al (87) and Flint et al (13). However, their findings are not supported by other authors (88).

Alveolar macrophages play a central role for the maintenance of the granulomatous process. Macrophage derived mediators (Interleukin-1, alveolar macrophage derived growth factor for fibroblasts, oxygen radicals etc.) (Fig.1) are suggested to be primarily responsible for fibroblast activation. Examining the stage of activation of BAL macrophages may be a sensitive indicator for enhanced fibroblast activity. Alveolar macrophages of patients with sarcoidosis express a typical pattern of maturity and subpopulations which can be stained with monoclonal antibodies (89, 90). Indices of alveolar macrophage activation correlated to intracellular Interleukin-1 activity (89).

Further and sequential BAL studies are necessary to give clinical proof and relevance to these very preliminary findings.

Are non cellular components of BAL fluid predictive ?

In past years significant research activity focused on the construction of the fibrotic pathway originating with activated macrophages that secrete effector substances which had been measured in BAL fluid or BAL in cell culture, such as Interleukin-1 (36) fibronectin (91, 92) growth factors (93) etc. that in turn can cause fibroblasts in culture to replicate and produce abnormal collagen (28, 92).

Alveolar macrophages in sarcoidosis are activated and challenged by maintenance of activated T-lymphocytes in the lung tissue. Enhanced lymphocyte activity is associated with significant spread of specific lymphokines which could be successfully measured in BAL fluid or in BAL cell culture like Interleukin-2 (34), Gamma Interferon (43,94). Specific alterations of the BAL fluid composition in patients of sarcoidosis like enhanced concentration of Albumin and Immunglobulin had been described (95, 96, 97, 98) and partly suggested as a marker of disease activity.

However, current efforts to quantitative soluble ingredients of BAL fluids has major logistic and technical obstacles. Today a completely reliable denominator or reference substance is not available. Attempts to use Albumin (99), methylenblue (100) or recently urea (101) are not commonly accepted.

In conclusion biochemical analysis of BAL fluid is an exciting field of research which elicites important details of the pathophysiology of the alveolar space but because of detailed problems of standardisation it should be restricted to research protocols.

CONCLUSION

In summary, monitoring patients with sarcoidosis longitudinally can be difficult because most patients experience varying degrees of activity and periods of remissions during the course of the disease.The usual physical signs, patient symptoms, radiographs, and simple pulmonary function tests, may not be sufficiently sensitive to detect subtle progression. Thus, tests that more closely examine the dieased lung, such as a periodic BAL, or noninvasively assess inflammation in the total lung, such as radioisotope scans, must be evaluated. Apparently, better and more sensitive tests are necessary to extract more kinetic and biochemical information from the BAL fluid and cells, and the overall approach to this analysis is changing, for cell counts alone have not been sufficient parameters. BAL should still be considered as an experimental procedure until its use is better established.

REFERENCES

1. Neville E, Walter AM, James DG (1983).Prognostic factors predicting the outcome of sarcoidosis. An analysis of 818 patients.
    Quart J Med New Series L 11; 208:525

2. James DG, Neville E, Turiaf J, Ballesti JP et al. (1976).A worldwide review of sarcoidosis. Ann NY Acad Sci 278:321

3. James DG, Jones Williams W (1985). Sarcoidosis and Other Granulomatous Disorders. Philadelphia:WB Saunders

4. Bell NH, Stern PH, Pantzer E, Sinhat K, Deluca HF (1979). Evidence that increased circulating 1.25 dehydroxy vitamin D in the probable cause for abnormal calcium metabolism in sarcoidosis. J Clin Invest 64:218

5. James DG (1986). ocular sarcoidosis. Ann NY Acad Sci; 456:551

6. Barter J (1986). NMR in Granulomatous Disorders. Sarcoidosis, 3:118

7. Fleming HA (1986). Cardiac sarcoidosis. Sem Resp Dis; 8:65

8. Flint K, Chir B, Johnson N (1967). Intrathoracic sarcoidosis.
    Sem Respir Dis; 8:41

9. Rosen Y, Amorosa JK, Moon S, Cohen S, Lyons HA (1977). Occurence of lung granulomas in patients with stage I sarcoidosis.Am J Roentgenol 129:1083-85

10. Klech H, Köhn H, Pohl W, Kummer F, Mostbeck A (1983). Aktivitätsdiagnostik der Sarkoidose. Wr Med Woschr 133:425-31.

11. Huang CT, Heinrich AE, Rosen Y, Moon S, Lyons HA (1979). Pulmonary sarcoidosis: Roentgenography, functional and pathologic correlations.
    Respiration 37:337-345

12. Klech H, Köhn H, Huppmann M, Pohl W (1987). Thoracic Imaging with [67]Gallium. Eur J Nucl Med 13: 24-36

13. Flint K, Leung KBP, Hudspith BN, Brostoff J, Pearce FL, James DG, Johnson N (1986). Bronchoalveolar mast cells in sarcoidosis: Increased numbers and accentuation of histamine release. Thorax 41:94-99

14. Huchon GJ (1986). Laboratory tests and radioisotopes studies to assess pulmonary fibrosis in sarcoidosis. Sarcoidosis 3:132-134

15. Renzi G, Dutton RE (1974). Pulmonary function in diffuse sarcoidosis. Respiration 31:124-136

16. Levinson RS, Metzger LF, Stanley NN, Kelsen SG, Altose MD, Cherniak NS, Brody JS (1977). Airway function in sarcoidosis. Am J Med 62:51-59

17. Klech H, Witek F, Köhn H, Pohl W (1983b). Pulmonary function tests compared to [67]Gallium scintigraphy and S-ACE for monitoring recurrent pulmonary sarcoidosis. Am Rev Respir Dis 127:4 (abstract)

18. Klech H, Witek F, Hubner M, Pohl W (1983c). Verlauf der Lungenfunktion bei pulmonaler Sarkoidose. Wr Med Woschr S 33; 74:23-24

19. Bouhuys A (1974). Breathing:physiology, environment and lung disease. Grune and Stratton,p:104-107

20. Studdy PR, James SG (1983). The specificity and sensitivity of serum angiotensin converting enzyme in sarcoidosis and other diseases:Experience in twelve centers in six different countries . In:Chretien J, Marsac J, Saltiel JC:Sarcoidosis; Paris:Pergamon Press p.332-334

21. De Remee RA, Rohrbach MS (1980). Serum angiotensin converting enzyme activity in evaluating the clinical course of sarcoidosis.Ann Int Med.92:361

22. Romer FK (1983). S-angiotensin converting enzyme (S-ACE) in hypercalcemia due to sarcoidosis and other disorders. In:Chretien J, Marsac J, Saltiel JC (eds):Sarcoidosis, Paris; Pergamon Press p.637

23. Perrin-Fayolle M, Pacheco Y, Harf R, Montagnon B, Biot N (1981). Angiotensin converting enzyme in bronchoalveolar lavage fluid in pulmonary sarcoidosis. Thorax 34:790

24. Stanilas-Leguern G, Leclerc P, Baumann FC, Mordelet-Dambrine M,Huchon GJ, Andreux JP, Marsac J, Rochemaure J, Chretien J (1983). Angiotensin converting enzyme in bronchoalveolar fluid and serum as indicators of spread of untreated sarcoidosis. In:Chretien J, Marsac J, Saltiel JC (eds).Sarcoidosis Paris, Pergamon Press ,p.

25. Klech H, Köhn H, Kummer F, Mostbeck A (1982). Assessment of activity in sarcoidosis. Chest 82:732-738

26. Rizzato G (1986b). Markers of activity. Sem Resp Dis 8:30-40

27. Rizzato G, Blasi A (1986a) .An European Survey on the Usefulness of [67]Ga Lung Scans in Assessing sarcoidosis experience in 14 Research Centers in seven different countries. Ann NY Acad Sci 465:463-478

28. Hunninghake GW, Garrett KC,Richardson HB, Fantone JC, Word PA, Rennard SI, Bittermann PB, Crystal RG (1984). Pathogenesis of the granulomatous lung diseases. Am Rev Resp Dis 130:476-496

29. Selroos O, Klockars M (1977). Serum lysozyme in sarcoidosis; evaluation of its usefulness in determination of disease activity. Scan J Resp Dis 58:110

30. Selroos O (1984). Value of biochemical markers in serum for determination of disease activity in sarcoidosis. Sarcoidosis 1:45-49

31. Pohl W, Hubner M, Riedl H, Legenstein E, Klech H (1985). Bedeutung von
     Serum Lysozym und S-ACE in Diagnostik und Verlaufsdiagnostik verschiedener
     Lungenerkrankungen. Wr Med Woschr 135, Suppl.90:24

32. Almenoff J, Skorron ML, Teirstein AS (1986). Thermolysin-like Serum Metallo-
     endopeptidase:A new marker for active Sarcoidosis that complements serum
     angiotensin converting enzyme . Ann NY Acad Sci 465:738-743

33. Köhn H, Woloszczuk W, Pohl W, Klech H (1986). Gamma Interferon and
     Neopterin as immunological markers for assessment of activity in sarcoidosis
     Sarcoidosis 3,2:156

34. Pinkston P, Bitterman BP, Crystal RG (1983). Spontaenous release of
     interleukin-2 by lung lymphocytes in active pulmonary sarcoidosis.
     N Engl J Med 308:793-800

35. Lawrence EC, Berger MB, Brousseau KP, Rodrigues TM, Siegel SJ, Kurman CC,
     Nelson DL (1987). Elevated Serum Levels of soluble Interleukin-2 Receptors
     in active pulmonary sarcoidosis. Relative specificity and association with
     hypercalcemia. Sarcoidosis 4:87-93

36. Hunninghake GW (1984). Release of Interleukin-1 by alveolar macrophages of
     patients with active pulmonary sarcoidosis. Am Rev Respir Dis 64:271-282

37. Low RB, Cutroneo KR, Davis GS, Giancola MS (1983). Lavage Type -III Pro-
     collagen N-Terminal Peptides in Human Pulmonary Fibrosis and Sarcoidosis.
     Lab Invest 48:755-759

38. Kirk J.ME, Bateman ED, Haslam PM, Laurent GJ, Turner-Warwick M (1984).
     Serum Type III procollagen peptide concentration in cryptogenic fibrosing
     alveolitis and its clinical relevance. Thorax 39:726-732

39. Bjermer L, Thunell M, Hällgren R (1986). Procollagen III peptide in broncho-
     alveolar lavage fluid: a potential marker of alter collagen synthesis
     reflecting pulmonary disease in sarcoidosis. Lab Invest 55:654-656

40. Bjermer L, Engström-Laurent, Lungren Rune, Rosenhall L, Hällgren R (1987).
     Hyaluronate and type III procollagen peptide concentrations in broncho-
     alveolar lavage fluid as markers of disease activity in farmers lung.
     Br Med J 295:803-806

41. Klech H, Hubner M, Pohl W, Köhn H, Riedl M, Legenstein E (1984). Lysozym
     und Prokollagen III, zwei neue Laborparameter zur Aktivitäts- und Verlaufs-
     diagnostik der Sarkoidose. Acta Med Austriaca 2,11:18

42. Pohl W, Klech H, Köhn H, Riedl M, Umek H, Kummer F (1987). Prokollagen III
     peptid is elevated in serum and BAL of patients with fibrosing lung dis-
     orders due to sarcoidosis, hypersensitivity pneumonitis and idiopathic
     pulmonary fibrosis. Manuscript in preparation.

43. Pohl W, Köhn H, Riedl M, Umek H, Hubner M, Rona G, Woloszczuk W,Klech H
     (1986). Procollagen III peptid and Gamma Interferon in BAL fluid in pat-
     ients with sarcoidosis and idiopathic interstitial fibrosis.Relations
     to other biological markers. Sarcoidosis 2:178

44. Line BR, Hunninghake GW, Keogh BA, Jones AE, Johnston GS, Crystal RG (1981).
     Gallium-67 scanning to stage the alveolitis of sarcoidosis:correlation with
     clinical studies, pulmonary function studies and bronchoalveolar lavage.
     Am. Rev Respir Dis 123:440-446

45. Huchon GJ, Berrisouk F, Barritoult LG, Venet A, Marsac J, Ronccayrol JC,
     Chretien J (1983). Comparison of bronchoalveolar lavage and gallium-67 lung
     scanning to assess the activity of pulmonary sarcoidosis.In:Chretien J,
     Marsac J, Saltiel JC (eds) Sarcoidosis and other granulomatous disorders.
     Pergamon Press, Paris,p.440-445

46. Beaumont D, Herry SY, Sapene M, Bourget P, Larzul JJ, DeLaberthe B (1982). Gallium 67 in the evaluation of sarcoidosis: correlation with serum angiotensin converting enzyme and bronchoalveolar lavage.Thorax 37:11-18

47. Baughman RP, Fernandez M, Bosken CH (1984). Comparison of gallium 67 scanning, bronchoalveolar lavage and serum angiotensin converting enzyme levels in pulmonary sarcoidosis. Am Rev Respir Dis 129:676-681

48. Fayman WA, Greenwald LV, Staton G (1984). Quantitative 67 gallium citrate lung imaging in sarcoidosis: comparison of three methods and correlation with bronchoalveolar lavage. AJR 142:683-688

49. Costabel U, Bross KJ, Fischer J, Guzman J, Matthys H (1983). Die Bedeutung der Helfer-T-Lymphozyten in der bronchoalveolären Lavage für die Aktivitätsbeurteilung der pulmonalen Sarkoidose.Prax Klin Pneumol 37:574-577

50. Havranek V, Klech H, Rona G, Hubner M (1983). Die bronchoalveoläre Lavage (BAL) bei pulmonaler Sarkoidose. Wr Med Woschr ;Suppl.133;75:42

51. Klech H, Köhn H, Pohl W, Kummer F (1984). Sensitivity and specificity of 67 Ga scanning, bronchoalveolar lavage (BAL) chest radiography and lung function tests (LFT) for assessment of activity in patients with pulmonary sarcoidosis. Respiration 46:1 (abstract).

52. Costabel U, Bross KJ, Guzman J, Nilles A, Rühle KH, Matthys H (1986). Predictive Value of Bronchoalveolar T cell Subsets for the Course of pulmonary sarcoidosis. Ann NY Acad Sci 465:418-426.

53. Coates G, O'Brodovich H (1986). Measurement of pulmonary epithelial permeability with 99m TC-DTPA Aerosol. Sem Nucl Med 16: 275-284

54. Köhn H, Klech H, König B, Mostbeck A (1987). Measurement of 99mTc-DTPA excretion in urine: a simple means for assessment of. lung epithelial permeability (LEP). Nucl Med 26:97

55. Rinderknecht J, Shapiro L, Krauthammer M, Toplin G, Wasserman K, Udzler JM, Effros RM (1980). Accelerated clearance of small solutes from the lung in interstitial lung disease. Am Rev Resp Dis 121:105-117

56. Dusser D, Mordelet-Dambrine M, Collignon MA, Barritoult L, Chretien J, Huchon G (1984). Permeabilite respiratoire determinee par la clairance d'un solute aerosolise et le lavage broncho-alevolaire dans les pneumopathies interstitielles. Bull Eur Physiopath Respir 20:223-227

57a. Jacobs MB, Baughman P, Hughes J, Fernandez-Ulloa M (1985). Radioaerosol clearance in patients with active pulmonary sarcoidosis.Am Rev Resp Dis 131: 687-689

57b. Jordana M, Dolovich M, Newhouse M (1987). Lung epithelial permeability in sarcoidosis. Sarcoidosis 4:116-121

58. Köhn H, Klech H, Pohl W, Mostbeck A (1987). Einsatz radioaktiver Aerosole in der Diagnostik von Lungenerkrankungen. Praxis Klin Pneumol.in press

59. Jones JG, Lewler P, Hulands G, Crowley JCW, Veaoll N (1980). Increased alveolar epithelial permeability in cigarette smokers. Lancet 1:66-68

60. Hedlund L, Friedman M, Effmann E, Puttman C (1981). Lung densitiy measurement by computed tomography. Am Rev Resp Dis 123:245

61. McFadden RG, Carr TJ, Word TE (1987). Proton Magnetic resonance imaging to stage activity of interstitial lung disease.Chest 92:31-39

62. Crystal RG, Reynolds HY, Kalica AR (1986). Bronchoalveolar lavage; the report of an international conference. Chest 90:122-131

63. Reynolds HY (1987). Stae of the art; Bronchoalveolar lavage. Am Rev Resp Dis 135:250-263

64. Haslam P (1984). Bronchoalveolar lavage. Sem Resp Med 6:55-70

65. Hunninghake GW, Gadek JE, Young RC Jr, Kawanami O, Ferrans VJ, Crystal RG (1980). Maintenance of granuloma formation in pulmonary sarcoidosis by T lymphocytes within the lung. N Engl J Med 302:594-598

66. Hunninghake GW, Crystal RG (1981). Pulmonary sarcoidosis, a disorder mediated by excess helper T lymphocyte activity at sites of disease. N Engl J Med 305:429-434

67. Rossi GA, Sacco O, Cosulich E et al (1984). Pulmonary sarcoidosis:excess of helper T lymphocytes and T cell subset imbalance at sites of disease activity. Thorax 39:143-149

68. Semenzato G, Chilosi M, Ossi E et al (1985). Bronchoalveolar lavage and lung histology: Comparative analysis of inflammatory and immunocompetent cells in patients with sarcoidosis and hypersensitivity pneumonitis. Am Rev Resp Dis 132:400-404

69. Campbell DA, Poulter LW, DuBois RM (1985). Immunocompetent cells in bronchoalveolar lavage reflect the cell populations in transbronchial biopsies in pulmonary sarcoidosis. Am Rev Resp Dis 132:1300-6

70. Klech H, Haslam P, Turner-Warwick M and 62 other contributors (1986). World Wide Clinical Survey on Bronchoalveolar Lavage (BAL) in Sarcoidosis. Experience in 62 centers in 19 countries. Sarcoidosis 3:113-122.

71. Keogh BA, Hunninghake GW, Line BR, Crystal RG (1983). The alveolitis of pulmonary sarcoidosis:Evaluation of natural history and alveolitis-dependent changes in lung function. Am Rev Resp Dis 128:256-65

72. Turner-Warwick M, Haslam P, McAllister U, Britton A, Lawrence R (1986). Do measurements of bronchoalveolar lymphocytes, Serum angiotensin converting enzyme and Gallium uptake help the clinician to treat patients with sarcoidosis (Sven Löfgren Memorial Lecture) Ann NY Acad Sci 465:387-94

73. Lawrence EC, Teague RB, Gottlieb MD, Jhingran SG, Lieberman J (1983). Serial changes in markers of disease activity with corticosteroid treatment in sarcoidosis. Amer J Med.74:747-56

74. Ceuppens JL,Lacquet LM, Marien G, Demedts .M, Van Den Eeckhout A,Stevens E (1984).Alveolar T-cell subsets in pulmonary sarcoidosis. Correlation with disease activity and effect of steroid treatment.Am Rev Resp Dis 129:563-8.

75. Israel-Biet D, Venet A, Chretien J (1986). Persistent high alveolar lymphocytosis as a predictive criterion of chronic pulmonary sarcoidosis. Ann NY Acad Sci 465:395-406

76. Chretien J, Venet A, Danel C, Israel-Biet D, Sandron D, Arnoux A (1985). Bronchoalveolar lavage in sarcoidosis.Respiration 49:222-230

77. Costabel U, Bross KJ, Rühle KH, Löhr GW, Matthys H (1985). Ia like Antigens on T-cells and their subpopulations in pulmonary sarcoidosis and in hypersensitivity pneumonitis.Am Rev Resp Dis 131:337-342

78. Rossi GA, Bitterman PB, Rennard SI, Ferrans VJ, Crystal RG (1985). Evidence for chronic inflammation as a component of the interstitial lung disease associated with progressive systemic sclerosis. Am Rev Resp Dis 131:612-7

79. Garcia JGN, Parhami N, Killam D, Garcia PL, Keogh BA (1986). Bronchoalveolar lavage fluid evaluation in rheumatoid arthritis. Am Rev Resp Dis. 133:450-4

80. Solal-Celigny Ph, Laviolette M, Hebert, Cormier Y (1982). Immune reactions in the lungs of asymptomatic dairy farmers. Am Rev resp Dis 126:964-967

81. Stoller JK, Rankin JA, Reynolds HY (1987). The impact of broncho-alveolar lavage cell analysis on clinicians diagnostic reasoning about interstitial lung disease. Chest 92:839-843

82. Klech (1986). Sarcoidosis, Differential Diagnosis. Sem Resp Med 8:72-94

83. Rudd EM, Haslam P, Turner-Warwick M (1980). Cryptogenic fibrosing alveolitis: relationship of pulmonary physiology and bronchoalveolar lavage to response to treatment and prognosis. Am Rev Resp Dis 124:1-8

84. Turner-Warwick M, Haslam P (1987). The value of serial broncho-alveolar lavages in assessing the clinical progress of patients with Cryptogenic fibrosing alveolitis. Am Rev Resp Dis 135:26-34

85. Roth C, Huchon GJ, Arnoux A, Stanislas-Leguern G. Marsac JH, Chretien J (1980). Bronchoalveolar cells in advanced pulmonary sarcoidosis. Am Rev Resp Dis 132:1060-1065.

86. Maffre JP, Tuchon E, Oury M (1987). Early neutrophil alveolitis in Löfgren syndrome. Abstract of XI. World Congress of Sarcoidosis Milan, Sept.1987, page 46.

87. Bjermer L, Thunell M, Hällgren R (1986). Mast cells in bronchoalveo-lar lavage (BAL) in patients with sarcoidosis. Sarcoidosis 3:182

88. Haslam PL, Dewer A, Butchers P, Primett ZS, Newman-Taylor A, Turner-Warwick M (1987). Mast cells , atypical lymphocytes and Neutro-phils in Broncho Alveolar Lavage in extrinsic allergic alveolitis. Comparison with other interstitial lung diseases. Am Rev Resp Dis 135:35-47

89. Klech H, Neuchrist C, Pohl W, Rona-Selnic G, Scheiner O, Sorg C, Knapp W, Luger Th, Kraft D (1987). Patterns of maturity in Broncho-alveolar lavage Macrophages in Sarcoidosis. Abstract of XI.World Congress of Sarcoidosis, Milan , Sept.1987, page 5

90. Ainslie GM, Poulter LW, DuBois RM (1987). Alveolar macrophage sub-populations and disease intensity in sarcoidosis. Abstract of XI. World Congress of sarcoidosis, Milan, Sept.1987, page 4

91. Bitterman BP, Rennard SI, Adelberg S, Crystal RG (1983). Role of fibronectin as a growth factor for fibroblasts. J Cell Biol 97:1925-32.

92. Rennard SI, Bitterman PB, Crystal RG (1984). Pathogenesis of fibrosis in the granulomatous lung diseases. Am Rev resp Dis 130:492-6

93. Bitterman PB, Adelberg S, Crystal RG (1983). Mechanisms of pulmonary fibrosis: spontaneous release of the alveolar macrophage derived growth factor in the interstitial lung disorders. J Clin Invest 72:1801-13.

94. Robinson BW, McLanore L, Crystal RG (1985). Gamma Interferon is spontaneously released by alveolar macrophages and lung T-lympho-cytes in patients with pulmonary sarcoidosis. J Clin Invest 75:1488-1495.

95. Rankin JR, Naegel GP, Schrader CE, Matthay RA, Reynolds HY (1983). Air-Space Immunoglobulin Production and Levels in Bronchoalveolar Lavage Fluid of Normal Subjects and Patients with Sarcoidosis. Am Rev Resp Dis 127:442-448.

96. Bauer W, Gorny MK, Baumann HR, Morell A (1985). T-Lymphocyte Subsets and Immunoglobulin Concentrations in Bronchoalveolar Lavage of Pa-tients with Sarcoidosis and High and Low Intensity Alveolitis. Am rev Resp Dis 132:1060-1065

482

97. Lawrence EC, Martin RR, Blaese RM et al (1980). Increased broncho-
     alveolar IgG secreting cells in interstitial lung diseases.
     N Engl J Med 302:1186-88.

98. Hunninghake GW, Crystal RG (1981). Mechanism of hypergammaglobulin-
     urie in pulmonary sarcoidosis. J Clin Invest 67:86-92

99. Davis GS, Giancola Ms, Costanza MC, Low RB (1982). Analyses of
     sequential bronchoalveolar lavage samples from healthy human volun-
     teers. Am Rev Resp Dis 126:611-6.

100. Baughman RP, Bosken CH, Loudon RG, Hurtubise P, Wesseler T (1983).
     Quantitation of bronchoalveolar lavage with methylene blue.
     Am Rev Resp Dis 128:266-70.

101. Rennard S. Basset G, Lecossier D, O'Donnell K, Martin P, Crystal RG
     (1986). Estimations of the absolute volume of epithelial lining
     fluid recovered by bronchoalveolar lavage using urea as as endo-
     genous marker of dilution. J Appl Physiol 60:532-8.

CLINICAL ASPECTS OF EXTRAPULMONARY SARCOIDOSIS

© 1988 Elsevier Science Publishers B.V. (Biomedical Division)
Sarcoidosis and other granulomatous disorders
C. Grassi, G. Rizzato, E. Pozzi, editors

SYNOVIAL SARCOIDOSIS IN CHILDREN. REPORT OF SIX CASES

F. Fantini,Gerloni V.,Murelli M.,Gattinara M.,Negro A.,Sciascia T.
Centre for Rheumatic Children, Chair of Rheumatology of the
University of Milan, Gaetano Pini Institute, Milan (Italy)

Synovial sarcoidosis (or sarcoid arthritis) constitutes a
special syndrome in infants and young children, which so closely
mimics juvenile rheumatoid arthritis (JRA) that differentiating the
two conditions in long-lasting disease is often impossible on
clinical grounds alone (1).
Since 1970 at our Centre in Milan 6 cases of synovial
sarcoidosis in children have been diagnosed (all by synovial
surgical biopsy), whose stories and findings are hereinafter
briefly reported.

CASE REPORTS

Case # 1. P.G. is a boy, now 24 years old. When 3 he presented a
diffuse slightly scaling rash and hand swelling with elevated ESR
and leukocytosis. A presumptive diagnosis of JRA was proposed and
steroids were administered. After steroid withdrawal
polytenosynovitis and polyarthritis with involvement of wrists,
knees, ankles, feet and hands with moderate pain and stiffness set
in. At age 5 the child was hospitalized: he presented also a
micropapular rash. A skin biopsy and a synovial biopsy were
performed and in spite of the presence of granulomas with giant
cells the diagnosis of JRA was retained and the child was put on
steroids and cyclophosphamide for about 1 year (25-50 mg a day).
Later oral steroids were discontinued and the boy was treated with
local steroids and NSAIDs. The boy entered our Centre when 10: he
presented a maculopapular rash, micropolyadenopathy, huge boggy
thenosynovitis of wrists and ankles, polyarthritis with effusion at
elbows, MCP and PIP joints, knees and feet. There was a slight ESR
elevation, both RF and ANA serology were negative. X ray pictures
showed diffuse osteoporosis, soft tissue swelling, finger and toe
subluxation and structural changes of several bones, in particular
widening of finger phalanges with spongialization of compact bone.
The boy underwent a thenosynovectomy at both ankles. The histology
of removed tissue showed the typical sarcoid granulomas. A lymph
node biopsy confirmed the diagnosis. A low-dose steroid treatment
(prednisone 5 mg) was started with beneficial effect on joint
symptoms. After 6 months the steroid treatment was discontinued and
short courses were administered when needed because of joint
symptoms. At age 13 the boy presented a cranial polyneuropathy with
dysphonia, dysphagia, facial palsy probably due to sarcoidotic
granulomatous basilar meningitis. A high-dose steroid treatment was
instituted (prednisone 2 mg/Kg/day) with almost complete remission
of neurological signs. Since then the patient has been on steroids,
with maintenance dosage of 15-10 mg prednisone on alternate days.
Tapering attempts have been followed by relapse of neurological
signs. Alternate day steroid regimen has been well tolerated: no
growth disturbances have been observed. The patient only rarely
presents a swollen knee or tendon sheath. An ophtalmologic check
showed some anterior lens opacities as sequelae of posterior
synechiae. Chest X rays never presented abnormalities. HLA
phenotype: A 9,w19(29); B 5,12(44); DR w6,X.

Case #2. C.C. is a boy, now 22. When 7 mild fever, weakness and swollen ankles occurred. Later persistent swelling of wrists and pain with functional impairment at both hands appeared. When first seen by us the patient was 10 years old. No skin lesions were present. A diffuse slight lymph node enlargement was appreciable. A boggy tendon sheath swelling was present at wrists and ankles; in addition there was a symmetrical polyarthritis involving the MCP, PIP and DIP joints with mild "bouttoniere" deformity. The ESR was moderately elevated, a slight hypergammaglobulinemia with increased IgG (1465 mg/dl) was present, RF and ANA serology were negative. The main finding of X rays was soft tissue swelling, moreover the hands showed osteoporosis and widening with spongialization of some metacarpals and phalanges. Chest X ray was negative and at that time an eye check showed no pathological changes. A tenosynovectomy of the right ankle was performed: the histologic examination showed the typical sarcoid granulomas. A low-dose steroid treatment was prescribed, but unfortunately the patient did not comply and was lost at follow-up. Recently the patient has been contacted by phone: on inquiry he explained that he has presented a severe bilateral uveitis which has been inadequately treated and now he is almost blind.

Case #3. M.N. is a boy, now 19. Since the age of 2 he presented follicular dyscheratosis. When 4 swollen wrists and ankles were noticed. At the age of 5 he presented eye redness and photophobia: an ophtalmologic visit revealed a severe picture of eye impairment with anterior and posterior synechiae and lens opacities. The child was hospitalized: a height and weight deficit and a polyarthritic condition were ascertained, a presumptive diagnosis of JRA was proposed. Elevated ESR and leukocytosis were recorded. The boy entered our Centre when 7: he presented a diffuse polyarthritis and polytenosynovitis with boggy tendon sheath effusion. Micropolyadenia was palpable. Leukocytosis was confirmed. RF and ANA serology were negative. X ray pictures showed mainly diffuse osteoporosis. Eye examination demonstrated a complicated cataract in both eyes. Surgical biopsy was performed on a tendon sheath and on a lymph node: both showed typical sarcoid granulomas. A low-dose steroid treatment was started. Surgery for complicated cataracts was performed but the eye condition went on worsening. The patient was lost at follow-up for a while. He reentered the hospital when he was 16: he was almost completely blind, his joint condition was poor and a marked muscle atrophy was also present. An intensive physiotherapy program was started and an alternate day steroid regimen was instituted (now deflazacort 12 mg on aa.dd.) with some functional improvement. Now he is 158 cm tall and weighs 39.5 Kg. X ray pictures show marked structural changes (especially brachymetacarpia) with some erosive features in the feet. No chest X ray changes have been observed.

Case #4. B.R. is a boy, now 17 years old. When 13 months old a scrotal granuloma was noticed: the biopsy showed a giant cell granuloma without caseum. A short time later a polysynovitis developed with generalized arthritis and boggy tendon sheath swelling. In spite of a synovial biopsy showing clear granulomatous sarcoid lesions, a presumptive diagnosis of JRA was proposed and the patient accordingly treated with steroids, gold salts and cytostatic drugs. A severe bilateral uveitis with rapidly evolutive eye impairment developed. When first seen by us the patient was 14, he presented polyarthritis with moderate pain and marked joint stiffness and limitation of movements, boggy effusions were present at wrists and ankles. The ophtalmologic visit showed phtisis bulbi on one side and complicated cataract at the other side. A micropolyadenopathy was present. He was 149 cm tall and his weight was 29.5 Kg. There were moderate ESR elevation, anemia, leukocytosis and hypergammaglobulinemia. RF and ANA serology were negative. X ray pictures showed diffuse osteoporosis, soft tissue enlargement, structural bone changes and some joint erosions and deformations. A low-dose steroid regimen was started (deflazacort 12 mg on aa.dd.) plus intensive physiotherapy with marked functional muscular and joint improvement. Now he is 160 cm tall and his weight is 48.5 Kg. No lung involvement. HLA phenotype: A 1,9(24); B 5,12(44); DR 3,4.

Case #5. M.M. is a little girl, now 6 year old. When 7 months old he presented a diffuse maculopapular rash; shortly later swelling of wrists, hands, ankles and knees with moderate pain and morning slowness appeared. A skin biopsy was inconclusive. The little girl was hospitalized in our Centre when 3 years old: she presented boggy tendon sheath swelling at wrists and ankles and a generalized polyarthritis with a marked height and weight deficit. There was a slight ESR elevation with leukocytosis (mainly lymph). RF and ANA serology were negative. Hand X rays showed structural bone changes (widening and periostosis of phalanges). An ophtalmologic visit detected only tiny endotelial pigmented precipitates on the cornea. The synovial surgical biopsy performed on the right hand extensor sheath revealed the typical sarcoid granulomas. An initially high-dose steroid regimen was started (6,methyl-prednisolone 12 mg/day) with marked functional joint improvement, which was later tapered until a maintenance dosage of 8 mg on alternate days, while the growth chart showed a complete height and weight recovery. HLA phenotype: A 9,w19; B 7,18(?); DR w6,7.

Case #6. M.T. is a girl, now 9 years old. When 6 ankle swelling with some walking difficulties were noticed. Some months later a symmetrical polyarthritis with involvement of hands and wrists and morning stiffness set in. The little girl was hospitalized: a presumptive diagnosis of JRA was proposed and a treatment with ASA was started. The ESR was slightly raised and a mild leukocytosis was recorded. When first seen by us the patient was 9 and her condition was stationary. Follicular dyscheratosis was diagnosed by the dermatologist. There persisted the bulking ankle tenosynovitis and the symmetrical upper extremity polyarthritis with moderately raised ESR and mild leukocytosis (mainly lymph). RF was negative, but ANA resulted slightly positive (1/80 on Hep2-cells). Hand X rays showed mild structural bone changes of some phalanges. A tenosynovectomy of right foot extensors was performed and at histology the sarcoid granulomas were demonstrated. No eye abnormality was observed. Chest X rays were normal. A low-dose steroid regimen was instituted (deflazacort 15 mg on aa.dd.) with beneficial effect on joints and general growth. HLA phenotype: A 1,2; B 5,18; DR 5,X.

DISCUSSION

Sarcoidosis of the synovium in children affects both tendon sheaths and joints and, since from a clinical point of view tenosynovitis is more striking than arthrosynovitis, we think that the term "synovial sarcoidosis" (SS) is more proper than "sarcoid arthritis" to define this condition.

Although a rare disease, SS in Italian children is not exceptional: during the period of time in which our 6 cases were observed, about 400 cases of JRA were diagnosed, so, according to our experience, the prevalence ratio between SS and JRA is about 0.015 (= 6/400).

Although in all cases the prevalent site of the disease was the synovium, in the majority of them the condition was multisystemic with involvement particularly of skin, eyes and lymph nodes (Table I). In most cases, sometimes notwithstanding a positive biopsy, the correct diagnosis was established only later on. Delay in diagnosis (#3 and #4) together with improper treatment (#2) seem to be the main causes of a poor prognosis, especially with regard to loss of sight. A rather surprising fact was that no patient showed clinical signs of lung sarcoidosis.

TABLE I. MAIN CLINICAL FEATURES OF REPORTED PATIENTS

Sex ratio M/F		4/2	
Onset age (yr)	mean	3.6	(range 0.8-7)
Diagnosis age (yr)	mean	8.7	(range 3-14)
Diagnosis delay (yr)	mean	5.0	(range 2-13)
Actual age (yr)	mean	16.2	(range 6-24)

Tenosynovitis	6/6	Polyneuritis	1/6
Polyarthritis	6/6	Lung involvement	0/6
Skin rashes	5/6	Joint disability	2/6
Eye involvement	5/6	Eye disability	3/6
Lymphnode involv.	4/6	Growth deficit	1/6

3 out of the 4 tissue-typed cases presented the B5 phenotype (against a control frequency of 21 %) (corrected chi-square = 4.122, $p < 0.05$, relative risk = 11.24): this same phenotype has been found associated with polyarticular onset seronegative juvenile chronic arthritis (2) and pauciarticular onset juvenile chronic arthritis with polyarticular course (3). These data suggest that also for sarcoidosis a genetic element of susceptibility could be important in conditioning the expression of the disease in children.

REFERENCES

1. North A.F.Jr., Fink C.W., Gibson W.M., Levinson J.E., Schuchter S.L., Howard W.K., Johnson N.H., Harris C. (1970) Am.J.Med. 48, 449

2. Hall P.J., Burman S.J., Barash J., Ansell B.M. XI European Congress of Rheumatology, Athens, 28th June-4th July 1987, Abstract F 488 - Clin. Exper. Rheumatology (1987) 5, suppl 2, 139

3. Fantini F. Unpublished observations

© 1988 Elsevier Science Publishers B.V. (Biomedical Division)
Sarcoidosis and other granulomatous disorders
C. Grassi, G. Rizzato, E. Pozzi, editors

ON THE EXISTENCE OF MICROANGIOPATHY IN SARCOIDOSIS

RIICHIRO MIKAMI, MORIE SEKIGUCHI, YOSHITADA RYUJIN, FUMIKO KOBAYASHI,
YOMEI HIRAGA, YUKIHIKO SHIMADA, ICHIRO MOCHIZUKI, SHIZUO TAMURA

Japan Sarcoidosis Research Committee, Clinical Research Center for Rheumato-
Allergology, National Sagamihara Hospital, Sagamihara City, 228 (Japan)

INTRODUCTION

In 1972, a 39-year-old female patient developed uveitis, bilateral hilar
lymphadenopathy and pulmonary lesions. During the previous ten years, she had
also developed pulmonary fibrosis, skin eruption, muscle weakness and proteinu-
ria. Biopsies revealed epithelioid granulomas in the skin and muscle, glomerulonephritis and arteriolar lesions in the kidney. The ocular fundi showed remarkable vascular changes. Since then, the authors began to pay much attention
to peripheral vascular changes. Our decade-long study regarding the changes in
the peripheral vasculature in various organs was recently introduced [1].
The purpose of this presentation is to briefly introduce our most recent research
regarding the systemic peripheral vascular changes and to describe our concept
on the existence of microangiopathy.

MATERIALS AND METHODS

Other than conventional histopathological diagnosis of sarcoidosis in target
organs, fundoscopic (n=63), bronchoscopic (n=130), and biopsy histopathologic
and electronmicroscopic examinations [skeletal muscle (n=29), cardiac muscle
(n=18), kidney (n=15), lung (n=7), peripheral nerve (n=1)]were carried out. In
all cases, more than 2 or 3 kinds of examinations in various organs were carried
out in each of the institutions of our group. Conventional methods were applied
in each study. For the statistical analysis, the data were analyzed and evaluated using chi-square test.

RESULTS (Figs. 1-7)

Typical signs of ocular sarcoidosis which include iritis, uveitis, string of
pearls and periphlebitis were found in 33 of the 63 cases (52%). Signs of microangiopathy (fig. 1) were seen in 58 cases (92%). They were string of pearls, 15
(24%); periphlebitis,14 (22%); parallel pipestem leakage or sheathing,24 (38%);
venous widening, engorgement of tortuosity, 22 (35%); and newly formed capillaries or abnormal course of vessels 31(49%). Nonspecific vascular reactions were
also observed in 61 (97%). Bronchoscopy revealed a network formation of small
blood vessels of the bronchial mucosa in 114 out of 130 sarcoidosis cases (88%),
but in only 5 out of 131 control cases (4%) with various other pulmonary
diseases (p<0.001). Fluorescence bronchial angiography clearly demonstrated the

490

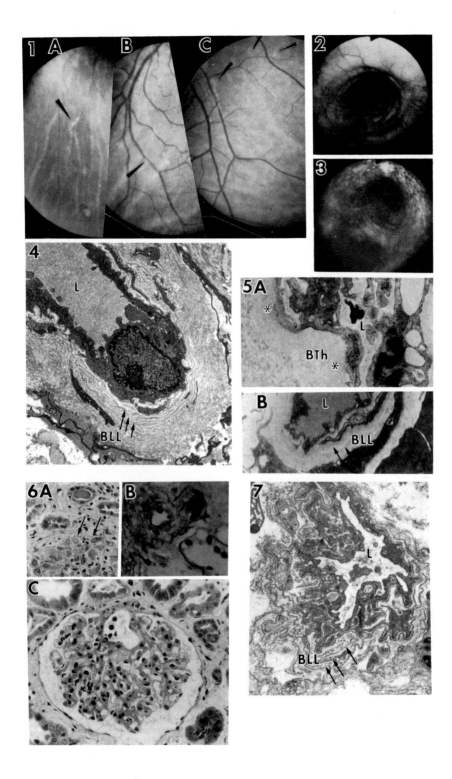

vascular network and signs of abnormal leakage from the vasculature in all 18 cases studied. Electronmicroscopic studies in a transbronchial lung biopsy(n=7) revealed basal lamina layering in small bronchi in 2/2 cases (100%) but no changes in the alveoli and respiratory bronchioles in all 7 cases (Fig. 2). In the skeletal muscle biopsy, sarcoid granulomas were found in 52% of the cases, and at sites where no granulomas were seen, perivascular fibrosis was noted very often. The EM in 20 cases revealed endothelial lesions in 55%, and basal lamina lesions in 60%, which consisted of thickening (25%), lamellation (15%) and irregularity (45%). Endomyocardial biopsy revealed the granulomas only in 4/18 cases (22%), but interstitial fobrosis was seen in all cases. Basal lamina layering (BLL) was observed in 14/18 cases (78%). Control biopsies in 20 cases with hypertrophic cardiomyopathy showed the BLL in 1/20 cases (5%)($p < 0.001$). In the 15 kidney biopsy cases, only 3 cases revealed the granuloma (20%) but anteriolar changes (vasculitis and intimal thickening) were seen in 12 (80%). Another important finding to be noted was glomerulopathy, which we saw in all 15 cases. The changes were interpreted as glomerulitis in 8, glomerulonephritis in 6 and hyalinization in 1 case. Among 10 cases where the kidney biopsies were performed, vascular changes in other organs were noted in ocular fundi in 9/10, skeletal muscle 5/6 and bronchoscopically observed network formation in 2/2 cases.

DISCUSSION

The following observations which we have made[1-7] may signify that systematic microangiopathy exists in sarcoidosis; 1. fundoscopically and bronchoscopically assessed peripheral vascular changes[3], 2. histopathologically assessed arteriolar thickening or perivascular fibrosis in various organs[1,2], 3. endothelial changes and basal lamina layering or thickening seen by electronmicroscope in

---

EXPLANATIONS OF FIGURES

1. Ocular fundi showing
   (A) increased vasculature showing exsudative signs.
   (B) signs of narrowing of the arteries.
   (C) string of pearls and foci of chorioretinal turbidity.

2. A bronchoscopic view showing network formation of small blood vessels.

3. Fluorescence bronchial angiogram demonstrating increased vascularity and leakage of dye.

4. Transbronchial lung biopsy showing basal lamina layering (BLL) of the capillaries in the small bronchi.

5. Skeletal muscle biopsy showing lamellation (BLL:A) and thickening(BTh:B) of the capillary basement menbranes.

6. Kidney biopsy showing a granuloma (A), arteriolar thickening (B) and glomerulopathy (C). A and C are taken from the same case.

7. Basal lamina layering in a endomyocardial biopsy specimen.

the skeletal or cardiac muscle[2,6], bronchus[5] and in the peripheral nerve. We also found a slightly different pathology, i.e., glomerulopathy[7]. This should not be called microangiopathy but the authors believe that a similar pathology is taking place as deposition of IgG was seen in the diseased site of the glomerulus and in the small arteries showing that there is some immune complex. Although the exact mechanism of the microangiopathic disorders is not well understood, it occurs independently of granulomatous disease.

SUMMARY

Systematic studies regarding the existence of microangiopathy in sarcoidosis have not appeared in the literature. We have paid special attention to the peripheral vasculature in various organs in our group study employing fundoscopic (n=63), bronchoscopic (n=130) and biopsy histopathologic and electron-microscopic examinations (skeletal muscle 29, cardiac muscle 18, kidney 15, and lung 7 cases, and peripheral nerve 1 case). Newly formed capillaries or abnormal course of vessels, parallel pipestem leakage or sheathing, venous or tortuosity and phlebitis and string of pearls in the ocular fundi, network formation of the small vessels in the bronchoscopy, arteriolar changes or perivascular fibrosis, endothelial changes and basal lamina layering or thickening of the capillaries were observed. The incidence of the above changes ranged from 78%-92% of the cases. Glomerular changes which were interpreted as glomerulitis or glomerulonephritis were seen in all kidney biopsy cases. It was noteworthy that the morphologically detected microangiopathic changes were essentially devoid of granulomatous changes. Therefore, in addition to systemic granulomatous disease, systemic microangiopathy should be included as part of the clinicopathological entity of sarcoidosis.

REFERENCES

1. Mikami, R et al. (1986) Heart and Vessels 2: 129-139

2. Mikami, R et al. (1981) In: Mikami R, Hosoda Y (eds) Sarcoidosis Univ of Tokyo Press, Tokyo PP 236-244

3. Kobayashi F (1981) ibid PP. 99-108

4. Hiraga Y et al. (1986) Ann Ny Acad S: 465: 731-737

5. Tamura S et al. (1985) Sarcoidosis 2: 68 (abstr.)

6. Sekiguchi M et al. (1985) Heart and Vessels Suppl 1: 45-49

7. Ryujin Y et al. (1985) Sarcoidosis 2: 65 (abstr.)

OPHTHALMIC CHANGES IN SARCOIDOSIS : A PROSPECTIVE STUDY OF 308 PATIENTS

M.R. ANGI, F. FORATTINI, °A. CIPRIANI, ^P. CAPELLI, "G. SEMENZATO
Departments of Ophthalmology, °Pneumology and "Internal Medicine, Padova
University School of Medicine, Padova; ^Department of Pathology, Verona
University School of Medicine, Verona, Italy.

INTRODUCTION

Sarcoidosis is a multi-system disease of unknown etiology, defined in the past
on clinical and histological grounds and more recently by a series of immunological parameters including the T lymphopenia associated with "in vivo" and "in
vitro" hyporesponsiveness in blood and enhanced immune responses at sites of
involvement (1). Sarcoidosis frequently involves the lungs, hilum-mediastinal
and peripheral lymph glands, skin, liver, spleen and bones. The frequency with
which the disease is localized in the eye and its adnexa is differently quoted
according to the means of instrumental investigation used (biomicroscopy, fluoro-
angiography, 67-Gallium scans), the type of study (prospective or retrospective),
the recruitment of cases (through General Doctors, Pneumologists, Internists or
Ophthalmologists) and also the patients' race: it is well known in fact that
ocular symptoms of Sarcoidosis are more common in Negroes than in Caucasians (2).

The aim of this work was to evaluate the prevalence and incidence of these
ocular symptoms and the response to therapy in 308 Italian patients affected by
Sarcoidosis examined over the past four years at the Ophthalmology Department
of Padua University.

MATERIALS AND METHODS

308 patients (146 men and 162 women aged 39 + 10 years and 44 + 13 years)
with biopsy-proven pulmonary, lymphnodal or cutaneous Sarcoidosis were studied.
The disease was first diagnosed from 6 months to 25 years (mean 7.7 years)
prior to admission to our Department. The diagnosis of Sarcoidosis was based
on consistent clinical features and histological findings; the activity of the
disease through broncho-alveolar lavage and 67 Gallium scans. In all cases the
biopsy material obtained from the lungs or lymphnodes showed characteristic
epithelioid cell granulomata without caseation; special stain for acid-fast
bacilli and polarized light failed to reveal organisms or foreign bodies in
the tissues.

Objective ophthalmic conditions were examined every 6 months, or more often
if necessary and always by the same team of doctors; the follow-up lasted from
9 months to 4 years (mean 2.9 years). The eye tests included measurement of
visual acuity and ocular pressure, the Schirmer I test to evaluate tear flow,

biomicroscopy of the conjunctiva and anterior segment to detect the presence
of nodules in the conjunctiva, iris or camerular angle or the presence of uveitis.
Examination of the posterior pole and retinal periphery was carried out by means
of indirect ophthalmoscopy and Goldmann lens with scleral depression. Biopsy of
the conjunctiva and fluorangiography were carried out on the basis of clinical
signs.

TABLE I

STAGING OF 308 ITALIAN PATIENTS AFFECTED WITH SARCOIDOSIS

Stage	Men	%	Women	%	Totals	%
0	7	4.8	11	6.8	18	5.8
I	82	56.2	82	50.6	164	53.2
II	44	30.1	59	36.4	103	33.4
III	13	8.9	10	6.2	23	7.5
Totals	146	100	162	100	308	100
Mean age (yrs)	39 $\pm$ 10		44 $\pm$ 13			
Range	20 - 66		22 - 66			

RESULTS

The data obtained on these patients is given in Table I. We found a slight
predominance of female patients over males among the cases we studied. The
majority of patients was aged between 30 and 50 years and we recorded no cases
in pediatric age nor aged over 66.

The prevalence and incidence of ocular changes in Sarcoidosis are given in
Table II and III. 17.5 % of cases had a positive Schirmer test and an abnormal
67-Gallium gain in the lachrymal gland region, indicating a current or previous
inflammation of the lachrymal glands. Seven cases of hypolacrimation occurred
in the course of the study. This hypolacrimation was symptomatic only in 4 cases:
3 patients affected with keratitis sicca, and one with a swelling in the outer
super-orbital region. The lack of subjective symptoms may be explained considering how the lipidic and mucous components of the lachrymal film, produced by
accessory glands situated on the conjunctival level, are not normally damaged
by sarcoidosis. The lachrymal film is therefore reduced in quantity but without
losing its lubricating capacity.

Conjunctival nodules were found in 91 cases; the biopsy, which was carried
out as a routine procedure to establish the nature of the suspected lesions
observed with the slit-lamp, confirmed the presence of sarcoid granulomata in
49 patients (15.9%), 9 of which became apparent in the course of the study. In

495

27 patients à biopsy of the conjunctiva was carried out even though there were
no lesions visible under the biomicroscope, and demonstrated the presence of
sarcoid granulomata in 3 cases. By comparison with the traditional histological
techniques, the immuno-histological and histochemical evaluations enabled us to
better detect the initial granulomatous lesions (3). In all the conjunctival
biopsies obtained, the predominant cells had the morphology of lymphocytes,
forming lymphoid infiltrates or surrounding granulomatous lesions. They consisted
mainly of T cells bearing the helper-related phenotype; the distribution of T
suppressor subsets appeared more restricted to the periphery of the granulomata
(Figure 1). Staining with alpha-naphtyl-esterase demonstrated the presence of
macrophagic aggregates, thus enabling us to distinguish between the initial
granulomas and the lymphatic follicles frequently found in conjunctival mucosa.

TABLE II
PREVALENCE OF OPHTHALMIC CHANGES IN 308 PATIENTS AFFECTED WITH SARCOIDOSIS

Signs	N. of cases	%	Onset	%
Hypolachrymation	54	17.5	-	
Conjunctival nodules	91	29.5	-	
Histologically verified conj. sarcoid granuloma	52	16.9	-	
Anterior uveitis	9	2.9	5	1.6
Vitreous opacities Perivasculitis/vasculitis Chorioretinitis	41	13.3	3	1.0
Panuveitis	1	0.3	-	
Optic nerv disease	1	0.3	-	

It is worth emphasising that anterior uveitis was rarely found in our patients:
this fact confirms and extends the findings of other Authors (4,5) and appears
to be due neither to a loss of cases in the course of the study nor to an incomplete eye test. On the other hand, the recruitment of patients, which in our
case was done through our colleagues in pneumology and internal medicine, may
have influenced the percentage of ocular lesions - which would have been higher
if a selection of cases had been identified by ophthalmologists.

The involvement of posterior segment (vitreous opacities, vasculitis, chorio-
retinitis) was apparent in 41 patients overall. Two patients had macular involvement which had given rise to a permanent reduction in visual acuity. In one
case there was a violent panuveitis, with a secondary detachment of the retina

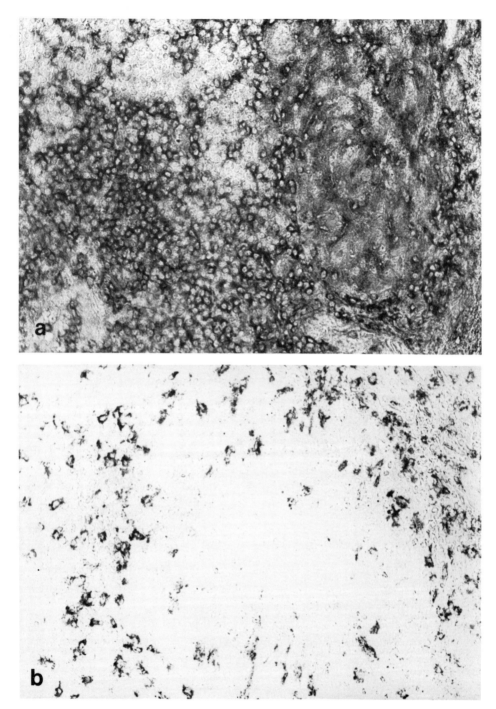

Figure 1. A conjunctival sarcoid granuloma immunostained for different T cell specific monoclonal antibodies. In a) Leu-3 reagent showing a large number of lymphocytes of helper-inducer phenotype around and within the granuloma. b) only a few Leu-2 suppressor-cytotoxic cells are found, mainly surrounding the granuloma.

and loss of sight; the corticosteroid therapy administered systemically and through retro-bulbar injections did not stop evolution of the disease. One case of optic disc swelling was reported together with a retinal vasculitis.

TABLE III

INCIDENCE OF OPHTHALMIC CHANGES DURING THE COURSE OF THE STUDY

Signs	N. of cases	%
Hypolachrymation	7	2.3
Conjunctival sarcoid granulomata	9	2.9
Anterior uveitis	4	1.3
Posterior uveitis	5	1.6
Panuveitis	1	0.3

In conclusion, the prevalence of ophthalmic changes found in this study was 19.8 % (61 cases), which is in agreement with data reported in other studies (4,5). The difference lies in the distribution of the ocular lesions, which in our experience proved mainly to involve the ocular adnexa, while in other studies (6,7) they more frequently involved the anterior uvea and the posterior segment.

The data obtained in this study further emphasize the utility of conjunctival biopsy in the clinical management of Sarcoidosis and also provide information on the ocular immunopathology of this disease: the close relationship between activated macrophages and T helper cells represents the event that triggers the formation of sarcoid granuloma in the conjunctiva as well as in other affected tissues (8).

REFERENCES

1. Angi MR, Cipriani A, Ossi E. et al. (1984) In: KM Saari (ed) Uveitis update Elsevier, Amsterdam, pp 337-343.

2. Merrit JC, Lipper SL et al. (1980) J Natl Med Assoc 72:347

3. Angi MR, Chilosi M, Agostini C et al. (1986) Bull Mem SFO 97:111-115

4. Karma A (1979) Acta Ophthalmol (suppl 141): 5-86

5. Bardelli AM, Barberi L, Lasorella G (1984) Boll Ocul 63:1119-1127

6. Obenauf CD, Shaw HE, Sydnor CF et al (1978) Am J Ophthalmol 86:648-655

7. James DG, Neville E, Langley DA (1976) Trans Ophth Soc UK 96:133-139

8. Semenzato G, Pezzutto A, Pizzolo G et al (1984) Clin Immunol Immunopathol 30:29-40.

PHOSPHOCALCIC METABOLISM, BONE QUANTITATIVE HISTOMORPHOMETRY AND CLINICAL
ACTIVITY IN 10 CASES OF SARCOIDOSIS

J. M. VERGNON[1], D. CHAPPARD[2], D. MOUNIER[1], A. EMONOT[1], C. ALEXANDRE[2]
1 - Department of pneumology, 2 - LBTO, University hospital St Etienne France

Phosphocalcic metabolism abnormalities are well known in sarcoidosis but
the frequency is diversely appreciated : the prevalence of hypercalciuria
reachs 60 % of the cases (1) while hypercalcemia is around 11 % (2). Several
recent studies (3,4,5) have demonstrated an extrarenal secretion of
1 α hydroxylase by sarcoid granuloma macrophages, which changes inactive
25 OH cholecalciferol in active 1-25 (OH)2 cholecalciferol (active vitamin D3).
It induces an increase of calcium intestinal absorption which is the more
important factor in the pathogenesis of hypercalcemia or hypercalciuria (6).
However 1-25 (OH)2 D3 also stimulates osteoclastic bone resorption which
may contribute to calcium changes (7). The aim of this study was to investigate
bone resorption in sarcoidosis using quantitative bone histomorphometry and
to correlate the results with the clinical activity of the disease.

PATIENTS AND METHODS
1) Patients
10 patients (2 males, 8 females, mean age 41.9 $\pm$ 10.7 Y) were included.
All patients presented an untreated histologically confirmed sarcoidosis. In
3 cases, it was a typical acute Loefgren Syndrom and in 7 cases, it was an
active thoracic sarcoidosis according to clinical, radiographic and functional
data. This activity was scaled in four groups. Low intensity : non evolutive
and asymptomatic sarcoidosis. Moderate intensity : moderate symptoms without
functional impairement. High intensity : acute symptoms without aggressive
impairement. Very high intensity : aggressive sarcoidosis, acute symptoms
and diffuse involvement. In 6 of these 10 cases, extrathoracic extension were
noted. Only one patient presented a bone osteolytic involvement.
2) Methods
- Bone biopsies were performed under local anesthesia, at the iliac crest.
The transiliac bone cores (8 mm in diameter) were immediately fixed and kept
at 4°C. Detailed procedures have been extensively described else-where (8,9)

. Total Trabecular Resorption Surfaces (TTRS) are expressed as a percentage of the total trabecular surfaces occupied by scalloped resorbed
surfaces (Howship lacunae).

Osteoclast number was measured at a magnification of x 100, using a semiautomatic image analyser. Only cells with tartrate resistant phosphatase acid activity and in close contact with the calcified bone surfaces were taken into account (10). The count was related to the trabecular surfaces (mm2). In Loefgren syndroms, the bone biopsy was performed around 2 months after the onset of symptoms. In the other cases, the biopsy was performed 18 $\pm$ 13.3 months after the first symptoms.

- Calcemia, calciuria, hydroxyprolinuria, 25 (OH) cholecalciferol, calcitonin and parathormone levels were measured at the time of the biopsy. 1-25 (OH)2 cholecalciferol levels could not be studied.

- The follow-up of the patients after the biopsy was 44.7 $\pm$ 26.1 months. The clinical status was appreciated on clinical, radiological and functional data as were measured calcemia and calciuria.

RESULTS

- Hypercalciuria was found in 4/10 patients associated with hypercalcemia in 3 of them. In these 3 cases, hypercalcemia was associated with hyperhydroxyprolinuria. Parathormone, calcitonin and 25-(OH) cholecalciferol levels were normal in all patients.

- Quantitative bone histomorphometry showed an increase of TTRS at 7.49 % $\pm$ 3.84 (normal values 3.6 % $\pm$ 1.1) with an increase of active osteoclasts per mm2 of trabecular bone : 6.57 $\pm$ 3.4 (normal values 3.83 $\pm$ 1.75). In hypercalcemic patients, bone resorption was significantly higher, (TTRS 12.1 $\pm$ 4.4 %) than in other patients (5.49 $\pm$ 0.58 %) p $<$ 0.01. In contrast, all other morphometric data (trabecular bone volume and osteoblastic parameters) were normal. In two patients (1/2 hypercalcemic), sarcoid granulomas were found in the marrow space. Some of these granulomas were surrounded by large TTRS and elevated osteoclast number.

- Correlations with clinical activity

In recent sarcoidosis (Loefgren syndroms), where the biopsies were performed a few days after the onset of the disease, no correlation was found between the high clinical level of activity and the bone histological disturbances. The regression of the disease occured in about 6 months. In the other cases, at the time of the biopsy, clinical activity was well correlated with TTRS, but not with the long term status of these patients, except when TTRS increase was associated with hypercalcemia : the follow-up showed a severe evolution with many recurrences in the first case (each time with concomittant increase of calciuria and hydroxyprolinuria), progressive sarcoid pulmonary fibrosis

in the 2nd case, renal lithiasis, renal failure, and steroid resistant hypercalcemia in the third case (but with good efficiency of cyclosporin A).

COMMENTS

Evidence of increased 1-25 (OH)2 cholecalciferol levels are found in sarcoidosis (3,4,5). The main biological effects of active vitamin D are the increase
of calcium absorption in the intestinal tract and the increase of calcium
resorption in bone by stimulating osteoclast activity (5,6). These 2 effects
can explain hypercalcemia, hypercalciuria and hyperhydroxyprolinuria in
sarcoidosis. Elevated TTRS on bone biopsies from sarcoidosis without increased
parathormone or 25-(OH) cholecalciferol are consistant with bone calcium
resorption, a biological effect of circulating 1-25 (OH)2 cholecalciferol. In
all cases, elevated TTRS are found, even in cases where phosphocalcic metabolism or active osteoclast count appeared normal. This dissociation between
these 2 ostoeclastic markers can have 2 explanations : first, osteoclast
count expresses a recent osteoclastic stimulation while TTRS increase reflects
a long standing stimulation (about 3 months). Secondly, TTRS increase seems
a more sensitive biological marker reflecting circulating 1-25 (OH)2 cholecalciferol levels than active osteoclast count. TTRS increase is well correlated
with clinical activity except in Loefgren syndroms where the duration of symptoms
is too short to increase TTRS. For instance in our active polyvisceral sarcoidosis, the probably high secretion of 1-25 (OH)2 cholecalciferol induces
a high bone resorption with TTRS increased hypercalcemia, hypercalciuria,
hyperhydroxyprolinuria. Hydroxyproline, a common aminoacid of bone collagen
is a good marker of bone resorption. These results are consistant with the
generally severe evolution of hypercalcemic sarcoidosis (11).
Moreover, this indirect effect of sarcoidosis on bones through vitamin D is
likely associated with local resorptive effect of sarcoid granuloma in bony
localisation. This is closely related to osteolytic lesions of myeloma in
which plasmocytes nodules are surrounded by osteoclasts ; some sarcoid granulomas (but not all of them) were surrounded by osteoclasts. The local stimulating agent of this osteoclastic activity (OAF) may be interleukine 1 (12)
or a tumor necrosis factor (13) secreted by macrophages.

CONCLUSION

This study shows that in active sarcoidosis, bone resorption plays an important
role in phosphocalcic disturbances and could reflect an increase of 1-25 (OH) D3
levels. Sarcoid granulomas in bone have an additional local osteoclastic stimulating effect. However performing a bone biopsy in patients with a common

502

sarcoidosis is questionable but biochemical parameters like calcemia, calciuria and hydroxyprolinuria are good biological markers of bone resorption and sarcoidosis activity (5). Thus a bone biopsy would appear usefull to understand the physiopathology of hypercalcemia and/or hypercalciuria and help the choice of antiosteoclastic agents other than steroids (ie : calcitonin, diphosphonates...)

REFERENCES

1. Golstein RA, Israel HL, Becker KL, Moore CF (1971). The infrequency of hypercalcemia in sarcoidosis. Am. J. med. 51 : 21-30

2. Studdy PR, Bird R, Neville E, James DG (1980). Biochemical findings in sarcoidosis. J. Clin. Pathol. 33 : 528-533

3. Adams JS, Gacad MA (1985). Characterization of 1α hydroxylation of vitamin D3 sterols by culture alveolar macrophages from patients with sarcoidosis. J. exp. med. 161 : 755-765

4. Mason RS, Frankel T, Chan YL, Lissner D, Posen S (1984). Vitamin D conversion by sarcoid lymph node homogenate. Ann. Intern. Med. 100 : 59-61

5. Meyrier A, Valeyre D, Bouillon R, Paillard F, Battesti JP, Georges R (1986). Different mechanisms of hypercalciuria in sarcoidosis. Correlation with disease extension and activity. Ann. N. Y. Acad Sci. 575-586

6. Zerwekh JE, Pake YC, Kaplan RA, Mc Guire JL, Upchurch K, Breslau N, Johnson R. (1980). Pathogenic role of 1α 25 dihydroxyvitamin D in sarcoidosis and absorptive hypercalciuria : different response to prednisolone therapy. J. Clin. Endocrinol. Metab. 51 : 381-386

7. Bell NH (1985). Vitamin D endocrin system. J. Clin. Invest. 76 : 1-6

8. Chappard D, Alexandre C, Camps M, Monthéard JP, Riffat G (1983). Embedding iliac bone biopsies at low temperature using glycol and methyl methacrylates. Stain Technol. 58 : 299-308

9. Chappard D, Alexandre C, Ponchon J, Riffat G (1984). Semiautomatic histomorphometry : Hist'os, hist'ocycline, hist'o clast : a versatile program series. Biol. Cell. 52 : 117 A

10. Chappard D, Alexandre C, Riffat G (1983). Histochemical identification of osteoclasts in undercalcified human bone biopsies. Reappraisal of a simple procedure for routine diagnosis. Bas Appl. Histochem. 27 : 75-85

11. Alberts C, Van den Berg H (1984). Calcium and phosphate metabolism in sarcoidosis. Adv. Exp. Med. Biol. 178 : 405-409

12. Abe E, Shiina Y, Miyaura C, Tanaka H, Hayashi T, Kanegasaki S, Saito M, Nishii Y, De Luca HF, Suda J (1984). Activation and fusion induced by 1-25 dihydroxyvitamin D3 and their relation in alveolar macrophage. Proc. Natl. Acad Sci. USA. 81 : 7112-7116

13. Bachwich PR, Lynch JP, Larrick J, Spengler M, Kunkel SL (1986). Tumor necrosis factor production by human sarcoid alveolar macrophages. Am. J. Pathol. 125 : 421-425

© 1988 Elsevier Science Publishers B.V. (Biomedical Division)
Sarcoidosis and other granulomatous disorders
C. Grassi, G. Rizzato, E. Pozzi, editors

DIAGNOSTIC SIGNIFICANCE OF TWO-DIMENSIONAL ECHOCARDIOGRAPHY IN SARCOID INFILTRATIVE CARDIOMYOPATHY

NESTOR ANGOMACHALELIS, ALEXANDER HOURZAMANIS

Department of Internal Medicine, University of Thessaloniki, George Papanikolaou General Hospital, Thessaloniki (Greece)

INTRODUCTION

Noninvasive qualitative estimation by cross sectional echocardiography of myocardial damage in sarcoid infiltrative cardiomyopathy has not been previously well recognized in the literature, although it has been presented relatively to certain types of primary myopathy or specific heart muscle disease[1,2].

The purpose of this study is to qualify Two-dimentional echocardiography (Two-D Echo), classify it's findings, describe the incidence of granulomatous infiltration of the heart and define the correlation with Technetium-99m-pyrophosphate myocardial imaging (Tc^{99m}-pyp)[3,4] in patients with systemic sarcoidosis.

MATERIAL AND METHODS

Thirty four selective patients, 11 males and 23 females (mean age $48,3 \pm 11,7$ years) with biopsy proven sarcoidosis and free of other cardiac pathology or systemic desease underwent a *qualitative* Two-dimentional echocardiogram[5] in various views. The majority number of these patients were undertaken a myocardial Tc^{99m}-pyp scintigraphy[6]. Two hours after an intravenous injection of 20 mCi of the radionuclide it's uptake was recorded in various positions and classified by computer analysis in 5 categories from 0 to 4 grades, depending on the activity in the myocardium.

RESULTS

The abnormal features of Two-D Echo were estimated as large or small, discrete, highly refractive echoes, atractoid in shape and classified in 2 categories from A to B grades as follows: *Grade A* represents massive, diffuse, large infiltrates of the most anatomic parts of the heart. *Grade B* represents smaller, segmental infiltrates of certain areas, especially the basal part of the ventricular septum[5,6] (Fig. 1$_A$). After exclusion of 2 patients (bad tracing) the results of the remaining 32 showed: 1. Abnormal echoes of *grade A* in 5 patients (15.62%), *grade B* in 23 patients (71.87%) and 4 normals (12.5%). The total incidence of abnormal echoes was 87.49%. 2. It is also revealed that IVS is the location of highest incidence and haviest infiltration (28 patients, 100%). 3. From the 27 patients (out of 32 studied), who underwent Tc^{99m}-pyp scintigraphy (Fig. 1$_B$), 23 had definitely positive myocardial uptake of the isotope (85.18%). 4. χ^2 test proved that there was strong statistical correlation between the results of Two-D Echo and radionuclide myocardial imaging.

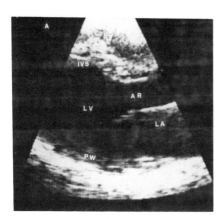
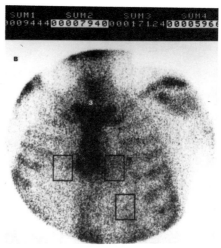

Fig. 1$_A$. Two-D echocardiogram (long axis) presents discrete, highly refractive echoes of the basal part of the septum B. Tc^{99m}-pyp myocardial scan showes increased isotope uptake > 2+ in ROI 1 (cardiac region).

CONCLUSIONS

We conclude that 1. These Two-D Echo features could be suggestive of granulomatous infiltrative cardiomyopathy. 2. Qualitative Two-dimentional echocardiography is a useful noninvasive modality for early identification of sarcoid cardiomyopathic patients.

REFERENCES

1. Goodwin FJ (1985): Heart Muscle Disease. Lancaster, MTP Press (Publishers) p. 146.

2. Tanaka M, Nitta S, Nitta K, Sogo Y, Yamamoto A, Katahira Y, Sato N, Ohkawai H, Tezuka F (1985): Non-invasive estimation by cross sectional echocardiography of myocardial damage in cardiomyopathy. Br. Heart J 53:137-152.

3. Angomachalelis Nest, Giannoglou G, Salem N, Patakas D, Louridas G. (1986): Radionuclide imaging in Cardiac Sarcoidosis by Technetium-99m-pyrophosphate. Sarcoidosis 3(2)169.

4. Angomachalelis Nest, Salem N, Giannoglou G, Patakas D, Louridas G. (1986): Myocardial Technetium-99m-pyrophosphate scintigraphy in the noninvasive diagnosis of infiltrative cardiomyopathy. X-World Congress of Cardiology, Washington. Abstract Book p. 176.

5. Valantine H, McKenna SW, Nihoyannopoulos P, Mitchell A, Foale R, Davies JM, Oakley MC (1987): Sarcoidosis: a pattern of clinical and morphological presentation. Br. Heart J. 57:256-63.

6. Forman BM, Sandler PM, Sacks AG, Kronenber WM, Powers AT (1983): Radionuclide Imaging in Myocardial Sarcoidosis. Chest 83(3):578-580.

VECTORCARDIOGRAPHY VERSUS ECHOCARDIOGRAPHY IN THE DIAGNOSIS OF SILENT MYOCARDIAL INVOLVEMENT IN SARCOIDOSIS

E. Giagnoni, L. Beretta, A.Sachero

Community Health Services - Chest Clinic - Cardiac Department - Milan (Italy)

Introduction

Up to date a good evidence of silent myocardial involvement in sarcoidosis has been obtained only by autoptical studies[1,2]. In order to detect any diagnostic marker of myocardial damage in vivo and to assess a score of risk, if possible, for symptomatic events, we have been performing a not invasive study on patients with pulmonary sarcoidosis.

Material and Methods

We have examined 139 patients (78 males, 61 females, ranged from 18 to 78 yrs of age) since January 1980 up to date, all with tissue confirmed sarcoidosis, asymptomatic and free from past or present history of cardiovascular and metabolic diseases. In all subjects we have looked for electrical markers of myocardial fibrosis (bites on vectorcardiographic traces) and we have performed an echocardiographic morphofunctional study to verify the correlation, if any, between electrical and anathomic or functional abnormalities. According to restrictive criteria[3] we have considered as "bite" on the vectorcardiographic traces an unexpected deviation of QRS loop-outline longer than 6 msec and higher than 0.1 mV, excluding those observed in the first and the last 15 msec.On M-Mode echocardiograms we measured the left ventricular dimensions, along with septum and posterior wall thickness, at end diastole and end systole, ejection fraction, percent fractional shortening of left ventricular internal dimensions, mean velocity of circumferential fiber shortening, percent systolic thickening of interventricular septum and left posterior wall, left atrium dimensions and right ventricle end diastolic diameter. Control values for echo parameters were obtained from normal subjects (observed in the same period)matched with cases for sex, age and body surface area.

Results

Bites in almost 1 plane were found in 49 subjects (35.2%) - against only 12% of controls - and in 2 or 3 planes in 22 (15.8%). When present in more than 1 plane bites were isocrone in 18 cases, suggesting a more reliable feature of myocardial scar tissue. The 98.5% of subjects with bites on vcg showed 1 or more echo parameters under or above 1 SD of normal mean values. The highest frequency of echo anomalies occurred when vcg bites were evidenced in 2 or 3 planes, the lowest when vcg trace was normal: left ventricle posterior wall end diastolic thickness in 68.2% vs. 48%, relative wall thickness in 50% vs. 27.3%, fractional shortening in 41% vs. 28.6%, right ventricle end diastolic diameter in 45.4% vs. 16.9%, left ventricle end systolic diameter in 41% vs. 27.3%. In the 59.7% of all cases 1 or more echo parameters were 2 SD under or above normal mean values.

Comments

In conclusion these data suggest silent myocardial involvement in a large number of cases, according to previous autoptical reports. Anathomic damage and functional abnormalities are detected by echocardiography with a higher frequency when vectorcardiographic trace shows an electrical picture of myocardial fibrosis. As a matter of fact, echocardiography reveals to have higher sensibility, probably because mild morphofunctional alterations are not always electrically detectable.
A long term follow up (in progress) will define whether these findings (in asymptomatic subjects) will have any predictive value for symptomatic events.

Acknowledgements

We acknowledge Mr.Francesco Maisto for technical assistance and Mrs. Corinna Santagostini for typing the manuscript.

References

1 - Longcope WT, Freiman DG (1952) A study of sarcoidosis based on a combined investigation of 160 cases including 30 autopsies from the Johns Hopkins Hospital and Massachussetts General Hospital Medicine 31:1-132

2 - Robert WC, McAllister HA, Ferrans VU (1977) Sarcoidosis of the heart. A clinicopathologic study of 35 necropsy patients (group I) and review of 78 previously described necropsy patients (group II) Am.J.Med. 63:86-108

3 - Obbiassi M. et Al. (1978) Presenza di bites nel vettorcardiogramma di una popolazione ad alto rischio coronarico G.Ital.Cardiol. 8: 1349-1356

© 1988 Elsevier Science Publishers B.V. (Biomedical Division)
Sarcoidosis and other granulomatous disorders
C. Grassi, G. Rizzato, E. Pozzi, editors

EVALUATION OF LUNG T-CELL SUBSETS IN UVEITIS PATIENTS WITH NORMAL CHEST ROENTGENOGRAMS

MINEHARU SUGIMOTO, MASAYUKI ANDO, HIRONORI NAKASHIMA, HIROTSUGU KOHROGI, SHUKURO ARAKI

The First Department of Internal Medicine, Kumamoto University Medical School, 1-1-1 Honjo, Kumamoto 860 (Japan)

INTRODUCTION

It is well known that uveitis is a major ocular complication of sarcoidosis. However, when confronted with uveitis patients with normal chest x-ray films, the differential diagnosis is so wide that some other evidences should be sought to establish a diagnosis of sarcoidosis. Recently, subclinical involvements of the lung have been described in patients with extrathoracic sarcoidosis and in patients with other granulomatous disease such as Crohn's disease (1-3).

The aim of this study was to investigate the pulmonary involvements in uveitis patients who did not show any radiological evidences of intrathoracic sarcoidosis.

MATERIALS AND METHODS

Subjects. Study populations consisted of 20 uveitis patients (3 males and 17 females, mean age: 28 ± 13 years), 11 patients with histologically verified pulmonary sarcoidosis (6 males and 5 females, mean age: 35 ± 15 years), 6 patients with hypersensitivity pneumonitis (1 male and 5 females, mean age: 45 ± 10 years) , and 10 healthy male nonsmokers (mean age: 27 ± 6 years).

Bronchoalveolar lavage (BAL). To obtain BAL cells, 150 ml of sterile saline was instilled in the right anterior basal bronchus in three aliquots, using a flexible bronchofiberscope (4).

Determination of T-cell subsets. T-cell subsets in blood and BAL fluids were determined by flow cytometry using monoclonal antibodies (OKT series) (5). Frozen sections of the lung tissues obtained by transbronchial lung biopsy were stained immunohistochemically for T-cell subsets.

RESULTS

Bronchoalveolar lavage studies revealed that 11 of 20 uveitis patients showed normal findings similar to those of healthy nonsmokers. As shown in Table 1, nine patients showed increased proportions of lymphocytes, OKT3+ and OKT4+ cells with elevated OKT4+:OKT8+ cell ratio in BAL fluids. Thus, BAL data were compatible with those of patients with pulmonary sarcoidosis, but different from those of patients with hypersensitivity pneumonitis who showed decreased ratio of OKT4+ and OKT8+ cells.

510

TABLE I

T-CELL SUBSETS IN BAL FLUIDS

Cases	Lymphocytes (%)	T-cell subsets		
		OKT3+(%)	OKT4+(%)	OKT4+/OKT8+
Uveitis (n=9)	40 ± 18	74 ± 4	65 ± 7	4.4 ± 2.5
Pulmonary sarcoidosis (n=11)	45 ± 13	81 ± 7	62 ± 13	5.5 ± 2.5
Hypersensitivity pneumonitis (n=6)	80 ± 16	86 ± 7	29 ± 12	0.6 ± 0.2
Controls (nonsmokers, n=10)	14 ± 3	49 ± 13	37 ± 14	1.9 ± 0.9

Transbronchial lung biopsy was performed in 9 uveitis patients with abnormal lymphocyte subsets in BAL fluids, demonstrating noncaseous epithelioid cell granuloma in 4 patients who showed a higher OKT4+:OKT8+ cell ratio.

Immunohistochemical studies of biopsied lung tissues showed many OKT3+ cells and OKT4+ cells with very few OKT8+ cells in the granulomas.

T-cell subsets and ACE levels in peripheral blood were within normal limit in all patients with uveitis (S-ACE: 15.2 ± 4.1 u/l).

DISCUSSION

This study demonstrated that BAL data in uveitis patients with normal chest roentgenograms were similar to those of active pulmonary sarcoidosis with bilateral hilar lymphadenopathy and/or pulmonary infiltrates, concerning increased proportions of lymphocytes and OKT4+:OKT8+ ratio in BAL fluids (6).

Wallert et al. described that there was an increased proportion of BAL lymphocytes with normal OKT4+:OKT8+ ratio in patients with extrathoracic sarcoidosis (2). In our study, 6 of 9 patients with an increased proportion of lymphocytes were associated with T-lymphocytosis and an elevation of OKT4+:OKT8+ ratio.

In conclusion, T-lymphocytosis with increased helper-inducer T-cells in BAL fluids could be a good marker for predicting the pulmonary involvements of sarcoidosis in uveitis patients with normal chest roentgenograms.

REFERENCES

1. Wallert B, Ramon P, Fournier EC, Tonnel AB, Voisin C (1982) Chest 82:553-5
2. Wallert B, Ramon P, Fournier EC, Prin L, Tonnel AB, Voisin C (1986) In: Johns CJ (ed), Tenth International Conference on Sarcoidosis and Other Granulomatous Disorders. Ann NY Acad Sci 465:201-210
3. Smiejan JM, Cosnes J, Chollet-Martin S, Soler P, Basset FM, Quintrec YL, Hance AJ (1986) Ann Intern Med 104:17-21
4. Sugimoto M, Nishi R, Ando M, Nakashima H, Araki S (1986) Jap J Med 25:135-143
5. Sugimoto M, Ando M, Nishi R, Nakashima H, Araki S (1986) Chest 89:517S
6. Hunninghake GW, Crystal RG (1981) N Engl J Med 305:429-434

© 1988 Elsevier Science Publishers B.V. (Biomedical Division)
Sarcoidosis and other granulomatous disorders
C. Grassi, G. Rizzato, E. Pozzi, editors

LONGITUDINAL STUDY OF OCULAR SARCOIDOSIS

ANNI KARMA
Department of Ophthalmology, University of Oulu, Finland

INTRODUCTION

Both the course and prognosis of pulmonary sarcoidosis have been studied extensively (1,2), but the long-term behaviour of ophthalmic sarcoid changes is not known. The purpose of this study was, in a prospective study, to investigate the course and outcome of sarcoidosis in the conjunctivae, lacrimal glands and intraocular tissues.

MATERIAL AND METHODS

In thorough ophthalmological examinations of an unselected group of 281 patients with histologically confirmed sarcoidosis, 79 patients showed one or more ophthalmic sarcoid changes as follows: Conjunctival granulomatosis confirmed by biopsy in 37 (46%), lacrimal gland affection assessed by decreased lacrimal secretion in 36 (46%), and uveitis in 22 (29%) patients. All except one patient had pulmonary changes and 55 (70%) patients had other extrathoracic manifestations, too (3).

The patients with uveitis were treated and followed until the inflammation subsided. Seventy-one patients (90%) were available in the follow-up study by the same ophthalmologist using the same protocol 5-16, mean nine years after the initial examination. A chest X-ray was also taken and angiotensin-converting enzyme (ACE) was measured.

RESULTS

Follow-up of uveitis. The sarcoid uveitis exhibited monophasic (9 patients), relapsing (9 patients) or chronic (4 patients) courses. One-fifth of the eyes lost useful vision (visual acuity $\leq$ 0.3).

Long-term outcome of ophthalmic changes. Thirty-three patients showed one or more ophthalmic changes at the follow-up examination (Table I). Thirty patients were assessed as totally recovered from sarcoidosis on a physical and radiologic basis, and eight patients had only chest X-ray changes. In 16 patients the ophthalmic manifestations were the only remaining sign of sarcoidosis. ACE was elevated in 53% (8/15) of these patients but in only 10% (3/39) of the remitted patients (p < 0.01 in χ^2-test).

TABLE I

SARCOID MANIFESTATIONS OF 33 PATIENTS WITH OPTHALMIC CHANGES AT FOLLOW-UP

Change	No. of patients	%	No. of patients with only ophthalmic change[2]
Conjunctiva[1]	13	39	5
Lacrimal gland	20	61	12
Uveitis	4	12	1
Lungs	17	51	

[1] Confirmed by biopsy in nine

[2] Two patients had both conjunctival and lacrimal gland disease

CONCLUSIONS

The uveal inflammation often subsided completely, but because of complications useful vision was lost in a considerable number of eyes. In chronic sarcoidosis affection of the conjunctivae and lacrimal glands was seen more frequently than uveitis.

The results of this study suggest that no phenomenon of isolated ocular sarcoid reaction exists. It is probable that a seemingly sole ocular or lacrimal gland sarcoidosis is always a residua of systemic sarcoidosis having been evident years earlier. The diagnosing of an isolated eye disease as sarcoidosis is difficult, but re-evaluation of earlier chest x-rays, measurement of ACE, and conjunctival biopsy may help to diagnose some of these cases.

REFERENCES

1. Smellie H and Hoyle C (1960) The natural history of pulmonary sarcoidosis. Quart J Med 29: 531-559

2. Johns CJ, Zachary JB, MacGregor MI, Curtis JL, Scott PP and Terry PB (1982) The longitudinal study of chronic sarcoidosis. Trans Am Clin Climatol Assoc 94: 173-181.

3. Karma A (1979) Ophthalmic changes in sarcoidosis. Acta Ophthalmol (Kbh) Suppl 141: 1-94.

© 1988 Elsevier Science Publishers B.V. (Biomedical Division)
Sarcoidosis and other granulomatous disorders
C. Grassi, G. Rizzato, E. Pozzi, editors

ANGIOTENSIN -CONVERTING ENZYME LEVELS IN TEARS AND SERA:
POTENTIAL PREDICTOR OF OCULAR SEQUELA IN NORTH CAROLINA AFRO-
AMERICANS

PAUL S. ELLISON, JR., M.D., JOHN C. MERRITT, M.D.

Within the southeastern United States ocular sarcoidosis
represents the most frequently diagnosed granulomatous uveitis.
Any clinical laboratory tool to help identify the subjects at
risk losing significant vision from its blinding sequela
(secondary glaucomas, retinopathy and corneal opacifications)
would greatly aid the clinical ophthalmologist.

Serum angiotensin-converting enzyme (ACE) levels are
elevated with sarcoidal disease activity. Our tear assay, a
modification of methods used to quantitatively determine
serum ACE,   is based on release of L-hippuric acid from a
synthetic tripeptide, hippuryl-L-histidyl L-leucine. The
hippuric acid in reflex tears is separated and quantitated by
reversed-phase high-performance liquid chromatography (HPLC).
The serum assay employes radiolabeled acylated tripeptide (^{3}H-
Hip-Gly-Gly) as a substrate and then measures the activity of
angiotensin-converting-enzyme by the amount of released ^{3}H-
hippuric acid.
Calculation: enzyme activity was determined by a modification
of the equation used by Shihabi and Scaro[1]. Enzyme ACE
activity in (u mol/min. gm) =

$$\frac{\dfrac{\text{peak height sample}}{\text{peak height internal}}}{\dfrac{\text{peak height standard}}{\text{peak height standard}}} \text{std. x 33.5 (umol/l)} \cdot \frac{\text{Tear weight (gm)}}{4.5 \times 10\ SL}$$

peak height standard std. x 15 minutes

Tears were obtained in 20 males (X ± S.E.= 20.7 ± 0.6 years)
and 16 females (X ± S.E. = 21.8 ± 0.6 years). 32 were permanent
residents of North Carolina with Virginia (2), South Carolina
(1), and Washington, D.C. (1) comprising the remaining population. Results derived from these (healthy) Afro-Americans
were evaluated. The mean tear ACE level for males was 1.53 ±
0.16 nmol/min. gm while females had a mean 1.55 ± 0.15 nmol/min.
gm. Results are displayed in table 1.

TABLE 1
TEAR ACE LEVELS IN HEALTHY AFRO-AMERICANS (n=70 eyes)

MALE	MEAN Nmol/min/gm	STANDARD ERROR	RANGE Nmol/min/gm
right eye	1.54	0.28	0.57 - 6.24
left eye	1.52	0.18	0.55 - 3.90
right & left	1.53	0.16	0.55 - 6.24

514

FEMALE	MEAN Nmol/min/gm	STANDARD ERROR	RANGE Nmol/min/gm
right eye	1.70	0.26	0.40 - 4.00
left eye	1.41	0.15	0.51 - 2.91
right & left	1.55	0.15	0.40 - 4.00

Corresponding serum levels of angiotensin converting enzyme were determined by the Ventrex radioimmunoassay kit. Sera from these 36 normal students was combined with 25 other normals derived from the Clinical Research Unit Labs, UNC School of Medicine to provide a range for normal values in North Carolina Afro-Americans.

Serum angiotensin converting enzyme in healthy North Carolina Afro-Americans: 38 males had mean ACE levels of (X ± S.D.) = 5.9 ± 2.0 activity units and 23 females: (X ± S.D.) = 5.6 ± 2.0 activity units. Tear ACE levels therefore may provide a useful index of ocular sarcoid activity prior to overt uveitis in susceptible subjects.

REFERENCE
1. Shihabi ZK and Scaro J: Liquid-chromatographic assay of angiotensin converting enzyme in serum. Clin. Chem. 27:1669-1671, 1981.

FINE NEEDLE ASPIRATION BIOPSY IN GRANULOMATOUS DISORDERS

J.J. ELO, H. JOENSUU AND P.J. KLEMI

Turku University Central Hospital
Departments of chest diseases, radiotherapy and pathology
SF-20520 Turku, Finland

INTRODUCTION

Fine needle aspiration biopsy is a commonly used screening method (1,2). The
main purpose of FNAB has been the differentiation of malignant and benign
lesions. Few studies have been published on FNAB in granulomatous disorders
(3,4).

At Turku University Central Hospital about 1500 FNABs have been done yearly,
but only very few granulomatous reactions have been seen. We report 21 cases
seen in cytological specimens during the years 1983-1986.

MATERIAL AND METHODS

There were 21 granulomatous reactions in FNABs from 21 patients, 16 (76%)
female, mean age 57 years. All had a palpable lesion, 18 had an enlarged lymphnode, and 3 an enlarged parotic gland. The method of FNAB was the same as described by Williams and Löwhagen (5). The same pathologist performed the aspirations and interpreted the cytological findings. Specimens were stained after
drying with May-Gruenwald-Giemsa staining. Special stainings were done for acid
fast bacilli and fungi.

The criteria for granulomatous reaction were single or clustered spindle
shaped, elongated epitheloid cells and Langhans-type Giant cells.

RESULTS

Seven patients had tuberculotic lymphadenitis, three were confirmed by histology, and three by positive mycobacterial culture. All responded favourably to
chemotherapy.

Five patients had sarcoidosis, two were confirmed by histology, one by positive Kveim test, and one by response to steroid treatment. All had clinical
picture typical for sarcoidosis (6).

Five patients had sarcoid reaction, a well known cell reaction to malignancy
(7,8). All patients had confirmed malignant disease in history, and no other
obvious reason for this type of reaction.

516

Granulomatous parotitis was seen in three patients, one was also confirmed by histology. There was no other etiology for this reaction, and all responded favourably to treatment with antibiotics.

One patient had a granulomatous reaction of inquinal lymphnode, soon after BCG-revaccination. This reaction is also known in the literature (9).

The cytological finding in all cases was very similar, in addition to epitheloid and giant cells there was necrotic, caseous material, and some neutrophils at the background of four tuberculous specimens, and many neutrophils, lymphocytes, and necrotic cell debris in two of parotitis specimens.

No complications were seen during or after FNAB.

CONCLUSIONS

Granulomatous disorders were easily diagnosed by FNAB. All diagnoses were further comfirmed by histopathology or by clinical and laboratory grounds. In all cases cytological diagnosis was for excluding malignancy, but no reliable suggestions could be made for spesific diagnosis.

FNAB is an easy, economical, and well accepted method, and we recommend it as a first line screening method also in granulomatous disorders.

REFERENCES

1. Oertel YC (1982) Fine-needle Aspiration: A Personal View. Laboratory Medicine 13:343-347.

2. Frable WJ (1983) Fine-needle Aspiration Biopsy A review Hum Pathol 14:9-28.

3. Selroos O (1976) Sarcoidosis of the Spleen Acta Med Scand 200:337-340.

4. Bailey MT, Akhtar M, Ali MA (1985) Fine-needle Aspiration Biopsy in the Diagnosis of Tuberculosis. Acta Cytologica 29:732-736.

5. Williams JS, Löwhagen T (1981) Fine-needle Aspiration Cytology in Thyroid Disease: Clinics in Endocrinology and Metabolism 10:247-266.

6. Scadding JG, Mitchell DN (1985) Sarcoidosis. Chapman and Hall Medical.

7. Gregorie H, Othersen H, Moore McK (1962) The significance of Sarcoid-Like Lesions in Association with Malignant Neoplasms, Am J Surg 104:577-586.

8. Hogsted T (1968) Sarcoid-Like Lesions (Epitheloid Cell Granulomatosis) of Regional Lymph nodes in association with Carcinoma of the Cervix Acta Radiologica 7:12-16.

9. Kobayashi Y, Komazawa Y, Kabayashi M, Matsumoto T, Sakura N, Ishikawa K, Usui T (1984) Presumed BCG Infection in a Boy with Chronic Granulomatous Disease, Clinical Pediatrics 23:586-589.

© 1988 Elsevier Science Publishers B.V. (Biomedical Division)
Sarcoidosis and other granulomatous disorders
C. Grassi, G. Rizzato, E. Pozzi, editors

A COMBINATORIAL ANALYSIS OF ^{67}Ga SCANNING OF THE HEAD AND THORAX IN THE DIAGNOSIS OF SARCOIDOSIS - THE PANDA SIGN

STEPHEN B. SULAVIK, DAVID WEED, RICHARD SPENCER, HOWARD SHAPIRO AND RICHARD CASTRIOTTA
Departments of Pulmonary and Nuclear Medicine, University of Connecticut School of Medicine, Farmington, Connecticut and Mt. Sinai Hospital, Hartford, Connecticut (U.S.A.)

INTRODUCTION

Clinical manifestations of lacrimal and salivary gland involvement in sarcoidosis has been known to occur since the earliest descriptions of Heerfordt and Bering. Since the advent of ^{67}Ga scanning, symmetric uptake within the lacrimal and parotid glands in sarcoidosis has been demonstrated. Though published scans have in addition demonstrated uptake in the submandibular glands as well, no specific significance has been paid to this finding. Also, there has been no effort to combine ^{67}Ga uptake findings of the head with those of the thorax in the diagnosis of sarcoidosis. The purpose of this study, therefore, was to determine, using bilateral symmetry as the cornerstone observation, whether ^{67}Ga uptake findings of a) the head alone, or b) combined with the thorax, would be useful in the diagnosis of sarcoidosis.

STUDY DESIGN

253 consecutive ^{67}Ga scans and appropriate clinical data represent the basic information from which this study was conducted. All ^{67}Ga scans were reviewed "blindly" by at least one nuclear radiologist and one pulmonary physician. Clinical data on all patients was reviewed by a pulmonary physician. Specific organ uptake of ^{67}Ga within the lacrimal glands and the salivary glands (parotid, submandibular) and the thorax (hilum, mediastinum and lung) was recorded and combinatorially analyzed for statistical significance. Clinical data included: age, sex and race; corticosteroid use; clinical activity; method of diagnosis; and chest x-ray stage.

RESULTS

General:

1) Of 253 scans, 185 were positive for head and/or thoracic ^{67}Ga uptake.

2) Diagnosis of 253 study patients: Non-pulmonary infection (137), hematologic and nonhematologic malignancy (40), sarcoidosis (36), COPD (13), renal disease (9), collagen vascular disease (CVD)(9), bacterial pneumonia (2), UIP (3), eosinophilic pneumonia (1), and AIDS (3).

Sarcoidosis:

1) Of 253 scans 21 demonstrated significant symmetric ^{67}Ga uptake within the

lacrimal, parotid and submandibular glands bearing a striking resemblance to the face of a Panda bear (Panda sign). Seven (7) of these patients had been irradiated for Hodgkins disease which included the head and neck. The remaining 14 patients had sarcoidosis. No patients in this group had clinically evident eye or salivary gland involvement. Three (3) of these sarcoidosis patients had no thoracic ^{67}Ga uptake and 12 were felt to be clinically active. In 14 of 36 sarcoidosis patients (38.8%), the Panda sign was present. No Panda sign was observed in the remaining 210 patients. Significantly, lacrimal and parotid uptake alone was noted in 14 non-sarcoidosis patients.

A combinatorial analysis of symmetric, increased lacrimal gland, salivary gland and thoracic ^{67}Ga uptake revealed the following three non-Panda patterns (N-PP) which were observed only in sarcoidosis patients (10 of 36): Uptake in a) lacrimals, hilum and parotids (5); b) lacrimals, hilum and lung (4); and c) lacrimals and hilum (1). No such patterns were observed in the remaining 210 patients. An histologic diagnosis of sarcoidosis was made in 26 of 36 patients (11 of 14 with a Panda sign). Excluding irradiated Hodgkins, the results of this study were highly significant for the diagnosis of sarcoidosis. The following contingency table summarizes our data from 246 patients.

TABLE 1

	Panda and N-PP	No Panda or N-PP
Sarcoidosis	24	12
Nonsarcoidosis	0	210

The relationship between sarcoidosis and the radiologic findings described is statistically significant well beyond the .0001 level with a sensitivity of 66.7% and a specificity of 100%.

In summary, within the design of this study: 1) The radiologic finding of a Panda sign with or without thoracic ^{67}Ga uptake is highly specific for sarcoidosis and may be especially helpful in instances of unusual clinical presentations. It is also suggestive of an active clinical process; 2) The combination of symmetric significant ^{67}Ga uptake of a) lacrimals, hilum and lung; b) lacrimals, hilum and parotids; and c) lacrimals and hilum, is also highly specific for sarcoidosis; 3) Further study to determine if there is any prevalence of these patterns in larger numbers of specific disease entities (e.g. Sjogren's/sicca syndrome, CVD, leukemia, and AIDS) is required; 4) Salivary gland biopsy is recommended for patients with the Sjogren's/sicca syndrome.

© 1988 Elsevier Science Publishers B.V. (Biomedical Division)
Sarcoidosis and other granulomatous disorders
C. Grassi, G. Rizzato, E. Pozzi, editors

GALLIUM 67 SCINTIGRAPHY IN THE LOCALIZATION OF SARCOIDOSIS

BY

DRS. V. LOPEZ-MAJANO[*], P. MUTHUSWAMY[@], & G. RENZI[°]
[*]NUCLEAR MEDICINE, AND [@]PULMONARY DISEASE DIVISION
COOK COUNTY HOSPITAL, CHICAGO, ILLINOIS[*@], NOTRE
DAME HOSPITAL[°], QUEBEC, CANADA (USA)

INTRODUCTION

The first localization of sarcoidosis described was in the skin, Mortimer's pernio and accepted by Besnier (1).
Successive authors found that sarcoidosis can affect any tissue of the body and this makes the diagnosis of sarcoidosis extremely difficult because of its polifacetic nature (2-3)
Thus the image of sarcoidosis is very diverse to the specialists; for a dermatologist any chronic skin lesion can be sarcoidosis and for an ophtalmologist sarcoidosis is the cause of many iritis (4). Arrhythmias can be the only anomaly present in cardiac sarcoidosis (5), and any abnormality in the chest radiograph should include sarcoidosis in the differential diagnosis, eventhough pulmonary localizations of sarcoidosis can co-exist with a normal chest radiograph (6). These systemic manifestations of sarcoidosis create a problem to the specialists who sometimes behave in front of a patient with sarcoidosis like the blind men describing an elephant; this makes necessary to have an objective method such as imaging of sarcoidosis with gallium 67 to locate the disease, to define its characteristics and to determine its activity.

SUBJECTS

355 patients had biopsy proven sarcoidosis and had increased serum angiotensin-converting enzyme (S.A.C.E.) levels. Many of them had respiratory symptoms.

METHODS

Time of study: 24-48 hours after I.V. injection of the 185 MBq (5 mCi) of gallium 67 citrate.
Technique: Tomoscintigraphy or whole body scan supplemented by spot scans.

RESULTS AND DISCUSSION

All the patients had abnormal increases in the gallium 67 uptake in different organs and the distribution of the active sarcoidosis can be seen in the whole body study.
The location of the disease process in order of decreasing frequency was: Lacrimal glands 70%, salivary glands 70%, nasal mucosa 67%, lungs 62%, peripheral lymphnodes 60%, hilar lymphnodes 38%, joints 16% and mediastinal lymphnodes 8%. The intensity of gallium 67 uptake was variable but always more than in the thigh; abnormal

520

gallium 67 uptake was present in the arms or legs of 8 patients.
Hepato-splenomegaly was present in 42 patients with increased gallium 67 uptake which indicated inflammation in these organs. This
location of the disease correlates with tissue findings in some cases
(7) but not always (8).
The gallium 67 uptake in active sarcoidosis is characterized by focal, well circumscribed, areas of gallium 67 uptake in salivary;
lacrimal glands, nasal mucosa and lymphnodes and diffuse gallium 67
uptake in the lungs, the gallium 67 uptake can be reversed by steroids
up to the point of normalization.
Systemic organ involvement with sarcoidosis studied by a non-invasive
method such as whole body gallium 67 scintigraphy was similar to that
found by some authors with tissue diagnosis but different of that
found by others, this is not surprising because the sarcoidosis can
prefer some areas to others which explains the variability in results.
Single photon emission computerized tomography with gallium 67 ob-
tains a three dimensional representation of the disease process and
this may help in differential the uptake in lungs from that in hila.
Magnetic resonance imaging demonstrates neoplastic lymphnodes but the
inflammed salivary glands of sarcoidosis were not well demonstrated (9).
Gallium 67 scintigraphy is the preferred noninvasive methodology used
to locate the distribution of sarcoidosis in the body and to determine
its activity.

REFERENCES

1. Besnier E: Lupus pernio de la face. Ann Derm Syph (paris).
    10:333, 1892.
2. Wagner JC.: Aetiological factors in complicated coal workers'
    pneumoconiosis. Ann N Y Acad Sci. 200:401, 1972
3. Jones Williams W.: Sarcoidosis-1977. Beitr Path. 160:325, 1977.
4. James DG, Neville E, Langley DA.: Ocular sarcoidosis. Trans
    Ophthalmol Soc (UK). 96:133, 1976.
5. Fleming HA, Bailey SM.: Sarcoid heart disease. J Roy Coll Phys
    (London). 15:245, 1981.
6. Lopez-Majano V, Muthuswamy P, Renzi G, Gupta B, and Dutton RE.:
    Gallium 67 scintigraphy and angiotensin I converting enzyme
    in the assessment of activity of pulmonary sarcoidosis. Proc
    10th Internat Conf Sarcoidosis, 1983
7. Brett Z.: Prevalence of intrathoracic sarcoidosis among eth-
    nic groups in London. In Levinsky L, Macholda F (eds): Proc
    5th Internat Conf Sarcoidosis. Praha, University Karlova,
    238, 1971.
8. Mames DG, Neville E, Siltzbach LE, Turiaf, Battesti JP, Sharma
    OP, Hosoda Y, Mikami R, Odaka M, Villar TG, Djuric B, Douglas
    A, Middleton W, Karlish AJ, Blasi A, Olivieri D, Press P.:
    A worldwide review of sarcoidosis. Ann N Y Acad Sci. 278:
    321, 1976.
9. Lopez-Majano V, Spigos D, Langer B, and Rhee R.: Nuclear
    magnetic resonance in the imaging of sarcoidosis. Presented
    to the U.S.A., N.M.R. Conference, 1987.

521

METHODOLOGY FOR GALLIUM 67 SCINTIGRAPHY IN SARCOIDOSIS

BY

DRS. P. SANSI[*], V. LOPEZ-MAJANO[*], AND P. MUTHUSWAMY[**]
*NUCLEAR MEDICINE AND PULMONARY MEDICINE DIVISIONS**
COOK COUNTY HOSPITAL, CHICAGO, ILLINOIS (USA)

INTRODUCTION

Sarcoidosis is a multisystemic disease and has diverse presentations which makes the diagnosis a little difficult. Gallium is being used to diagnosis active sites of involvement (1).
Whole body can be imaged by gallium scintigraphy using a gamma camera aligned to a moving table and tomographic camera (2).
The purpose of this study is to compare the efficacy of gallium scanning by two whole body scanning techniques in detecting various sites of active sarcoidosis.

MATERIAL AND METHOD

Radiopharmaceutical: The standard adult intravenous dose of about 5 mCi of 67 Gallium citrate (175 MBq) was used in all patients.

Equipment: The tomographic camera system was used to study the distribution of gallium in one hundred patients (PTS).
Another group of one hundred patients were studied using a large-field camera with a medium energy collimator, aligned with a whole body moving table (WBMT). 24 or 48 hours whole body images, using 3 peaks of gallium 67 (93, 184, 296 KeV) in the auto mode, were obtained. Anterior and posterior whole body images, along with spots of the chest in the anterior and posterior views were done.

RESULTS AND DISCUSSION

The results of each group of 100 patients studied by WBMT and PTS are shown in Tables I and II.

TABLE I

	Nasal Mucosa	Lacrimal Glands	Salivary Glands	Medias-tinum	Lungs	Hila
PTS	35	40	38	17	52	23
WBMT	35	41	52	34	39	39

TABLE II

	Lymphnodes				Soft Tissue	
	Axilla	Neck	Abdomen	Inguinal	Legs	Arms
PTS	4	5	12	13	10	1
WBMT	5	4	1	4	19	14

A total of 253 sites of increased gallium activity were picked up by PTS and 282 sites by WBMT respectively. Lung activity showed a diffuse pattern frequently. Rarely focal lesions were seen. Abdominal and inguinal lymphnodes

522

were better seen with PTS as compared to WBMT. The delineation of contour and number of lymph nodes was better demonstrated by PTS. This correlates with Staab and McCartney's (2) observations.

WBMT picked up more positive sites in salivary glands, mediastinum, hila, legs, and arms. There was no significant differences in sites of nasal mucosa, lacrimal glands, axilla or neck by either technique.

Chest spots were positive in 93 patients. They were frequently essential in obese patients. This is most likely because these patients need higher doses, (adjusted according to the body surface area), have increased background activity and the location of lesions in deep (deeper than the WBMT or PTS can resolve).

Lymphnode involvement occurs in majority of sarcoid patients. Total sites picked up were 113. Hilar and mediastinal lymphadenopathy is most common and was seen in 113 sites by both techniques. Gallium scan was most useful in demonstrating abdominal lymph nodes which were clinically unsuspected.

Diffuse skin activity was seen in 44 patients. These findings may be non-specific at times as muscle or skin biopsies were not performed to separate the two.

The triad of increased activity in salivary glands, lacrimal glands along with nasal mucosa was the most frequently encountered observation. This was observed in 36% by PTS and in 42% patients by WBMT. Parotid glands may be involved unilaterally or bilaterally or as a spectrum of multisystem disease. These findings along with lung activity are suggestive of sarcoidosis.

The diagnosis of suspected sarcoidosis is made by histological demonstration of non-caseating granuloma along with increased levels of SACE (3). The sites of biopsy are chosen by the help of gallium scans. The biopsy, SACE and typical gallium distribution in salivary glands, nose, and lung are conformity of active sarcoidosis. WBMT and PTS are instrumental in locating areas of active sarcoidosis throughout the body. Gallium scintigraphy is conventionally used in the diagnosis (4), in sequential assessment of activity of pulmonary sarcoidosis and in delineating the sites of involvement in sarcoidosis. PTS and WBMT were found to be equally effective for detecting the various sites of active sarcoidosis. Chest spots were helpful in most patients especially in obese patients.

REFERENCES

1. McKusik KA, Soin JS, Ghiladli A, et al.: (1973) Gallium 67 accumulation in pulmonary sarcoidosis. JAMA 223:688.

2. Staab EV, and McCartney WH.: (1978) Role of gallium 67 in inflammatory disease. Sem Nucl Med 8:219-234.

3. Muthuswamy P, Lopez-Majano V, Rangiwala M, Trainor WD.: (1987) Serum angiotensin converting enzyme (SACE) activity as an indicator of total granuloma local and prognosis in sarcoidosis. Accepted for presentation to 11th International Congress of Sarcoidosis.

4. Rohatgi PK, Singh R, and Vieras F.: (1987) Extrapulmonary localization of gallium in sarcoidosis. Clin Nucl Med 12:9-16.

ASSESSMENT OF SARCOID ACTIVITY

ASSESSMENT OF SARCOID ACTIVITY: STATE OF ART

J. CHRETIEN

Clinique des Maladies Respiratoires et INSERM U.214 - Hôpital Laennec - 42, Rue de Sèvres, 75007 Paris

The term activity (active disease, active sarcoidosis, sarcoidosis in activity) is currently in wide use for sarcoidosis and is to be found in various publications and in clinical practice. Nevertheless, as previously underlined (1, 2), such a term is not clearly defined. Despite the current use it represents a sort of waste basket where plural notions and meanings are confusedly mixed-up. Unfortunately to many authors active sarcoidosis implies a necessity for treatment with corticosteroids. It has not been proven that steroid treatment is either necessary or beneficial in such conditions except in cases with specific indications such as important organ involvement (i.e., posterior uveitis, cardiac or nervous system involvement, severe and progressive lung function deterioration, etc.). All the large series in various countries, including our own with a 15-year follow-up on some of the patients, demonstrate that sarcoidosis is often a benign disease (3, 4, 5, 6). Spontaneaous regression is frequent and 60 to 70% of sarcoidosis Type I or Type II spontaneously recover in 2 or 3 years. Other chronic forms are stable and do not require permanent steroid treatment or, for that matter, any treatment. We had suggested at the last international meeting that activity be considered and defined as the maintenance of granuloma formation, or of granuloma production, sarcoidosis being characterized by multisystem granuloma formation of unknown mechanism. This activity does not necessarily imply serious general involvement and should not lead to unnecessary corticosteroid treatment. We will consider this term rather in the sense of a predictive criterion and as a therapeutic guideline expressing the maintenance of granuloma formation and possible spreading of the disease towards still unaffected organs or systems. Various criteria have so far been proposed in this way, including clinical criteria and biological criteria which are the markers of the persistance and possibly the extent and aggravation of the disease.

1. As far as the clinical criteria of the so-called sarcoidosis activity are concerned, many signs and symptoms have been proposed by different authors and exhaustive lists have been published (7). In practice, 2 groups may be isolated: those which identify with the usual clinical picture of the disease, being

related with general inflammatory syndroms such as Erythema nodosum, or polyarthralgiae; and those which concern the prognosis of the disease, either local prognosis (such as posterior uveitis, cardiac, renal or nervous system involvement) or general prognosis (such as skin lesions or splenomegaly symptomatic of chronic and severe sarcoidosis). Even a clinical activity index has been proposed in a cooperative group to evaluate in numerical terms the clinical picture and assess the prognosis is scoring the clinical data (8).

2. Biological criteria are probably more interesting and many studies have been devoted to this in recent years. Due to the uncertainty of prognosis in sarcoidosis many biological markers have been studied and compared. The meaning of the various markers is different: some are related to the inflammation and granuloma formation in general such as Ga scan or disturbance in calcium metabolism, whereas some concern more specifically a cell line of the granuloma. This is the case for angiotensin converting enzyme (ACE) and lysozyme (L) which concern macrophage, or $\beta 2$ microglobulin which is generally considered as a marker of lymphocyte activation. On the other hand, some markers are related to the development of fibrosis. In fact, some markers may reflect several biological processes for instance both specific cell number in granuloma and cell replication or cell activation; also for lymphocyte or macrophage simultaneous activation.

For practical reasons biological markers may be classified into 3 groups: (1) Biochemical markers in serum and other biological fluids (e.g. angiotensin converting enzyme); (2) Isotopic markers (e.g. 67 Ga scan); and (3) Immunological cell markers (e.g. lymphocyte count in BAL). For each of these we shall try to consider the following aspects: (a) Theoretical measuring; (b) technical principes of determination; (c) sensitivity and specificity; and finally, (d) practical value on the basis of the previous items and in relation to the cost and the feasibility namely the acceptability by the patient and the more or less invasive procedure.

BIOCHEMICAL MARKERS

Inflammatory processes and granuloma formation and proliferation within the lung or within the other involved organs may be responsible for enzymatic activity expressed by biochemical markers (9). They are determined in blood or in other fluids, or both. Among the most commonly used, some are related to cell activation: macrophage activity and transformation into epithelioid and giant cells, or lymphocyte activity. Others are related to metabolism or granuloma such as calcium metabolism, collagen metabolism. They will be successively considered.

Angiotensin Converting Enzyme (ACE)

ACE determination is probably the most widely used test in the follow-up of sarcoid patients (7). This enzyme, a peptidyl-dipeptidase, or Kininase II converts angiotensin I, an inactive decapeptide, into angiotensin II and inactivates bradykinin (9). Its molecular weight is approximately 150,000. It is inhibited by a large number of natural synthetic peptides and drugs used in treatment of hyptertension and even proposed in the treatment of sarcoidosis such as Captopril which has a pronounced inhibitory capacity. ACE is mainly found in the endothelial cells in pinocytic vesicles on the luminal surface, but also in other fluids and organs (renal tubuli, intestinal microvilli and brain).

The assay commonly used for ACE determination is the spectrophotometric method of Cushman and Cheung which has been modified to some extent by Lieberman (10, 11, 12) and optimised with further partial improvement (9). In sarcoidosis, ACE is detected in alveolar macrophages and at the surface of epithelioid cells and consequently may reflect the development and extent of the granuloma.

Serum activity of ACE is, in an adult, independent of sex, age, smoking habits, ethnicity, horary and regimen. ACE is normally higher in children. It may be observed as a familial phenomenon (9). ACE is primarly determined in serum (SACE) and the majority of sarcoid patients have elevated values but with variations in the proportion of increased SACE and mean values due to heterogeneity of the series (7, 9, 10, 11, 12, 13, 14). This heterogeneity concerns the type, site and intensity of clinical symptoms, the duration of the disease and particularly the presence and duration of intercourse, the treatment (with or without steroids), etc.

In patients with acute sarcoidosis and erythema nodosum, SACE may be normal. The increased activity may be delayed after the onset of disease and the small number of granuloma present at this stage probably explains these unexpected results, the level of SACE increase depending on the extent of the lesions and especially of the active granulomas. The same explanation is given for the lower incidence of SACE abnormal values with Type I sarcoidosis on chest X-ray compared to Type II and III in several series. Nevertheless, correlations between X-ray types and SACE have been reported as variable. A significant change of SACE may be found when parenchymal abnormalities change on roentgenogram whatever the stage. Correlations of SACE with abnormalities in lung function (degree and nature) are also debated.

On the other hand, and as a general rule, the degree of extrapulmonary lesions is correlated with SACE values. SACE is frequently elevated in sarcoid patients with hypercalcemia and declines parallely. Steroid therapy influences the level of SACE with a certain delay after the onset of the treatment but a minimum dose of prednisone is required to obtain a SACE normalization. After discontinuation of steroid treatment, a transient increase of SACE may be observed before a final normalization. Even inhaled corticosteroids (Budesonide) without addition of systemic steroids may lead to SACE normalization (15). In spontaneous recovery of sarcoidosis, without steroids, even previously persistent SACE for a long tissue may normalize (9). The sensitivity and specificity of SACE may be evaluated through extensive references including comparative results in sarcoid patients, control healthy group and control group with other diseases (13, 14). The sensitivity was found to be approximately 60% with 95% confidence limits (14).

Despite the rise of SACE in a large variety of diseases such as miliary tuberculosis, atypical mycobacteriosis, asbestosis, silicosis, Beryllium disease, Gaucher's disease, the specificity is around 90% with a predictive value of 90%. Despite the theoretical partial restrictions resulting from the above notions SACE is well accepted by the patients, and is easily and reliably measurable. Finally, its cost is low and, on the whole, it is a convenient and practical marker of activity.

What about the determination of ACE other than in serum? It has been proposed in fact in tears (16, cerebrospinal fluid (CSF) (17, 18) and mainly in BAL fluid (LACE) (19, 20). With ocular lesions ACE may increase in tears and decrease with steroid treatment. In CSF, ACE follows the clinical course, in particular the outcome of neurological symptoms. ACE is increased in BAL fluid and a good correlation exists between SACE and LACE, and also between LACE and lymphocytosis in BAL. LACE may be more sensitive than SACE (21). In fact the ACE determination in such different conditions is mainly of theoretical interest and ACE assays in other biological fluids than serum are of low practical value.

Other Markers of Cell Activity

Among the other biochemical markers of cell activity, some may be related to macrophage activity and be close to SACE, while some are considered as markers of lymphocytic activity.

Among the former group belong, seryum lysozyme, carboxypeptidase N and Thermolysin-like neutral metalloendopeptidase.
(a) Serum lysozyme (SL) (= muramidase) is a low molecular weight bacteriolytic enzyme present in many cells but found mainly in cells of the mononuclear phagocytic system (MPS), including epithelioid cells, and in polymorphonuclears. SL increases in diseases involving such cells especially when their number increases (22). SL values are independent of age, sex and smoking habits but not of renal function.

An increases of lysozyme rate in serum and urine (UL) has been confirmed in sarcoidosis in all forms and stages (23). The values are higher with Type II sarcoidoses and in pateints with subjective symptoms, and also in those with extrathoracic lesions. SL decreases in patients who improve but may persist in patients with inactive disease (23).

As a marker of activity, SL has a high sensitivity similar and even superior to SACE (24) and serial determination of SL may be more useful than a single measurement: changes in the SL concentrations accompany clinical changes and although seldom may even precede them. Unfortunately SL specificity is low: abnormal values have been reported in many other diseases inlcuding those resembling sarcoidosis. Lysozyme is also produced by bronchial mucosal cells and lysozyme determination is irrelevant to BAL fluid.

Finally, the determination of lysozyme has little practical interest.

(b) Carboxypeptidase (N) (CPN) or Kininase I has biochemical properties similar to those of ACE, inactivating bradykinine, anaphylatoxin and finbrinopeptides. Compared to ACE the sensitivity of CPN is lower (< 20%) whereas the specificity is higher (> 90%) (25). CPN activity may be unchanged despite clinical improvement and compared to ACE the follow-up of CPN appears to be of little value in the management of pateitns with sarcoidosis.

(c) Thermolysin-like neutral serum metalloendopeptidase (STME) has recently been identified in human serum (22). Its concentration is significantly elevated (8.23 nM/ml/min) in sarcoid patients versus healthy controls (2.68). The functions of this enzyme are not clearly defined but like ACE it is a membrane-bound metallopeptidase which is abundant in lung, but the two enzymes are distinct.

STME has been proposed (22) routinely as a marker of disease activity and has been compared to SACE. Significant differences have been reported between sarcoidosis considered as active versus inactive. The sensitivity of STME was 43% and the specificity 83% with a positive predictive value of 77%. When used concurrently with SACE the sensitivity and specificity improve.

Nevertheless, further studies are needed to determine the prognostic significance of TME and its clinical usefulness.

Among markers related to lymphocyte activation, β2 microglobulin (β2 M) in serum and BAL fluid has been extensively studied in sarcoidosis (9, 27, 28, 29, 30).

It is a low molecular weight protein of about 20,000 daltons binding to HLA antigen on cell membranes, not specific of lymphocytes but increasing in serum in lymphoproliferative disorders. It may indicate lymphocyte activation in high concentrations with normal renal function, and β2 M may be used as a marker in a disease such as sarcoidosis where granuloma production results in an initial accumulation and activation of lymphocytes at different sites (2, 27). Determination of β2 M may be performed in serum and BAL (9, 28, 30). Conflicting results have been reported concerning the value of β2 M determination as a biological maker of activity and its comparison to other markers. The following points may be stressed:

* Increase of β2 M values in serum correlates with active dsiease, relapses and acute forms.

* There is no correlation between serum and BAL fluid determination of β2 M.

* Correlation between SACE and β2 M in serum is variable according to the different series. The differences seem related to the mechanism of the granuloma formation (9).

* Also for the correlations between β2 M and SACE and LACE or BAL lymphocytosis, conflicting data have been reported.

Finally, the specificity of the test is very low; it does not give more information than the clinical picture and SACE. Nevertheless, increasing lymphocytic activation remains an indicator for frequent clinical follow-up examinations (9) and consequently may have a certain predictive value to recurrences or relapses of the disease.

Adenosine deaminase is another marker of lymphocyte activity. Adenosine deaminase (ADA) is necessary for the differentiation of lymphoid cells particularly (but not specifically) for T lymphocytes. The serum ADA may consequently relfect lymphocyte activity in sarcoidosis and has been considered as a marker of the disease activity. But the sensitivity of the test is low and further studies are needed to define its theoretical and practical value and its place in sarcoidosis (9).

Trascobalamine II (TC II) may be increased in serum of sarcoid patients as in other lymphoproliferative or immune disorders (9) and may be considered to be closely related to the lymphocyte activity markers. Correlationship has been found with serum lysozyme but not with SACE and TC II may be normal in very active sarcoidosis. Finally, determination of serum TC II is neither specific nor sensitive and its measurement is of limited value (9).

Neopterin (N), which is more interesting, is a pyrazinopyrimidine comound derived from guanosine triphosphate which represents a precursor of biopterin (31). It is an essential cofactor in neurotransmitter synthesis. N determination in blood and urine has been proposed as an index of immune response in patients with various conditions involving the cellular immune system. N is involved in the activation of lymphocytes: activated T cells at the site of sarcoid inflammation release increased amounts of Interferon which induces an increased production of N in macrophages (31). N is measured by radioimmunoassay. Increased serum levels (31) and urinary excretion (32) have been reported in sarcoidosis in relation with the intensity of alveolitis and activation of T4 cells.

In serum, normal values are 2.3-8.3 mmol/l. Serum N (SN) level is significantly elevated both in inactive and active sarcoidosis but increases with clinical activity (31). Urinary excretion is also related to clinical activity.

The correlation between serum levels of N and other markers, biochemical and clinical, is not yet well defined. Incomplete correlation was found between SACE and SN and a single N determination seems to be of limited value due to a lack of specificity, the compound being affected by other factors such as viral infections (31). Further studies are needed to assess the precise place of such a marker.

Collagen Metabolism Alterations

The disturbance of pulmonary function is one of the most preoccupying features in sarcoidosis. This evolution is often unpredictible and it is most important to recommend corticosteroid treatment for stopping the fibrosing process and for preventing functional degradation. The markers of altered collagen metabolism may be measured in that way in serum, BAL fluid or urine. Among them four have been proposed and, strictly speaking, these, are indirect indexes iof collagen abnormal production and turn-over rather than activity markers:

(1) Collagenase in seruma and in BAL fluid. (2) Type III procollagen N-terminal peptide. (3) Hyaluronic Acid (Hyaluronate) in BAL fluid. (4) Fibronectin in BAL fluid.

(1) In sarcoidosis an increase in the activity of collagenase has been noted in serum (9). It results, probably not exclusively, in macrophage activation. Serum collagenase might be correlated to SACE. Collagenase in the lower respiratory tract may be correlated with fibrosing processes (33) and may be measured in BAL fluid (34) but the correlation of the increase with a fibrosing process remains debatable and the value of such a marker seems to be low (9).

(2) Type III procollagen N terminal peptide could be a marker of collagen secretion and the level may be compared between serum and BAL fluid (35, 9) but the practical interest of such a test, namely in BAL fluid, is still debatable.

(3) The production of hyaluronic acid is stimulated in experimental granulomatosis and has been measured in BAL fluid in sarcoidosis (36). Its determination compared to serum level seems interesting but its practical value needs further studies.

(4) Fibronectin (F) is a large glycoprotein present in plasma and tissues with different functions namely to mediate the biding of fibroblasts to collagen and to serve as a chemoattractant for fibroblasts. It is assumed that F may be correlated to the development of fibrosis. F has been measured in BAL fluid and is significantly greater than that in normal subjects (37). In practice the

532

fibronectin determination remains only of theoretical interst and its usefulness in clinical practice is not yet assumed in important series.

Disorders of Calcium Metabolism

Sarcoidosis hypercalcemia and hypercalciuria have long been recognized as symptomatic. Hypercalciuria may occur in all types and stages of sarcoidosis without influence of age, sex, race or environment.

The frequency of such abnormalities is still controversial but probably low (from 4 to 11% according to the series) (9). The variations depend partly on the method used for dosage and on the type of patient recruitment. Hypercalciuria is more frequent than hpercalcemia.

Recently it has been demonstrated that the distorsion of calcium metabolism results from an endogenous overproduction of an active vitamine D metabolite: 1.25-dihydroxyvitamin D or calcitriol (38). The source of the metabolite is extrarenal and several studies have demonstrated that alveolar macrophages and sarcoid granulomas are these extrarenal sources (39).

Calcitriol level seems to be correlated with the development and extent of sarcoidosis and consequently hypercalcemia and hypercalciuria may be considered as biochemical markers of active sarcoidosis but the sensitivity of such a marker is likely to be low and it is not absolutely specific: calcitriol production may be observed in sarcoid-like granulomas of other conditions.

ISOTOPIC MARKERS

Gallium (67Ga) is practically the only isotopic procedure used for global evaluation of sarcoidosis activity. Fixation by sarcoid granuloma has been extensively studied in recent years as an index of the extent at different sites and of the permanence of inflammation process and granuloma formation (40, 41, 42, 43, 44, 45).

Gallium fixation has been qualified as a marker of sarcoid activity, in particular as an index, assessing the degree of T lymphocytes alveolitis (40). Different quantitative scoring methods are used to improve the precision of the method (41, 45) but with a still debatable accuracy. An in vitro 67Ga lung index has also been proposed (46, 47). 67Ga activity may be assessed in BAL fluid (48). Prospective clinical studies and correlations with other indexes such as SACE and cell counts of T lymphocytes in BAL have been performed. A collective experience of 14 clinical groups was presented at the previous international conference on sarcoidosis (45).

The following aspects were considered: (1) methods used for the most reliable score, (2) sensitivity and specificity respectively compared to X-ray imaging, BAL fluid cell count, SACE and clinically evident signs and symptoms, (3) evolution under steroid therapy, (4) appropriate doses and cost of the method. From the various publications it can be assumed that 67Ga is neither specific nor useful for sarcoid diagnosis, but rather for assessing the extent of the diseases at different sites and for the degree of granuloma activity in those sites.

Repeated 67Ga scan is more sensitive than chest radiography and clinical symptoms but no comparison has been made with lung CT scan in sarcoidosis. 67Ga scan is roughly correlated with functional lung abnormalities at least if simultaneously performed, but the predictive value of 67Ga is poor. 67Ga is not a good sensitive index for therapy (43). Nevertheless Ga scan may sometimes help take therapeutical decisions by separating the respective part of fibrosis and granuloma in lung sarcoidosis. The correlations between Ga index and other parameters, the so-called activity indexes, are still debated, in particular with the BAL lymphocyte cell count and with histological score index (49).

Finally, 67Ga scan is still considered as a valuable non-invasive method for: (1) assessing the extent and, to a lessor degree, the degree of inflammatory process, (2) choosing the preferential site for BAL or guiding for lung biopsy, (3) following the therapeutic response. However, 67Ga scan is a test lacking specificity. It necessitates exposure to radiations if repeated and mainly, it is expensive despite the suggestions of more appropriate techniques. In conclusion 67Ga scan has a limited value in the management of sarcoidosis (44).

IMMUNOLOGICAL CELL COUNTS AND CELL MARKERS

In sarcoidosis the distribution of the cell population in blood and BAL fluid may serve in the diagnosis and management of the disease. The study of lymphocyte subsets, in BAL fluid by membrane markers or monoclonal antibodies, compared with those of normal subjects shows that T cells are significantly increased ($84 \pm 1\%$ in our won series) with an increased ratio of T helper ($58 \pm 14\%$) to T suppressor cells ($25 \pm 13\%$) and a significant increase in activated T cells (50). This alveolar lymphocytosis have been considered as the direct reflection of alveolitis and there has been considerable enthusiasm in the past ten years about the use of BAL including repeatitive BAL in assessing disease activity, prognosis and therapeutic management (50, 51). Even a threshold has been suggested, introducing the concept of high alveolitis intensity (i.e. lymphocytes > 28% of the total cell count).

In fact many experienced centers restrict themselves to this range of values (41, 50, 51, 52, 53): the degree of lymphocytosis in BAL fluid at the time of diagnosis for predicting the outcome of the disease and consequently for assessing a rational basis for treatment is also controversial. Lymphocytosis at sequential BAL examinations could be more significant. After 12 months of follow-up, persistent high lymphocytosis might be of predictive value (50), but

534

finally all the schemas based only on BAL lymphocyte counts, even on serial lavage lymphocyte counts (total lymphocyte count and T4/T8 ratio), are not reliable enough for disease management.

If high intensity alveolitis at the first examination or at sequential examination may suggest a more probably deterioration in lung functions, many examples exist of patients with a high degree of alveolitis in terms of lymphocytosis, who finally recover without steroids or who have a chronic, benign sarcoidosis. In view of this, despite the fact that BAL may complete the diagnositic procedure of sarcoidosis and give theoretically valuable information on the disease, the practical interest of this method for disease management has probably been overestimated in recent years. As a single criterion, the value of the total lymphocytes and lymphocytes subsets count in BAL is low in terms of sensitivity and specificity.

Other immunocytological considerations, based on peripheral blood tests or BAL fluid, have recently been suggested as possible indexes of disease activity:
* Comparative studies of T4/T8 ratio in blood and BAL fluid.
* BAL immunoglobulin content and BAL histamine release (54) in the above two media.
* In vitro tests with cell cultures (55).
* Phagocytic activity for alveolar macrophages (56).
* Cell-cell interactions, namely Il 1 production by alveolar macrophages (57) or spontaenous release of Il 2 by T cells, etc.
Neither the significance nor the reliability, in terms of predictive value and therapeutic guidelines, have so far been clearly demonstrated in any such parameters or biological features despite their theoretical interest.

CONCLUSIONS

As it can ben seen many papers have been devoted in the past ten years to the criteria of the so-called "activity" in sarcoidosis. Among these criteria SACE, 67Ga scan and immunologic cell counts in BAL fluid, appear to be preferential. They have been compared, in several series, between themselves and to other indices (40, 41, 51, 58, 59, 60, 61, 62, 63). In fact, 2 points explain the divergence and sometimes the conflicting conclusions in the evaluation of the different methods.
(1) Each determination, for instance Ga scan, SACE or BAL may refelct different aspects of the disease process (i.e. granuloma formation, inflammatory process in general, activation of different cells, etc.). The only term of activity in fact covers different meanings under the mask of an aparent unit.
(2) Many problems in our understanding of disease activity arise from the absence of a precise definition of this concept. Sophistication of several criteria

contrasts with the lack of precision and the variety of content and interpretation of the term activity. While currently we discuss about the specificity or the sensitivity of a marker, we have not as yet defined the sense, the limits and the specificity of the term "activity".

In conclusion, we will reiterate what we proposed during the last international conference: preference should be given to the terms predictive criteria and therapeutic guidelines instead of the term activity, and the value of such indices should not be assessed by reference to the notion of activity but by reference to sequential studies with a sufficiently long follow-up. Only such follow-up can help assess the validity of each criterion in both treated and untreated groups of patients. Furthermore, in sarcoid pateints assessing the value of the different criteria, such as the degree of extrathoracic lesion, and the overall duration of the disease should be more precise (64). Despite much recent increase in our knowledge, sarcoidosis remains a mysterious and complex disease and may have plurifactorial causes. In such a context, above all, we need unequivocal, clear and precise definitions.

REFERENCES

1. De Labarthe B, Chretien J. Les indices d'activité de la sarcoldose. Ann Med Interne 1987,132:221-224.

2. Chretien J, Venet A, Israel-Biet D, Clavel F, Sandron D. Summary statement of disease activity assessment. 10th Int Conf in Sarcoidosis and other Granulomatous Disorders. Ann NY Acad Sci 1986,465:479-481.

3. Chretien J, Stanislas-Leguern G, Saltiel JC, Huchon G, Marsac J. Course and treatment of sarcoidosis in 350 patients. A follow-up study for ten yeras. In: Sarcoidosis. Jpn Med Res Found, eds, Univ of Tokyo Press pub. 1 vol 1984:301-314

4. MacFarlane JT. Prognosis in sarcoidosis. Brit Med J 1984,288:1557-1558.

5. Hillerdal G, Nou E, Osterman K, Schmekel B. Sarcoidosis: Epidemiology and prognosis. A 15 year European study. Am Rev Respir Dis 1984,130:29-32.

6. Reich JM, Johnson RE. Course and prognosis of sarcoidosis in a nonreferrral setting. Analysis of 86 patients observed 10 years. Am J Med 1985,78:61-67.

7. James DG, Jones-Williams W. Sarcoidosis and other granulomatous disorders. W.B. Saunders. Philadelphia, PA 1985, 1 vol.

8. Simon MR, Desai SG, Lee KK, James KE, Cummiskey J, Daniele RP, Lieberman J, Israel HL. Method for the derivation of clinical and laboratory indices in relation to disease activity and outcome in sarcoidosis. A projective non randomized study. Chest 1986,89:138-140.

9. Selroos OBN. Biochemical markers in sarcoidosis. Clin Lab Sci 1986,24:185-216.

10. Lieberman J. Elevation of serum angiotensin-converting enzyme (ACE) level in sarcoidosis. Am J Med 19675,59:365-372.

11. Lieberman J. The specificity and nature of serum angiotensin-converting enzyme (serum ACE) elevation in sarcoidosis. Ann NY Acad Sci 1976,278:488-497.

12. Lieberman J. Sarcoidosis. J Lieberman, ed. Grune and Stratton publ 1 vol. 1985:145-159.

13. Studdy PR, James DG. The specificity and sensitivity of serum angiotensin converting enzyme in sarcoidosis and other diseases. Experience in twelve centers in six different countries. In: J Chrétien, J Marsac, JC Saltiel, eds. Sarcoidosis and other granulomatous disorders, Paris, 1983:332-344.

14. Romer FK. The level of angiotensin converting enzyme as indicator of 2 year prognosis in untreated pulmonary sarcoidosis without erythema nodosum. Acta Med Scand 1982,211:293-295.

15. Selroos O. Use of budesonide in the treatment of pulmonary sarcoidosis. Ann NY Acad Sci 1986,465:713-721.

16. Sharma OP, Vita JB. Determination of ACE activity in tears. A non invasive test for evaluation of ocular sarcoidosis. Arch Ophthalmol 1983,101:559-561.

17. Okansen V, Gronhagen-Riska C, Fyhrqvist F, Somer H. Systemic manifestation and enzyme studies in sarcoidosis with neurologic involvement. Acad Med Scand 1985, 218:123.

18. Chan Seem CP, Norfok G, Spokes EG. CSF angiotensin-converting enzyme in neurosarcoidosis. Lancet 1985,i:456-457.

19. Lanzillo JJ, Fanburg B. Angiotensin-converting enzyme in bronchoalveolar lining fluid. Lancet 1979,i:1199-1200.

20. Mordelet-Dambrine M, Stanislas-Leguern GM, Huchon GJ, Baumann FC, Marsac JH, Chretien J. Elevation of the bronchoalveolar concentrations of angiotensin-converting enzyme in sarcoidosis. Am Rev Respir Dis 1982,126:472-475.

21. Perrin-Fayolle M, Pacheco Y, Harf R, Montagnon B, Biot N. Angiotensin-converting enzyme in bronchoalveolar lavage fluid in pulmonary sarcoidosis. Thorax 1981,36:790-792.

22. Almenoff J, Skovrow ML, Teirstein AS. Thermolysin-like serum metallo endopeptidase. A new marker for active sarcoidosis that complement serum angiotensin converting enzyme. Ann NY Acad Sci 1986,465:738-743.

23. Klockars M, Selroos O. Elevad muramidase levels in histiocytic medullary reticulosis. N Engl J Med 1976,294:901-902.

24. Gronhagen-Riska C, Selroos O. Angiotensin converting enzyme IV changes in serum activity and in lysozyme concentrations as indicators of the course of untreated sarcoidosis. Scand J Resp Dis 1979,60:337-344.

25. Selroos O, Klockars M. Serum lysozyme in sarcoidosis. Evaluation of its usefulness in determination of disease activity. Scand J Respir Dis 1977,58:110-116.

26. Rohatgi PK, Ryan JW. Serum angiotensin converting enzyme (SACE) and Carboxypeptidase N (CPN) activities in sarcoidosis and other chronic lung diseases (abstract). Am Rev Respir Dis 1982,125,suppl:115.

27. Mornex JF, Revillard JP, Vincent C, Deteix P, Brune J. Elevated serum B2 microglobulin levels and Clq-binding immune complexes in sarcoidosis. Biomedicine 1979,31:210-213.

28. Mornex JF, Biot N, Pacheco Y, Perrin-Fayolle M, Vincent C, Revillard JP. Beta 2 microglobulin level in serum and bronchoalveolar lavage fluid from patients with sarcoidosis. In: Sarcoidosis and other granulomatous disorders. J Chretien, J Marsac, JC Saltiel eds 1 vol 1983, Paris Pergamon Press, 372-377.

29. Parrish RW, Williams JD, Davies BH. Serum B2-microglobulin and angiotensin converting enzyme activity. In: Sarcoidosis and other granulomatous disorders. J Chretien, J Marsac, JC Saltiel eds 1 vol 1983, Paris Pergamon Press, 366-371.

30. Morishita M, Torii Y, Ichimura K, Takada K, Suzuki M, Ina Y, Aoki H, Sugiura T, Yamamoto M. Serum and bronchoalveolar lavage level of beta-2 microglobulin in patients with sarcoidosis. In: Sarcoidosis and other granulomatous disorders. J Chretien, J Marsac, JC Saltiel eds 1 vol 1983, Paris Pergamon Press, 383-388.

31. Eklund A, Blashke E. Elevated serum Neopterin levels in sarcoidosis. Lung 1986,164:325-332.

32. Lacronique J, Traore BM, Auzeby A, Soler P, Venot A, Pre J, Regnard J, Marsac J, Touitou Y. Follow-up study of pulmonary sarcoidosis: Interest of urinary neopterin. Am Rev Respir Dis (abstract):A548.

33. Gadek JE, Kelman JA, Fells G, Weinberger SE, Horwitz AL, Reynolds HY, Fulmer JD, Crystal RG. Collagenase in the lower respiratory tract of patients with idiopathic pulmonary fibrosis. N Engl J Med 1979,301:737-742.

34. O'Connor CM, Power C, Ward K, Fitzgerald MX. Collagenase in the lower respiratory tract of patients with sarcoidosis (abstract). Am Rev Respir Dis 1987,135:A-28.

35. Watanabe Y, Yamaki K, Yamakawa I, Takagi K, Satake T. Type III procollagen N-terminal peptides in experimental pulmonary fibrosis and human lung disease. Eur J Respir Dis 1985,67:10-16.

36. Hallgren R, Eklund A, Engstrom-Laurent A, Schmekel B. Hyaluronate in bronchoalveolar lavage fluid: A new marker in sarcoidosis refelcting pulmonary disease. Br Med J 1985,290:1778-1781.

37. Rennard SI, Crystal RG. Fibronectin in human bronchopulmonary lavage fluid. Elevation in patient with interstitial lung disease. J Clin Invest 1982,69:113-122.

38. Sharma OP. Hypercalcemia in sarcoidosis. The puzzle finally solved. Arch Intern Med 1985,145:626-627.

39. Adams JC, Singr FR, Sharma P, Hayes MJ, Vouros PM, Holic MF. Isolation and structural identification of 1,25-dihydroxyvitamin D3 produced by cultured alveolar macrophages in sarcoidosis. J Clin Endocrinol Metab 1985,60:960-96.

40. Line BR, Hunninghake GW, Keogh BA, Jones AE, Johnston GS, Crystal RG. Gallium-67 scanning to stage the alveolitis of sarcoidosis: Correlation with clinical studies, pulmonary function studies and bronchoalveolar lavage. Am Rev Respir Dis 1981,123:440-446.

41. Beaumont D, Herry JY, Sapene M, Bourgnet P, Larzul JJ, De Labarthe B, Gallium-67 in the evaluation of sarcoidosis: Correlation with serum

angiotensin-converting enzyme and bronchoalveolar lavage. Thorax 1982,37:11-18

42. Huchon GJ, Berrissoul LG, Barritault LG, Venet A, Marsac J, Roucayrol JC, Chretien J. Comparison of bronchoalveolar lavage and Gallium-67 lung scanning to assess the activity of pulmonary sarcoidosis. In: Sarcoidosis and other granulomatous disorders. J Chretien, J Marsac, JC Saltiel eds 1 vol 1983, Paris Pergamon Press, 440-445.

43. Niden AH, Mishkin FS, Salem F, Thomas Jr AV, Kamdar V. Prognostic significance of Gallium lung scans in sarcoidosis. Ann NY Acad Sci 1 vol. C Johnson-John ed. NY 1986:435-443.

44. Israel HL, Gushue GF, Park CH. Assessment of Gallium-67 scanning in pulmonary and extrapulmonary sarcoidosis. ANN NY Acad Sci 1 vol. C Johnson-John ed. NY 1986:455-462.

45. Rizzato G, Blasi A. A European survey on the usefulness of 67 Ga lung scans in assessing sarcoidosis. Experience in 14 research centers in seven different countries. Ann NY Acad Sci 1 vol. C Johnson-John ed. NYU 1986:463-478.

46. Braude AC, Cohen R, Rahmani R, Hornstein A, Klein M, Meindok HO, Chamberlain DW, Rebuck AS. An in vitro Gallium-67 lung index for the evaluation of sarcoidosis. Am Rev Respir Dis 1984,130:783-785.

47. Van Maarsseveen A, Alberts C, van der Schoot J, van Royen E, Hens C, Mullink H, de Groot J. Radionuclides in detecting active granuloma formation. Ann NY Acad Sci 1 vol. C Johnson-John ed. NY 1986:427-434.

48. Trauth HA, Heims K, Schubotz R, Von Wichert P. Gallium-67 activity in bronchoalveolar lavage fluid in sarcoidosis. Ann NY Acad Sci 1 vol. C Johnson-John ed. NY 1986:444-454.

49. Whitcomb ME, Dixon GF. Gallium scanning, bronchoalveolar lavage and the national debt. Chest 1984,85:719-721.

50. Chretien J, Venet A, Danel C, Israel-Biet D, Sandron D, Arnoux A. Bronchoalveolar lavage in sarcoidosis. Respiration 1985,48:222-230.

51. Daniele RP, Elias JA, Epstein PE, Rossman MD. Bronchoalveolar lavage: Role in the pathogenesis, diagnosis and management of interstitial lung disease. Ann Int Med 1986,102:93-108.

52. Turner-Warwick M, McAllister W, Lawrence R, Britten A, Haslam PL. Corticosteroid treatment in pulmonary sarcoidosis: Do serial lavage lymphocyte counts, serum angiotensin converting enzyme measurement, and Gallium-67 scans help management. Thorax 1986,41:903-913.

53. Ward K, Odlum C, O'Connor C, Van Breda A, Fitzgerald MN. BAL T lymphocyte helper/suppressor cell ratio does not predict subsequent change in pulmonary function in sarcoidosis (abstract). Thorax 1987,42:225.

54. Casale TB, Trapp S, Wood D, Zehr B, Hunninghake GW. Elevated bronchoalveolar lavage fluid (BAL) histamin levels in interstitial lung diseases and assoicated with disease activity (Abstract). Am Rev Respir Dis 1987,135 suppl:A29.

55. Arnoux AG, Jaubert F, Stanislas-Leguern G, Danel C, Chretien J. In vitro granuloma-like formations in bronchoalveolar cell cultures from patients with sarcoidosis. Ann NY Acad Sci 1 vol. C Johnson-John ed. NY 1986,465:183-192.

56. Clavel F, Laval AM, Venet A, Cayrol E, Chretien J. Alveolar macrophage phoacytosis in sarcoidosis. The role of activated lymphocytes. Ann NY Acad Sci 1 vol. C Johnson-John ed. NY 1986,465:110-121.

57. Kleinhez ME, Fujiwara H, Rich EA. Interleukin-1 production by blood monocyte and bronchoalveolar cells in sarcoidosis. Ann NY Acad Sci 1 vol. C Johnson-John ed. NY 1986,465:91-97.

58. Hunninghake GW. Role of alveolar macrophage and lung T-cell derived mediators in pulmonary sarcoidosis. Ann NY Acad Sci 1 vol. C Johnson-John ed. NY 1986,465:42-90.

59. Klech H, Kohn H, Kummer F, Mostbeck A. Assessment of activity in sarcoidosis sensitivity and specificity of 67-Gallum scintigraphy, serum ACE levels, chest Roentgenography, and blood lymphocyte subpopulation. Chest 1982,82:732-738.

60. Schoenberger CI, Line BR, Keogh BA, Hunninghake GW, Crystal RG. Lung inflammation in sarcoidosis. Comparison of serum angiotensin converting enzyme levels with bronchoalveolar lavage and Gallium-67 scanning assessment of the T lymphocyte alveolitis. Thorax 1982,37:19-25.

61. Selroos O. Value of biochemical markers in serum for determination of disease activity in sarcoidosis. Sarcoidosis 1984,1:45-49.

62. Rizatto G. Markers of activity of sarcoidosis. Sarcoidosis 1985,2:12-15.

63. Staton Jr GM, Gilman MJ, Pine JR, Fajman WA, Check IJ. Comparison of clinical parameters, bronchoalveolar lavage, Gallium-67 lung uptake, and serum angiotensin converting enzyme in assessing the activity of sarcoidosis 1986,3:10-18.

64. Selroos O, Kockars M. Relation between clinical stage of sarcoidosis and serum values of angiotensin converting enzyme and Beta 2-microglobulin. Sarcoidosis 1987,4:13-17.

65. Sanguinetti CM, Montroni M, Balbi B, Prete M, Gasparini S, Rossi GA. Does activity of pulmonary sarcoidosis depend on disease duration? A comparison between bronchoalveolar lavage, scintigraphic, radiologic and physiologic parameters. Sarcoidosis 1987,4:18-24.

MAGNETIC RESONANCE IMAGING IN SARCOIDOSIS

B.G. LANGER,[*+] V. LOPEZ-MAJANO,[*] R. RHEE,[*] D.G. SPIGOS[*+]

[*]COOK COUNTY HOSPITAL AND [+]UNIVERSITY OF ILLINOIS HOSPITAL, CHICAGO,
ILLINOIS

INTRODUCTION

A variety of examinations exist for the evaluation of sarcoidosis.
In addition to the conventional chest film, the gallium scan has for
some time been recognized as a detector of salivary gland, pulmonary, and hilar sarcoidosis (1-3). Magnetic resonance imaging is a
modality with great diagnostic potential, the extent of which is
just beginning to be tapped. This study was undertaken to determine
whether MRI could add information or contribute to the diagnostic
specificity of the current diagnostic workup.

MATERIALS AND METHODS

Nineteen patients with clinical evidence of sarcoidosis were examined using conventional chest radiographs, ^{67}Ga scans, and magnetic
resonance imaging. ^{67}Ga-citrate uptake scans were performed conventionally with appropriate views of the mediastinum, pulmonary parenchyma, and head and neck. MRI examinations of the salivary glands
were obtained using a 1.5T superconducting magnet (General Electric
Signa, Milwaukee, Wisconsin) with head imaging coil. The images
were obtained using either a 256x256 or 256x128 imaging matrix.
When the 256x256 matrix was used one excitation was aquired, when
the 256x128 matrix was used two excitations were aquired. Sections
obtained were three to five millimeters thick and both partial saturation (TR = 300-600msec, TE = 25msec); and spin-echo (TR = 2000-
2500msec, TE = 20-25msec/70-80msec) images were aquired. Axial and
sagittal imaged were obtained in all cases and in selected cases
coronal images were aquired. As a criterion for inclusion in the
study all patients had strongly positive gallium uptake in at least
two of the salivary glands. MRI examinations were compared to a
control group of 10 patients made up of five normal volunteers and
five patients whose salivary glands were included in MRI examinations performed for other reasons.

The same equipment was used to obtain MRI examinations of the
chest. As a criterion for inclusion in the study, the nine patients
examined with chest MRI had pronounced ^{67}Ga uptake in the hila. Six

of the chest examinations were performed without cardiac gating.
When cardiac gating capability become available, it was used for the
remaining three patients. A variety of sequences were used (TR 500-
2000, TE 20-80 for chest imaging. A matrix of 256x128 was used and
two excitations were aquired. Axial images were aquired in all
cases. Sagittal and coronal sections were obtained in selected
cases.

RESULTS

MRI, ^{67}Ga, and plain film examinations were reviewed. The salivary gland MRI examinations were compared both to the gallium scans
and to the MRI examinations of the control group with particular
attention to size, signal intensity, and signal homogeneity (Fig. 1,
2).

SIZE - The normal parotid glands ranged in sized from 2.2-4.1cm(x=
3.2) in AP dimension, 4.4-5.0cm(x=4.9) in superior to inferior
dimension, and 1.2-3.0cm(x=2.5) in transverse dimension. The parotid glands of the sarcoidosis patients ranged in size from 2.9-5.0cm
(x=3.5) in AP dimension, 3.0-6.0(x=4.6) in superior to inferior
dimension, and 1.8-3.3cm(x=2.6) in transverse dimension.

The normal submandibular glands ranged in size from 1.6-3.0cm(x=2.
2) in AP dimension, 1.5-2.5cm(x=2.1) in superior to inferior dimension, and 1.1-2.5cm(x=1.7) in transverse dimension. The submandibular glands of the sarcoidosis patients ranged in size from 1.5-3.3cm
(x=2.3) in the AP dimension, 1.5-3.3cm(x=2.4) in superior to inferi-
or dimension, and 1.2-2.8cm(x=1.9) in the transverse dimension.

SIGNAL INTENSITY

All imaged glands, both submandibular and parotid, both in the
sarcoidosis patients and in the control group were judged to exhibit
2+ signal intensity on all imaging sequences. The following grading
system was used: for T1 and proton density images 0 = intensity of
air/bone, 1 = intensity greater than air and less than or equal to
muscle, 2 = intensity greater than muscle but less than fat, 3 = intensity greater than or equal to fat. For T2 images 0 = intensity
of air/bone, 1 = intensity greater than air and less than or equal
to muscle, 2 = greater than muscle and less than fluid, 3 = greater
than or equal to fluid.

SIGNAL HOMOGENEITY

In all normal cases the salivary glands were judged to be of homo-

genous MRI signal. In nine of the ten sarcoidosis patients the
salivary glands were judged homogenous in MRI signal. In a single
sarcoidosis patient the MRI signal of both the parotid and submandibular glands was judged nonhomogenous.

In the chest MRI revealed the hilar enlargement detected by other
modalities in all cases. As has been shown elsewhere,[4,5] the multiplanar capabilities of MRI can provide accurate anatomic detail
(Fig. 1-3). The hilar enlargement was not quantified as enlargement
itself was used as a criterion for inclusion in the study. In all
cases the enlarged nodes were judged to have a 2+ signal intensity
on all imaging sequences and all cases the signal intensity was
judged homogenous.

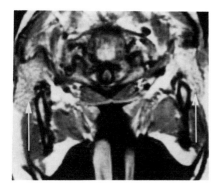 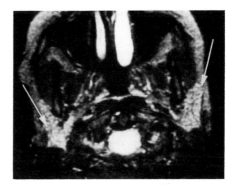

Figures 1 (TR=2000, TE=20) and 2 (TR=2000, TE=80). Axial images revealing the parotid glands (arrows) of a 36 year old female with
systemic sarcoidosis and intense salivary gland uptake on gallium
scan.

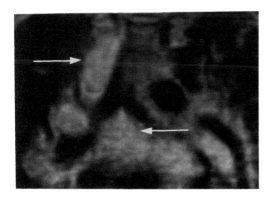

Fig. 3 (TR=1395, TE=20) coronal image revealing extensive mediastinal adenopathy (arrows) in a 30 year old female with intense
mediastinal uptake on gallium scan.

DISCUSSION

The parotid and submandibular glands of both normal patients and those with sarcoidosis exhibited a wide variation in size. Although the upper limit of gland size seen in the sarcoidosis group was slightly higher than that seen in the normal group, this difference was minimal.

There was no demonstrable difference in signal intensity between the glands of the sarcoidosis patients and those of the control group. Although in a single case the salivary glands of a sarcoidosis patient were judged nonhomogenous, no consistent differences between the two groups could be appreciated.

In the chest, although all hilar enlargement identified using other modalities was also imaged using MRI, the signal characteristics were nonspecific. Although MRI has undeniable advantages giving multiplanar[4,5] and cross-sectional images in this series, no findings specific to sarcoidosis were seen in the salivary glands or chest.

ACKNOWLEDGEMENTS

We would like to thank Cyndy Gonzalez for her cooperation in preparing this manuscript.

REFERENCES

1. Van Heerden PDR, Klopper JF. Diagnosis of sarcoidosis with gallium-67. Radiology 1981; 140:870.

2. Lubat E, Kramer EL. Gallium-67 citrate accumulation in parotid and submandibular glands in sarcoidosis. Clin Nucl Med 1985; 10:593.

3. Weiner SN, Patel BP. ^{67}Ga-citrate uptake by the parotid glands in sarcoidosis. Radiology 1979; 130:753-5.

4. O'Donovan PB, Ross JS, Sivak ED, O'Donnell JK, Mearcy TF. Magnetic resonance imaging of the thorax: the advantages of coronal and sagittal planes. AJR 1984; 143:1183-1188.

5. Webb WR, Jensen BG, Gamsu G, Sollitto R, Moore EH. Coronal Magnetic resonance imaging of the chest: normal and abnormal. Raddology 1984; 153:729-735.

LONG-TERM FOLLOW UP OF Ga^{67} SCANS AND BAL LYMPHOCYTES IN UNTREATED
SARCOID PATIENTS. A WORLDWIDE STUDY FROM 9 CENTRES IN 7 DIFFERENT
COUNTRIES

G RIZZATO[1] (Milan), C ALBERTS (Amsterdam), F BADRINAS (Barcelona),
A CIPRIANI (Padua), P DELAVAL (Rennes), M GRANATA[2] (Milan), T IZUMI
(Kyoto), M PERRIN-FAYOLLE (Lyon), P ROHATGI (Washington), T SHARKOFF
(Cottbus)

Niguarda Hospital, Milan, Italy: 1: Sarcoidosis Clinic, 2: Medical
Physics Dept

INTRODUCTION

In 1984 R DeRemee (1) asked: "Do bronchoalveolar lavage (BAL) and
Gallium give more accurate prediction of course than does the Chest
Roengtenographic stage ?". In 1985 M Turner Warwick et al (2) have
shown that during treatment serial BAL, Ga^{67} and ACE are not consistently more sensitive methods by which to monotor patients with
sarcoidosis than are serial measurements of Chest X ray and lung
function tests; such measurements may however prove useful in individual cases when simple clinical measurements are discordant and
additional indications of possible activity are needed. In 1984 we
have started the present retrospective and prospective study on sarcoid patients followed up for a minimum of 12 months; in order to
evaluate the natural history of the disease and the natural changes
of parameters, only untreated patients were admitted to the study;
the difficulty of finding long term followed up untreated patients
has been overcome putting together the data resulting from 9 different centres (Tab 1)

MATERIAL AND METHODS

Only untreated patients with histologically proven sarcoidosis
and with a minimum follow up of 12 months were admitted to the stud
y. The study was only retrospective in some patients and prospective in others, both retrospective and prospective in most. If a
patient at any time needed therapy, his data were included into the
study only up to the beginning of therapy, provided one year had
passed from the first observation. Spirometry, $D_L co$, Chest X ray
were serially studied together with Ga lung scan and/or BAL. Most
patients had both Ga and BAL serial studies , but some could be included only in the Ga or in the BAL study. Serial Ga scans could be
carried out more frequently than serial BAL studies probably due to
low compliance of patients versus BAL. Tab 2 shows the patients ad-

TABLE   1

PARTICIPATING CENTRES

City	Hospital	Authors
Amsterdam	Vrije Universiteit	C Alberts
Barcelona	Hospital de Bellvitge "Princeps d'Espanya"	F Badrinas, F Manresa, P Romero, B Rodriguez Sanchon, M Ramos, Y Ricart, A Clarvana
Cottbus	Dept of Lung Disease, BKH	T Sharkoff, W Weidig
Kyoto	Chest Disease Research Institute	T Izumi
Lyon	Hopital Sainte Eugenie, St Genis Laval	M Perrin-Fayolle, Y Pacheco, B Coppere, B Tavot, R Harf, D Azzar
Milan	Ente Ospedale Niguarda	G Rizzato, F Spinelli, L Allegra
Padua	Complesso Convenzionato Ospedale-Università, USSL 21	A Cipriani, G DiVittorio, G Festi, A Tommasini, D Casara, G Semenzato, R Zambello, L Trentin
Rennes	Centre Hospitalier Université	P Delaval, P Bourget, C Pencole Nouveau, N Goarant B Desrues, J Kernec, J Herry
Washington	Veterans Administration Medical Center, Pulmonary Division	PK Rohatgi

TABLE 2

PATIENTS

Stage	Ga Study	BAL Study
0	7	2
I	89	22
II	44	20
III	21	9
Total	161	53
Steroids	27 (16.7%)	6 (11.3%)

mitted to the BAL and Ga studies, grouped according to the radiological stage of the first Chest X ray; in some of them the follow up was interrupted due to the need of steroids. The mean follow up period was 27 $\pm$ 19 months (range 12-140) for patients admitted to the Ga study and 22 $\pm$ 12 months (range 12-64) for patients admitted to the BAL study

The dose of Gallium injected ranged from 1.5 mCi (Milan and Cottbus) to 5 mCi (Washington); mean dose was 2.5 mCi, only the centre of Washington used a dose over 3 mCi; scoring method was subjective in some centres and semiquantitative in others. Improvement or worsening was assessed on the basis of the serial gammacamera images.

The study on BAL fluid was limited to cellularity: a lymphocyte percentage over 28 was assumed expression of high intensity alveolitis, while low intensity alveolitis was assumed when lymphocytes were between 15 and 28 percent. BAL was assumed worsening if a subject passed from low to high intensity alveolitis or from no to low or high intensity alveolitis; BAL was assumed improving if changes were observed from high to low intensity alveolitis of from low alveolitis to no alveolitis.

For forced vital capacity good laboratories mantain the variation due to measurement error between repeated measurements in normal subjects at approximately 3%, but the variations are wider for FEV_1 and $D_L co$ and wider in abnormal patients. Moreover an unexplained drift over time occurs in even the most experienced laboratories and must be borne in mind in the interpretation of results (3). In order to reduce this error two arbitrary levels of change of $\pm$ 10% or $\pm$ 20% (in respect of the first value) have been used to define change of VC or of FEV_1 ; the limits used for $D_L co$ were $\pm$ 15% and $\pm$ 25%

RESULTS

A. Ga STUDY

According to the time course of Ga lung scan, the 161 patients were grouped in 7 different groups (Tab 3)

TABLE 3

TIME COURSE OF Ga LUNG SCAN IN 161 PATIENTS

	First Ga scan	Ga scan in the follow up	n	mean follow up (months)
1	Negative	Negative	25	25 $\pm$ 21
2	Negative	Positive	15	30 $\pm$ 14
3	Hylar positive	Negative	57	23 $\pm$ 14
4	Hylar positive	Hylar positive	20	36 $\pm$ 30
5	Hylar positive	Lung uptake	17	30 $\pm$ 22
6	Lung (or hylar and lung) uptake	Improvement	11	29 $\pm$ 14
7	Lung (or hylar and lung) uptake	No improvement	16	20 $\pm$ 9

A_1. GROUPING PATIENTS ON THE BASIS OF THE RESULT OF THE FIRST SCAN

  1. Patients with initially negative Ga scan (Tab 4)

   Taking into consideration the 40 patients (Groups 1 and 2 of Tab 3) with initially negative Ga lung scan, we have observed the follow up of single parameters and compared the results using the chi square test (Tab 4): in the long term (28 months) Ga lung scan appears more sensitive than spirometry or diffusion, but no more sensitive in respect of Chest X ray.

Table   4

LONGITUDINAL OBSERVATIONS IN 40 PTS WITH INITIALLY NEG Ga LUNG SCAN

Mean follow up : 28 .0 ± 19.9 months

Test	Ga^{67} scan	FEV$_1$		VC		D_L co		Chest
		≥ 20%	≥ 10%	≥ 20%	≥10%	≥ 25%	≥ 15%	X ray
Unchanged (or Improved)	25	37	35	39	34	39	34	25
Worse	15	3	5	1	6	1	6	15
P*		.003	.020	.0002	.040	.0002	.040	n.s.

* chi square test versus Ga^{67} scans

In the long term Ga^{67} appears more sensitive than spirometry or diffusion, but no more sensitive in respect of Chest X ray.

---

  2. Patients with only hylar uptake at the first scan (Tab 5)

   94 Patients (Groups 3, 4 and 5 of Tab 3) had only hylar uptake at the first scan; during the follow up Ga scan improved in 57, worsened in 17 and was unchanged in 20. Again at the chi square test (Tab 5) Ga lung scan appears more sensitive than spirometry or $D_L$co but no more sensitive than radiology.

  3. Patients with lung uptake at the first scan (Tab 6)

   27 Patients (Groups 6 and 7 of Tab 3) had lung uptake at the 1st scan, that improved in 11 during the follow up. The chi square test

TABLE 5

LONGITUDINAL OBSERVATIONS IN 94 PTS WITH ONLY HYLAR
UPTAKE AT THE FIRST SCAN
Mean follow up : 27.6 ± 20.8 months

Test	Ga^{67} scan	FEV$_1$		VC		D$_L$co		Chest X ray
		≥20%	≥10%	≥20%	≥10%	≥25%	≥15%	
a) improved	57	15	32	15	21	13	28	47
b) unchanged	20	76	53	77	65	74	53	23
c) worsened	17	3	9	2	8	7	13	24
P * a vs. b.	<-------------------------------------- <.001 --- >							n.s.
b vs. c	<-------------------------------------- <.001 --- >							n.s.
a vs.c	< ------------------------------------- n.s. --- >							n.s.

* chi square test vs. Ga^{67}scans

Ga appars more sensitive than spirometry or D$_L$co but no more
sensitive than radiology

TABLE 6

LONGITUDINAL OBSERVATIONS IN 27 PTS WITH LUNG
UPTAKE AT THE FIRST SCAN

Mean follow-up : 23.4 ± 12.4 months

Test	Ga^{67} scan	FEV$_1$		VC		D$_L$co		Chest X ray
		≥ 20%	≥ 10%	≥ 20%	≥10%	≥ 25%	≥15%	
Improved	11	1	4	1	3	5	9	7
Unchanged (or Worse)	16	26	23	26	24	22	18	20
P *		.003	n.s.	.003	.029	n.s.	n.s.	n.s.

* Chi square test vs. Ga^{67}scans

Ga appears more sensitive than spirometry only if the limit is choosen ≥ 20%. No
more sensitive than diffusion or radiology.

shows (Tab 6) that Ga appears more sensitive than VC, but no more sensitive than $D_L$co or radiology. In respect of FEV_1, Ga appears more sensitive only when the limit of FEV_1 changes is chosen $\geqslant$ 20% while the significance is lost at the level of $\geqslant$10%.

A_2. GROUPING PATIENTS ON THE BASIS OF TIME COURSE OF Ga SCAN

1. Patients with improving or unchanged Ga lung scan (Tab 7)

We have researched (Tab 7) when Chest X ray or spirometry or $D_L$co were worsening without simultaneous worsening Ga lung scan. Taking into consideration the $\geqslant$10% level for spirometry and the $\geqslant$15% level for $D_L$co, this behaviour was observed in 39 of 129 patients or 30.2% Thus in 30% of patients there is a worsening that is not seen on Ga lung scan. The most frequent worsening parameter is Chest X ray : 13.2% of patients showed worsening Chest X ray with improving or unchanged Ga lung scan.

TABLE 7A

LONGITUDINAL OBSERVATIONS IN 129 PATIENTS
WITH IMPROVING OR UNCHANGED Ga SCAN

First scan	n	Worsening of other indices
Negative	25	8 pts (32%)
Hylar uptake	77	21 pts (27%)
Lung uptake	27	10 pts (37%)
Total	129	39 pts (30%)

TABLE 7B

WORSENING
INDICES

Chest X ray	17 pts (13.2 %)
$D_L$co	16 pts (12.4 %)
VC	12 pts (9.3 %)
FEV_1	11 pts (8.5 %)

2. Patients with worsening Ga lung scan (Tab 8)

TABLE 8 A

LONGITUDINAL OBSERVATIONS IN 32 PATIENTS
WITH WORSENING Ga LUNG SCAN

First scan	n	Improving of other indices
Negative	15	5 pts (33.3 %)
Hylar Uptake	17	3 pts (17.6 %)
Total	32	8 pts (25 %)

TABLE 8 B

IMPROVING INDICES

VC	5 pts (15.6 %)
$D_L$co	2 pts (6.2 %)
FEV_1	2 pts (6.2 %)
Chest X ray	0

In 8 of 32 patients with worsening Ga lung scan the behaviour of other parameters showed at least the improvement of one of them; thus in 25 % of patients there is an improvement that cannot be seen at the Ga scan. The improving parameter is in most cases VC (Tab 8 B).

B. BAL STUDY

According to the time course of BAL results, patients were grouped in 7 different groups (Tab 9)

TABLE 9

TIME COURSE OF T LYMPHOCYTES % IN BAL FLUID - 53 PATIENTS

	First BAL	Follow up	n	mean follow up (months)
1	≤14	≤14	18	24 ± 13
2	≤14	>14	8	18 ± 7
3	14 ≤ T lymphocytes ≤ 28	≤14	5	30 ± 11
4	14 ≤ T lymphocytes ≤ 28	unchanged	5	14 ± 2
5	14 ≤ T lymphocytes ≤ 28	>28	3	34 ± 21
6	>28	≤28	10	19 ± 9
7	>28	>28	4	13 ± 1

B_1. GROUPING PATIENTS ON THE BASIS OF THE RESULT OF THE FIRST BAL

1.Patients without alveolitis at the first BAL (Tab 10)

TABLE 10

LONGITUDINAL OBSERVATIONS IN 26 PTS WITHOUT ALVEOLITIS AT THE FIRST BAL

Mean follow up : 22.4 ±11.9 months

Test	BALs	FEV1		VC		D L co		Chest
		≥ 20%	≥ 10%	≥ 20%	≥ 10%	≥ 25%	≥ 15%	X ray
Unchanged	18	24	18	26	23	26	25	25
Worse	8	2	8	0	3	0	1	1
P*		.046	n.s.	.007	n.s.	.007	.027	.027

* chi square test vs. BALs

BAL appears more sensitive in respect of spirometry only when evaluating changes ≥ 20%. BAL appears also more sensitive than Chest X ray and diffusion.

552

26 patients with this condition were followed up for 22.4 ± 11.9
months: in 8 of them an alveolitis appeared during the follow up.
At the chi square test BAL appears more sensitive than Chest X ray
and diffusion; in respect of spirometry BAL appears more sensitive
only when evaluating FEV_1 or VC changes ≥ 20 %.

2. Patients with low intensity alveolitis at the first BAL (Tab 11)

13 patients with this condition were studied in a follow up of
23.8 ± 16.9 months; a worsening alveolitis was observed in 3 patients only , so that no significant differences could be observed
in respect of chest X ray or respiratory function data. An important consideration is that with so low a number of patients it is
difficult to obtain significant differences at the statistical
study

TABLE 11

LONGITUDINAL OBSERVATIONS IN 13 PTS WITH LOW INTENSITY ALVEOLITIS AT THE FIRST BAL

mean follow up : 23.8 ± 16.9 months

Test	BALs	FEV1		VC		$D_L$co		Chest
		≥ 20%	≥10%	≥ 20%	≥ 10%	≥ 25%	≥15%	X ray
Improved or Unchanged	10	12	10	13	11	13	12	11
Worse	3	1	3	0	2	0	1	2
P*		n.s.	n.s.	n.s.	n.s.	n.s.	n.s.	n.s.

* chi square test vs. BALs

3. Patients with high intensity alveolitis at the first BAL (Tab 12)

14 patients with this condition were studied in a follow up of
28.1 ± 12.5 months. While lymphocytes improved in 10 patients, chest
X ray improved in 4 only, so that BAL appears more sensitive than
chest X ray in evaluating changes. No significant differences could
be shown in respect to $D_L$co, while in respect of spirometry BAL was
more sensitive only considering changes ≥ 20 % .

TABLE 12

LONGITUDINAL OBSERVATIONS IN 14 PATIENTS WITH HIGH INTENSITY ALVEOLITIS AT THE FIRST BAL

Mean follow up : 28.1 ± 12.5 months

Test	BALs	FEV1		VC		D_L co		Chest
		≥20% ≥ 10%		≥20% ≥10%		≥ 25% ≥15%		X ray
Improved	10	1	5	0	6	5	7	4
Unchanged or Worse	4	13	9	14	8	9	7	10
P*		.001	n.s.	.0004	n.s.	n.s.	n.s.	.058

* chi square test vs. BALs

B_2. GROUPING PATIENTS ON THE BASIS OF TIME COURSE OF LYMPHOCYTOSIS

1. Patients with improving or unchanged lymphocytosis (Tab 13)

In 42 over 53 patients lymphocytes percentage did not worsen during the follow up, however in 12 of these 42 (28.4 %) a worsening of at least an other index could be observed; thus, similarly to the Ga study, in around 30 % of patients there is a worsening that cannot be seen at the BAL.

TABLE 13 A
LONGITUDINAL OBSERVATIONS IN 42 PTS
WITH IMPROVING OR UNCHANGED BAL

1st BAL	n	Worsening of other indices
negative	18	4 pts (22 %)
low intensity alveolitis	10	3 pts (30 %)
high intensity alveolitis	14	5 pts (36 %)
Total	42	12 pts (29 %)

TABLE 13 B
WORSENING INDICES

Chest X ray	3 pts (7 %)
VC	5 pts (9%)
FEV_1	7 pts (17%)
$D_L$co	4 pts (10%)

2. Patients with worsening lymphocytosis (Tab 14)

In 11 patients over 53, lymphocytosis did worsen during the follow up; in 2 of the above patients (18 %) an improvement of at least one of the other parameters was observed in spite of worsening BAL.

554

TABLE 14 A

LONGITUDINAL OBSERVATIONS IN 11 PTS
WITH WORSENING BAL

First BAL	n	Improving of other indices
No alveolitis	8	2 pts (25 %)
Low intensity alveolitis	3	0
Total	11	2 pts (18 %)

TABLE 14 B
IMPROVING INDICES

VC	2 patients
FEV_1	2 patients
$D_L co$	1 patient
Chest X ray	1 patient

DISCUSSION

We have studied only untreated patients, and this is an important
limitation because the most impaired patients - where probably
changes during the follow up are more striking and significant -
must be treated in most cases so that they are not included in our
study. In other words we have probably selected a population that is
not representative of all the wide range of patients with sarcoidosis. In making this choice we have also considered that the natural
history of the disease and the natural changes of parameters cannot
be studied when a treated population is included into the study. In
spite of this limitation, our longitudinal study shows usefulness
and limits of Ga lung scan and of BAL.

With few exceptions Ga lung scan appears more sensitive than spirometry or $D_L co$ but no more sensitive than Chest X ray in this long
term follow up of 27 months. In a former multicentre study (4) we
have shown in a group of 183 untreated patients studied for 3-9
months that Ga was more sensitive than Chest X ray in detecting
changes, in the brief term follow up of around 6 months; in 35 patients with early improvement of Ga and with unchanged X ray, further observations were available in the long term, and in 68.8 % of
them we had observed a late improvement on X ray. The present study
confirms that the better sensitivity of Ga lung scan versus chest
X ray is lost when the study spans over the long term period.

Furthermore, in spite of the better sensitivity of Ga lung scan
over spirometry, the limits of Ga scan are clear in Tables 7 and 8:
in 30 % of patients with improving or unchanged Ga lung scan, there
is the worsening of at least an other parameter (VC or FEV_1 or $D_L co$
or Chest X ray), and in 25 % of patients with worsening Ga lung scan
there is an improvement of at least one of the above parameters.
These variations could be due to the unexplained drift over time of

555

respiratory function data (3), however also in our former multi-centre study (4) we have observed in a group of 179 untreated patients with negative scans that other signs of clinical activity could be shown in 51 of them (28.5 %): this was not a follow up observation but a single observation; now the follow up study confirms that Ga evaluation of clinical activity differs from other parameters in around 30 % of patients and this is probably the most important limit of Ga lung scan.

The evaluation of lymphocytosis on BAL fluid cannot be conclusive in our study due to the low number of patients in some Tables. In spite of this limitation BAL appears more sensitive than Chest X ray and spirometry when FEV_1 or VC changes over 20 % are taken into consideration; the better sensitivity over $D_L co$ appears in the only group with a number of patients over 20 (Tab 10). However Tables 13 and 14 show that BAL has the same limitation as Ga lung scan: nearly 30 % of patients with improving or unchanged BAL show a worsening of at least one of the other parameters studied (VC, FEV_1, $D_L co$, or Chest X ray) and nearly 20 % of patients with worsening BAL show an improvement of at least one of the other parameters.

All the above changes confirm that in the long term follow up the correlation between Ga, BAL, spirometry, $D_L co$ and chest X ray is not simple because the above parameters express different phenomena and different changes that occur in different phases of the granulomatous process. However the following conclusions can be drawn by our study:
1) both Ga and BAL appear more sensitive than spirometry and $D_L co$
2) BAL appears also more sensitive than chest X ray
3) neither Ga nor BAL are a golden test because in around 30 % of patients they fail to detect an improving or worsening situation

REFERENCES

1. DeRemee RA (1984) The alveolitis of pulmonary sarcoidosis. Am Rev Respir Dis 129 : 343
2. Turner Warwick M, McAllister W, Lawrence R, Britten A, Haslam PL (1986) Corticosteroid Treatment in Pulmonary Sarcoidosis: do serial lavage lymphocyte counts, serum ACE measurements, and Ga-67 scans help management ? Thorax 41: 903-913
3. Becklake MR (1986) Concepts of Normality Applied to the Measurement of Lung Function. Am J Med 80: 1158-1164
4. Rizzato G, Blasi A (1986) A European Survey on the Usefulness of [67]Ga Lung Scans in Assessing Sarcoidosis. Experience in 14 Research Centres in Seven Different Countries. In: C J Johns: Tenth International Conference on Sarcoidosis and Other Granulomatous Disorders.Annals New York Acad Sc 465: 463-478

MAST CELL—DERIVED MEDIATORS IN PULMONARY SARCOIDOSIS

ANTONIO MIADONNA, ALBERTO PESCI*, ALBERTO TEDESCHI, ENNIO LEGGIERI,

GIUSEPPINA BERTORELLI*, MARCO FROLDI, DARIO OLIVIERI*, CARLO ZANUSSI

Istituto di Medicina Interna, Malattie Infettive e Immunopatologia, Università
di Milano, *Clinica Pneumologica, Università di Parma, Italia

INTRODUCTION

Activated T helper lymphocytes and macrophages have been found in the pulmonary
lesions of sarcoidosis (1, 2). Since both cells have been shown to release
factors with histamine-releasing activity (3, 4), we decided to investigate if
mast cells could be involved in the pathogenesis of pulmonary sarcoidosis.
Therefore the concentrations of histamine (a typical mast cell-derived mediator)
and leukotrienes C4 and B4 were evaluated in bronchoalveolar lavage (BAL) fluids
from patients affected with pulmonary sarcoidosis.

MATERIAL AND METHODS

Subjects

Thirty patients (22 females, ages ranging 16-67 years, mean age 40 years),
affected with pulmonary sarcoidosis,were included in the study. The diagnosis
was based on the presence of clinical symptoms and typical roentgengram features.
Only one patient was a smoker. The control group consisted of 10 subjects
(7 females, ages ranging 30-57 years, mean age 45 years), undergoing bronchoscopy
for routine diagnostic purposes. Six subjects were smokers and none was atopic.
The fiberoptic bronchoscopy in these cases was normal.

Bronchoalveolar lavage and cell counts

BAL was performed with 3 x 50 ml aliquots of prewarmed (37°C) saline solution,
which was instilled into the lingula or the right middle lobe. The lavage fluid
was gently aspirated, filtered on a single layer of surgical gauze, and centrifuged at 800 g for 10 min, to separate cellular and non cellular components.
The cell-free supernatant was divided in aliquots and stored at -80°C until
assayed. The cell pellet was utilized for total and differential cell counts
(performed with methyl violet and May-Grunwald-Giemsa stainings). Mast cells were
counted by Alcian blue-safranin staining.

Characterization of T cell subpopulations in bronchoalveolar lavage fluids

T cell subsets were characterized by Leu monoclonal antibodies (Becton Dickinson,

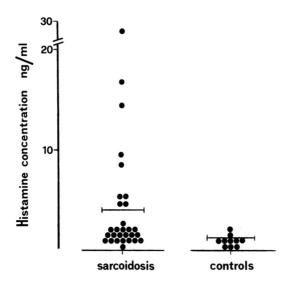

Fig. 1. Histamine levels in bronchoalveolar lavage fluids from 30 patients affected with pulmonary sarcoidosis and 10 controls.

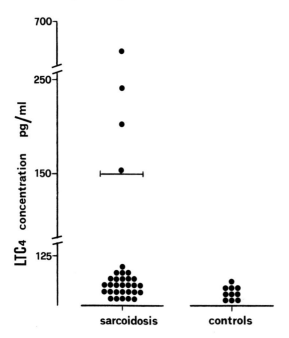

Fig. 2. Leukotriene C4 concentrations in bronchoalveolar lavage fluids from 30 patients affected with pulmonary sarcoidosis and 10 controls.

CA), using an indirect immunofluorescence technique. Leu 3 and Leu 2 antibodies were employed for the investigation.

Determination of albumin and IgG concentrations

Albumin and IgG levels in BAL fluids were measured by simple immunodiffusion in agar plates (LC Partigen, Behring, FRG).

Evaluation of histamine and leukotrienes C4 and B4 concentrations

Histamine was measured in BAL fluids by an automated fluorometric technique, modified from Siraganian (5). Leukotrienes C4 and B4 were evaluated by radio-immunoassay, using commercially available kits (Amersham, UK).

RESULTS

Total and differential cell counts

Recovery of total cells and differential cell counts results are reported in the table. The percentage of BAL mast cells in patients affected with sarcoidosis was significantly higher than in normal controls ($1.0 \pm 0.2\%$ vs. $0.3 \pm 0.5\%$; $p < 0.05$).

Characterization of T cell subpopulations

Leu 3/Leu 2 ratio was elevated in all patients with pulmonary sarcoidosis. The data are reported in the table.

Albumin and IgG concentrations

Albumin and IgG levels in BAL fluids of patients affected with pulmonary sarcoidosis are illustrated in the table. IgG/albumin ratio was significantly higher in the patient population than in controls (0.96 ± 1.1 vs. 0.31 ± 0.04; $p < 0.02$).

Mediators assays

Histamine level in patients with sarcoidosis ranged between 0.1 and 28.4 ng/ml, with a mean value of 4.1 ± 6.3 ng/ml. Control histamine concentration never exceeded 1.8 ng/ml (mean value 0.9 ± 0.3 ng/ml). Histamine levels correlated with Leu 3/Leu 2 BAL lymphocyte ratio ($r = +0.50$; $p < 0.05$) and with mast cell counts ($r = +0.52$; $p < 0.05$). Conversely, no correlation was found between histamine concentration and total cells, lymphocytes and macrophages counts, and IgG/albumin ratio.

Leukotriene C4 value was elevated in 4 patients with sarcoidosis, and ranged between 150 and 650 pg/ml. In healthy controls leukotriene C4 was always undetectable.

No leukotriene B4 was found either in patients or in controls.

TABLE I

Histamine, leukotriene C4 (LTC4) and albumin levels, IgG/albumin and Leu 3/Leu 2 ratios, total cells, lymphocytes and macrophages numbers in BAL fluids from patients with pulmonary sarcoidosis

Patient	Histamine (ng/ml)	LTC4 (pg/ml)	Albumin (mg/dl)	IgG/Alb. (mg/mg Alb.)	Leu 3/ Leu 2	Cells/ ml x 10^3	Lymp./ ml x 10^3	Macroph./ ml x 10^3
R.I.	0.76	<125	20.41	0.39	5.3	232	104	122
P.S.	14.65	<125	5.60	0.62	19.0	328	51	275
C.C.	5.40	150	61.60	0.35	3.5	152	83	57
D.D.	0.83	<125	10.79	0.81	8.7	224	90	129
S.R.	1.27	<125	76.19	0.72	3.1	496	164	297
M.D.	0.70	650	23.88	0.87	18.8	304	149	145
F.M.	1.50	<125	9.50	0.77	3.7	272	43	224
B.C.	28.40	200	10.70	1.10	20.5	264	84	176
F.L.	1.80	<125	13.97	0.72	4.6	200	46	152
B.G.	0.90	<125	12.47	0.54	8.6	392	50	329
V.A.	0.10	<125	17.91	0.69	7.3	272	62	206
M.O.	9.70	<125	8.90	0.39	3.1	158	27	119
L.R.	1.00	<125	44.95	0.34	5.5	388	116	271
P.G.	0.70	<125	12.47	0.37	16.0	336	91	241
R.A.	0.70	<125	11.73	0.44	8.1	172	38	131
C.G.	2.25	<125	12.47	0.59	6.1	152	30	120
A.E.	0.90	<125	10.18	0.28	2.3	123	28	89
C.G.	0.90	<125	13.56	0.78	9.7	336	148	181
F.L.	0.60	<125	6.89	n.d.*	17.2	n.d.	n.d.	n.d.
B.S.	0.60	<125	10.20	0.54	8.0	352	39	309
S.A.	1.20	<125	7.55	0.76	6.0	224	49	172
M.F.	17.00	<125	2.57	4.07	14.3	432	207	220
C.S.	1.30	<125	2.00	5.39	4.2	272	95	160
A.A.	5.10	<125	n.d.	n.d.	4.3	285	210	72
G.M.	n.d.	<125	28.4	1.98	n.d.	492	118	369
S.I.	4.80	<125	17.0	0.38	n.d.	270	90	182
F.A.	1.30	<125	9.5	1.05	n.d.	64	14	43
A.E.	8.60	<125	23.5	0.69	n.d.	256	154	92
P.T.	1.30	240	21.0	0.90	22.7	536	289	196
S.A.	4.80	<125	n.d.	n.d.	4.3	500	305	173
Mean ±	4.10	149.6	18.0	0.96	9.0	292.5	102.5	181.1
S.D.	6.31	97.7	16.8	1.1	6.2	120.9	75.5	83.1

*n.d. not done

DISCUSSION

Our findings showed increased numbers of mast cells and increased levels of free histamine in BAL fluids from patients with pulmonary sarcoidosis. The percentage of mast cells and the histamine concentration did not correlate with total cell counts, lymphocyte counts and IgG concentration. Conversely, a significant correlation was found between histamine concentration and Leu 3/Leu 2 ratio, a marker of disease activity. Measurable amounts of immunoreactive leukotriene C4

were detected in BAL fluids of four patients with sarcoidosis, while no leukotriene C4 could be found in BAL fluids from controls. This mediator could be
generated from mast cells, even if it can be released also by activated macrophages. Leukotriene B4 was always undetectable in BAL fluids either from
patients or from controls.

These results support the hypothesis that mast cells can be actively involved in
the pathogenesis of pulmonary sarcoidosis. The finding of high histamine levels
in BAL fluids from patients with high Leu 3/Leu 2 ratios suggest a possible link
between lymphocyte activation and mediator release from mast cells. It is
becoming increasingly evident that human lymphocytes, as well as macrophages
(3, 4), can generate factors which can modulate mast cell function and induce
histamine release. Since pulmonary sarcoidosis is characterized by an alveolitis
with a mononuclear cell infiltrate, consisting mainly of activated helper T
cells and macrophages, it is conceivable that mast cells could also be involved
and play a pathogenetic role through the release of potent inflammatory mediators. Flint and coworkers (6) reported an increased number of BAL mast cells in
patients with sarcoidosis; moreover the IgE-mediated releasability of these
cells was enhanced. Haslam et al. (7) found higher lavage histamine levels in
patients with x-ray evidence of upper lobe contraction and parenchimal involvement. Other authors (8, 9) did not observe an increased mean histamine level in
BAL fluids from patients with sarcoidosis, even if they detected an increased
number of mast cells. These differences can perhaps be explained by the
different selection of the patients.

In conclusion, we suggest that histamine assay in BAL fluid may be an additional
and useful parameter for the assessment of disease activity in pulmonary
sarcoidosis.

REFERENCES

1. Hunninghake GW, Garrett KC, Richerson HB, Fantone JC, Ward PA, Rennard SI,
   Bitterman PB, Crystal RG (1984) State of art: pathogenesis of the granulomatous
   lung diseases. Am Rev Respir Dis 130: 476-496

2. Crystal RG, Hunninghake GW, Gadek JE, Keogh BA, Rennard SI, Bitterman PB (1981)
   In: Chretien J, Marsac J, Saltiel JC (eds) Sarcoidosis and other granulomatous
   disorders. Pergamon Press, Paris, pp 13-35

3. Thueson DO, Speck LS, Lett-Brown MA, Grant JA (1979) Histamine releasing
   activity (HRA). I. Production by mitogen or antigen-stimulated human
   mononuclear cells. J Immunol 123: 626-632

562

4. Schulman ES, Liu MC, Proud D, Mac Glashan DW, Lichtenstein LM, Plaut M (1985) Human lung macrophages induce histamine release from basophils and mast cells. Am Rev Respir Dis 131: 230-235

5. Siraganian RP (1974) An automated continuous flow system for the extraction and fluorometric analysis of histamine. Anal Biochem 57: 283-294

6. Flint KC, Leung KBP, Hudspith BN, Brostoff J, Pearce FL, Geraint-James D, McI Johnson N (1986) Bronchoalveolar mast cells in sarcoidosis: increased numbers and accentuation of mediator release. Thorax 41: 94-99

7. Haslam PL, Cromwell O, Dewar A, Turner-Warwick M (1981) Evidence of increased histamine levels in lung lavage fluids from patients with cryptogenic fibrosing alveolitis. Clin Exp Immunol 44: 587-593

8. Agius RM, Godfrey RC, Holgate ST (1985) Mast cell and histamine content of human bronchoalveolar lavage fluid. Thorax 40: 760-767

9. Rankin JA, Kaliner M, Reynolds HY (1987) Histamine levels in bronchoalveolar lavage from patients with asthma, sarcoidosis and idiopathic pulmonary fibrosis. J Allergy Clin Immunol 79: 371-377

© 1988 Elsevier Science Publishers B.V. (Biomedical Division)
Sarcoidosis and other granulomatous disorders
C. Grassi, G. Rizzato, E. Pozzi, editors

ELEVATION OF SERUM TYPE III PROCOLLAGEN N-TERMINAL PEPTIDE LEVELS IN THORACIC

SARCOIDOSIS:A POSSIBLE INDEX FOR FIBROBLAST ACTIVITY

MAURIZIO LUISETTI[1],CARLO APRILE[2],LUISA BACCHELLA[2],VIRGINIA DE ROSE[1],VITTORIA PEONA[1],

ERNESTO POZZI[3]

[1]Istituto di Tisiologia e Malattie dell'Apparato Respiratorio,Università di Pavia
[2]Servizio di Medicina Nucleare,Fondazione Clinica del Lavoro,Pavia;[3]Cattedra di
Fisiopatologia Respiratoria,Università di Torino(Italy).

INTRODUCTION

Thickening of the pulmonary interstitium(which is the morphologic feature of

diffuse interstitial fibrosis)is due to uncontrolled deposition of collagen by

hyperactive fibroblasts(1).Although diffuse fibrosis is not a significant problem

in thoracic sarcoidosis(the evolution towards fibrosis is rather rare),many me-

diators,produced mainly by alveolar macrophages(interleukin-1,fibronectin,immune

interferon and AMDGF)(2),have been found able to influence the fibroblast activi-

ty during the granulomatous phase of the disease.

In spite of these observations,the in vivo quantification of fibroblast activity

(in this and in other diffuse pulmonary diseases)remains a problem.Recently a ra-

dioimmunoassay of a cleavage product of type III procollagen has been described;

this assay allows to determine the serum levels of the N-terminal peptide(PCP)

which is cleaved by a specific extracellular peptidase(3).This parameter has been

useful in monitoring acute and chronic liver diseases(4)and high levels have been

found in cases of idiopathic pulmonary fibrosis(5),while in sarcoidosis only pre-

liminary and sometimes discordant results are available at this time(6-10).

In this paper we present the results obtained in a large series of patients

with sarcoidosis and other interstitial pulmonary diseases.

MATERIALS AND METHODS

Subjects.Subjects were divided into 5 groups:a)32 patients with thoracic sarcoi-

dosis recently diagnosed by biopsy,not receiving corticostreoid treatment;b)22

patients of the above group who received prednisone for not less than 4 weeks;c)

15 subjects with non-sarcoid diffuse pulmonary fibrosis(nsDPF),consisting of pul-

monary histiocytosis X(1 case),collagen vascular disorder(4 cases),chronic hyper-

sensitivity pneumonitis(2 cases),idiopathic pulmonary fibrosis(8 cases).All of these cases were recently diagnosed and none had received corticosteroids;d)4 cases of bronchial asthma who required corticosteroid treatment;e)15 healthy controls.Subjects with known liver sarcoid and those with high transaminase,alkaline phosphatase or bilirubin levels and those with altered renal function were excluded.

Radiographic staging and assessment of sarcoidosis activity.The radiographic stage of sarcoidosis was determined according to DeRemee(11);the disease activity was assessed by BAL T-lymphocyte count,Ga67 lung scan(12)and S-ACE colorimetric assay(13).

Serum PCP assay.This was performed using the kit Ria-Gnost Prokollagen III Peptide(Boehringwerke,West Germany),according to Rhode et al(14).Variations among kits were always less than 25%,and intrakit differences did not exceed 8%.All measurements were performed in duplicate.

RESULTS

Table I shows the data concerning the subjects with sarcoidosis and those with nsDPF who had not been treated with corticosteroids.

TABLE I
SERUM PCP (ng/ml)IN UNTREATED SARCOIDOSIS AND IN nsDPF

	Healthy controls (no.15)	Untreated sarcoidosis (no.32)	Untreated nsDPF (no.15)
$\bar{x}$	15	20.35*	25.642**
+SD	5.71	7.46	13.215

* $p < 0.025$ Vs controls
** $p < 0.001$ Vs controls

In both of these groups values are significantly higher than in normal subjects. We found no correlation with usual markers of sarcoidosis activity in patients with this disease(data not shown),while there seems to be a correlation with the radiologic extension of the granulomatous process(table II).

During treatment with prednisone there was a dramatic drop in PCP levels in patients with sarcoidosis,while in the 4 asthmatic subjects(i.e.without any pathological alterations of fibroblasts function)high dosage cortisone therapy did not significantly alter PCP lavels(table III).

TABLE II
RELATIONSHIP BETWEEN SERUM PCP LEVELS(ng/ml) AND RADIOLOGIC STAGE OF THORACIC
SARCOIDOSIS IN UNTREATED PATIENTS

	Stage I (no.10)	Stage II (no.15)	Stage III (no.7)
x̄	17.402	28.18*	18.47
±SD	10.134	11.923	7.436

* p < 0.02 Vs stage I and stage III

TABLE III
SERUM PCP(ng/ml)DURING STEROID THERAPY

	Untreated sarcoidosis (no.22)	Treated sarcoidosis[1] (no.22)	Untreated asthma (no.4)	Treated asthma[2] (no.4)
x̄	21.418	9.955*	7.9	5.37**
±SD	9.861	5.022	2.53	1.67

1 prednisone 0.75-1 mg/Kg/day for at least 28 days
2 methylprednisolone 1 mg/Kg/day i.v. for 10 days
* p < 0.001   ** p > 0.05

DISCUSSION

These data seem to suggest the following observations:

a) high serum PCP levels can be found in the course of thoracic sarcoidosis and nsDPF;

b) in sarcoidosis these values are not correlated with the markers of alveolitis nor with S-ACE levels,but rather with the radiologic extension of the granulomatous process;

c) when fibrosis predominates(stage III)PCP levels tend to drop;this is in contrast to the values obtained in the course of nsDPF(which is actually a very heterogeneous group and therefore not very useful for comparison);

d) in sarcoidosis PCP levels would seem to reflect an increased functional activity of pulmonary fibroblasts during a florid granulomatous phase of the disease;

e) prednisone treatment,suppressing fibroblast activity,reduces serum PCP levels;

f) this cross-sectional study does not clarify the clinical usefulness of PCP determination in sarcoidosis,but preliminary data on long term longitudinal observation appear to be more promising.In two cases of relapse of the disease(one due to insufficient doses of prednisone and one 3 months after the end of treatment) PCP levels increased several months before the worsening of the chest-X rays;in one case of spontaneous improvement of chronic sarcoidosis PCP levels returned to normal 6 months before improvement of chest-X rays and normalization of S-ACE.

AKNOWLEDGEMENTS

Partially supported by a grant of the Italian National Research Council,contract no.86.00440.44

REFERENCES

1. LAURENT GJ(1986) Thorax 41:418

2. HUNNINGHAKE GW,GARRETT KC,RICHERSON HB et al(1984) Am.Rev.Respir.Dis.130:476

3. KIVIRIKKO KI,MAJAMAA K(1985) In:Fibrosis,Ciba Foundation Symposium 114, Pitman,London,34

4. BOLARIN DM,SAVOLAINEN ER,KIVIRIKKO KI et al(1984) Eur.J.Clin.Invest.14:90

5. KIRK JME,BATEMAN ED,HASLAM PL et al(1984) Thorax 39:726

6. LOW RB,CUTRONEO KR,DAVIS GS,GIANCOLA MS(1983) Lab.Invest.48:755

7. ASAI M.,YAMAMOTO M.,TAKADA K et al(1986) Sarcoidosis 3:156(abs.FC 14)

8. PERRINE-FOYOLLE M,BARBIER Y,BARBIER M et al(1986) Sarcoidosis 3:157 (abs.FC 15)

9. POHL W,KOHN H,RIEDEL M et al(1986) Sarcoidosis 3:178 (abs.PP 64)

10. LUISETTI M,APRILE C,BACCHELLA L et al(1986) Sarcoidosis 3:178 (abs.PP 66)

11. DEREMEE RA (1985) In:Lieberman J(ed) Sarcoidosis,Grune & Stratton,Orlando, 117

12. KEOGH BA,HUNNINGHAKE GW,LINE BR,CRYSTAL RG (1983) Am.Rev.Respir.Dis.128:256

13. PEONA V ,NONIS A,GUALTIERI G,LUISETTI M (1986) Medicina Toracica 8:33

14. RHODE H,VARGAS L,HAHN E et al (1979) Eur.J.Clin.Invest.9:451

THE CLINICAL APPLICATION OF BRONCHOALVEOLAR T-CELL SUBSETS IN THE FOLLOW-UP
OF PULMONARY SARCOIDOSIS

M.G. PERARI, G. CARRIERO, P. ROTTOLI, L. ROTTOLI, A. COLLODORO, °G. COVIELLO,
S. BIANCO
Institute of Respiratory Diseases, Siena University, Siena, Italy
°Radiology Unit, Sclavo Hospital, Siena, Italy.

INTRODUCTION

Today, there is still much discussion on the usefulness of BAL in the
clinical management of sarcoidosis. Controlled trials are required to
assess its validity in this disease. Previously, we have reported that, in
our experience, the % of lymphocytes in BAL has no prognostic value. However, in most of the patients, a correlation has been found between the % of
alveolar lymphocytes and the clinical evolution, especially in patients with
pulmonary sarcoidosis. The subtyping of lymphocytes with monoclonal antibodies (OKT3, OKT4, OKT8) has been performed to see if the T cell ratio
(CD4/CD8) was more sensitive in predicting the outcome of the disease.

PATIENTS AND METHODS

Bronchoalveolar lavage (BAL) was performed as previously described (1).
Twenty-six patients with pulmonary sarcoidosis were studied. Diagnosis
was confirmed by biopsy and/or Kweim test. Eight patients were classified
radiologically in Stage I, 12 in Stage II and 6 in Stage III. A score
based on x-ray alterations, respiratory function (PFR, DLCO) and immunological and biochemical tests (SACE, Lisozyme, circulating immunocomplexes,
immunoglobulins, T cell subsets) was given to each patient: 5 points for
x-ray variations, 2 points for changes in respiratory function, 2 points
for DLCO (total variations 10% when compared to previous examination), 2
points for SACE (serum angiotensin converting enzyme) and 1 point for
variations of each of the other biochemical and immunological parameters.
A positive or negative score was given according to the improvement or
deterioration of each individual parameter.

Carrying out algebraic sums of the partial scores, the patients were
divided into improved (Group "I") with a final score   3 and unimproved
(Group "U") with a final score of /3. According to this classification,
16 patients were placed in Group I and 5 patients in Group U. Statistical
analysis was performed using the Student's t test for paired data and
Fisher's test.

RESULTS

The average helper/suppressor ratio (CD4/CD8) was 2.7 ± 0.42 (M $\pm$ SE) in Group I (improved) and 3.9 ± 0.86 in Group U (unimproved). This difference was not statistically significant (Student's t test). We subdivided the patients according to whether the CD4/CD8 ratio was above or below 3. This value represented the M + 2SD in healthy control subjects (Table 1). A comparison between the average values in these two groups was statistically significant (1.72 ± 0.2 vs 4.54 ± 0.35, P $/0.01$). The two groups did not differ, however, in percentage values of alveolar lymphocytes (A.Ly)(41.35 ± 4.8 vs 38 ± 4.2, N.S.). In the group of patients with CD4/CD8 $/3$, the number of subjects with a favourable prognosis (3/12) was similar to that of patients with CD4/CD8 > 3 (2/9).

TABLE I

	$CD4^+/CD8^+$		
	$/$ 3	> 3	P
°$CD4^+$	44.00 ± 2.9	65.8 ± 1.8	$/0.01$
°CD8+	29.90 ± 2.5	17.7 ± 1.0	$/0.01$
$CD4^+/CD8+$	1.72 ± 0.2	4.54 ± 0.35	$/0.01$
°A.Ly	41.35 ± 4.8	38.0 ± 4.20	N.S

° = percentage (M̄ $\pm$ SE)   A.Ly = Alveolar Lymphocytes
Student's t test

If the cases are divided on the basis of the percentage of A.Ly, taking 25% (the average percentage of A.Ly in all our patients with sarcoidosis) as the parameter of reference, no difference was found either in the values of the CD4/CD8 ratio (A.Ly > 25% vs A.Ly $/25\%$; 2.9 ± 0.3 vs 2.3 ± 0.8) or as regards the prognosis. Moreover, taking into consideration the treated patients (Prednisone: 30-40 mg as attack therapy dose with total treatment lasting more than 6 months) and those untreated in Groups I and U, the values of the CD4/CD8 ratio do not give any indication of the response to therapy. The statistical analysis (Fisher's test) does not, in fact, show significant differences.

When the patients are subdivided according to the radiological stage, the analysis of the CD4/CD8 ratio shows a significant difference (P < 0.05) between Stage III and Stage I (4.58 ± 0.6 vs 1.83 ± 0.5) and between Stages I + II and Stage III (2.67 ± 0.4 vs 4.58 ± 0.6), whereas the difference between Stages I and II is not significant (1.83 ± 0.5 vs 3.12 ± 0.4). A difference has also been shown in the average percent of A.Ly between Stages

I and III (52.9 ± 6 vs 30.3 ± 3.8; P /0.05)(Table 2).   Figure 1 shows the
distribution of the patients in the various stages, on the basis of a CD4/
CD8 ratio above or below 3.   We found no significant correlation between
the percentage of A.Ly and CD4/CD8 values, between serum levels of ACE and
the percentage of A.Ly, between SACE values and OKT4[+] and OKT8[+] lymphocytes,
or between SACE values and CD4/CD8 ratio.

Table 2

	ALVEOLAR LYMPHOCYTES	CD4[+]/CD8[+]
STAGE I	52.9 ± 6.0	1.83 ± 0.5
STAGE II	40.9 ± 6.1	3.12 ± 0.4
STAGE III	30.3 ± 3.8	4.58 ± 0.6
(M ± SE)		

Statistical analysis: Student's t test

A.Ly	CD4[+]/CD8[+]	
St. I vs St. III p /0.05	St. I vs St. III	P /0.05
	St. I + St. II vs St. III	P /0.05

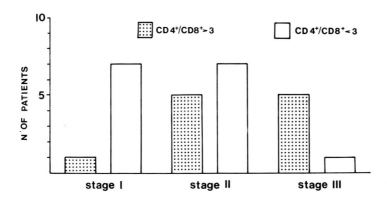

Figure 1   Distribution of Patients in the various stages, on the basis
of a CD4/CD8 ratio above or below 3

570

CONCLUSIONS

The following conclusions can be drawn from these results:

1. The helper/suppressor ratio (CD4/CD8) is of no prognostic value;
2. The CD4/CD8 ratio gives no indication of the response to therapy;
3. The percentage of A.Ly is of no prognostic value;
4. Dividing the patients into two groups on the basis of the average percentage (25%) found in all our sarcoidosis cases (A.Ly / or > 25%), no difference can be seen in the average values of the CD4/CD8 ratio;
5. There is a significant difference in the CD4/CD8 ratio between Stage III and Stages I + II; does the presence of ileomediastinic lymph nodes influence the helper/suppressor ratio? Are the "activated" lymph nodes capable of maintaining the helper/suppressor balance in loco?
6. Patients at Stage III have the highest CD4/CD8 ratios and the lowest A.Ly percentage; this could constitute the clinical picture in chronic forms of the disease.

The data so far obtained do not seem to provide precise indications for considering the outcome of sarcoidosis. It is generally rather difficult to find a single parameter able to predict the prognosis of a disease. Therefore, we think that BAL may contribute, together with other conventional measurements, to the clinical management of sarcoidosis. It is necessary to combine the results of many different groups, in order to obtain sufficient data for a better understanding of the clinical value of BAL in sarcoidosis.

REFERENCE

1. Carriero G, Rottoli P, Rottoli L, Perari MG (1984) Allergol et Immuno-Pathol 12,5:377-382

© 1988 Elsevier Science Publishers B.V. (Biomedical Division)
Sarcoidosis and other granulomatous disorders
C. Grassi, G. Rizzato, E. Pozzi, editors

GALLIUM-67 LUNG SCAN IN THE EVALUATION OF PULMONARY SARCOIDOSIS

ROSARIO SCAGLIONE, GASPARE PARRINELLO, GIUSEPPE CAPUANA, GIUSEPPE
LICATA

Institute of Clinical Medicine, Chair of Medical Theraphy (Head Prof. G. Licata)
University of Palermo (Italy).

INTRODUCTION

Several studies have recently suggested that Gallium-67 lung scan is an useful tool for sarcoidosis diagnosis and a sensitive predictor index of sarcoidosis activity (1-7). In fact a significant correlation between Ga-67 accumulation and serum lysozyme and angiotensine converting enzyme (widely used as markers of sarcoidosis activity) have been observed (6-7). Moreover a significant correlation between Ga-67 uptake and a specific test of alveolitis activity, as lymphocyte counts in bronchoalveolar lavage fluid, has been well documented too (1).

Our study was carried out to evaluate the utility of Ga-67 lung scan both in activity monitoring and in therapeutical follow up of the pulmonary sarcoidosis.

MATERIAL AND METHODS

Scintigraphy was performed in 15 patients (9 males and 6 females ranging from 25 to 52 years of age) with pulmonary sarcoidosis and in 10 control subjects.

The diagnosis of sarcoidosis was based on clinical and radiographic data and confirmed by transbronchial biopsy. The patients, according to Ellis and Renthal classification (8), were grouped in the following stages:- stage I: patients with hilar bilateral lymphadenopathy alone (n=6); -stage II: patients with hilar lymphadenopathy and pulmonary involvement (n=5); -stage III: patients with parenchimal fibrosis without lymphadenopathy (n=4). The control subjects suffered from a variety of diseases not located in the chest (abdominal mass, thyroid neoplasm, lymphoma and abscess). All the subjects were informed about the purpose of the study and gave previously their consent. Lung scintigraphy was performed 24, 48 and 72 h. after i.v. injection of 2 mCi of Ga-67 citrate, using Elscint Pho Camera with dycomette computer. In each patient anterior and posterior views of the chest were analyzed. For both views a standard area were selected around both hili and around the pheripheri of both lungs and counts rate were automatically detected by computer. These counts were divided by the time of measu-

572

rement of each view (3 min.) and reported as counts/area/min. at 48 h.

Moreover Ga-67 lung scan was repeated after 6 months of corticosteroid treatment (Prednisone from 10 to 50 mg daily related to extension or severe symptomatic sarcoidosis).

RESULTS

Our results are presented in Table I and they show: 1) an evident increment of Ga-67 counts/area/min. in patients with sarcoidosis in comparison with control group. This behaviour is relative to anterior and posterior view and to both hili and to both lungs; 2) in 6 patients at stage I hilar and lung values were clearly increased compared with those found in control group (p<0.001); 3) in 5 patients at stage II hilar values were similar to those of patients at stage I, while lung values were much higher than in stage I (p<0.001); 4) in 4 patients who were classified at stage III values did not differ from those of stage II; 5) after corticosteroid treatment an evident reduction of hilar and lung values have been observed. These values, even if higher, did not differ significantly from those of control group.

CONCLUSION

Ga-67 lung scan has recently become a major diagnostic tool for assessing disease activity in pulmonary sarcoidosis (2-5). Our study has demonstrated that this method is able both to discriminate patients with sarcoidosis from normal subjects and to evaluate activity stage of disease. In fact the patients at stage I show a significantly increase of Ga-67 uptake in comparison with control subjects.

The patients at stage II and III show a lung activity values higher than lung activity values at stage I. The mean hilar activities were instead like in stages I, II and III. Therefore actually it seems that changes in lung activity provide the most relevant information on disease activity in the course of pulmonary sarcoidosis rather than hilar values (9), but, while it is suitable to differentiate stage I from stage II or III of sarcoidosis, appears instead very difficult to discriminate patients at stage II from those at stage III. Moreover the clear effects of corticosteroid theraphy on Ga-67 uptake promise that this method can be an useful and sensitive parameter to sarcoidosis therapeutical follow up.

In conclusion our findings suggest that Ga-67 uptake is an useful non invasive method both for staging clinical activity and for evaluating therapeutical effects in patients with pulmonary sarcoidosis.

TABLE I

GALLIUM-67 UPTAKE (counts/area/min.-mean $\pm$SD) IN CONTROL SUBJECTS AND IN PATIENTS WITH SARCOIDOSIS.

Patients	Left Hilus	Right Hilus	Left Lung	Right Lung
Controls (n=10)				
Anterior view	3555+770	3908+333	3047+204	2694+352
Posterior view	3508+431	4136+328	3297+241	3135+305
SARCOIDOSIS				
Stage I (n=6)				
Anterior view	7058+433	7367+556	4546+318	4405+379
Posterior view	7517+507	7994+518	4394+381	4684+403
Stage II (n=5)				
Anterior view	6723+325	7172+356	5900+309	6139+325
Posterior view	7205+334	7366+314	6075+318	6379+349
Stage III (n=4)				
Anterior view	6796+517	7339+403	5661+381	5161+303
Posterior view	6930+525	7063+372	5674+355	5727+293
After corticosteroid treatment (n=15)				
Anterior view	4524+637	4271+711	3774+541	3578+497
Posterior view	4763+619	4966+694	3532+609	4566+517

REFERENCES

1. Line BR, Hunninghake GW, Jones AE, CrystalRG (1981) Am Rev Respir Dis 123:440-46

2. Fajman WA, Greenwald LV, Staton G (1984) J Radiol 142:683-88

3. Johnson DG, Johnson SM, Harris CC, Coleman RE (1984) Radiology 150:551-56

4. Alberts C, Van der Schoot JB, Groen AS (1981) Eur J Nucl Med 6:205-12

5. Van Unnik JG, Van Royen EA, Alberts C (1983) Eur J Nucl Med 8:351-53

6. Alberts C, Van der Schoot JB, Roos CM (1982) Eur J Resp Dis 5:315-21

7. Lieberman J, Nosal A, Sastre A, Mishkin S (1983) Chest 84,5:522-28

8. Ellis K, Renthal G (1962) A J R 88:1070-83

9. Beaumont D, Herry JY, Le Cloirec J (1982) Eur J Nucl Med 7:41-43

URINARY NEOPTERIN FOR ASSESSING THE FOLLOW-UP OF PULMONARY SARCOIDOSIS.

J. LACRONIQUE*, B.M. TRAORE*, A. AUZEBY**, P. SOLER***,

Y. TOUITOU**, J. MARSAC*.

*Département de Pneumologie, Hôpital Cochin, Paris 75014

**Laboratoire de Biochimie, Faculté Pitié-Salpetrière, Paris 75013

***Inserm U 82, Paris 75018

INTRODUCTION

Active pulmonary sarcoidosis is characterized by a spontaneous release of Gamma-interferon by alveolar macrophages and lung T-lymphocytes (1) and by an enhanced antigen presentation process (2). Background studies on pteridines have indicated that Neopterin is a marker of T-cell immune-mediated activation in vivo (3) and that it is released in vitro from human mononuclear cells under control of gamma-interferon secreted from activated T-cells (4). We therefore hypothesized that urinary neopterin could represent a marker of the activity of the disease in patients with sarcoidosis.

We undertook a preliminary study in 45 patients with biopsy proven sarcoidosis. Our preliminary data (5) showed that, regardless of activity of the disease, urinary neopterin was increased in patients with pulmonary sarcoidosis as compared to normal subjects. Patients who met clinical criteria of active disease or patients with laboratory evidence of activity assessed by high alveolar OKT-4 positive lymphocytosis recovered from bronchoalveolar lavage (ALY from BAL), and positive 67-Gallium Scan index (67-Ga) had significantly higher urinary neopterin than patients without clinical or biological active disease.

PATIENTS AND METHODS

1) <u>Patients and study design</u>

Among sarcoidosis patients included in our preliminary study, a follow-up study was undertaken to determine whether the measurement of urinary Neopterin could help in the management of such patients. We studied 15 subjects with pulmonary sarcoidosis (8 females and 7 males, 34 ± 10 yr). Disease activity was assessed by clinical examination, chest roentgenograms and pulmonary function tests initially (T1) and then after a period (T2) of 24 ± 14 months (range 10 to 59). Different patterns of evolution were assessed allowing to separate patients into 3 groups of clinical evolutivity : Group 1 characterized by worsening of the disease (n =3) ; Group 2 : stability (n = 5) ; Group 3 : improvement (n = 7).

Contemporarily to the clinical pattern of evolution, ALY from BAL, 67-Ga and serum angiotensin converting enzyme (SACE) were assessed at T1 and T2 and compared to the urinary neopterin values .

2) <u>Assessment of disease activity.</u>

We considered as clinically active patients in whom fever, loss of weight, increasing shortness of breath, erythema nodosum, any worsening picture on Chest roentgenograms or any additional sarcoid lesion occured during the three preceeding months. Laboratory evidence of activity included ALY from BAL (> 30% of total cells) in BAL, positive 67-Ga (index > 20) and increased SACE (> 60 U/ml).

3) <u>Urinary Neopterin measurement</u>

Neopterin measurement was performed on a sample of the first early morning urine by reversed-phase HPLC according to the method described by Hausen et al. (6). Results are expressed as the ratio of μmol urinary Neopterin / mol urinary creatinine (UN, mean ± SEM).

577

RESULTS (see table 1)

In Group 1, (n = 3) clinically characterized by a worsening course, the mean values of all biological markers were above the normal range at T1 and T2. The values for UN were significantly increased at T1 (1068 ± 463) and at T2 (922 ± 261), more than five fold those of normal subjects (126 ± 5, n = 45, p < 0,001).

In Group 2, (n = 5) in whom patients showed clinical stability, mean values of biological markers were increased at T1, but only slightly for 67-Ga and SACE. At T2, all of them remained stable.

In Group 3, (n = 7) where patients showed an improvement mean values of all biological markers where increased at T1 ; mean values of 67-Ga, SACE, and UN returned to normal at T2. The fall from T1 to T2 was significant only for UN and for absolute number of OKT-4 cells.

Comparison between Group 1 and Group 3 for each parameter did not show any significant difference at T1 for none of them. At T2, UN was the only parameter different between Group 1 and Group 3 (p <.05).

TABLE 1

URINARY NEOPTERIN IN THE THREE GROUPS OF SARCOIDOSIS PATIENTS

Period	group 1 worsening (n=3)	group 2 stability (n =5)	group 3 improvement (n=7)
T1	1068 ± 463	447 ± 102	506 ± 107
T2	922 ± 261	359 ± 65	249 ± 43

DISCUSSION

No consensus exists between authors about criteria to assess the activity of the disease with the current parameters, and there is some need to find new parameters able to assess accurately this activity.

We first showed (5) that urinary neopterin is increased in patients with active sarcoidosis. In spite of the relatively small number of patients studied our present study shows that, follow-up of UN parallels the clinical assessment of evolutivity. Comparison between UN and the current biological parameters of activity indicates that UN and ALY from BAL are the only parameters to fall significantly in patients whose disease improve. Morever, UN is the only one showing a significant difference at T2 between group 1 and group 3.

We conclude that urinary neopterin may represent an accurate and sensitive biological marker of evolution in patients with pulmonary sarcoidosis, to be conveniently used for the follow-up of such patients.

REFERENCES

1- Robinson BWS, McLemore TL, Crystal RG (1985) Gamma interferon is spontaneously released by alveolar macrophages and lung T lymphocytes in patients with pulmonary sarcoidosis. J Clin Invest 75 : 1488-1495

2- Venet A, Hance AJ, Saltini C, Robinson BWS, Crystal RG (1985) Enhanced alveolar macrophage-mediated antigen-induced T lymphocyte proliferation in sarcoidosis. J Clin Invest 75 : 293-301

3- Huber C, Fuchs D, Hausen A, Margreiter R, Reibnegger G,Spielberger M, Wachter H (1983) Pteridines as a new marker to detect human T cells activated by allogeneic or modified self major histocompatibility complex (MHC) determinants. J Immunol 130 : 1047-1050

4- Huber C, Batchelor JR, Fuchs D, Hausen A, Lang A, Niederwieser D, Reibnegger G, Swetly P, Troppmair J, Wachter H (1984) Immune response- associated production of neopterin. Release from macrophages primarly under control of interferon-gamma. J Exp Med 160 : 310-316

5- Lacronique J, Auzeby A, Barbosa MLA, Valeyre D, Soler P, Venot A, Marsac J et Touitou Y (1986) Urinary Neopterin as a new marker of lympho cytic alveolitis in pulmonary sarcoidosis Am Rev Respir Dis 133 : A-24

6- Hausen A., Fuchs D., König K., Watcher H. (1982) Determination of Neoterine in human urine by reversed-phase high-performance liquid chromatography J Chromatog 227 : 61-70

PROGNOSTIC ASSESSMENT OF BAL AND GALLIUM 67 SCAN IN SARCOIDOSIS LESS THAN 2 YEARS AFTER THE ONSET

MASAHIKO YAMAMOTO[1], MASAHARU NODA[1], YUTAKA HOSODA[2], YOHMEI HIRAGA[3], TAKATERU IZUMI[4], TERUO TACHIBANA[5], KIYOSHI SHIMA[6] and ATSUHIKO SATO[7]

Japan Sarcoidosis Committee, 1: 2nd Dpt. Inter. Med., Nagoya City Univ., Medical School, Mizuho-Cho, Mizuho-Ku, Nagoya 467 (Japan) 2: Radiation Effects Research Found. 3: JNR Sapporo Hosp. 4: Kyoto Univ. 5: Osaka Pref. Hosp. 6: Kumamoto City Hosp. 7: Hamamatsu Univ.

INTRODUCTION

There are still many discussions that BAL lymphocytosis and positive Gallium 67 lung scan at the early stage of sarcoidosis could predict the outcome of the disease, although, these data were accepted as the markers of the activity of the disease.

In this study, prognostic values of BAL and Gallium 67 lung scan performed at less than 2 years lapse since the presumed onset of sarcoidosis were assessed.

MATERIAL AND METHODS

One hundred and forty-four cases of sarcoidosis from 26 institutes over Japan were studied. The eligible criteria were; 1) histologically proven cases, 2) less than 2 years (86% less than 6 months) since the presumed onset of the disease, 3) 1 year or more (69% 2 years or more) followed-up after BAL or Gallium study, 4) no corticosteroids and 5) known smoking history.

BAL was analysed only for non- and ex-smokers.

Patients characteristics were as follows; male 60, female 84, mean age 37.2 ± 15.2; type 0 7, I 77, II 55, III 5; without extrapulmonary lesions 70, with 1 lesion 60, with 2 lesions 14; %VC less than 80% 9/121, FEV1%, less than 75% 13/121, DLC0% less than 80% 32/78.

RESULTS

Chest X-rays cleared in a significantly higher rate ($p < 0.05$) in those who had BALF lymphocytes less than 20% (62%) than those who had 20% or more (32%) (table 1).

Chest X-rays cleared in 9 out of 18 cases (50%) with BALF T-lymphocytes less than 28%, while in 18 out 48 cases (38%) with 28% or more, and there was a significant difference ($p < 0.05$) between them.

T 4/8 ratio had no correlation with X-rays.

Pulmonary functions were not correlated with BAL results.

Chest X-rays cleared in a significantly higher rate ($p < 0.05$) in those who had no lung Galluim uptake (45%) than in those who had it (23%) (table 2).

Pulmonary functions were not correlated with Gallium results.

TABLE 1

BALF LYMPHOCYTES % AND THE COURSE OF X-RAYS AT THE END OF THE STUDY

Lymphocytes	X-rays/Cleared	Improved	Unchanged	Worsened	Total
< 20%	8 (62%)	3 (23%)	1 (8%)	1 (8%)	13 (100%)
20% ≦	22 (23%)	13 (19%)	26 (38%)	8 (12%)	69 (100%)

TABLE 2

GALLIUM LUNG UPTAKE AND THE COURSE OF X-RAYS AT THE END OF THE STUDY

Ga lung uptake	X-rays/Cleared	Improved	Unchanged	Worsened	Total
Without	35 (45%)	12 (15%)	23 (29%)	8 (10%)	78 (100%)
With	9 (23%)	17 (43%)	10 (25%)	4 (10%)	40 (100%)

Chest X-rays cleared in a significantly higher rate ($p < 0.05$) in those who had 30% or more decrease in second BALF lymphocytes % to the first BALF (42%) than in those who had no decrease (10%) (table 3).

Chest X-rays cleared in a significantly higher rate ($p < 0.01$) in those who had a decrease in Gallium uptake in the second scan (53%) than those who had no decrease (7%) (table 4).

As a conclusion, BAL and Gallium lung scan revealed prognostic values in sarcoidsis especially in serial examinations.

TABLE 3

CHANGES OF LYMPHOCYTES % IN THE SECOND BALF AND THE COURSE OF X-RAYS

Lymphocytes %	X-rays/Cleared	Improved	Unchanged	Worsened	Total
Decreased	10 (42%)	4 (17%)	8 (33%)	2 (8%)	24 (100%)
Not decreased	2 (10%)	5 (25%)	9 (45%)	4 (20%)	20 (100%)

TABLE 4

CHANGES OF GALLIUM UPTAKE IN THE SECOND SCAN AND THE COURSE OF X-RAYS

Changes of Ga uptake	X-rays/Cleared	Improved	Unchanged	Worsened	Total
Decreased	10 (53%)	4 (21%)	5 (26%)	0	19 (100%)
Not decreased	1 (7%)	3 (20%)	7 (47%)	4 (27%)	15 (100%)

© 1988 Elsevier Science Publishers B.V. (Biomedical Division)
Sarcoidosis and other granulomatous disorders
C. Grassi, G. Rizzato, E. Pozzi, editors

INCREASED PROCOAGULANT ACTIVITY OF BRONCHOALVEOLAR LAVAGE CELLS
IN PATIENTS WITH SARCOIDOSIS: RELATIONSHIP TO STEROID TREAT-
MENT, FORCED VITAL CAPACITY, GALLIUM UPTAKE, AND BRONCHOALVEOLAR
LAVAGE PERCENT LYMPHOCYTES

R. Perez[1], G. Staton[1], M. Kidd[1], Check[2]
Emory University School of Medicine, Atlanta GA USA. 1: Dept.
of Medicine; 2: Dept. of Pathology.

INTRODUCTION

The procoagulant activity (PCA) of activated macrophages in
sarcoidosis is elevated (1). This may lead to net fibrin
deposition which has been postulated to be an early event of
pulmonary fibrosis (2). Measurement of PCA, alone or in
combination with other parameters of disease activity, could be
of prognostic value and allow optimal therapy decisions.

We measured bronchoalveolar lavage (BAL) cell PCA in patients
with steroid treated and untreated sarcoidosis compared to that
of normal volunteers and correlated PCA with other measures of
disease activity - forced vital capacity (FVC), gallium uptake,
and BAL per cent lymphocytes.

MATERIALS AND METHODS

BAL cells: Cells lavaged from the lungs of sarcoidosis
patients in the years 1982-1984 and cryopreserved (RPMI-1640/10%
DMSO) at -70°C in 12 X 75 mm Nunc tubes (Becton Dickinson, U.S.A.)
were reconstituted in three wash steps. In the first step, RPMI-
1640/20% FCS was used to thaw the cells in a 37°C water bath.
After spinning at 400 G X 5 min. at 4°C, 1 c.c. of RPMI-1640/10%
FCS containing 0.1 mg. of DNAse (Sigma, U.S.A.) was used to
disrupt cell clumps. A second wash in RPMI-1640/10% FCS was done
to clear the DNAse followed by a cell count and third wash. The
cells were finally adjusted to a concentration of 1.33 X 10^6
cells/ml. in PBS/33% RPMI-1640 for PCA assay. BAL cells collected
in mid-1984 from normal volunteers were processed in the same way.

PCA Assay: Prepared BAL cells were lysed by freeze-thawing (-
70°C to 37° C) and sonication (Bransonic-32, Smith Kline) for 5
minutes. Procoagulant activity was recorded as a clotting time
using a single-step plasma coagulation assay normalized to rabbit-
brain thromboplastin (American Dade, Puerto Rico). 75 ul of test
lysate (10^5 cells) were added to 75 ul of normal saline. After a

3 minute incubation, 75 ul of 20 mM $CaCl_2$ was added rapidly and the time to fibrin clot formation was measured in a coagulation timer (Fibrometer, Becton Dickinson). The shorter the clotting time, the greater the PCA.

Clinical Measures of Disease Activity: Pulmonary function testing and gallium-67 lung scans were done within one-to-two months of BAL. BAL cell differentials were performed on slides prepared by cytocentrifugation.

RESULTS

Patients had a significantly elevated PCA (reduced clotting time) as compared to normals (p=0.004; fig. 1). Treated patients tended to have less PCA than those that were untreated (p=0.06). Two patients had measurements before and after steroids. Both showed a decrease in PCA (55 to 81 seconds and 59 to 77 seconds) even though only one patient improved in FVC (69% predicted to 86% predicted vs. 64% predicted to 61%). Increased PCA tended to correlate with lower FVC (p=0.03; fig. 2), but did not correlate with gallium-67 uptake (r=0.07) or the per cent BAL lymphocytes (r=0.24).

PCA (clot time +/- 1 SEM) of BAL cells from normal vs sarcoidosis patients

PCA (as clotting time) vs FVC in Sarcoid Patients

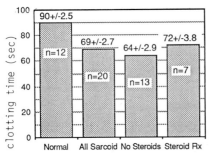

Fig. 1. Faster clotting time indicates greater PCA.

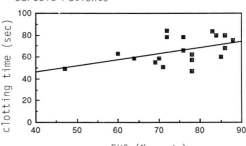

Fig. 2. Tendency for correlation of PCA to FVC; r = 0.48.

DISCUSSION

Current methods used to assess the activity of sarcoidosis are hampered by the cumulative effects of the disease and may not reflect the activity at any given time. Efforts to understand the pathogenesis of this and other interstitial lung diseases at the cellular and molecular level should yield more sensitive

methods of assessment. Measurement of BAL cell PCA offers a
relatively simple way to look at a critical event that may lead
directly to pulmonary fibrosis. The mechanism involves the
extrinsic coagulation cascade centered about the production of
tissue factor activity by the macrophages (3). The fact that
steroids can abrogate this activity (4) makes PCA a logical
choice with which to follow treatment response.

In this preliminary report, we found that sarcoidosis patients
had a significantly higher PCA (i.e. lower clotting times) in
their BAL cells than normals. Steroid treated patients tended to
have a lower PCA than untreated patients which may or may not
prove to be significant. Since the BAL were not collected under
a specific protocol, treatment criteria were not specified, and
follow-up was not reported, we can not speculate further on the
significance of our findings. With the possible exception of
FVC, other measures of disease activity did not correlate with
PCA. The relation to FVC may reflect the effects over time to
fibrin deposition and fibrosis on pulmonary mechanics. We are
currently developing a protocol designed to examine the interplay
between procoagulant and fibrinolytic activities on the
pathogenesis and outcome in patients with sarcoidosis and other
interstitial lung diseases.

ACKNOWLEDGEMENTS
This work was supported in part by the American Lung
Association of Georgia and the Carlyle Fraser Heart Center.

REFERENCES
1. Chapman, H.A., et. al. Abnormalities in the pathways of
alveolar fibrin turnover among patients with interstitial
lung disease. Amer Rev Respir Dis 1986;133:437-443.

2. Chapman, H.A., et. al. Human alveolar macrophages synthesize
factor VII in vitro: possible role in interstitial lung
disease. J Clin Invest 1985;75:2030-37.

3. Edgington, T.S. et. al. "Cellular pathways and signals for
the induction of biosynthesis of initiators of the coagulation
cascade by cells of the monocyte lineage," in Mononuclear
Phagocytes ed. Ralph van Furth. The Hague, Martinus Nijhoff,
1985.

4. Muhlfelder, T.W., et. al. Glucocorticoids inhibit the
generation of leukocyte procoagulant (tissue factor) activity.
Blood 1982;60:1169-72.

© 1988 Elsevier Science Publishers B.V. (Biomedical Division)
Sarcoidosis and other granulomatous disorders
C. Grassi, G. Rizzato, E. Pozzi, editors

BRONCHOALVEOLAR LAVAGE IN PATIENTS WITH ERYTHEMA NODOSUM

KEVIN WARD, C ODLUM, C O'CONNOR, A VAN BREDA, MUIRIS X FITZGERALD

Dept. of Medicine, University College Dublin, Elm Park, Dublin 4, Ireland

INTRODUCTION

There have been widely conflicting results from studies of the prognostic value of bronchoalveolar lavage (BAL) T lymphocyte (Tlymph.) count and T-lymphocyte helper (TH) : T lymphocyte suppressor (TS) ratio (TH : TS) in patients (pts.) with pulmonary sarcoidosis. This study examines those BAL cellular indices in pts. presenting with erythema nodosum (EN); an association known to have a good prognosis.

METHODS

Patients

Histologically proven sarcoid pts. with EN were arbitrarily divided into 2 groups. 1) Acute EN: patients who presented with acute EN and who had BAL performed within 2 months of acute lesions; n = 23 ; stage 1 = 12, stage 2 = 11 ; mean 29 yrs. 2) Resolved EN: patients who had presented initially with EN and who had BAL between 2 and 6 months afterwards n = 9 ; stage 1 = 6, stage 2 = 3 ; mean 33 yrs.

For comparative purposes we report the TH : TS ratio in a further 42 newly diagnosed sarcoid pts.; 16 with acute uveitis, 8 asymptomatic with abnormal chest x-rays and 22 with respiratory symptoms.

Results from a control group of 12 subjects are also included.

Bronchoalveolar lavage

BAL was performed in a standardized fashion. Lavage volume was 180 mls in 60 ml aliquots. Recovered cells were subtyped by monoclonal antibodies (Becton Dickinson).

RESULTS

There was no difference between the groups in age, cigarette consumption, BAL volume recovered, total number of cells recovered or BAL cellular concentration. Table 1 shows the Tlymph. profiles for both groups. Chest x-ray stage of disease does not appear to influence the % Tlymph. or the TH : TS ratio. In the acute EN group the mean Tlymph. % was 47 (SD 16) in stage 1 and 30 (SD 10) in stage 2. Similarly there was no difference in the TH : TS ratio; stage 1 12.9 (SD 13) and stage 2 11.2 (SD 12).

TABLE 1

T lymphocyte profiles in pts. with EN (mean +- SD)

	Acute EN (n=23)	Resolved EN (n=9)	Control (n=12)	p
T lymphs. %	39 (16)	11 (13)	10 (5)	p <.02
T helper %	33 (15)	7 (11)	5 (3)	p <.01
T suppressor %	5 (5)	5 (3)	6 (6)	
T helper:				
T suppressor ratio	12 (13)	1.2 (1.2)	1.3 (1)	p <.001

In acute EN Tlymph., mainly of the T helper celltype, predominate; the T helper : suppressor ratio is also high.

FIGURE 1

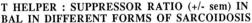
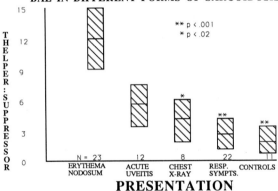

T HELPER : SUPPRESSOR RATIO (+/- sem) IN BAL IN DIFFERENT FORMS OF SARCOIDOSIS

DISCUSSION

This report confirms that the lymphocytosis associated with sarcoidosis is predominantly a TH lymphocytosis. The proliferation of TH cells is at its highest in patients with acute presentations of sarcoid. Yet despite the intensity of the immunological response associated with acute EN this presentation of sarcoid is recognised as being the most benign form of the disease. The TH:TS ratio and the total Tlymph. count are virtually normal in the resolved EN group; this implies the pleocytosis usually rapidly return to normal. Thus high Tlymph. counts and TH : TS ratios should be assessed in the context of the clinical setting. Any study of the prognostic value of BAL cellular subtypes should control for the nos. of patients with recent EN or acute uveitis.

© 1988 Elsevier Science Publishers B.V. (Biomedical Division)
Sarcoidosis and other granulomatous disorders
C. Grassi, G. Rizzato, E. Pozzi, editors

THE ROLE OF BRONCHO-ALVEOLAR LAVAGE IN PREDICTING THE OUTCOME OF PULMONARY SARCOIDOSIS

N.M. FOLEY, K. TUNG, A.P. CORAL, *D.G. JAMES and N.McI. JOHNSON
Middlesex and *Royal Northern Hospitals, London, U.K.

SUMMARY

Many studies have suggested a role for broncho-alveolar lavage (BAL) cell counts in predicting the functional or radiological outcome of pulmonary Sarcoidosis. (1- 5). We have prospectively studied 52 patients with biopsy-proven sarcoidosis, and found that a high initial lymphocyte count was of no prognostic value with regard to subsequent deterioration in CXR or DLCO, but did correlate with improvement in FVC. Almost all newly-diagnosed patients had a high lymphocyte count, even when CXR was normal. Repeat BAL showed no correlation between change in lymphocyte or neutrophil counts and changes in radiological or functional measurements. Patients with a initial high BAL lymphocyte count were more likely to require corticosteroid treatment over the following two years, but not necessarily for pulmonary involvement.

PATIENTS AND METHODS

52 patients were recruited consecutively from a Sarcoid Clinic.29 male, 23 female. Mean age 42 years (range 18-62). 22 Caucasian, 20 Black, 10 Asian. Mean duration of disease was 54 months (0-240) at onset of study. 10 were newly-diagnosed. The mean follow-up period was 24.75 months (10-39). All patients had B.A.L., pulmonary function tests and chest x-ray at the onset of the study period. These were repeated at 6 months in 31 patients, and all tests but B.A.L. were performed in all patients at the end of the period.

Clinical data at the initial assessment were as follows: CXR Stage 0 - 12 patients, Stage 1 - 10 patients, Stage 2 - 16 patients, Stages 3 and 4 - 7 patients each, mean ILO profusion score 5.16. Pulmonary function tests; FVC mean 82% predicted, DLCO mean 68%. Mean BAL cell counts were ; lymphocytes 32%, neutrophils 7%.

Patients were also defined as having high or low-intensity alveolitis (HIA or LIA) at the outset of the study, on the basis of BAL lymphocyte count. 30% lymphocytes was used as the cut-off point. 32 patients had HIA , including 9 of the 10 newly-diagnosed cases. 20 patients had LIA.No patient was on corticosteroid treatment initially. 21 patients were treated during the follow-up period, 3 of these for pulmonary disease alone. Treatment decisions were uninfluenced by BAL findings.

RESULTS

No statistically significant correlation was found between initial lymphocyte count and either initial or change in CXR stage, ILO score or DLCO. Initial lymphocyte count did correlate positively with change in FVC (Fig.1). Neutrophil counts did not correlate with any other clinical parameter. Repeat BAL at 6 months was of no clinical value, as change in lymphocyte and neutrophil count did not correlate with changes in CXR stage, ILO score, FVC or DLCO.

Patients with High Intensity Alveolitis showed a greater improvement in FVC and ILO score than did those with initial Low Intensity Alveolitis (Figs. 2 and 3). This improvement was seen both in the treated and untreated patients in this group. 15 patients in the HIA group (47%) required corticosteroid therapy , compared with 6 in the LIA group (33%).

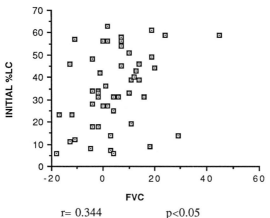

r= 0.344   p<0.05

Fig.1 Each point represents one patient. There is a significant correlation between an initial high lymphocyte count and an improvement in FVC over the follow-up period (mean 24.8 months)

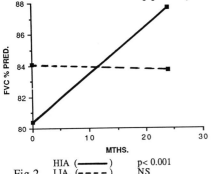

HIA (———)   p< 0.001
Fig.2 LIA (- - - -)   NS

Patients with High Intensity Alveolitis (HIA) show a significant improvement in FVC over a 25 month follow-up period, while those with Low Intensity Alveolitis (LIA) do not.

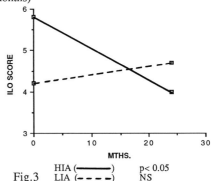

HIA (———)   p< 0.05
Fig.3 LIA (- - - -)   NS

This diagram represents the change in ILO profusion score in both groups of patients over the same period. The HIA patients improve significantly, the LIA do not.

REFERENCES

1. Carreiro G (1984) Allergol. et Immunopathol. 12, 5: 337 - 382

2. Keogh BA, Hunninghake GW, Line BR, Crystal RG (1983) Am Rev Respir Dis;128: 256-265

3. Baughman RP, Fernandes M, Bosken CH, Mantil J, Hurtubise P (1984) Am Rev Respir Dis; 129: 676-681

4. Lin YH, Haslam PL, Turner-Warwick M (1985) Thorax; 40: 501-507

5. Turner-Warwick M, McAllister W, Lawrence R, Britten A, Haslam PL (1986)Thorax; 41: 903-913

© 1988 Elsevier Science Publishers B.V. (Biomedical Division)
Sarcoidosis and other granulomatous disorders
C. Grassi, G. Rizzato, E. Pozzi, editors

589

CIRCULATING MONOCYTES FROM PATIENTS WITH SARCOIDOSIS EXPRESS CELL SURFACE LAMININ

MASAYUKI NISHIMURA[1], TETSUYA KOGA[1], KENICHI MATSUBA[2], NOBUAKI SHIGEMATSU[2]
Dept. of Dermatology, Med. Inst. of Bioregulation, Kyushu Univ., Beppu[1] and
Research Inst. of Dis. of Chest, Faculty of Med., Kyushu Univ., Fukuoka[2] (Japan)

INTRODUCTION

Laminin (LN) and fibronectin (FN) are present on the surface of mouse macrophages (1), and these cell surface molecules have been considered to play an important role in host defence (2). LN binds to circulating monocytes (CM) and macrophages via specific receptors (2, 3). Recently we demonstrated immunohistologically LN-positive intravascular mononuclear cells and macrophages in the sarcoid granulomas (unpublished data). The findings suggest that cell surface glycoproteins of blood derived mononuclear leukocytes might be involved in human granulomatous diseases. In this study, we examined ultrastructural localization of LN and FN on CM, and quantified LN- or FN-positive CM in patients with sarcoidosis and compared to those in patients with lung tuberculosis and in normal subjects.

MATERIAL AND METHODS

SUBJECTS

Ten patients with sarcoidosis, 11 with lung tuberculosis and 10 normal subjects of both sexes with ages ranging from 20 to 60 were included.

IMMUNOCYTOCHEMISTRY

Mononuclear cells were isolated from heparinized venous blood by Ficoll-Conray density gradient centrifugation, and prefixed in periodate-lysine-paraformaldehyde. Localization of LN and FN was examined at light and electron microscopic levels using immunogold-silver staining and preembedding immunogold staining.

FLOW CYTOMETRY

Percentages of cell surface LN or FN positive CM were determined with a laminar flow cytometer (Spectrum III, Ortho, USA) after indirect immunofluorescent staining. Monoclonal antibodies used: anti-LN rat (Immunotech, France); anti-human plasma FN mouse (Takara Shuzo, Japan). Statistical analysis: by Student's t-test.

RESULTS

In the immunogold-silver preparation, CM reacting with anti-LN antibody had numerous brownish granules. Electron microscopically, gold deposits for LN located randomly on cell surfaces of CM (Fig. 1). Immunocytochemically FN was not identified. Mean percentage of LN-positive CM was higher ($p < 0.05$) in patients with sarcoidosis than those in patients with tuberculosis and in normal subjects, whereas few CM express FN in any group of subjects (Table 1).

590

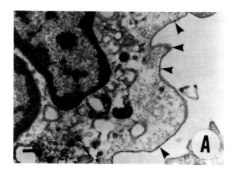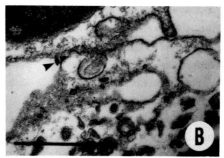

Fig. 1. Gold deposits (►) located singly or in a small group on the monocyte cell surface (A), and were seen in an aggregated form at the portion where a lymphocyte adhered (B).

TABLE 1

PERCENTAGES OF LAMININ- OR FIBRONECTIN-POSITIVE CIRCULATING MONOCYTES

Subjects (Number)	Sarcoidosis (10)	Tuberculosis (11)	Normal subjects (10)
Laminin-positive monocytes	37.4 ± 32.0*	11.1 ± 10.1	4.6 ± 3.6
Fibronectin-positive monocytes	2.0 ± 1.7	1.5 ± 0.8	2.2 ± 2.6

* mean ± standard deviation %

DISCUSSION

The precise role of LN in mononuclear phagocyte system in granulomatous diseases is not clear at present. Our findings suggest that cell surface LN take part in a monocyte-lymphocyte interaction, and that an elevated percentage of LN-positive CM is involved in the pathogenesis of sarcoidosis.

ACKNOWLEDGEMENTS

Dr Hynda K Kleinman (NIH, USA) kindly provided anti-LN rabbit antibody for the immunocytochemical study. This work was supported in part by a Grant-in-Aid for Cooperative Research (No 61300006) from the Ministry of Education, Science and Culture of Japan.

REFERENCES

1. Wicha MS, Huard TK (1983) Exp Cell Res 143: 475
2. Brown EJ (1986) J Leukocyte Biol 39: 579
3. Huard TK, Malinoff HL, Wicha MS (1986) Am J Pathol 123: 365

ASSESSMENT OF DISEASE ACTIVITY IN PULMONARY SARCOIDOSIS :
A CLINICO-PATHOLOGICAL CORRELATION

D.J. ROSSOUW, J.R. JOUBERT and CAROL C. CHASE
Departments of Pathology and Internal Medicine, University of
Stellenbosch Medical School and Tygerberg Hospital, Pulmonary
Research Group of South African Medical Research Council,
P.O. Box 63, TYGERBERG 7505, Republic of South Africa.

INTRODUCTION

While in some patients there is no doubt about disease activity, the assessment of active lung disease remains a major problem.[1,2,3] The objective of this study was therefore to correlate the morphological index of active disease in open lung biopsies with individual indirect markers and combinations of markers of disease activity in patients with pulmonary sarcoidosis.

MATERIAL AND METHODS

Open lung biopsies were studied in 30 patients of all population groups (mean age = 36; 19 females 11 males).   Clinical
evidence of pulmonary disease, extrapulmonary manifestations,
values and signs of parenchymal involvement on chest radiography
were considered as "clinical" activity.   Gallium-67 uptake, biochemical determinations (SACE; serum α_1 and γ-globulin values)
and analyses of broncho-alveolar lavage fluids (total and differential lymphocyte counts) were interpreted as "laboratory" evidence of activity.   Lymphocyte subsets (helper/suppressor ratios) were determined in frozen tissue sections, lavage fluid
and peripheral blood cells using monoclonal antibodies.

RESULTS

The combined clinical and laboratory index of activity showed a
significant correlation (p < 0,01) with the histological assessment of active disease (Fig. 1) but no indirect marker on its own
were helpful.   Table I demonstrates compartmentalization of
helper-lymphocytes in pulmonary sarcoidosis.   The mean T_4^+:T_8^+
ratio in 5 patients with high intensity alveolitis (lavage lymphocytes > 20%) was significantly higher than in 5 patients with low
intensity alveolitis (5,6 vs 2,2), indicating the importance of
T-helper/inducer lymphocytes in active lung disease.

592

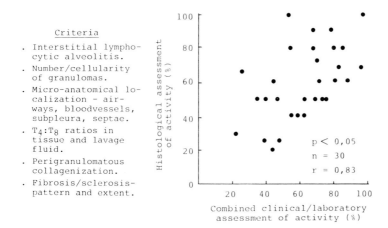

Criteria
. Interstitial lympho-
  cytic alveolitis.
. Number/cellularity
  of granulomas.
. Micro-anatomical lo-
  calization - air-
  ways, bloodvessels,
  subpleura, septae.
. T_4:T_8 ratios in
  tissue and lavage
  fluid.
. Perigranulomatous
  collagenization.
. Fibrosis/sclerosis-
  pattern and extent.

Fig. 1.   Graph to illustrate the correlation between histological index of activity and combined clinical and laboratory
assessment of disease activity in pulmonary sarcoidosis.

TABLE I

T_4^+:T_8^+ LYMPHOCYTE RATIOS IN OPEN LUNG BIOPSIES, BRONCHO-ALVEO-
LAR LAVAGE FLUID AND PERIPHERAL BLOOD

| | | Normal Control Subjects | Pulmonary Sarcoidosis | | Cryptogenic Fibrosing Alveolitis |
			Untreated	Treated	
Tissue	mean	-	**3,9**	-	**1,7**
	range		1,0-7,0		1,0-2,0
	n		10		4
Lavage	mean	**1,8**	**3,6** *	**1,3**	**1,2**
	range	0,3-2,1	0,5-5,7	0,6-1,9	0,3-2,6
	n	6	12	7	5
Blood	mean	**1,7**	**1,6**	**1,9**	**0,9**
	range	0,6-2,6	0,1-2,1	0,5-4,9	0,1-1,4
	n	7	12	7	5

* T_4^+:T_8^+ ratio statistically significant higher than lavage
values of control subjects ($p < 0,05$);   blood values in sarcoidosis ($p < 0,01$) and lavage values after 9 months prednisone
treatment.

REFERENCES

1.   Crystal RG et al (1981): Annals of Internal Medicine 94:73-94.

2.   Benatar, SR et al (1985): S Afr Med J 67(3):73-75.

3.   Rizzato G (1986): Seminars in Respiratory Medicine 8(1):30-40.

SPONTANEOUS SECRETION OF HYDROGEN PEROXIDE BY ALVEOLAR MACROPHAGES OF PATIENTS WITH SARCOIDOSIS

ROBERT P. BAUGHMAN, SUSAN STROHOFER, ELYSE E. LOWER

Department of Medicine, University of Cincinnati Medical Center, Cincinnati, Ohio, USA.

INTRODUCTION

Alveolar macrophages (AM) from patients with sarcoidosis have been shown to secrete several factors spontaneously, including inter-leukin-1 and interferon (1). We studied AM retrieved by broncho-alveolar lavage (BAL) from nonsmoking sarcoids compared to AM from smoking and non-smoking controls. The amount of hydrogen peroxide (H_2O_2) released by the AM spontaneously or after stimulation by phorbol myristate acetate (PMA) was measured. The cells retrieved by BAL were also characterized using beta-galactosidase (BG) histo-chemical staining. The presence of BG on the surface of the cell membrane is seen in older, activated macrophages (2).

MATERIALS AND METHODS

A total of 39 subjects was studied including 14 nonsmoking sarcoid patients, 10 nonsmoking controls, and 15 smoking controls. H_2O_2 re-lease was measured using a previously described technique (3). BAL fluid aliquots were spun in a cytocentrifuge to prepare slides for subsequent staining. Slides were stained for differential counts with a modified Wright-Giemsa stain and BG using a modified tech-nique described by Yarborough et al (3,4). The disease activity in sarcoid patients was assessed by gallium scanning and lymphocyte percentage and subpopulation in the BAL fluid.

RESULTS

AM from the nonsmoking controls did not release detectable amounts of H_2O_2 spontaneously, but when these AM were stimulated with PMA, they released 54.6 ± 6.9 nm $H_2O_2/10^6$ AM (Mean$\pm$S.E.M.). AM from the smokers released detectable amounts of H_2O_2 spontaneously (52.9 ± 7.9 nm $H_2O_2/10^6$ AM, compared to nonsmokers, $p<0.01$) H_2O_2 production in-creased more when these AM from smokers were stimulated with PMA (92.1 ± 10.1 nm $H_2O_2/10^6$ AM). The 14 nonsmoking sarcoid patients also released detectable amounts of H_2O_2 (52.4 ± 19.1 nm $H_2O_2/10^6$ AM, com-pared to nonsmokers, $p<0.01$) which also increased when stimulated with PMA (73.3 ± 13.5 nm $H2O2/10^6$ AM).

The percentage of AM positive for BG by histochemical staining was lowest for the nonsmokers (median = 0%, range 0-9%)and highest for the smokers (median=8%, range 0-36%, compared to nonsmokers, p<0.01). For the sarcoid patients, the percentage of AM positive for BG was significantly less than the smokers (median=3, range 0-14%, compared to smokers, p<0.05).

The results of spontaneous H2O2 production by AM from the sarcoid patients was compared to other assessments of disease activity. No significant correlation was found between H2O2 release and the percentage of lymphocytes in the BAL fluid (R=0.15), the ratio of T4:T8 lymphocytes in the BAL fluid (R=0.26), or gallium uptake by the lung (R=0.22).

CONCLUSION

Recently, it has been emphasized that the severe pulmonary fibrosis in sarcoidosis is a relatively rare but significant event. It has been suggested that assessment of lymphocyte activity may be inadequate to predict who will develop fibrosis. Interest has therefore changed to the AM, since several factors released by the AM may cause fibrosis (1). This study measured one factor released by AM when stimulated and found high spontaneous levels in nonsmoking patients with active sarcoidosis. The histochemical staining studies would suggest a different subpopulation of AM are secreting H2O2 in the sarcoid group compared to the smokers' group (2). The measurement of H2O2 release by AM may provide important new information about AM response in sarcoidosis.

REFERENCES

1. Thomas PD, Hunninghake GW (1987) Current concepts of the pathogenesis of sarcoidosis. Am Rev Respir Dis 135:747-760.

2. Bursuker J, Rhodes JM, Goldman R (1982) B-galactosidase - an indicator of the maturational stage of mouse and human mononuclear phagocytes. J Cell Physiol 112:385-390.

3. Baughman RP, Corser BC, Strohofer S, Hendricks DE (1986) Spontaneous hydrogen peroxide release from alveolar macrophages of some cigarette smokers. J Lab Clin Med 107:233-237.

4. Yarborough DJ, Meyer OT, Dannenberg AM, Pearson B (1967) Histochemistry of macrophage hydrolases. III. Studies on B-galactosidase, B-glucaronidase, and aminopeptidase with indolyl and napthyl substrates. J Reticuloendothel Soc 4:390-408.

PROGNOSTIC VALUE OF ACE, LYSOZYME and PULMONARY LYMPHOCYTOSIS IN SARCOIDOSIS : RESULTS OF MULTICENTRIC PROSPECTIVE STUDY.

R. HARF, N. BIOT, M. PERRIN FAYOLLE and THE EMMEAMS COOPERATIVE STUDY GROUP[*].
Service de Pneumologie, CENTRE HOSPITALIER LYON SUD,
69310 PIERRE BENITE - FRANCE

Over recent years, several biological markers for assessing activity of sarcoidosis have been described. Up to there, medical management of the disease was based on clinical, radiological and spiromectric survey and an interesting point was to know if these new informations could be helpful in the survey and the prognosis of the patients.

Therefore in 1980 a multicentric prospective study was undertaken concerning 3 markers already well documented by numerous clinical and experimental investigations : lysozyme (LZ), angiotensin converting enzyme (ACE) and lymphocytosis (L) in BAL fluid.

MATERIAL AND METHODS

From january 1980 till september 1983, 212 patients with histological proof, giving consent, and without contraindication to the foreseen investigations were recruted in 10 hospitals chest departments in various parts of FRANCE.

1.The protocol included following investigations at 6 months interval :
- standard chest X ray,
- determination of lung diffusion capacity,
- BAL with fiberoptic material,
- veinous blood puncture,

2.L was measured in each of the participating centers whereas 10 ml of serum and 50 ml of supernatant were deep frozen before being sent to the central laboratory (N. BIOT P.D).

ACE was assessed by the method of Friedland and Silverstein, LZ by the microbiological technique with micrococcus lysodeicticus.

BAL was concentrated 10 times before enzyme determination.

3. Chest X ray were red by 3 independant trained physicians according to the international classification and also by comparaison of 2 successive pictures. In case of disagreement, consensus was obtained after consultation.

* : J. BRUNE (LYON), J.P. GUERIN (LYON), C. BRAMBILLA (GRENOBLE),
D. CHAVEZ (GRENOBLE), F. PATTE (POITIERS), J. BOTTA (POITIERS), P. DE
LABARTHE (RENNES), P. DELAVAL (RENNES), G. COURTY (BORDEAUX), K. THAK
(TOULOUSE), P. LEOPHONTE (TOULOUSE), P. GODARD (MONTPELLIER).

4. Statistical analysis :

Measure of the predictive value of the various parameters was done in 2 ways : the first using punctual informations at inclusion, the second using the changes observed at 6 months interval. All patients had an end point statement : were considered as cured those who were free from any clinical and radiological signs and without treatment.

As multiple linear regression did not isolate predictive factors we used a segmentation method (Belson) in order to find dichotomous explicative variables.

RESULTS

1) Characteristics of the patients at inclusion.

The 212 patients (112 men $\pm$ 100 women) had a mean + sd age of 35,5 $\pm$ 11,6 years. 38 were smokers. Mean duration of the disease was 1.4 years (0-13). At inclusion 107 were symptomatic and 11 received oral steroids. Radiological stage was 0 in 2, I in 43, II in 156 and III in 11.

Biological data : L percentage was 36 $\pm$ 20. SACE was 56,8 $\pm$ 24,6 nmol/ml/mn. (N $<$ 40), SLZ 12,4 $\pm$ 6,7 ng/ml (N $<$ 11). BALACE 1 $\pm$ 1.2 nmol/ml/mn (N $<$ 0,8).

2) Predictive value of parameters at inclusion.

The major prognostic factor is the disease duration : at the end of the survey 55 % of recent diseases ($\leq$ 1 year) are cured and only 5 out of 32 with a disease duration $>$ 3 years. From the 11 stage III only 1 became free from disease. Biological data are shown on figure I..

% of " cured "		ALL	Dur $\leq$ 2 yrs	Dur $>$ 2 yrs
L	$<$ 15 %	65 ⌐	71 ⌐	33 ⌐
	15 - 60	46 *	52,4 *	15 n.s
	$>$ 60 %	32 ⌐	33 ⌐	25 ⌐
SL Z	$\leq$ 15 ng/ml	51,7 ⌐*	56,4 ⌐*	26,3 ⌐ n:s
	$>$ 15 ng/ml	34 ⌐	39 ⌐	39 ⌐
SACE	$\leq$ 60 ng/ml/mn	48,4 ⌐	54 ⌐ n:s	15 ⌐ n:s
	$>$ 60	44,7 ⌐	48 ⌐	25 ⌐
BALACE	$<$ 0,5 ng/ml	58,1 ⌐ n:s	66,7 ⌐*	14 ⌐ n:s
	$>$ 0,5 ng/ml	43,1 ⌐	47,6 ⌐	20 ⌐

3) Prédictive value of 6 months inteval changes. Main results are shown on the following table :

CX	I	I	U or W	W
L	↓ (decrease)	↑ or ↕ (increase or unchanged)		↑ (increase)
% cured	76	54	54 38	25

CX	I	U or W	I	U or W
SACE	↓ or ↕ (decrease or unchanged)	↓ (decrease)	↑ (increase)	↑ (increase)
% cured	73,5	L↓ 56 L↑ / 72 10	42	23,5

CX	I	I	W
SLZ	↓ (decrease)	↕ or ↑ (unchanged or increase)	↕ or ↑ (unchanged or increase)
% cured	73,5	55,5	27

CX	I	I	W
BALACE	↓ (decrease)	↕ or ↑ (unchanged or increase)	↕ or ↑ (unchanged or increase)
% cured	78	60	39

CX = Chest x ray
U = unchanged
B = improved
W = worsened
↑ = increase : I
↕ = Unchanged: U
↓ = Decrease : D

DISCUSSION

Nobody believes anymore that the intensity of BAL lymphocytosis or an increased level of SACE are predictive for the course of sarcoïdosis. However the present study shows that it is possible to descriminate between patients group with better or poorer prognosis. The predictive value of the studied markers seems of interest among newly diagnosed patients : except for SACE, the prognosis at inclusion is linked with the level of the marker. Modifications observed at 6 months either increase the prognostic value of radiological or clinical changes when they go in the same direction or at the contrary reduce them when they are opposite.

MARKED ELEVATION OF SERUM ANGIOTENSIN CONVERTING ENZYME ACTIVITY - CLINICAL CORRELATES

HL ISRAEL, H PATRICK, JE GOTTLIEB, RM STEINER

Division of Pulmonary and Critical Care Medicine, Department of Medicine, Jefferson Medical College, 1025 Walnut Street, Philadelphia, Pennsylvania 19107, U.S.A.

Serum angiotensin converting enzyme (ACE) activity is raised in 50 to 60% of patients with active sarcoidosis. Although the cellular origin appears to be monocytes/ macrophages (1,2), the tissue origins of circulating ACE enzyme have not been identified despite numerous clinical studies. Unable to demonstrate a correlation of ACE activity with pulmonary, mediastinal or extrathoracic sites of involvement, most investigators have concluded that the elevations are related to the total body "granuloma load" (3,4).

We have studied the clinical and laboratory findings in 60 sarcoidosis patients whose ACE activity was markedly elevated [above 189 nm/ml/min; normal = 44-125 using ^{3}H-hippuryl-glycyl glycine (5)], in the hope that the sources of enzyme production in such patients might be more evident. The 60 patients, 12 white and 48 black, were not receiving corticosteroids. Sixty sarcoidosis patients with ACE activity below 190 served as controls and were matched for age, sex, and race. All patients had "active" sarcoidosis as demonstrated by recent histologic evidence of granuloma formation; not all patients had clinically "active" disease requiring treatment. Marked elevation of serum ACE [HI-ACE] was not related to age and sex but was more frequent in black patients. HI-ACE was associated with increased frequency and intensity of chest x-ray involvement [Table 1]. Extrathoracic involvement was similar except for hepatic [35%] and splenic [10%] dysfunction. HI-ACE was not related to the total body "granuloma load" since in 17 patients it occurred in patients with localized ocular, lymph node/salivary gland or skin sarcoidosis. In these cases, HI-ACE was often transient, at times subsiding in a few days on corticosteroids or in a few weeks without therapy. Forty patients with HI-ACE versus 22 controls improved on administration of prednisone with a decline in ACE; in 6, HI-ACE recurred within days or weeks of lapse of 5-10 mg daily doses, indicating extraordinary sensitivity of ACE activity to small doses of prednisone. Ten patients with HI-ACE versus 3 controls failed to respond to tolerable doses of prednisone and supplementary chlorambucil was given. Ten patients with HI-ACE versus 35 controls improved and ACE declined without therapy, indicating that HI-ACE has some prognostic value (Table 1).

The vagaries of ACE production and metabolism in sarcoidosis are as puzzling as the etiology of the disease. HI-ACE is noted more often with liver and spleen involvement, may be exquisitely sensitive to corticosteroids, but is sometimes due to intractable sarcoidosis. Elevated ACE activity is also noted in patients with non-granulomatous hepatic dysfunction (6,7), confirming our observations that ACE activity does not reflect total body "granuloma load". However, HI-ACE has some value in predicting the need for treatment and the response.

Table 1 - X-Ray and Clinical Features

X-Ray Stage		ACE > 189 # of Patients: 60	ACE < 190 # of Patients: 60
0		5	4
I		15*	27
II & III		40*	29
Profusion:	1-9	30	26
" "	10-18	10*	3

Clinical Features

Extrathoracic Involvement		
Liver	21*	4
Eyes	15	13
Skin	10	8
Nodes & salivary glands	8	8
Spleen	6*	0
Hypercalcemia	5	1

Treatment		
None	10*	35
Steroids	40	22
Chlorambucil	10*	3

*Significant [p<0.05] difference by Chi square or Fisher's exact test

REFERENCES

1. Conrad AK, Rohrbach MS (1987) An in-vitro model for the induction of angiotensin converting enzyme in sarcoidosis. Amer Rev Resp Dis 135:396-400

2. Okabe T, Yamagata K, Fujisawa M, et al. (1985) Increased angiotensin converting enzyme in peripheral blood monocytes from patients with sarcoidosis. J Clin Invest 75:911-914

3. Selroos OBN (1986) Biochemical markers in sarcoidosis. CRC Crit Rev Clin Lab Sci 24:185-216

4. Rizzato, G (1986) Markers of activity. Sem in Resp Med 8:30-40

5. Ryan JW, Chung A, Ammons C, Carlton ML (1977) A simple radioassay for angiotensin converting enzyme. Biochem J 167:501-504

6. Matsuki K, Sakata, T (1982) Angiotensin converting enzyme in diseases of the liver. Amer J Med 73:549-551

7. Johnson DA, Diehl AM, Sjogren MH, et al. (1987) Serum angiotensin converting enzyme activity in evaluation of patients with liver disease. Amer J Med 83:256-260

Supported in part by NIH Clinical Investigator Award K08-HL01488

© 1988 Elsevier Science Publishers B.V (Biomedical Division)
Sarcoidosis and other granulomatous disorders
C. Grassi, G. Rizzato, E. Pozzi, editors

ANGIOTENSIN CONVERTING ENZYME (ACE) INHIBITORS IN SARCOIDOSIS SERA WITH MARKEDLY ELEVATED ACE ACTIVITY

H PATRICK, JW GRAY, KJ SHEPLEY, HL ISRAEL

Division of Pulmonary and Critical Care Medicine, Department of Medicine, Jefferson Medical College, 1025 Walnut Street, Philadelphia, Pennsylvania 19107, U.S.A.

Recent reports indicate the presence of angiotensin converting enzyme [ACE] inhibitors of unknown origin circulating in plasma and serum (1,2) which can mask elevated ACE activity. Although conventional assays designed to measure pharmacologic ACE inhibitors such as captopril, enalapril and lisinopril fail to detect these natural inhibitors (3), the natural inhibitors express greatest ACE inhibition at low sample dilutions thereby permitting detection using serial dilution assays.

Using serial dilution assays, we studied 42 sera from sarcoid patients with markedly elevated ACE activity [above 189, normal range 44-125 nm/ml/min], 56 sera from sarcoid patients who were matched for age, sex and race but with ACE activity below 190 and 15 sera from normals with ACE=44-125. The clinical aspects of the two groups of active sarcoidosis patients have been described separately (4). ACE activity was measured by a modified Ventrex ACE radioassay system (5) utilizing ^{3}H-hippuryl-glycyl-glycine. This assay is linear up to 275 nm/ml/min as determined using purified human ACE samples which contain no inhibitors (6), and incorporates HEPES buffer which avoids pH fluctuations and resulting underestimates of activity. Our tests of the Lieberman spectrophotometric assay (7) indicated that its phosphate buffer, susceptible to pH fluctuations, caused errors depending on the dilution factor and type of diluent. All sera were assayed at the standard 1:5 and also at 1:10, 1:20, 1:40 and 1:80 dilutions. For samples exceeding assay linearity at 1:5 dilution, the 1:10 dilution was considered standard and a 1:160 dilution included. Our purified human ACE and normal serum with and without the addition of lisinopril acted as controls. To quantitate the inhibitors, we first defined "inhibitor free" ACE activity for each sample as the activity one dilution below the dilution where the increase in ACE activity was less than 10%. Then, comparing "inhibitor free" ACE activity versus the activity at the standard dilution provided a semi-quantitative measure of the inhibitors, i.e., a sample with a larger increase in activity would contain more inhibitors.

As shown in Table 1, all sample groups, including the normals, displayed mean increases in activity. The largest increase occurred in the group of sarcoid sera with ACE activity >189 even though three of these sera requiring standard dilutions of 1:10

had their inhibitor content underestimated. We conclude that naturally occurring ACE inhibitors are common in sera assayed by our technique and are present in greatest quantities in sarcoidosis patients with markedly elevated ACE activity. The origin and clinical significance of these inhibitors capable of altering ACE activity remain to be elucidated while a convenient inhibitor assay is sorely needed. We are presently investigating the comparison of ACE immunologic level (concentration) with ACE enzymatic level (activity) as an indirect inhibitor assay.

TABLE 1

	n	ACE Activity, Mean (nm/ml/min)		% Change	p vs. Normal
		Standard Dilution	"Inhibitor Free"		
Normal, ACE=44-125	15	75	104	+42%	-
Sarcoid, ACE=44-125	26	86	120	+41%	N.S.
Sarcoid, ACE=126-189	30	148	216	+46%	N.S.
Sarcoid, ACE>189	42	239	417	+76%	<0.01

REFERENCES

1. Lieberman J, Sastre A (1986) An angiotensin-converting enzyme (ACE) inhibitor in human serum: increased sensitivity of the serum ACE assay for detecting sarcoidosis. Chest 90:869-875

2. Hazato T, Kase R (1986) Isolation of angiotensin converting-enzyme inhibitor from porcine plasma. Biochem Biophy Res Comm 139:52-55

3. Shepley K, Rocci ML, Patrick H, Mojaverian P (in press) An optimized fluoroenzymatic assay for the determination of angiotensin converting enzyme inhibitors in biological fluids. J Pharm and Biomed Anal

4. Israel HL, Patrick H, Steiner RM, Gottlieb JE (in press) Marked elevation of serum angiotensin converting enzyme - clinical correlates. Presented at XI World Congress on Sarcoidosis and other granulomatous disorders

5. Ryan JW, Chung A, Ammons C, Carlton ML (1977) A simple radioassay for angiotensin converting enzyme. Biochem J 167:501-504

6. Patrick H, Shepley KJ, Scuitto E, Gray JW (1987) Affinity purification of human angiotensin converting enzyme from small volume samples. Fed Proc 46:1963

7. Lieberman J (1976) Elevation of serum angiotensin converting enzyme level in sarcoidosis. Am J Med 59:365-372 and (1976) erratum 60:A23

Supported in part by NIH Clinical Investigator Award K08-HL01488.

© 1988 Elsevier Science Publishers B.V. (Biomedical Division)
Sarcoidosis and other granulomatous disorders
C. Grassi, G. Rizzato, E. Pozzi, editors

SERUM ANGIOTENSIN-CONVERTING ENZYME (SACE) ACTIVITY AS AN IN-
DICATOR OF TOTAL BODY GRANULOMA LOAD AND PROGNOSIS IN SARCOI-
DOSIS

PETHAM P. MUTHUSWAMY*, VINCENT LOPEZ-MAJANO**, MOIN RANGINWALA*,
WILLIAM D. TRAINOR*

Division of Pulmonary Medicine* and Division of Nuclear Medicine**
of Cook County Hospital and the University of Illinois College of
Medicine at Chicago. 1835 W. Harrison St. Chicago, IL. 60612

The relationship between the level of serum angiotensin converting enzyme (SACE) and the total body granuloma load in patients
with sarcoidosis was studied in two groups using SACE levels and
total body gallium 67 scans. The study group consisted of 22
patients with SACE levels $\geq$ 100 U/ml (EH-SACE GROUP) and the control
group consisted of 24 patients consecutively diagnosed to have
sarcoidosis in a one year period with SACE level of $<$ 80 U/ml. The
roentgenographic features of the two groups are shown in table I.

TABLE - I

STAGE	SACE $\geq$ 100 (n=21) %	SACE $<$ 80 (n=24) %	p value
I	9	4	NS
II	68	42	NS
III	23	58	0.03

Based upon gallium 67 scans, the average number of organs involved in the EH-SACE group was 3.9±1 compared to 2.3±1 in the
control group (p $<$ 0.0001). The incidence of extra pulmonary organ
involvement in the EH-SACE group was 2.2±1 organs compared to
1.0±0.8 in control group (p $<$ 0.0002). The SACE level was correlated
with the number of organs involved for all patients with sarcoidosis
(r=.55; p $<$ .0001).

The total body granuloma load as assessed by gallium 67 scintigraphy in the two groups are shown in table II.

TABLE - II

Gallium uptake by organs	SACE ≥ 100 (n-22) %	SACE < 80 (n-24) %	p value
Nasal mucosa, salivary and lacrimal glands	95	66	NS
Lungs	90	83	NS
Intrathoracic nodes	68	37	0.01
Marked hepatomegaly	27	0	0.02
Marked splenomegaly	32	4	0.01
Joints	32	8	NS
Skin, soft tissue, muscles	22	4	NS
Extrathoracic nodes	18	20	NS

Following corticosteroid therapy for 39±41 weeks the SACE dropped to 64±45 units in the EH-SACE group. But it took only 13±10 weeks to normalize the SACE level to 27±9 units in the control group. The EH-SACE group patients were followed for 114±64 weeks and 73% of them still have active sarcoidosis requiring repeated cycles of corticosteroid therapy, while after 42±23 weeks of follow up only 10% of patients from the control group were still on therapy.

The clinical characteristic of the two groups of patients are shown in table III.

TABLE - III

Characteristic	SACE ≥ 100 (n=22)	SACE < 80 (n=24)	p value
1. Age yr.	32±9	34±11	NS
2. Male	10	12	NS
3. Female	12	12	NS
4. SACE-pre-steroid therapy	125±33	43±17	0.001
5. Steroid therapy in weeks	39±41(17)	13±10(16)	0.03
6. SACE-post-steroid therapy	64±45(17)	27±9(16)	0.004
7. Total number of organs with significant gallium 67 uptake	3.9±1	2.3±1	0.0001
8. Number of extrathoracic organs with significant gallium 67 uptake	2.2±1	1.0±0.8	0.0002

CONCLUSION:

Our study shows that in patients with sarcoidosis the SACE activity correlates well with the total body granuloma load as assessed by gallium 67 scans; SACE level appears to be an useful indicator of severity of disease, response to therapy and prognosis.

ACTIVITY ASSESSMENT AND TREATMENT DECISIONS. OUTLOOK

HL ISRAEL, JE GOTTLIEB, H PATRICK, RM STEINER

DIVISION OF PULMONARY AND CRITICAL CARE MEDICINE, JEFFERSON
MEDICAL COLLEGE, THOMAS JEFFERSON UNIVERSITY, PHILADELPHIA, PA

In their Summary Statement on Disease Activity Assessment,
presented at the 10th International Conference on Sarcoidosis,
Chrétien and his associates proposed that the next conference use
the terms predictive criteria and therapeutic guidelines instead
of the term activity, since there is no real consensus as to the
precise meaning of the latter term (1). We have followed this
recommendation and in order to assess the sensitivity and
specificity of the predictive criteria in common use, have
compared clinical, radiologic and biochemical findings in
sarcoidosis patients requiring treatment and in those observed
without therapy.

MATERIALS AND METHODS

We have tabulated data on 336 cases of sarcoidosis examined in
the 2 year interval between August 1, 1985 and July 31, 1987 at
Thomas Jefferson University Hospital (TJUH), comprising 216 black
and 120 white patients. In each case, a decision was made (1) to
inaugurate or continue corticosteroid therapy or (2) to observe
without therapy. Asymptomatic patients were not treated; in
symptomatic patients, the decision was based on severity of
symptoms and physical findings, and by chest roentgenograms,
automated clinical biochemical measurements (SMA-12), and serum
angiotensin converting enzyme (ACE) levels. Patients with
respiratory symptoms had measurement of spirometry and diffusing
capacity. Gallium-67 scans were obtained when indicated as aids
to diagnosis or for distinguishing granulomatous from fibrotic
pulmonary infiltrates.

We divided the patients into 3 groups based on the following
criteria: 1) 130 "new" patients were seen for the first time at
TJUH. The other 206 "old" cases had been earlier seen at TJUH,
and comprised 2) 86 under treatment with corticosteroids, and 3)
120 not under treatment, 59 who had never received medication and

61 who had been treated in the past, but had received no corticosteroids in the prior 12 months.

Of the new patients, 60 were treated (Table I). No asymptomatic patient was treated, and patients with parenchymal disease (Types II and III) were more often treated - but there was no difference between treated and observed patients in extent of pulmonary disease, serum ACE activity and frequency of extrapulmonary involvement. A significant difference in radiologic findings was observed between the 60 treated patients and the 70 who were observed. Type 0 and I roentgenograms were present less often in treated patients (Table II), that is, patients with pulmonary infiltrates (Types II and III) were more often treated.

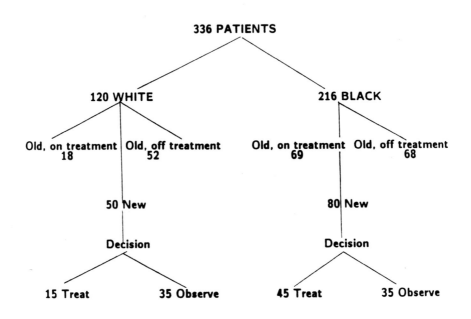

Figure 1. Treatment decisions in 336 sarcoidosis patients
Thomas Jefferson University Hospital
August 1985 - July 1987

TABLE I

ACTIVITY MARKERS IN 130 NEW CASES
RELATED TO TREATMENT DECISION

	TREAT	OBSERVE
Number of Patients	60	70
ACE	134.2	130.1
X-Ray Stage: 0/I	*26	*47
II/III	*34	*23
Profusion: 1-9	28	21
10-18	6	2
Respiratory Symptoms	31	17
Extrathoracic "	29	32
None	*0	*21

*Significant differences by chi-square test

TABLE II

PREDICTIVE VALUE OF ACTIVITY MARKERS
RELATED TO DECISION TO TREAT SARCOIDOSIS

	SENSITIVITY	SPECIFICITY	POSITIVE PREDICTIVE VALUE
Race - B	74%	51%	.56
Sex - F	64%	44%	.49
ACE> 124	48%	44%	.42
Any Symptoms	100%	30%	.54
Stage II/III X-Ray	58%	68%	.60

TABLE III

ACTIVITY ASSESSMENT AND TREATMENT DECISION BY RACE

130 NEW CASES

	WHITE	BLACK
Number of Patients	52	78
ACE	*111.2	*145.7
X-Ray Stage: 0/I	30	43
II/III	22	35
Profusion: 1-9	17	32
10-18	5	3
Respiratory Symptoms	18	30
Extrathoracic "	19	42
None	*15	*6
Treated	*15	*44
Observed	*37	*35

*Significant differences by chi-square test

TABLE IV

GALLIUM 67 SCANS ORDERED IN PATIENTS 1985-1987

PATIENT CATEGORY	NUMBER OF PATIENTS	NUMBER OF SCANS	NUMBER MISLEADING
New	130	39	2
Old, on treatment	86	6	0
Old, not on treatment	120	14	0
TOTAL	336	59	2

The severity of parenchymal disease as reflected in the profusion of radiologic densities were similar in treated and observed patients.

Table II summarizes the positive predictive values for selecting treatment of the "activity" indicators we have assessed. Since only symptomatic patients were treated, symptoms showed a high correlation with treatment although many patients with symptoms were not treated. Serum ACE activity, race, sex and pulmonary infiltrates showed no significant correlation with symptoms requiring treatment.

Although serum ACE activity, race, sex and pulmonary infiltrates were of little assistance in the treatment decision, erythema nodosum proved a specific predictor of rapid recovery without therapy. Onset with erythema nodosum was rather infrequent in Philadelphia, but as in Europe, heralded a favorable prognosis. Erythema nodosum was the mode of onset in 7 new white and 2 black patients. Eight of the nine recovered rapidly without corticosteroids, while one white patient developed hypercalcemia and required prednisone for 5 months. None had subsequent relapse.

Race. The racial distribution of new patients permitted a comparison of activity markers and treatment decisions in black and white patients (Table III). Black patients more often required treatment and there was a greater proportion of asymptomatic onsets in white patients. The mean serum ACE activity was significantly higher in black patients (145 vs. 101, $p<.05$), who also had marked elevations (>189 nm/ml/min) more often than white patients (2). Mean ACE values were 101 in treated whites and 115 in observed whites compared to 144 in treated and 146 in observed black patients. Of the 52 white patients 18 had predominantly respiratory symptoms, 19 had extrathoracic symptoms, and 15 were asymptomatic. Of the 78 black patients, 30 had predominately respiratory symptoms, 42 had extrathoracic manifestations, and 6 were asymptomatic. Treatment was considered indicated for 16 (31%) new white patients, and 44 (56%) new black patients. Treatment was required for 8 (16%) white patients and for 23 (52%) black patients with predominately respiratory symptoms; for 8 (14%) whites with extrathoracic disease and 20 (45%) black patients with extrathoracic disease.

There was no significant difference in chest x-ray patterns between the races. White and black patients had a similar distribution of the radiologic stages; 30 white patients (58%) had Type 0-I roentgenograms, while 43 (55%) of black patients had no parenchymal disease. Parenchymal disease was seen in 45% of black patients, and 42% of white patients. Profusion was 9 or less in 32 black patients and in 17 white patients, and was greater than 9 in 3 black, and 5 white patients.

Gallium-67. Fourteen "old" patients not on corticosteroid therapy had gallium scans ordered, usually in perplexing or unusual problems in assessing whether relapse had occurred (Table IV). Gallium-67 scans were ordered in 38 "new" patients as an aid to diagnosis, especially as a guide to selection of biopsy sites. It was occasionally difficult to differentiate granulomatous from fibrosed pulmonary infiltrates, and scanning was used for this purpose. Gallium scanning was not employed in fresh cases of sarcoidosis to assess the need for treatment.

Pulmonary function. Pulmonary function tests, performed in all patients with respiratory symptoms, usually showed typical patterns of restriction and impaired diffusing capacity in patients with pulmonary infiltrates. However, various other patterns were also observed, as well as striking disparities such as intense Gallium-67 uptake in the lungs of patients with normal function.

Relapse. It has been our clinical impression that serial ACE activity measurements are useful in assisting detection of relapse in sarcoidosis. In an attempt to assess the value of ACE for this purpose, we tabulated the frequency of relapse in the patients observed in the 2 year interval 1985-87 (Table V). Relapse was distinguished from progression under treatment, and was defined as requiring re-institution of systemic therapy, so that development of small skin sarcoids or flares of uveitis controllable by local medication were not regarded as a relapse for the purposes of this study.Relapse proved to be common, not only among patients whose medication lapsed through lack of compliance; it was surprisingly frequent when medication was discontinued by the patient's physician. Relapse was rare in patients not under treatment, occurring in only 4 of the 120 patients in this category.

TABLE V
ACCURACY OF TREATMENT DECISIONS 1985-87

Category	Total Number	Number Observed	Number Later Treated	Number RX Stopped	Number Relapses
New	130	64	6	22	10
Old, on treatment	86	-	-	32	22
Old, off treatment	120	116*	0	0	0
White	120	86	1**	20	10**
Black	216	94	5**	34	22**
TOTAL	336	180	6	54	32

*Four patients required treatment

**Significant difference by chi-square test

Relapses followed cessation of corticosteroid therapy - whether given a few months or many years - in 10 (45%) of 22 "new" cases and in 22 (69%) of 32 "old" patients (Table V). Serum ACE activity was of little help in making the decision to stop treatment, nor was ACE of assistance in detecting the need for resumption of treatment, having only 63% sensitivity and 63% specificity for this purpose. Relapse following a decision to stop corticosteroids was slightly more frequent among black patients, but was a major problem in both races. The patterns of relapse were similar in both races, most often involving the respiratory tract - but exhibiting a wide variety of systemic manifestations (Table VI), indicating the limited role of radiologic examination and pulmonary function study for detection of relapse.

DISCUSSION

Our decisions to institute or continue corticosteroid therapy were, we believe, conservative ones. In no case was treatment instituted in asymptomatic patients, while symptomatic patients were treated only if objective laboratory evidence of dysfunction supported the decision. Abnormal radiologic and nuclear scan changes or ACE elevations were not by themselves indications for the start of treatment.

The decision to continue treatment in 1985-87 was based on similar considerations, with the additional philosophy that corticosteroids should be discontinued for a period of observation of new patients when it appeared that the treatment had not been appropriately instituted. Among the 130 "new" patients examined, 60 had corticosteroids started or continued, and 70 were observed without therapy. This decision proved erroneous in

TABLE VI

RELAPSES AFTER CESSATION OF THERAPY
1985-87

Major Site of Recurrence	22 Black Patients	10 White Patients
Respiratory	10	5
Ocular	5	1
Musculoskeletal	1	1
Hepatic	2	0
Hypercalcemia	0	2
CNS	1	0
Peripheral Gland	2	0
Cardiac	0	1
Skin	1	0

a relatively small number, i.e., corticosteroids were later started or resumed in 1 white and 5 black patients (Table V). This evidence supports our use of the treatment decision as the standard by which the clinical value of laboratory markers of "activity" can be assessed.

The chest roentgenogram has long been employed as a guide to treatment decisions, with Type I disease often considered not requiring therapy and Type II and III disease often justifying corticosteroid administration. Our data gives little support to this view. There was no significant difference in sensitivity of Type 0, I, or II/III roentgenograms in selecting patients for treatment. Among the patients with parenchymal disease, profusion of radiologic densities bore no relationship to the decision to start therapy or to continue it in patients already on medication.

Serum angiotensin converting enzyme levels were measured on virtually every visit. ACE measurements proved to have low sensitivity (48%) and specificity (44%) as an indicator of the need for treatment. We have reported at this meeting (2) a study of 60 patients with extremely high ACE levels (greater than 189 nm/ml/min). Such extreme elevations were more common in black patients and in those with hepatosplenomegaly, and a majority of such patients required corticosteroid therapy. The response to therapy was unpredictable, however. In most cases there was prompt response to minimal dosage. Ten patients were corticosteroid failures and required cytotoxic agents, while at the other extreme 10 patients recovered without therapy.

We have had the clinical impression that ACE levels are chiefly valuable in detecting relapse if performed serially when corticosteroid discontinuation is deemed appropriate. However, among the 32 patients in whom discontinuation was followed by relapse requiring re-institution of therapy, serial ACE activity was of little practical value in detecting relapse.

Our judgments as to the need for treatment may appear to be reasonably accurate in new patients, but our experience indicates that our judgment in discontinuing therapy is appallingly deficient. It has seemed a reasonable clinical practice in chronic sarcoidosis controlled by minimal (5 mgm daily) doses of prednisone to stop therapy at 18 to 24 month intervals. In some cases arthralgia and vague systemic or respiratory symptoms appear, which are often difficult to determine whether due to anxiety or relapse of sarcoidosis, while in others radiologic, pulmonary function and biochemical changes quickly corroborate recurrence. Unfortunately, there are no markers to guide the decision to stop medication, since the indicators of activity are suppressed by even small doses of prednisone. Trial and error has proven the only way to test when corticosteroids can be stopped, and long experience had taught us not to stop medication too soon. It was, therefore, astonishing to discover in the present analysis that despite long clinical experience and coupled with generous use of ACE, chest x-rays and other appropriate tests - that in the 54 cases in which medication was stopped by a physician, we were wrong more often than right. It is evident that low dose corticosteroid therapy can result in suppression of symptoms, serum ACE activity and gallium uptake for years, with recurrence evident from 1 to 12 months after cessation of these minimal doses. What is sorely needed is a marker of activity that is not suppressed by the same small dose of corticosteroids that suppresses symptoms.

The greater severity of sarcoidosis in black patients is shown by the markedly greater number who were regarded as needing corticosteroid therapy, 56% compared to 30% in white patients. Prednisone failure requiring chlorambucil supplementation was observed in 21 of the 216 black patients reviewed in this study and 3 of the 120 white patients. Total blindness developed in 2 black young men and the sole death, from respiratory failure, occurred in a black woman. It might be expected that the "activity" indices would be vastly higher in black patients. In fact, neither the roentogenographic pulmonary changes in black patients nor clinical manifestations were greater; although serum angiotensin converting enzyme activity was higher in black patients, it was not related to need for treatment.

Thus, the activity markers so intensively studied in recent years added little to clinical evaluation in respect to treatment decisions. Many investigators have come to a similar conclusion (3-5), but infer that what is needed are more sensitive indicators. We draw the opposite conclusion: the initial intensity of inflammation in sarcoidosis does not determine the severity of the local damage or the extent of systemic dissemination. This is illustrated by Valeyre et al. (6) who demonstrated intense alveolitis by bronchoalveolar lavage in patients with erythema nodosum who recovered without treatment.

The search for sensitive indicators of activity had as a premise the belief that corticosteroid therapy applied early and vigorously enough could alter the outcome of the disease. Six controlled studies of corticosteroid treatment of sarcoidosis have demonstrated no significant advantage (7-12) even after prolonged therapy (8-12). If the action of corticosteroids in sarcoidosis is merely suppressive rather than curative, there is little point to the search for earlier or more sensitive indicators of the inflammatory process. It is time to divert our investigational talents elsewhere - to exploration of the factors that really do determine the outcome of sarcoidosis, such as erythema nodosum, race and extrathoracic spread (13).

SUMMARY

In an effort to assess the sensitivity, specificity and predictive value of the methods in clinical use for estimation of "activity" of sarcoidosis, clinical, radiologic and biochemical findings in 336 patients recently seen at Thomas Jefferson University Hospital have been analyzed. Among 130 patients evaluated for the first time, 60 required treatment and 70 were observed. The decision to treat was related to presence of symptoms and of pulmonary infiltrates in the chest roentgenogram, but extent of pulmonary infiltrates, serum angiotensin converting enzyme (ACE) activity, extrapulmonary manifestations and sex had little or no predictive value. The activity markers in black and white patients were compared in order to determine whether they reflected the racial difference in outcome of the disease. Mean serum ACE was higher in black patients who more often had marked elevations (>189 nm/ml/min). Treatment was more often required for black (56%) than white patients (31%). There was no significant difference between the races in chest roentgenographic changes, or in patterns of extrathoracic involvement.

616

Relapse proved to be infrequent among 120 patients previously
treated or observed at TJUH who had been off corticosteroids at
least 12 months. Among patients currently on corticosteroid
therapy, relapse proved to be extremely frequent following
attempts to terminate therapy: treatment had to be resumed in 32
(59%) of the 54 instances in which physicians stopped treatment.
Indicators of "activity" were useless as a predictor of relapse,
since all activity markers were suppressed by the same small dose
of corticosteroids that suppressed symptoms. Attempts to devise
more sensitive or specific markers to predict the need for
treatment and the likelihood of relapse are unlikely to be
successful, since there is increasing evidence that the ultimate
outcome of sarcoidosis is determined not by the initial intensity
of pulmonary inflammation, but by race and other constitutional
factors.

REFERENCES

1. Chrétien J, Venet A, Israel-Biet D, Clavel F. (1986) Summary
    statement on disease activity assessment. Ann NY Acad Sci
    465:479-481

2. Israel H, Patrick H, Gottlieb JE, Steiner RM (1988) Marked
    elevation of serum angiotensin converting enzyme - clinical
    correlates. Proc 11th Int Conf on Sarcoidosis and other
    granulomatous diseases

3. Delaval P, Pencole C, Bourquet P, Genetet N et al (1987)
    Predictive value of serum angiotensin converting enzyme,
    bronchoalveolar lavage, T-lymphocyte subsets and gallium-67
    lung scan in pulmonary sarcoidosis Am Rev Resp Dis 135: #4,
    Part 2, p A397

4. Niden AH, Mishkin FS, Salem F, Thomas AV Jr et al. (1986)
    Prognostic significance of gallium lung scans in
    sarcoidosis. Ann NY Acad Sci 465:435-443

5. Turner-Warwick M, Haslam PL, McAllister W, Britton A et al.
    (1986) Do measurements of bronchoalveolar lymphocytes and
    neutrophils, serum angiotensin converting enzyme, and gal-
    lium uptake help the clinician to treat patients with sar-
    coidosis? Ann NY Acad Sci 465:387-394

6. Valeyre D, Saumon G, Georges R, Kemeny JL et al (1984) The
    relationship between disease duration and noninvasive pul-
    monary explorations in sarcoidosis with erythema nodosum. Am
    Rev Resp Dis 129:938-943

7. Israel HL, Fouts DW, Beggs RA (1973) A controlled trial of
    prednisone treatment of sarcoidosis. Am Rev Respir Dis
    107:609-614

8. Harkleroad LE, Young RL, Savage PJ et al. (1982) Pulmonary sarcoidosis. Long-term follow-up of the effects of steroid therapy. Chest 82:84-87

9. Selroos O, Sellergren TL (1979) Corticosteroid therapy of pulmonary sarcoidosis. A prospective evaluation of alternate day and daily dosage in stage II disease. Scand J Respir Dis 60:215-221

10. Eule H, Weinecke A, Roth I (1986) The possible influence of corticosteroid therapy on the natural course of pulmonary sarcoidosis. Ann NY Acad Sci 465:695-701

11. Yamamoto M, Saito N, Tachibana T et al (1980) Effects of an 18 month corticosteroid therapy to stage I and stage II sarcoidosis patients (a control trial) in Chretien J, Marsac J, Saltiel JC (eds): Sarcoidosis and Other Granulomatous Disorders. Paris Pergamon Press pp 470-474

12. Zaki MH, Lyons HA, Huang CT et al (1987) Corticosteroids in sarcoidosis: A five-year controlled therapeutic follow-up study. NY State J Med 87:496-499

13. Israel HL, Karlin P, Menduke H, Delisser OG (1986) Factors affecting outcome of sarcoidosis. Influence of race, extrathoracic involvement, and initial radiologic lung lesions. Ann NY Acad Sci 465:609-618

TREATMENT

TREATMENT OF PULMONARY SARCOIDOSIS
STATE OF THE ART

MARGARET TURNER-WARWICK

The Cardiothoracic Institute, Brompton Hospital, Fulham Road, London SW3
6HP.

INTRODUCTION

In spite of substantial advances in our scientific understanding concerning the immunological features of sarcoid granulomata (1), the abnormal features observed in bronchoalveolar lavage fluids (2) knowledge of markers of activity such as serum angiotensin converting enzymes in blood (3) and gallium scans (4), the controversies about when and how to treat patients with pulmonary sarcoidosis remains unresolved.

The reasons for this are not hard to find. In general, pulmonary sarcoidosis is a self limiting benign condition (5). When irreversible lung damage occurs, it tends to develop very slowly (although there are many notable exceptions). Thus, unless meticulous follow up is planned as a routine, the unfortunate minority of patients with lung damage tend to present late in the course of disease and often to physicians other than those initially responsible for diagnosis. Treatment at this stage is often too late (6).

The perspectives expressed in this State of the Art summary are my own current views; I realise fully that many are still contentious and others unproven.

WHY IS CORRECT MANAGEMENT IMPORTANT?

Although irreversible lung damage affects only some 10% of all patients with parenchymal lung involvement, the consequences for them are serious and sometimes fatal. Pulmonary hypertension is a rare but life threatening complication. Irreversible fibrosis resulting in life threatening aspergillomas, respiratory failure or recurrent severe bronchial infection are all very serious conditions, and are particularly disasterous when affecting individuals in their 30's and 40's.

MISUNDERSTANDINGS ABOUT SARCOIDOSIS

The problem is made worse by the fact that owing to its generally benign course, follow up care by physicians is often sketchy and unsystematic. This practice is largely based on the widely held view that there is no need to take the condition seriously unless the patient develops respiratory symptoms. The problem is compounded by many large scale but short term studies where corticosteroids have been used for over relatively short periods of time and then discontinued. These results are often quoted as evidence to demonstrate that progression of disease is no different in treated and untreated groups of patients (6). It is however illogical to treat a condition known to be active over much longer periods than that of treatment and then to expect modulation of the final outcome. The influence of long term management has been limited to a small number of uncontrolled studies; for example in caucasians (7)(17) and in blacks (8).

Communication about the facts of sarcoidosis are also not yet agreed. For example, the radiographic stages of sarcoidosis are not used in the same way throughout the world. Some view 'stages' as a shorthand descriptive term of the radiographic abnormality present. Some imply that patients necessarily progress from one stage to another - which is by no means invariable. Some even imply that stage III is synonymous with pulmonary fibrosis; this has the implication that this stage must be irreversible which is patently not the case. It is often not appreciated that fibrotic destruction of the lung can be seen in stage II as well as stage III. Further, staging includes no indication of the severity of the parenchymal shadows - yet there is good evidence that the extent of reversibility of shadowing following corticosteroid treatment is dependent in part on the severity of the profusion score at the start of treatment (Fig 1)(9)

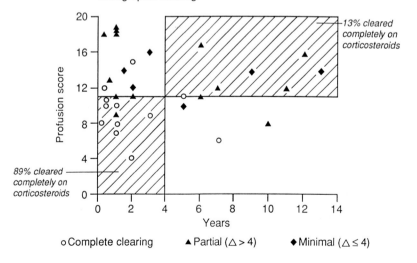

Sarcoidosis

Duration, radiographic profusion score + extent of radiographic clearing

o Complete clearing   ▲ Partial (△ > 4)   ◆ Minimal (△ ≤ 4)

TWO SCHOOLS OF THOUGHT ON MANAGEMENT

School I

Their views can be summarised as follows:

1. Sarcoidosis is generally a benign self limiting condition, often showing spontaneous resolution. This is generally agreed.

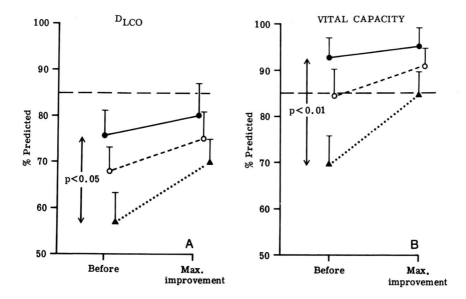

Fig. 2. Lung function before and after maximum radiographic improvement after corticosteroids in three groups of patients:

●——● those achieving complete radiographic resolution.
o-----o those with incomplete radiographic resolution.
▲.....▲ those with incomplete resolution and residual evidence of linear shadows and lung contraction.

624

2. Treatment with corticosteroids may result in unwanted side effects. This is also undeniable but is less likely when only small doses of steroids are effective in controlling activity of disease.

3. If fibrosis is going to develop it will do so in spite of steroids. There is no good evidence for this except in cases managed with steroids for arbitrary and limited periods and in doses which do not maintain optimal clearing of the chest radiograph or they are started, only when the disease is very advanced (7).

4. There is nothing to be lost by waiting for the patient to develop the symptoms of breathlessness or substantial deterioration of their lung function. Evidence from our own studies show that irreversible changes can indeed occur in asymptomatic patients (9) and that once the lung function is substantially impaired, especially the DL_{co}, even in asymptomatic patients, radiographic changes are more likely to be irreversible (Fig 2).

School II

Their case rests on the following principles:

1. Preservation of lung architecture can be achieved better by treating asymptomatic patients with persisting radiographic shadows who have failed to resolve spontaneously over approximately 9-12 months.

2. Radiographic parenchymal shadows reflect lung pathology of various types such as granulomas, lymphocytic infiltrates, fibrosis and linear atelectasis.

3. The longer shadows persist, the less likely they are to resolve completely with treatment. (See Fig 1).

4. The greater the perfusion scores the less likely treatment will result in complete clearing.(Fig 1)

5. It is better for the patient to have a normal structure and function of the lung preserved as far as is measurable.

6. It is possible to restore to normal (or optimal improvement) and maintain a maximally improved radiograph and lung function by titrating the dose of steroids against simple measurements (i.e. high quality chest radiographs and lung function).

7. The dose necessary to achieve this is often small e.g. 10 mg daily or less (7). In our experience alternate day regimen is often feasible.

8. There is good evidence that using this system, steroids may be withdrawn eventually without relapse, even when treatment to maintain optimal improvement has been necessary over periods of several years (7)(8).

Of some 600 patients seen in the Edinburgh series(7), 260 received steroids and in the majority treatment was discontinued within two years (80% without relapse). On the other hand 37 patients required treatment for more than three years. 13 (35%) received treatment for persisting radiographic abnormality and could be withdrawn without deterioration after a mean of 6.7 years. In 4 the chest radiograph returned to normal but in 9 there was minimal fibrosis. In 15 patients (41%) treated mainly for persisting radiographic abnormality, prednisone needed to be continued (to the point of follow up) to prevent relapse. The mean duration of treatment at assessment was 9.6 years. The maintenance dose to prevent relapse was 10 mg or less in all patients. The chest radiograph at review was normal in 2, moderate in 6 and severe in only 1. In 9 patients (24%) treatment was begun only after the development of dyspnoea and with the established evidence of fibrosis at the time. Treatment was continued to the follow up date with a mean of 9.8 years. All of these patients are severely disabled. Four have died. Clearly treatment was started too late and only at a very advanced stage of disease.

The proof of the advantage of School II

A really long term trial to see how far irreversible damage to the lung can be prevented by treating patients earlier in the course of disease in doses adequate to maintain an optimally improved radiograph and lung function still needs to be performed. Large numbers will be needed because many patients will have self limiting disease. The duration of observation will need to be extended over at least ten years, probably longer. The definitive scientific study will therefore be hard to design. It will certainly be exceedingly difficult to maintain. In the meantime physicians continue to argue and while they do so a minority of patients will develop serious life threatening complications of sarcoidosis.

Other methods of treatment

Selroos has provided (10) preliminary data to suggest that inhaled corticosteroids may be effective in treating sarcoidosis and a preliminary study has suggested an oral steroid sparing effect in relapsing patients (11).

A number of uncontrolled studies have reported the use of immunosupprassents such as azathioprine or cyclophosphamide but in the authors limited experience these are often not convincingly effective in improving the chest radiograph when corticosteroids have failed.

Some preliminary studies using Cyclosporin A have not proved useful in spite of their anticipated value on theoretical grounds.

Recent Studies

'Activity' of various individual cellular components of a granuloma is not necessarily synonymous with progression towards irreversible destruction of the lung architecture.

Attempts to identify markers which more reliably predict those cases with a tendency to progress to fibrosis and develop irreversible changes (before they have occurred) have not so far been successful. It was suggested that those patients with bronchoalveolar lavage total T lymphocytes of greater than 28% and a positive 67 gallium scan would progress (12), but there are too many progressive cases with normal lymphocytes (9) for this to be reliable in individual patients (Fig 3).

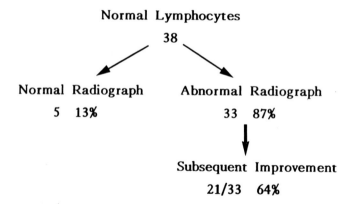

Normal Lymphocytes and Radiographic Change

Normal Lymphocytes

38

Normal Radiograph   **Abnormal Radiograph**

5   13%   **33   87%**

Subsequent Improvement

21/33   64%

Irreversible changes and fibrotic contraction as well as impaired lung function has been found to be associated with higher neutrophil counts (13)(Fig 4) but this correlation is found after the event and is too late to be used as a predictive marker.

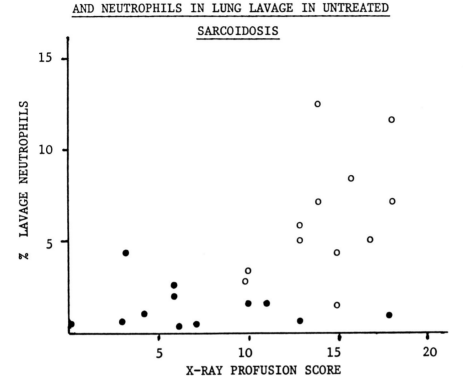

THE RELATION BETWEEN RADIOGRAPHIC PROFUSION SCORE
AND NEUTROPHILS IN LUNG LAVAGE IN UNTREATED
SARCOIDOSIS

With (o) and Without (●) Contraction

A maintained increase in Helper T cells has been identified in deteriorating patients whereas where there is a change towards suppressor T cells, patients remit spontaneously (14). However, again it must be recognised that there are a considerable number of patients with continuingly active disease who can be improved by steroid treatment but in whom lymphocyte counts in lavage fluid are entirely normal.(Fig 4) Whether markers of fibrogenesis such as procollagen peptides will prove to be a more useful predictive marker awaits further study. Thus currently the newer markers of activity have not proved to be sufficiently reliable to identify those cases which will fail to

628

resolve spontaneously and which will progress to architectural destruction of the lung. One of the central difficulties in this area is the fact that sarcoidosis can be highly active over limited periods of time and yet clear completely, whereas those cases destined to progress with more fibrosis may have a more insidious onset and evidence of 'activity' may be much less florid (15).

CONCLUSIONS

The reasons for divergent views on the management of pulmonary sarcoidosis are not hard to identify.(16)

The proof of the correctness of the policy of maintaining an optimally improved x-ray and lung function using steroids in asymptomatic patients remains lacking and because of this many patients are allowed to develop life threatening irreversible changes before treatment is attempted. A logical if unproven scheme is suggested as a feasible way of limiting the irreversible damage to the lung. Perhaps the onus should lie with those who do not subscribe to School II to justify their policy of withholding treatment in patients with persisting abnormal chest radiographs and who choose to deny their patients this potential protection.

REFERENCES

1. Munro CS, Campbell DA, Mitchell DN, DuBois RM, Cole PJ, Poulter LW. Lymphocyte and macrophage phenotypes in the lesions of sarcoidosis: are there two pathological processes? Thorax 1986; 41 231-232.

2. Crystal RG, Roberts WC, Hunning Lake GW, Gadek JE. Fulmer JD, Line BR. Pulmonary Sarcoidosis - a disease characterized and perpetuated by activated lung T Lymphocytes. Ann. Int.Med. 1981 94 73-94.

3. Lieberman J. A New confirmatory test for Sarcoidosis. Ann.Rev. Resp.Dis. 109: 743 1974

4. Line BR, Hunninghake GW, Keogh BA, Jones AE, Johnston GS, Crystal RG. 67 gallium scanning to stage alveolitis of sarcoidosis: correlation with clinical studies, pulmonary function studies and broncho alveolar lavage. Ann. Rev. Resp. Dis.(1981) 123 440-6.

5. Scadding JG, Mitchell DM. Sarcoidosis 1986. Second edition published by Eyre & Spottiswoode.

6.   Israel HL, Fonts DW, Beggs, RA. A controlled trial of prednisone
     treatment of sarcoidosis. Ann. Rev.Resp. Diseases 1973 **107** 609-

7.   Middleton WG, Douglas AC. Prolonged corticosteroid therapy in
     pulmonary sarcoidosis. Eighth International Conference on Sarcoidosis
     and other granulomatous disease. Ed. W Jones Williams; Brian H
     Davies 1980 632-647.

8.   Johns CJ, MacGregor MI, Zachary JB, Ball WC. Extended experience in
     the long term corticosteroid treatment of pulmonary sarcoidosis. Ann.
     NY Acad.Science 1976 **278** 722.

9.   Turner-Warwick M, McAllister W, Lawrence R, Britten A, Haslam PL.
     Corticosteroid treatment in pulmonary sarcoidosis. Do serial lavage
     lymphocyte counts, serum angiotensin converting enzyme measurements
     and ^{67}gallium scans help management? Thorax 1986 **41** 903 - 913.

10. Selroos O. (1987) Use of budesonide in the treatment of pulmonary
     sarcoidosis. Ellul-Micaleff R, Lam WK, Toogood JH (Eds) Advances in
     the use of inhaled corticosteroids. Excerpta Medica, Hong Kong, pp
     188-197

11. Morgan AM, Turner-Warwick M (1986) European Conference on
     Sarcoidosis and other Granulomatous Diseases. Vienna Ed Klech (in
     press)

12. Keogh B, Hunninghake GW, Crystal RG. Therapeutic decisions in
     sarcoidosis, prospective use of BAL and ^{67}gallium scanning. Ann.
     Review Respiratory Disorders 1980 **121** 151A.

13. Lin YH, Haslam PL, Turner-Warwick M. Chronic Pulmonary Sarcoidosis:
     relationship between lung lavage cell counts, chest radiograph and
     results of standard lung function tests. Thorax 1985 **40** 501-507.

14. Costabel U. European Conference on Sarcoidosis and other
     Granulomatous Diseases. Vienna Ed. Klech (in press)

15. James DG, Jones Williams W. Sarcoidosis and other Granulomatous
     Diseases. W B Saunders Co, London 1985

16. De Remee RA (1977). The present status of treatment of pulmonary
     sarcoidosis. A house divided. Chest **71** 388.

17. Hoyle C, Smyllie H, Leak D. Prolonged treatment of pulmonary
     sarcoidosis with corticosteroids. Thorax 1967 **22** 519.

REDUCING OSTEOPOROSIS IN CHRONIC LONG-TERM STEROID THERAPY: USEFULNESS OF
CALCITONIN

G.RIZZATO[1], G.TOSI[2], C.MELLA[3], L.MONTEMURRO[1], D.ZANNI[2], S.SISTI[3]
E. O. Niguarda, Milan, Italy. 1: Sarcoidosis Clinic; 2: Medical Physics Dept;
3: Radiology Dept.

ABSTRACT

Evaluating Bone Mineral Content (BMC) through computed tomography we have
shown (1) that osteoporosis is far more frequent than previously suspected in
chronic sarcoid patients treated with Prednisone (PD). Osteoporosis could perhaps be reduced associating Calcitonin. To evaluate this hypothesis, we have
studied BMC in 31 chronic sarcoid patients requiring steroids: 13 of them took
PD 14.3 $\pm$ 7.6 mg/ day per 15.5 $\pm$ 3.5 months, and 18 of them took equivalent
doses of other steroids per 12.1 $\pm$ 4.0 months. Four of 13 patients taking PD
and ten of 18 taking other steroids were given salmon Calcitonin (sCT), 100 U
i.m. injection daily for one month, then every two days for all the time of the
study. Thus in total we had 14 patients protected with sCT (per 12.36 $\pm$ 4.2
months) vs 17 unprotected. The two groups with and without sCT were matched for
age, sex and length of steroid therapy, while the initial BMC averaged 89.5 $\pm$
24.2 in the sCT group versus 121.4 $\pm$ 25.2 in the group without sCT (p<.005);
moreover sCT group was treated with around 30% lower doses of steroids. At the
end of the study we have calculated for each subject the mineral loss in percent of initial value (ML%): ML% averaged 13.4 $\pm$ 2.9 in the group without sCT
and -1.2 $\pm$ 3.9 in the sCT group (p<.01). In spite of the bias due to the different initial BMC and dose of steroids we think that sCT may be useful for reducing the risk of osteoporosis. In order to overcome the problems of compliance in long-term therapy with i.m. injections, we are presently evaluating the
usefulness of nasal spray sCT.

INTRODUCTION

In glucocorticoid-induced osteoporosis the histological study of trabecular
bone has revealed a reduction in bone formation probably due to a direct inhibition of osteoblastic function. Moreover glucocorticoids increase bone resorption probably through inhibition of intestinal calcium absorbtion with a secondary increase in parathyroid hormone secretion. Last but not least, Lo Cascio et
at (2) have shown a suppressive effect of chronic glucocorticoid treatment on
circulatory calcitonin. Using Quantitative Computed Tomography (QCT) of vertebral spongiosa in sarcoid patients treated with prednisone, we have observed

(1) that osteoporosis occurs in over 70% of long term prednisone treated sarcoid patients, a percentage far higher than previously reported (3). The delet-
erious effects of corticosteroids on trabecular bone can be diminished by simultaneous administration of calcitonin (4, 5). Aim of the work is to evaluate the
usefulness of salmon Calcitonin (sCT) in long term prednisone treated sarcoidosis.

MATERIAL AND METHODS

Vertebral Cancellous Mineral Content (VCMC, expressed in mg/cm^3 K_2HPO_4
eq) has been studied through QCT and calibration phantom as previously
described (1). The studied population included 31 patients with histologically
proven sarcoidosis, mostly chronic, all with active disease needing long term
therapy: age, sex, initial VCMC (before giving Calcitonin) are described in
Table 1. Mean age of the women was 56.2 ± 6.7 (sCT protected) vs 51.6 ± 10.0
(unprotected): the difference was not significant $(p > .05)$. Patients were
treated for over 1 year with prednisone or other steroids; 14 of them were
protected with sCT, 100 U i.m. injections daily for the first month and every
two days for all the time of the study. Dose of steroids given and duration of
therapy are presented in Table 2. VCMC was evaluated at the entry into the
study and over one year later. In each patient, the mineral loss at the end of
the study was expressed in percent of the initial value according to the formula

$$ML\% = (VCMC_{initial} - VCMC_{final}) \times 100 / VCMC_{initial}$$

TABLE 1

31 SARCOID PATIENTS NEEDING LONG TERM THERAPY

	No Calcitonin	Calcitonin	P
n	17	14	
Males	8	6	n.s.
Females	9	8	n.s.
(Postmenopausal Females)	(7)	(7)	n.s.
Age	43.59 ± 13.9	49.28 ± 10.5	n.s.
Initial VCMC	121.4 ± 25.2	89.50 ± 24.2	<.005
Months of therapy	14.5 ± 4.4	12.36 ± 4.2	n.s.
Prednisone	9	4	
Other steroids	8	10	

RESULTS

Results of single patients are expressed in Figure 1. Figure 2 shows ML % vs
time separately in the 14 patients protected with sCT and in the 17 unprotected

While no mineral loss was observed in patients protected with sCT a significant mineral loss was shown in the 17 unprotected patients and this difference is statistically significant (p<.01).

TABLE 2
DOSE OF STEROIDS*

	n	mg/day	Months of Therapy	Total Dose(g)	P
Prednisone	9	16.03 ± 8.4	15.88 ± 4.0	7.17 ± 3.2	n.s.
Prednisone+sCT	4	10.62 ± 4.5	14.75 ± 1.7	4.73 ± 2.2	
OS	8	15.40 ± 4.7	12.93 ± 4.6	5.97 ± 2.0	n.s.
OS + sCT	10	12.02 ± 5.9	11.40 ± 4.6	4.11 ± 2.5	

* for Other Steroids (OS) the equivalent Prednisone dose is given

DISCUSSION

  Two bias may be identified in our study:
1) Initial VCMC was lower in the group treated with sCT: further mineral loss is less likely in a population starting with lower VCMC and this difference could explain the different behaviour of the two populations of Figure 2.

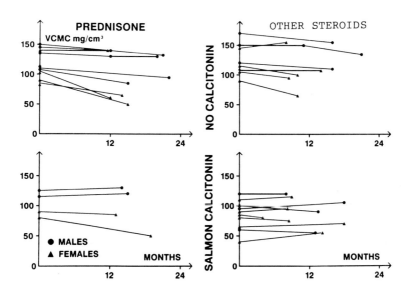

Figure 1. VCMC versus time in 4 steroid treated populations. Two groups were protected with sCT.

However taking into consideration a more homogeneous group of patients from Figure 1, i.e. only patients with initial VCMC between 80 and 120 mg/cm^3 (n=8 sCT protected, 9 unprotected), the same usefulness of sCT may be shown: ML% averaged -0.3 + 6.9 in sCT protected group and -20.1 + 13.0 in unprotected group (p<.005); these two populations were matched not only for age, sex, length and total dose of therapy, but also for initial VCMC (averaging 100.8 + 13.1 in sCT protected group versus 101.0 + 10.1 in unprotected, with p>.05).

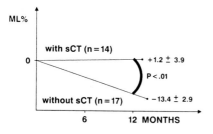

Figure 2. ML% vs time in two sarcoid populations both treated with steroids, one protected with sCT, one unprotected. Mean values (+ s.e.) of ML% are significantly different.

2) Another important point is the total dose of steroids: Table 2 shows that prednisone treated population took 4.73 + 2.2 g versus 7.17 + 3.2 in the population treated with prednisone plus calcitonin: even if the difference was not significant, sCT protected population took a dose of prednisone 34.03% lower in respect of unprotected population: similarly, in the population taking other steroids, the dose of steroid was 27.08% lower (difference again not significant).

Figure 2 shows that the corticosteroid induced osteoporosis no longer occurs in a population protected with sCT. The managing of glucocorticoid induced osteoporosis has received up to now only minor attention; morever a recent work suggests to avoid Vitamin D in this form of osteoporosis (6). Thus, in spite of the two above bias of our study, we conclude that sCT is useful and should be given to sarcoid patients with corticosteroid-induced osteoporosis. Similarly, Pasero et al (5), have concluded that Calcitonin appears the only practical help available at this time for patients with corticosteroid induced osteoporosis. Another important decision should be to give calcium-sparing deflazacort (7) and not prednisone. The problem of avoiding long-term i.m. injections could perhaps be resolved giving sCT nasal spray and we are presently evaluating the usefulness of this treatment.

REFERENCES

1. Rizzato G, Tosi G, Mella C, Zanni D, Sisti S, Loglisci T (1987):
   Researching Osteoporosis in Prednisone Treated Sarcoid Patients.
   Sarcoidosis 4: 45-48

2. Lo Cascio V, Adami S, Avioli LV, Cominacini L, Galvanini G, Gennari C,
   Imbimbo B, Scuro LA (1982): Suppressive Effect of Chronic Glucocorticoid
   Treatment on Circulating Calcitonin in Man. Calcif Tissue Int 34: 309-310

3. Baylink DJ (1983): Glucocorticoid-Induced Osteoporosis. New Engl J Med
   309: 306-308

4. Ringe JD, Steinhagen-Thiessen E (1985): Treatment of Corticosteroid-
   Induced Osteoporosis with Salmon Calcitonin. In: Second International
   Conference on Osteoporosis. Masson Italia, 1986

5. Pasero G, Gennari C, Di Munno O, Agnusdei D, Montagnani M (1985):
   Prevention of Glucocorticoid-Induced Osteopenia by Calcitonin in:
   Pecile A: Calcitonin 1984. Excerpta Medica, Amsterdam, 1985: 315-323

6. Schwartzmann MS, Franck W (1987): Vitamin D Toxicity Complicating the
   Treatment of Senile, Postmenopausal and Glucocorticoid-Induced
   Osteoporosis, Am J Med 82: 224-230

7. Avioli LV (1986): Concluding Remarks in: Avioli LV, Gennari C, Imbimbo B:
   Glucocorticoid Effects and their Biological Consequences: Advances in
   Glucocorticoid Therapy. Excerpta Medica, Amsterdam: 209-211

FURTHER EXPERIENCES WITH INHALED BUDESONIDE IN THE TREATMENT
OF PULMONARY SARCOIDOSIS

OLOF SELROOS

Mjölbolsta Hospital, SF-10350 Mjölbolsta (Finland), Department
of Chest Diseases, University Hospital, and Department of Clinical Research, AB Draco, P.O. Box 34, S-22100 Lund (Sweden)

INTRODUCTION

Systemic corticosteroids may cause side-effects. Inhaled bu-
budesonide, BUD, (600-1200 µg x 2) can replace oral steroids -
partly or totally - in patients with stage II-III pulmonary sarcoidosis and without causing side-effects (1-4). However, the
initial improvement is slower with BUD than with high dose
treatment with oral steroids (1). In order to improve the initial response we have tested a combination of BUD and oral steroids for the first 2-3 months but used only BUD for the maintenance treatment. The results have been compared to findings
obtained in an age and sex matched group of patients treated
with oral corticosteroids throughout.

MATERIAL AND METHODS

Patients

Group A. Ten sarcoidosis patients for the BUD part of the
study. They all had parenchymal lesions with or without enlargement of the hilar lymph nodes. They fulfilled criteria neces-
sitating treatment with corticosteroids: troublesome respiratory symptoms, impaired lung function (DL_{CO} <70% of predicted,
VC <75% of predicted and/or an abnormal pressure-volume curve),
or progressive or unchanged radiographic picture 6-12 months
after diagnosis. Nobody had earlier received corticosteroids.

Group B. Ten age and sex matched patients (historical controls) with a similar picture of pulmonary sarcoidosis and
treated only with oral steroids served as controls. They fulfilled the same criteria for starting treatment.

Table I shows data of the two groups. The spleen findings
represent positive fine-needle aspirations in patients without
splenomegaly.

TABLE I

Patient data at start of treatment

Group	n	Male/ Female	Age	(range)	Subj.resp. symptoms	Extrapulm.sarcoi- dosis diagnosed
A	10	4/6	44.3	(32-61)	6	4*
B	10	4/6	42.8	(27-63)	5	5**

*   skin (2), spleen (1), liver (1)

** URT and hypercalcaemia (1), spleen (2), uveitis (1), skin (1)

Treatment

Group A. Methylprednisolone 32 mg/d for 2 w, 16 mg/d for 2 w, 8 mg/d for 4-8 w and all the time together with BUD (Pulmicort^R, Spirocort^R) 1600 μg/d via a 750 ml spacer (Nebuhaler^R). Thereafter only BUD in individually adjusted doses, 800-1600 μg/d, up to 18 months.

Group B. Oral corticosteroids according to the clinical routine: usually prednisolone 40 mg/d for 2 w, 30 mg/d for 2 w, 20 mg/d for 4-8 w and thereafter tapering the dose to a maintenance dose of 7.5-10 mg/d. In some patients equivalent doses of methylprednisolone were used.

RESULTS

Drug therapy according to the original scheme

Group A. 6/10 patients were treated with BUD only during the maintenance phase. In 2 cases oral steroids were added at 6 and 12 months respectively and 2 patients received 3- and 4-month courses with oral drugs during the follow-up.

Group B. 5/10 patients were treated according to the plan. In the other 5 the dose had to be increased in various ways during the follow-up.

Chest radiographs

Table II shows the chest radiographic findings. Compared to the initial pictures the improvement rate was quite similar in the two groups. Clear radiographic deteriorations occurred in 4 cases in each group. Despite deteriorations no picture became worse than the initial radiographic finding.

TABLE II

Chest radiographic findings during the follow-up compared to
the initial findings in group A (n=10) and group B (n=10)

Radiographic state	Follow-up time in months							
	2-3		6		12		18	
	A	B	A	B	A	B	A	B
Unchanged	2	1	1	1	1	1	1	1
Slightly improved	5	7	2	3	3	4	1	2
Markedly improved	3	2	6	6	5	3	6	4
Normal	0	0	1	0	1	2	2	3

Vital capacity

Two patients per group had an initial VC <75%. At the first
follow-up a 5% mean increase was noted in both groups. On the
whole, the individual VC values seen at 3 months were maintained
up to 18 months.

Uptake of ^{67}Gallium in the lungs

The initial uptake was visibly increased in all 12 patients
tested. At follow-up the uptake in group A was unchanged in 3
and reduced in 5. In group B the corresponding figures were
1 and 3.

Serum ACE

The level of S-ACE mean values decreased in a similar fashion
in both groups. The decreases were statistically significant
compared to the starting values at all points in both groups
except the 6-month value in group A. No statistically significant differences were noted between the groups. The results are
shown in Table III.

TABLE III

Serum ACE mean values (range). Normal range 25-80 U/mL

Group	Initial value	Follow-up time in months			
		2-3	6	12	18
A	90.4 (46-124)	72.8 (46-112)	77.0 (54-93)	71.6 (49-96)	66.1 (51-82)
B	91.0 (38-115)	73.0 (42-93)	71.2 (40-98)	73.7 (46-89)	70.5 (53-86)

640

Plasma cortisol

Before therapy p-cortisol values were within the normal
range (190-700 nmol/L) in the 16 tested patients. At 3 months
a drop in p-cortisol >100 nmol/L (122-354) was seen in all but
2 patients. During the maintenance phase normal values were
seen in group A (n=10) except in one patient on a methylprednisolone (12 mg/d)-BUD (1600 µg/d) combination, whereas 4/10 patients in group B had abnormally low values.

Advese drug experiences

One BUD patient reported hoarseness. Candidiasis was not
found. Body weight and appearance remained normal in group A
whereas 2 group B patients became cushingoid, 3 developed skin
acne, 1 an abnormal glucose tolerance and 1 arterial hypertension.

DISCUSSION

A combination therapy of oral and inhaled steroids resulted
in an expected improvement within the first 3 months of treatment. In some patients BUD was enough for the maintenance
therapy. The overall results indicated equal efficacy with the
two treatment regimens. The highest BUD dose, 1600 µg/d, corresponds to 5 mg prednisolone from a systemic side-effect point
of view. It is therefore not surprising that fewer systemic
side-effects were seen in patients using BUD than in patients
on oral steroids. BUD in individually adjusted doses can be
used alone, or combined with a low dose of oral steroids for
the maintenance treatment of pulmonary sarcoidosis. BUD should
not be used for treatment of extrapulmonary lesions. The results are not applicable to other inhaled steroids because of
differences in lung pharmacokinetics and systemic potencies.

REFERENCES

1. Selroos OB (1986) Ann N Y Acad Sci 465:713-721
2. Selroos O (1987) In: Ellul-Micallef R, Lam WK, Toogood JH
    (eds) Advances in the use of inhaled corticosteroids. Ex-
    cerpta Medica, Hong Kong, pp 188-197
3. Selroos OB (1987) Amer Rev Respir Dis 135/2:A349
4. Morgan AD, Johnson MA, Kerr I, Turner-Warwick M (1987)
    Amer Rev Respir Dis 135/2:A349

© 1988 Elsevier Science Publishers B.V. (Biomedical Division)
Sarcoidosis and other granulomatous disorders
C. Grassi, G. Rizzato, E. Pozzi, editors

CORTICOSTEROID THERAPY OF PULMONARY SARCOIDOSIS (PS): EFFICACY AND TOLERABILITY OF
DEFLAZACORT (DFZ) vs PREDNISONE (PR).

G.VELLUTI*, O.CAPELLI*, L.AZZOLINI*, E.PRANDI*, A.FONTANA*, M.O.GUAGLIANONE**,
C.DRAGONETTI**.

*Cattedra e Divisione di Tisiologia e Malattie dell'Apparato Respiratorio. Uni-
versità di Modena - Italy   **Direzione Medica Gruppo Lepetit S.p.A. Milano Italy

INTRODUCTION

Deflazacort (DFZ), an oxazoline derivative of prednisolone, is a new synthetic
calcium-sparing and bone-saving corticosteroid agent, known to retain the same
anti-inflammatory activity of the parent compound (1). Aim of this pilot study
was to evaluate efficacy and tolerability of DFZ in comparison with those shown
by prednisone (PR) in the treatment of pulmonary sarcoidosis (PS).

MATERIAL AND METHODS

Twenty-one patients - 10 "fresh cases" (FC, because never treated before) and
11 retreated cases (RC) previously corticosteroid-treated - 12 males and 9 females, mean age 37 ± 2.3 (S.E.M.) yrs have been admitted to the study and randomly
treated with DFZ (10 pts) at mean daily dose of 16 ± 2.0 (S.E.M.) mg for a mean
period of 187 ± 21.9 (S.E.M.) days (FC:4 pts and RC:6 pts), or with PR (11 pts) at
mean daily dose of 15 ± 1.7 mg for a mean period of 237 ± 44.2 days (FC:6 pts and
RC:5 pts). The treatment scheme has been adjusted according to the initial clinical status, the therapeutic response and the drug tolerability. PS was initially
defined according to chest x-ray assessment at basal time and controlled during
treatment and between 3-12 months after the end of treatment.

In all 21 pts bronchoalveolar lavage (BAL) was performed before and between
3-12 months after treatment, to observe the modification in number of alveolar
cells, lymphocytes percentage and total proteins considered to be valid parameters for the evaluation of alveolitis severity (2,3,4). Moreover serum angiotensin converting enzyme (ACE) was also measured before and after therapy to com-.
plete the assessment of treatment's response.

Homogeneity between groups at the start of the study was statistically tested.
Between treatments (DFZ and PR) within group (FC and RC) comparison was performed

642

by means of Student's t test for unpaired samples (significant level $a = 0.05$).

RESULTS

The pulmonary radiological picture controlled between 3-12 months after treatment became normal in 3 out of 4 of the FC treated with DFZ and in all 6 cases
treated with PR. In the RC some improvement was observed in both groups of treat-
ment-pulmonary infiltrated area and hiliar lymph nodes were reduced of about 20-
30% - but without relevant differences among them. DFZ and PR have demonstrated
to be equally effective for the rapid improvement of the following symptoms:
cough, dispnoea, arthralgia, fever,asthenia and eritema nodosum, initially present with variable frequency in 20 out of 21 pts. As far as BAL and serum ACE are
concerned, DFZ and PR have shown to be equally active in reducing the number of
cells, percentage of lymphocytes, total proteins value and serum ACE level. Among
the RC 2 out of 5 cases in PR group and 3 out of 6 cases in DFZ group had a clinical relapse. Both treatments have been well tolerated, adverse events were mild
and more frequent with PR than with DFZ - PR:moon facies 6 cases, pyrosis 3,
C.N.S. 4, edema 2, acne 1, hypertension 1, hepatomegalia 1, menstrual disturbances
1; DFZ: moon facies 2, pyrosis 3, C.N.S. 2, acne 1, weight gain 1 - some pts have
more than one event.

DISCUSSION AND CONCLUSION

In spite of the small number of pts with acute and chronic PS treated in this
pilot study, DFZ has demonstrated to be endowed with a comparable efficacy regarding PR for the control of the symptoms, the improvement of the chest x-ray
picture, BAL finding and serum ACE.

Although this finding need to be confirmed in controlled studies with large
number of patients, it is reasonable to think that DFZ is an active and safe corticosteroid for the treatment of acute and chronic PS.

REFERENCES
1. Nagat C et al (1986) J.Bone Min.Res. (S-1):1
2. Velluti G et al (1983) Respiration 44:403-410
3. Velluti G et al (1984) Respiration 46:1-7
4. Thomas PD, Hunninghke GH (1987) Am Rev Respir Dis

STEROID AEROSOLS IN SYSTEMIC SARCOIDOSIS IN INDIA

SAMIR K GUPTA

Sarcoidosis Unit, The Calcutta Medical Research Institute and Institute for Respiratory Diseases, Calcutta.

INTRODUCTION

Since the introduction of steroid aerosols in India, these were in extensive use, mostly for the treatment of bronchial asthma[1]. Since these drugs have excellent local action, a comprehensive study was undertaken to see if these act well on cases of sarcoidosis in Indian subjects.

MATERIALS AND METHODS

During the past 10 years, steroid aerosols (mostly beclomethasone dipropionate, BDP) have been used in a dose of 800 - 1600 ug per day in two divided dosage to use as a substitute for oral steroids in sarcoidosis cases, who were not seriously ill.

None of the patient had less than 3 months treatment and most used aerosol between 6 months to 2 years continuously. Records of a total of 88 epidoses of treatment were available, when this report was compiled. 46 patients had initial oral steroids while 42 were treated with steroid aerosols.

Improvement was measured by lessening of signs and symptoms, lowering of ESR, improved VC and biochemical findings, lowering of SACE values and clearing of chest Xray. Good results indicated improvement in at least 4 of the parameters.

RESULTS

Steroid aerosols, on analysis (Table 1) appeared to be less effective than oral steroid to control most of the analysed parameters (29 episodes) and to be somewhat more useful in controlling pulmonary symptoms than in the previous group; even so it was less effective than oral steroid (13 episodes).

DISCUSSION

Steroid aerosol (BDP), in the dosage used, had very little systemic action. Hence it could not give much relief to the general condition and non-pulmonary systemic manifestations.

Oral steroids are cheaper, easier to administer, act faster and give a quick sense of well being. In comparison, aerosols are costlier, difficult to administer and cause problem to keep patients under supervision, act slower and often give unpleasant burning sensation in mouth. There was no incidence of 'thrush' in the oral cavity with BDP in Indian subjects, as compared to

644

West[1].

It is concluded that steroid aerosol cannot be a suitable substitute in multi-system diseases like sarcoidosis. Patients well controlled on oral steroid could, however, be weaned off to steroid aerosol in a few cases. Hasty withdrawals caused steroid-withdrawal symptoms in addition to features of relapse of sarcoidosis. In nearly one third, relapse occurred within 3 months of switching over to steroid aerosols.

TABLE I

COMPARATIVE STUDY OF ORAL/STEROID AEROSOL IN 88 EPISODES : ANALYSIS OF PARAMETERS

Parameters	CS*	L/S**	L.node	Joint	Skin	Eye	CXR***	Lungs
Oral Steroids	Good	Good	Poor	Good	Good	Poor	Good initially	Good
Steroid Aerosol N = 42	Poor	Poor	Poor	Poor	Poor	Poor	Poor	Poor, but symptoms, fairly controlled

*CS   = Constitutional symptoms.
**L/S = Liver spleen.
***CXR = Chest Xray.

REFERENCES

1. Gupta Samir K, Mitra K. The present status of steroid aerosol. J Assoc Phys India 33 : 720, 1985.

2. Gupta Samir K, Mitra K, Chatterjee, S, Chakravarty SC. Sarcoidosis in India. Br J Dis Chest 79 : 275, 1985.

3. Brogden R. Factors which may affect the response to inhaled steroids. In : Steroids in Asthma : A reappraisal in the light of inhalation therapy, Auckland,ADIS press p 154, 1983.

SPARING HOSPITALIZATIONS AND STEROIDS: THE ROLE OF A SARCOIDOSIS CLINIC IN ITALY

LIDIA MONTEMURRO* FERNANDO DURANTE, LUCIA CASTRIGNANO, TERESA LOGLISCI
Sarcoidosis Clinic, E.O. Niguarda, Milan, Italy

INTRODUCTION

Hospitalization is a source of high costs for Public Administration. In 1986 Braham et al (1) have shown that 50% of the inpatients of the New York Hospital-Cornell Medical Center were previously enrolled in the clinic system.With this in mind,we analysed all the charts of the patients seen in our Sarcoidosis Clinic during last years in order to detect if something like that occurs also in our Hospital.Moreover our epidemiological study is concerning geographic provenience of our patients and therapy given.

MATERIAL AND METHODS

In the period January 1,1979 to March 31,1986 we have seen 444 patients,but it has been possible to recover and study only the charts of 332 of them. 262 (over 332) had a histologically proven sarcoidosis, the other 70 had a clinical diagnosis of very likely sarcoidosis.In this population biopsy had been refused or considered too at risk. Data concerning geographic provenience and steroid treatment have been reviewed in all the 332 patients. In 175 of them, seen in the period January 83-March 86, we have also collected data about admission to Hospital and mean length of hospitalization. Steroid therapy was given in our Clinic according to our protocol (2), in brief evaluating sarcoid activity and functional impairment and treating only patients with functional impairment plus clinical activity.

RESULTS

1. Geographic provenience

77% of our patients came from Lombardia (our region), the other 23% came from the other italian regions. (Fig. 1)

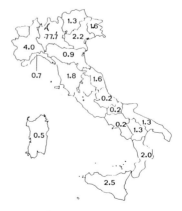

Fig. 1. Geographic provenience of our
        patients (in percentage)

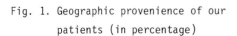

* Milan prize winner for authors under 35 years.

2. Hospitalizations

Table 1 shows that admissions to Niguarda Hospital have been 21 versus 129 elsewhere.Mean length of stay at Niguarda was 12.4+6.3 days versus 36.9+15.8 days in other Hospitals.

TABLE 1

SARCOID HOSPITALIZATIONS: JANUARY 1983 TO MARCH 1986.

Patients	175		
- Outpatients	25		
- Admitted to hospital	150	Niguarda Hospital	21
		Other Hospitals	129
Mean length of stay (days)		Niguarda	12.4+ 6.3
		Other Hospitals	36.9+15.8

3. Therapeutic decisions

Table 2 shows the therapeutic decisions.We have given therapy to 144(43.4%)of 332 sarcoid patients in our centre and on the basis of our protocol we should have treated only 48 of the 111 patients treated elsewhere.

TABLE 2

THERAPEUTIC DECISIONS:JANUARY 1979 TO MARCH 1986

1. Therapy given to 144/332 patients (43.4%) in our centre
2. Patients treated elsewhere before reaching our centre: 111
   Our decision had been to treat 48 of them only (43.2%)

DISCUSSION

In the period January 83-March 86 sarcoid hospitalizations have been 150 (Tab.1)but 21 of them only to our Hospital;the other 129 patients have been admitted elsewhere nearly always before reaching our centre and were sent us when the diagnosis of sarcoidosis was proven.Furthermore:the two groups were matched for age,sex and initial Chest X ray stage,however mean length of stay at Niguarda Hospital was lower than in other Hospitals(12.4+6.3 days vs 36.9+15.8). The elsewhere longer period is due in most cases to the pre-biopsy work-up that we carry out on outpatients(versus inpatients elsewhere).Thus -first conclusion- Sarcoidosis Clinic appears a strong tool permitting to avoid unnecessary hospi- talizations in Italy.

TABLE 3
SPARING MONEY*

1. REDUCING THE LENGTH OF STAY IN HOSPITAL
   - Difference Niguarda/Other Hospitals: 24.5 days per patient
   - 24.5 days x 21 patients admitted = 514.5 days (total days in 39 month)
   - Days / 12 months: 158.3
   - Money saved / year: 45,907,000 Italian Liras
2. AVOIDING UNNECESSARY HOSPITALIZATIONS
   - (175 patients x 30% x 36.9 days) = 173,000,000 Italian Liras/year
3. TOTAL
   1 + 2 = 218,907,000 Italian Liras/year

---

* Estimated Cost of 1 hospitalization day = 290,000 Italian Liras

Table 3 shows that we spare 24.5 days per patient, that means 45,907,000 Italian Liras per year. This is only a rough underestimation of the real advantage because we have also avoided to admit to hospital a wide number of patients (probably around 30%); so the total saving is about 219 millions/year(Table 3). Furthermore: if simply the other Hospitals had limited the admissions to 12.4 days instead of 36.9, a further saving of 129 x 24.5 x 290,000 = 916,545,000 Italian Liras had been obtained over 39 months, that means 282,013,000 Italian Liras/year. But again this is an underestimation because many patients were admitted elsewhere without a steady indication. We were not prepared to analyse in detail the problem of the costs, that began to emerge, with our surprise, only when data were on the Table. We will analyse better this problem in a further step of our study.

111 patients had been treated elsewhere before reaching our Centre and in most cases we tapered that therapy, because unnecessary. We also reviewed the reasons why therapy was given elsewhere and on the basis of our protocol we have drawn the conclusion that our decision had been to treat 48 of them only. Thus-second conclusion - steroid therapy in Italy is given to many patients without a steady indication.

ACKNOWLEDGEMENTS
We thank Prof. G. Rizzato for permitting this study on his patients and for his useful suggestions.

REFERENCES
1. R.L. Braham et al. (1986). Closing the Clinics? Am J Med. 80: 71-76
2. G. Rizzato (1987) Sarcoidosis, R. Rakel:Conn's Current Therapy. WB Saunders: Philadelphia, 157-159.

THERAPEUTIC TRIAL OF PULMONARY SARCOIDOSIS WITH SULFATHIAZOLE: A POSSIBLE ETIOTROPIC TREATMENT

A.GIOBBI, G.MARTIGNONI, E.MIRADOLI

Institute for Social Respiratory Diaseases - Community Health Services of Milan

Introduction

According to the hypothesis of a mycobacterial etiology of sarcoidosis, we started to treat the new cases of pulmonary sarcoidosis (PS), detected in our institute from 1985, with a drug with some anti-mycobacterial activity, but usually not included in TB treatments. We opted for Sulfathiazole at the daily dosage of 50 mg/Kg in three separate administrations, for a period of three months.

Patients

Since then, we have been observing 40 patients, at different stages:
-   29 patients at first stage, with bilateral hilar limphadenopaty (BHL);
-   7 patients at second stage, with pulmonary infiltrations;
-   4 patients at third stage, with pulmonary fibrosis

Ten cases out of 40 (25%) didn't enter the study because of refusal or spontaneous interruption of the trial.

As a control group we used the 60 cases of PS detected in our institute in the period of time immediately preceding the start of the therapeutic trial.

The two groups were comparable as for sex, mean age and staging.

Results

As far as clinico-radiologic features are concerned, the effectiveness of a drug, expecially in a short follow-up, must be evaluated upon the number of patients showing a regression of radiologic findings and upon the regression time.

In this respect, we compared the group A (treated patients) and the group B (untreated patients). Group A showed a complete regression of radiologic features in 25 patients (83.3%), while group B showed this result only in 28 cases (46.7%). Five cases were unchanged in group A (16.4%), and 29 in group B (48.3%). Moreover, no patients showed a progression of the disease in the treated group, against 3 (5%) in the control group.

Among the 25 recovered cases from group A, radiologic findings completely disappeared within 3 months in 18 patients (72%), while after the three month observation only 4 cases (14%) out of 28 recovered from group B showed a complete regression.

Differences are statistically significant in both observations
($P < 0.001$).

Conclusions

The results of this trial show the effectiveness of Sulfathiazole in the treatment of Sarcoidosis.

This seems even more supported by the lack of reappearances of lesions, as usually observed straight after the break of the corticosteroid treatments in the recovered patients, particularly in the short term.

Therefore the therapeutic efficacy of Sulfathiazole looks to be owed to a mechanism different from the usual anti-inflammatory and temporary action of corticosteroids. It is reasonable to think that Sulfathiazole works directly against the pathogenic agent, because of the speed of action and the recovery stability.

EFFECT OF TREATMENT OF SARCOIDOSIS IN INDIA

SAMIR K GUPTA, SUBIR K DUTTA, KOUSHIK MITRA, MANOJ ROY

Sarcoidosis Clinic, The Calcutta Medical Research Institute and Institute for Respiratory Diseases, Calcutta

In the Western World, controversy rages[1] as to whether treatment should be given to asymptomatic bulk of cases with hilar adenopathy (stage-I disease). The situation faced by sarcoidologists in India is quite different. In the absence of MMR surveys almost all the diagnosed patients are symptomatic when they seek medical help, and treatment is mandatory[2]. The present paper deals with the effect of treatment in 124 cases of biopsy proven sarcoidosis, observed between 1-15 years, following diagnosis.

MATERIAL AND METHODS

A total of 314 courses of treatment was analysed - these include the initial treatment and treatment of relapses. Indications for treatment were standard recommendations.[2,3]

Either steroids (S) or non-steroidal drugs (NS) were used during treatment. No case received less than 3 months treatment and most cases had 6 months - 2 years with probing interruptions, after 6-12 months.

Steroid used was usually prednisolone in the dose of 0.3-0.6 mg/kg/day. Non-steroidal drugs, used in pairs, were either a) chloroquin phosphate (250 mg with a chloroquin base of 155 mg), thrice daily; b) Oxyphenbutazone 100 mg, thrice daily or c) N-phthalyl anthranilic acid, 400 mg thrice daily.

In addition most NS patients received later beclomethasone dipropionate, a locally acting steroid aerosol in the dosage of 400-1600 ug daily, when pulmonary symptoms were also present.[4]

The parameters of good improvement has been described elsewhere.[4]

RESULTS

Steroid showed better response than NS drugs in reducing constitutional symptoms, hepatosplenomegaly, arthralgia, cardiac, skin and eye lesions, SACE and lung - changes (in the latter condition, NS also caused good relief). Lymphadenopathy had poor response to both S or NS drugs.

DISCUSSION

Most of the general or constitutional symptoms responded much quicker to steroids than to NS drugs. However, skin manifestations like maculo - papular lesion, lupus pernio or erythema induratum, subcutaneous nodules etc. responded equally and extremely well to NS drugs. Pruritus was controlled better by steroids.

652

Initial satisfactory results in both groups were temporary. Radiological clearing in chest was slow and progressive fibrosis gradually appeared in most cases, whether treated with S or NS. Unlike in the West, most of the hilar adenopathy cases i.e. Stage I disease progressed to Stage II or III. Pulmonary streaky shadows rarely showed complete clearing in either group[5]. SACE showed a more rapid fall on steroidal drugs. Several biochemical abnormalities like hypergammaglobulinaemia, hypercalcaemia tended to relapse or at times did not respond well to treatment.

TABLE I

RESULTS, FOLLOWING   TREATMENT WITH STEROID/NON-STEROIDAL DRUGS IN SARCOIDOSIS

Clinical features		Good results (S)	Good results (NS)
CS*	(291)	79% (130)	41% (161)
Pulmonary	(287)	86% (123)	37% (164)
Liver/spleen	(126)	48% (66)	23% (60)
Cardiac	(48)	69% (48)	not used
Skin	(67)	71% (33)	78% (34)
CXR**	(296)	58% (130)	29% (166)
SACE	(237)	64% (148)	38% (89)
Pulmonary function	(273)	30% (140)	21% (133)

*CS   = Constitutional symptoms
**CXR = Chest Xray
S   = Steroids
NS   = Non-steroids

REFERENCES

1. DeRemee RA. The present status of treatment of pulmonary sarcoidosis : a house divided. Chest 1977, 71 ; 388-392.

2. James DG, Jones William W.Sarcoidosis & Other Granulomatous Disorders,London, WB Saunders, 1985, 222-232.

3. Gupta Samir K, Mitra K, Chatterjee, S, Chakravarty SC. Sarcoidosis in India. Br J Dis Chest 1985 : 79, 275-283

4. Gupta Samir K. Steroid aerosols in systemic sarcoidosis in India : In : Proceedings of the 11th International Conference on Sarcoidosis, Milan, in press.

5. Gupta Samir K, Sharma Surendra K.Radiological pulmonary changes in sarcoidosis : a modification of International staging system. In : Proceedings of the 11th International Conference on Sarcoidosis, Milan, in press.

THE ORALLY ACTIVE ANGIOTENSIN-CONVERTING ENZYME INHIBITORS IN SARCOIDOSIS

S.PANAYEAS[1], A.MICHALOPOULOS[2], C.TSIROYIANNIS[3], A.PAPAPASCHALI[4],
N.SIAFAKAS[3], S.PAPADOPOULOS[1]
a: SOCIAL SECURITY FOUNDATION: Subdivision of Athens, Greece:
 1:Pathology Dept; 2:Out patients Dept of Cardiology;
b: EVANGELISMOS Hospital, Athens, Greece:
 3:Diseases of the Chest Dept; 4:Lab. of Biochemistry

SUMMARY

The effect of an ACE inhibitor in active and inactive sarcoidosis has been studied in comparison with control subjects not receiving the drug. The evaluation was based on complete clinical and laboratory examination of each patient including also determination of ACE values as an index indicating activation of the disease.

It was found that oral treatment of few months with 50 mg of Captopril daily can reduce or normalize the high blood pressure (a positive sign of activation of sarcoidosis) and improve or eliminate subjective complaints in patients with active sarcoidosis not accompanied with hypertension. It can also improve or normalize some laboratory parameters including ACE in patients with active sarcoidosis. No significant side effects were observed during the treatment period of 6 months although longer periods of observation involving also patients with more serious forms of sarcoidosis (lupus pernio, cardiac, renal, occular and C.N.S. localization of the disease) are necessary to establish such a treatment.-

KEY-WORDS: ACE-inhibitors, Captopril, Blood pressure, Sarcoidosis.

INTRODUCTION

Cumulated data from International bibliography indicate that a high percentage (up to 85%) of patients with active sarcoidosis have increased values of ACE in body fluids or secretions (SACE, TACE, LACE, Salivary or Spleen ACE) as compared with a low percentage (10%) with increased values found in inactive disease.

Based on the above observations we have studied in our patients the effect of an ACE inhibitor and the results were recorded not only for hypertension but also for the remaining manifestations and parameters of sarcoidosis.-

MATERIALS AND METHODS

A total of 2I patients with sarcoidosis and 4 normal controls
participated in the study. Most of the patients had well documented systemic sarcoidosis recorded previously in the files of the
Department of Pathology of Greek Social Security Foundation, Subdivision of Athens. The remaining patients came to the out patient's Department of the above Organization complaining for crises
of arterial hypertension or showing other signs and symptoms relative to the unknown-underlying sarcoidosis.

Table I shows the classification of patients and controls in
groups and subgroups.

TABLE I
THE GROUPS AND SUBGROUPS OF SUBJECTS

	A	B	C	D	T o t a l
a	6	3	3	2	I4
b	3	3	3	2	II
T o t a l	9	6	6	4	25

A: Patients with hypertension and active sarcoidosis.
B: "   without   "   but with   "   "
C: "   "   "   with inactive   "
D: Normal Controls (from the same social environment).
a: Subjects receiving the drug and
b: "   not   "   "   "

In I2 patients with sarcoidosis and 2 normal controls who received
Captopril the dose of the drug was 25 mg b.i.d. for 3-6 months.

All subjects had a complete clinical and laboratory examination
before during and after the treatment period.

RESULTS

In all patients with active sarcoidosis and hypertension (group
Aa) the blood pressure was normalized within 6 months of therapy.

In addition a great percentage of patients had a substantial
improvement of the signs and symptoms of active disease inclunding
also some laboratory haematological or biochemical abnormalities
and the values of ACE in the serum.

Similar improvement was also noticed in biochemical and enzymatic parameters of group Ba patients after treatment. while no
change or deterioration was noticed in groups Ca and Da.-

The effectiveness of the drug and the improvement of ACE-activity (months of Captopril therapy / mean values of ACE in the serum) is indicated by Table II.

TABLE II
MONTHS OF CAPTOPRIL / EFFECT ON SACE

	Aa	Ab	Ba	Bb	Ca	Cb	Da	Db	M e a n s
Drug	4.3	–	5	–	3	–	3	–	4
SACE	II.9	I4.I3	I2.2	I4	8.26	9.26	8.2	I0.5	II

Method of assay of SACE-LIBERMAN /Normal values $I0^{\pm}5$ ($\male$), $8^{\pm}4$ ($\female$).

DISCUSSION

From the literature seems that no proper attention has been given to hypertension as an expression of activation of sarcoidosis and not either in the exclusive use of ACE-inhibitors, like Captopril, as a treatment of choice in patients with this condition.

The improvement of patient's subjective complaints, accompanied by a feeling of good health, the reduction of SACE values, the normalization of blood pressure and of preexisting haematological and biochemical abnormalities, strongly suggest a pathogenetic relationship between hypertension and preexisting inactive sarcoidosis.-

CONCLUSION

Based on the results of our study and the possibility of deterioration of arterial hypertension in patients with active sarcoidosis we consider ACE-inhibitors as the drugs of choice for the treatment of at least the hypertensive crises, seen in these patients.

Although the number of patients in our study is relatively small there is also evidence for the improvement of other clinical and laboratory parameters of the active disease.-

ACKNOWLEDGEMENTS

We wish to thank Squibb Pharmaceutical Co. for kindly providing Capoten (Captopril) and for financial support for this study.-

REFERENCES
I. Mizuno K. et al (I983): Tohoku J. Exp. Med.; I40 / I (I07-I08)
2. Ueda T. et al (I983): Proc. 9th Internat. Conf. Sarcoidosis. Paris, Pergamon Press, p 475.-

© 1988 Elsevier Science Publishers B.V. (Biomedical Division)
Sarcoidosis and other granulomatous disorders
C. Grassi, G. Rizzato, E. Pozzi, editors

THE TREATMENT OF SARCOIDOSIS   OUTLOOK

RAMIRO ÁVILA

Departamento de Pneumologia, Faculdade de Ciencias Médicas, Hospital de Pulido
Valente, 1700 Lisboa

I would like to invite you for a short trip through what has been said during
this session with the aim of taking some ideas and conclusions for further
investigations in this field.

In fact the three questions one can raise after Professor Turner Warwick's
Conference are why, when and how to treat Sarcoidosis and I think we do not yet
have a definitive answer.

We do not yet have the ability to predict which patients will improve
spontaneously and which will develop fibrosis. So, for many, like Dr. Gupta,
treatment must be given with the aim of preventing irreversible lesions
regardless of the presence or absence of symptoms. For others, treatment does not
alter the course of the disease but it is helpful in alleviating symptoms.

To give you an idea of what has been said I would like to show some of the
results of an epidemiological survey we performed and which will support our
doubts.

We studied 274 cases of sarcoidosis (125 males and 149 females) being 267
Caucasians, 6 Africans and 1 Indian, with a mean age of 35 years (range 10-75
years). Eighty-five were non-smokers and 15% smokers. Fourteen percent were
detected by routine X-ray, 35% presented with respiratory symptoms, 26% with
systemic, 26% with dermatological and 23% with bone and joint complaints. Forty-
one percent were in Stage I, 31% in Stage II, 15% had no respiratory
manifestations and 14% were in Stage III.

With respect to lung function tests it is important to stress that 20% had a
restrictive defect and 6% an obstructive one. Ten percent had a combined defect.
DCO was low in 38% of the cases and 62% also had a low static compliance. Sixty-
seven percent of the patients were treated with only corticosteroids.

As far as the evolution of the disease was concerned there was no significant
difference irrespective of whether the patients had been subjected to treatment
or not.

These results once again leave us without a firm answer to the first question
- Why to treat Sarcoidosis. However, the results obtained by Dr. Hosoda and
co-workers and shown in a Poster, will, perhaps, in the near future, give us a
definitive answer to this question.

Regarding the methods used for assessing activity and the need for therapy,
although during this Congress many approaches have been presented, clinical

symptoms, chest-X-ray and lung function tests are still the most commonly employed techniques for taking a decision about treatment.

Various drugs have been used in the treatment of Sarcoidosis. During this session many important papers have been presented on this subject and I would like to stress the importance of corticosteroids.

As we said before, we look forward to the results from the International Controlled Clinical Trial on Prednisone Therapy in Pulmonary Sarcoidosis, bearing however, in mind the idea given by Dr. Velluti and co-workers of using Deflazacort and of Drs Selroos and Gupta and co-workers, of using inhaled Budesonide. The effect of new drugs, like orally active angiotensin converting enzyme inhibitors of Dutinulan 8-15 or, even, Sulphathiazole, must be extensively studied and we hope that the authors of the Posters on this subject will continue with their studies in order to give us additional results. Bearing in mind the side effects of corticosteroids it seems important to stress the results obtained by Dr. Rizzato and co-workers not only on giving Calcitonin to their patients, but also, as said before, Deflazacort. The same applies to the use of Budesonide.

On the other hand, I would like to draw your attention to the Poster of Dr. Loglisci and co-workers on avoiding hospitalization and steroids.

With regards to the starting dose, maintenance dose, schedule of administration (daily, alternate-day, single or divided) and duration of treatment with corticosteroids (3, 6, 12, 18 months; guided by indices of activity; until remission; variable), in fact we once again, hope that the International Controlled Clinical Trial on Prednisone Therapy in Pulmonary Sarcoidosis of Dr. Hosoda and co-workers will give some answer to this question.

Finally, I would like to draw your attention to the results presented by Professor Turner-Warwick concerning the methods of assessing the response to therapy and stress the point that the new methods are not more sensitive than serial Chest-X-rays and lung function tests.

To conclude, I would like to say that this Session has been very interesting and important but our trip must continue until the moment we have a precise criteria for the treatment of Sarcoidosis and ideal methods for alleviating the symptoms of our patients.

OTHER GRANULOMATOUS DISORDERS

© 1988 Elsevier Science Publishers B.V. (Biomedical Division)
Sarcoidosis and other granulomatous disorders
C. Grassi, G. Rizzato, E. Pozzi, editors

661

GRANULOMAS IN THE DIAGNOSIS OF SARCOIDOSIS. STATE OF THE ART

W JONES WILLIAMS

University of Wales College of Medicine, Pathology Department, Llandough
Hospital, Penarth, South Glamorgan, (United Kingdom)

The finding of multisystem epithelioid cell granulomas for pathologists and
should be for clinicians,is a mandatory criterion for the diagnosis of
sarcoidosis[1]. Academically it is easy for the pathologist to demand
biopsies from all possible sites, but for the clinician this is often
impractical. I feel that at least one site requires biopsy proof and would
accept that clinical involvement of other systems or organs would then
suffice. This was one of the advantages of the Kveim Siltzbach test which
though not now as widely used, did provide confirmatory evidence.

Dependant on the clinical findings, we must therefore consider all possible
biopsy sites. Though the differential diagnosis may vary with the affected
site and organs, theoretically all possible known causes of sarcoid
granulomas must be excluded. It is not enough to send tissue in formalin;
whenever possible all biopsy material requires culturing, especially for
Mycobacteria tuberculosis. Recent advances in immunological markers though
not yet of diagnostic value, may become so and require preservation of frozen
material. Electron microscopy may also be required.

Before discussing the differential diagnosis of granulomas in sarcoidosis,
their nature must be defined. The granulomas consist of focal aggregates of
pale staining (Eosin positive) modified macrophages - epithelioid cells.
These often fuse to form characteristically Langhans' (tuberculous) and
sometimes foreign body type giant cells. Interspersed between and around the
epithelioid cells are lymphocytes, now identified as predominantly central T
helper cells and peripheral T suppressor cells. B lymphocytes and
eosinophils are not a feature. Central necrosis and caseation is usually
absent or rarely may be present to a minimal extent. With ageing the
granulomas are infiltrated with fibroblasts with deposition of reticulin and
collagen. Care must be taken to distinguish denatured 'hyalinised' collagen
from necrosis. Of particular interest is that though the granulomas may
aggregate into larger masses, they maintain their individuality as distinct
from tuberculosis when fusion takes place, particularly around caseation.
Intra-cellular inclusion bodies may be found, particularly in old lesions,
including Schaumann, asteroid and Hamazaki-Wesenburg bodies. Though not

diagnostic of sarcoidosis the presence of Schaumann bodies in focal scars are a marker of preceeding granulomas.

LUNG

In the majority of patients with sarcoidosis the main site of involvement is within the chest (88%) [2] with hilar lymphadenopathy and/or pulmonary involvement. How then can we obtain material from the chest for histology? Mediastinoscopy is the best method for obtaining ample material but is now less popular and superceded by the less invasive techniques of fibro-optic bronchoscopy. For the histologists, transbronchial biopsies suffer from the severe limitation of specimen size which can partly be offset by sampling as many areas as possible. The technique has certainly shown that the bronchial involvement is far more common than previously thought. Direct needle lung biopsy (Nordenstrom) is seldom of value in sarcoidosis as very few cases show nodules large enough for radiographic identification. Here, we are not concerned with bronchoalveolar lavage as it does not provide tissue and its diagnositc value is still not fully established.

Infections. As with any other organ tuberculosis is in the forefront, in particular miliary tuberculosis, hence the importance of culturing all specimens. Depending on locality other infections, particularly fungi such as histoplasmosis and aspergillosis must be identified. Granulomas in histoplasmosis may mimic tuberculosis and sarcoidosis but the organism is readily identifiable by silver stains as rounded basophilic double countered bodies of nuclear size, particularly found in giant cells. Histoplasmosis can occur outside endemic areas such as the US Mid West and the first case recorded in Britain [3] affected cervical lymph nodes, in a patient a year after complete recovery from sarcoidosis! We have recently seen an interesting example in Cardiff.

Case Report - Histoplasmosis. A 37 year old Asian male who had moved from Kenya to the UK 15 years previously, presented with signs and symptoms of diabetes. He was found to have hepatomegaly with a normal chest x-ray. Liver biopsies showed portal tract inflammation with poorly formed granulomas but no identifiable organisms. He left hospital against advice and without a definitive diagnosis though tuberculosis and sarcoidosis were considered. Six months later he collapsed and died at home following a short flu like illness.

At autopsy the lungs and hilar glands appeared normal and
the only abnormalities were bilateral caseous destruction of
both adrenals with one calcified liver nodule. Microscopy
showed several loose granulomas in the lung and portal tracts
but with no identifiable organisms. The adrenals showed
extensive necrosis with macrophages containing Histoplasma
capsulatum (Fig. 1).

The case illustrates the difficulties of identifying
causative organisms in granulomas. Histoplasma were very few
and only found in the adrenals.

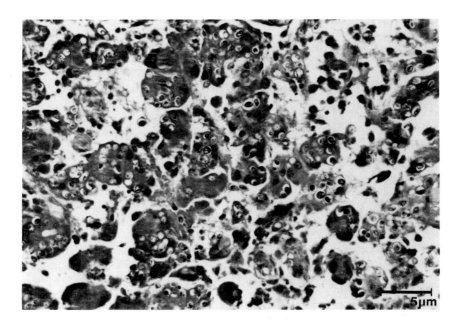

Fig. 1. Loose macrophage foci containing Histoplasma Dubosii.

Invasive Aspergillosis, usually seen in severely immunosuppressed patients as a fulminent terminal infection, results in diffuse and focal pneumonitis, often affecting normal lung. The usual histological features include numerous eosinophils, necrosis and easily identified fungi, often with vascular invasion and widespread dissemination. Rarely it is associated with granulomas.

It is important to recognise Bronchocentric Granulomatosis (BCG) as a separate entity from sarcoidosis. The disease is nearly always confined to the lungs but has been reported to co-exist with systemic diseases, such as rheumatoid arthritis [4]. The disease is characterised by necrotising rheumatoid like granulomas centred on the bronchiole commonly caused by aspergillosis. In some cases fungi cannot be found, so the granulomas may be a reaction to other chronic intraluminal inflammatory agents associated with bronchial obstruction. This would explain those cases with asthma, precipitins and eosinophilia from those without these stigmata [5].

Vasculidities. The rare entity of Necrotising Sarcoidal Granulomatosis (NSG) though sometimes difficult to distinguish from sarcoidosis [6] is identified by necrotising granulomas centred on blood vessels. Extra-pulmonary involvement is extremely rare. Occasionally NSG may however be difficult to separate from localised Wegener's Granulomatosis (WG). The features of WG are easily distinguished from sarcoidosis as focal granulomas are exceptional. The lesions show extensive necrosis, mainly centred on blood vessels and consist of a mixture of macrophages with peculiar (Wegner's) giant cells often with polymorphs and plasma cells. Similarly Churg and Strauss granulomatosis (CSG) is identified by extensive eosinophilic infiltration, centred on vessels with only loose collections of macrophages and absent granulomas.

Metal Lung Disease. Despite its rarity, chronic beryllium disease is a continuing threat to exposed workers particularly in the metal industry. The granulomas are identical to those of sarcoidosis but the accompanying alveolitis is far more conspicuous. Histochemical identification of beryllium in the tissue sections is of little value and bulk tissue analysis is often unsatisfactory due to limited amount of available tissue. The recent development of laser mass spectrometry analysis on tissue sections is of diagnostic value as beryllium is not present in normal lung or in the granulomas of sarcoidosis[7]. 'In vitro' beryllium induced lymphocyte transformation is also of diagnostic value, as it is seldom positive in beryllium workers without disease and negative in sarcoidosis[8].

It has recently been confirmed that inhalation of Titanium can result in sarcoid like granulomas of the lung[9]. It can be distinguished from sarcoidosis by the identification of contained Titanium particles using x-ray (EDAX) or laser (LAMMS) analysis. It was previously suggested[10] and recently confirmed that these patients also show in vitro lymphocyte transformation to Titanium and hence hypersensitivity[9]. It is surprising that the entity has not been more often recognised as titanium is so widely used in various alloys.

Aluminium has long been recognised as a cause of pulmonary fibrosis in bauxite smelters (Shaver's disease). Recently a case of Aluminium granulomatosis has been described in a patient exposed to Aluminium oxide powder. As well as identifying Aluminium in the lesion by EDAX analysis (confirmed by LAMMS with exclusion of Be) both peripheral blood and lavage lymphocytes showed in vitro transformation. Of further interest was the excess of T helper cells in broncholavage specimens, therefore closely mimics sarcoidosis and might be used as an experimental model[11].

Dental technicians may be exposed to a large variety of metals, in particular cobalt - chromium alloys, Beryllium, Titanium, Nickel, Silica and others. The resulting interstitial fibrosis and occasional silicotic like lesions are distinguishable from sarcoidosis but focal macrophage aggregates may be a source of confusion. The diagnosis may be established by x-ray analysis (EDAX) of the contained particles while the LAMMS technique will in addition detect Beryllium[12].

Extrinsic Allergic Alveolitis. Though long recognised as a granulomatous disease induced by inhaled allergens e.g., Farmer's lung disease, from inhalation of fungi from mouldy hay, an increasing number of other causes are now recognised. These range from protozoa in air conditioner lung, to penicillin in cheese washer's lung[13]. All are characterised in the acute disease by classical sarcoid like granulomas with prominent alveolitis. The diagnosis requires a history of exposure and the finding of circulating precipitins to the causative antigen. The histological diagnosis may be suspected by recognising the peribronchial distribution of the granulomas.

Miscellaneous. Pulmonary Talc Granulomatosis may result from intravenous drug abuse, using crushed tablets containing talc, and closely mimic sarcoidosis including raised SACE, lavage lymphocyte counts, positive Gallium scans and nodular radiological lesions[14]. However the histological diagnosis is made obvious by the finding of birefringent talc cystals within non-caseating granulomas. Occasionally the disease follows talc inhalation as seen in a local "deranged" sufferer from rheumatoid arthritis who thought the cure was talc baths, using 10 packs a day!

Exogenous lipid pneumonia may result from inhalation of oily droplets from nasal spray or from accidental inhalation in habitual liquid paraffin takers.

The resulting reaction shows collections of fat laden macrophages and giant cells which, to the unwary, may appear granulomatous. A recent report has shown the advantage of infra red spectrometry over histochemistry in distinguishing exogenous from endogenous fat resulting from bronchial obstruction[15].

Histiocytosis X (Eosinophilic granuloma) is often included in the differential diagnosis. Histologically it bears little or no resemblence to sarcoidosis. True focal granulomas are absent, foam cells with the characteristic Langerhan's bodies[16] are diagnostic and eosinophils are often prominent.

LYMPH NODES

Peripheral lymphadenopathy is found in 27% of patients with sarcoidosis[17] and form a ready source for biopsy proof. Before the bronchoscopy era 'blind' scalene node biopsy was common practice.

Infections. Again, it is important to exclude tuberculosis. The finding of Ziehl Neilson positive mycobacteria within the sections may be conclusive but is often negative in the most confusing cases of non caseating granulomas. Culture is always mandatory. Sarcoidosis is suspected by the presence of discrete granulomas involving a whole gland, tuberculous granulomas usually coalesce and often involve only part of the gland. In indiginous areas, lepromatous leprosy is distinguished by the presence of giant leprae cells teaming with mycobacteria while the more sarcoid like picture of tuberculous leprosy lymph node involvement is exceptional.

Bacterial infections, such as Brucellosis, Yersinia, Francisella Tularense rarely cause sarcoid like granulomas but should be looked for in problem cases. However, Toxoplasmosis, though characteristically producing isolated, three or five macrophage clusters - starry sky appearances; occasionally results in sarcoid like granulomas.

Organic and Inorganic Particulates. Silica and silicate granulomas in glands draining old injuries may be distinguished by the finding of birefringent crystals using polarised light. More exceptional are silicone granulomas in glands draining joint prosthesis but the foreign material is identified as faintly refractile intracellular granules.

Crohn's Disease. Identical sarcoid granulomas are found in about 20% of cases but only in association with the affected bowel disease.

Neoplasia. Sarcoid like granulomas in glands draining tumours occur as a result of degenerate tumour products and present no real problem. More confusion however may arise in Hodgkin's disease when granulomas may be found admixed with tumour and sometimes in non tumourous glands. The presence of eosinophils should alert the pathologist to look for tumour elsewhere [18]. Isolated granulomas within tumours are also a feature of seminomas, dysgeminomas and pinealoma.

ALIMENTARY SYSTEM

Intestinal. Intestinal involvement in sarcoidosis is exceptionally rare. The main cause of intestinal granulomas - Crohn's disease - does not usually present any diagnostic problem and isolated second class granulomas such as in diverticulitis are easily distinguished.

Liver. Of the many causes of liver granulomas, sarcoidosis is the commonest, 54%[19]. Primary biliary cirrhosis (PBC) is one of the main differential diagnosis (19%). As distinct from the random distribution of granulomas in sarcoidosis those of PBC are clearly centred on bile ducts with biliary obstruction and cirrhosis. Though considered to be distinct from sarcoidosis overlap cases do occur[20]. Bronchoalveolar lavage changes of subclinical alveolitis have been recorded associated with both PBC and Crohn's disease[21].

Case Report - Alimentary. A 63 year old female complained of progressive dyspnoea with fatigue, weight loss and puritis. She had tender hepato-megaly with bilateral pulmonary reticulo-nodular shadowing, Mitochondrial antibodies, positive with raised enzymes, normal SACE, negative Mantoux and Kveim test. Liver biopsy showed micronodular cirrhosis with granulomas centred on damaged bile ducts. Transbronchial biopsies showed poorly formed granulomas (Fig 2).

Diagnosis - "Overlap" PBC and Sarcoidosis.

SKIN

Skin involvement, when present (18%) forms a ready source for biopsy. It is usually a sign of chronicity and commonly associated with bone lesions. Repeat biopsies of an affected site, such as lupus pernio, will indicate response to treatment. The curious association of sarcoid lesions in old scars is well documented. The development of swelling or redness in a previously white, avascular, scar may be the first indication of disease and is useful confirmatory evidence in suspect chest lesions. Granulomas in scars however are most often a reaction to foreign material. The commonest skin granulomas are a reaction to degenerate cholesterol rich debris from a

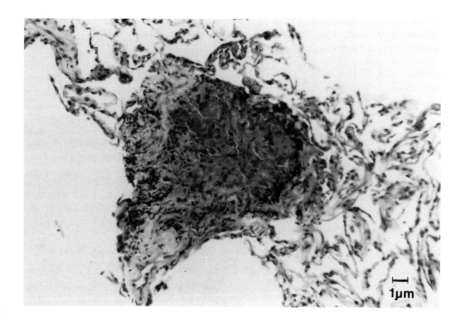

Fig. 2. "Second class" lung granulomas in Primary Biliary Cirrhosis

ruptured sebaceous cyst. Exogenous material such as talc, silica particularly after road injuries, displaced hairs e.g., pilonidal sinus and suture material should be excluded. Of other skin diseases with sarcoid like granulomas, the commonest is rheumatoid/rheumatic nodules (RA). The granulomas of RA however, show prominent central necrosis and instead of focal granulomas characteristic surrounding pallisade of histiocytes with occasional giant cells.

Metal granulomas may also cause confusion, in particular beryllium[22], and up to recently zirconium containing deodorants.

URINARY TRACT

Malakoplakia. The rare entity of malakoplakia though primarily found in the bladder, may affect any part of the urinary tract. The characteristic sheets of macrophages with contained calcified Michaelis-Gutmann bodies, bear a resemblance to epithelioid cells and Schaumann bodies, but true focal sarcoid type granulomas are absent. The cause is considered to be protracted coliform infection[23].

MALE GENITAL TRACT

Sarcoidosis, though very rarely, may affect any part of the male genital tract. Clinically it may be confused with epididymitis which may present as bilateral hard craggy masses [24], a feature of about 1/3 of patients, or testicular tumours. Histologically the disease must be distinguished from tuberculosis, though exceptional in the testis, from sperm granulomas and from local sarcoid like lesions related to tumours. Sperm granulomas are identified by the finding of central sperm remnants surrounded by epithelioid cells and are increasingly found as a complication of vasectomies. Sarcoid type granulomas are common in testicular seminoma, up to 40%, sometimes associated with extensive fibrosis, and probably a reaction to lipids derived from degenerate spermatocytic cells.

In the prostate, granulomas may also be a complication of previous operations though more like rheumatoid granulomas than classical sarcoid[25].

BREAST

Involvement of the breast is an unusual manifestation of sarcoidosis. Banik et al[26] have recently recorded a single, well substantiated case with associated BHL, raised SACE and a positive Kveim test with granulomas within a fibroadenoma. Such lesions must be distinguished from the common leaking duct granuloma and granulomatous mastitis[27]. Granulomatous lobular mastitis is a disease of young women often following pregnancy and lactation and characterised by a lobular distribution. It is thus distinguished from the more common local granulomatous reaction to cholesterol rich duct contents. Sarcoid like granulomas may also be seen in relation to the breast carcinoma.

FEMALE GENITAL TRACT

Sarcoidosis of the uterus and appendages is a rare occurrance with only about eight recorded cases in endometrium, myometrium and fallopian tubes[28]. Tuberculosis on the other hand not infrequently affects the tubes, but is rarely found in the endometrium. Due to menstruation granulomas are often immature and without caseation. As in other sites, it is essential to stain for M. tuberculosis but though tuberculosis is known to exist at other sites the bacilli may not be found. Giant cell granulomas may also be due to foreign material such as talc, often in conjunction with intra-uterine contraceptives (coil).

Tuberculosis of the fallopian tubes used to be common, often associated with extensive caseation. Localised tubal granulomas, sometimes with conchoidal bodies also occur as part of salpingitis isthmica nodosum and must not be confused with Schaumann bodies; the hallmark of end stage sarcoidosis.

The last illustrative case reminds us that we all have much to learn about the many and varied presentations of sarcoidosis.

Problem Case. Female, aged 60, presented with a past history of myocardial infarction and clear chest radiographs (1983). A year later she complained of mild dyspnoea and wheezing and diagnosed as chronic bronchitis. In 1985 increasing dyspnoea but still no radio-logical changes. She died in 1986 from respiratory failure with weight loss, marked clubbing, palmar erythema, abnormal liver function tests and bilateral diffuse pulmonary shadowing. The clinical diagnosis was ? alveolar cell carcinoma.

At autopsy she had bilateral upper zone honey-comb lung; hepatic fibrosis but no cirrhosis. The lungs, liver and hilar glands showed numerous fresh and hyalinised granulomas.

Having covered only a few of the problems encountered by an overzealous granulomatous pathologist, the message is clear - "use every means to exclude known causes before diagnosing sarcoidosis".

REFERENCES

1.   James DG, Jones Williams W (1985) Sarcoidosis and Other Granulomatous Disorders. W B Saunders, Philadelphia, Series No 24, Major Problems in Internal Medicine, pp 17

2.   James DG, Jones Williams W (1985) Sarcoidosis and Other Granulomatous Disorders. W B Saunders, Philadelphia, Series No 24, Major Problems in Internal Medicine, pp 39

3.   Symmers W St C (1956) Histoplasmosis contracted in Britain: A case of histoplasmosis lymphadenitis following clinical recovery from sarcoidosis. Brit Med J ii:786-790

4.   Bonafede RP, Benatar SR (1987) Bronchocentric Granulomatosis and Rheumatoid Arthritis. Br J Dis Chest 81:197-201

5.   Jones Williams W (1986) Bronchocentric granulomatosis: Letters to the Case. Path Res Prac 181:624-625

6.   Gibbs AR, Jones Williams W, Kelland D (1987) Necrotising Sarcoidal Granulomatosis. Sarcoidosis, (in press)

7.   Jones Williams W, Kelland D (1986) A new aid for the diagnosis of chronic beryllium disease: Laser Ion Mass Analysis (LIMA). J Clin Path 39:900-901

8.   Jones Williams W, Williams WR (1983) Value of lymphocyte transformation test in chronic beryllium disease and potentially exposed workers. Thorax 38:41-44

9.   Redline S, Barna BP, Tomashefski JF et al (1986) Granulomatous disease associated with pulmonary deposition of titanium. Brit J Industr Med 46:652-656

672

10. Shigematsu N, Matsuba K, Watanabe K et al (1980) A Granulomatous lung disease produced by Titanium. In: Jones Williams W, Davies BH (eds) Sarcoidosis. Alpha and Omega Press, Cardiff, pp 728-733

11. DeVuyst P, Dumortier P, Schandene L et al (1987) Sarcoid like granulomatosis induced by Aluminium dusts. Amer Rev Resp Dis 135: 493-497

12. Morgenroth K, Kronenberger H, Michalke G et al (1985) Morphology and pathogenesis of pneumoconiosis in dental technicians. Path Res Pract 179:528-536

13. James DG, Jones Williams W (1985) Sarcoidosis and Other Granulomatous Disorders. W B Saunders, Philadelphia, Series No 24, Major Problems in Internal Medicine, pp 65

14. Farber HW, Fairman RP, Glasier FL (1982) Talc Granulomatosis: Laboratory findings similar to sarcoidosis. Am Rev Resp Dis 125:258-261

15. Corrin B, Crocker PR, Hood BJ et al (1987) Paraffinoma confirmed by infra-red spectrometry. Thorax 42:389-390

16. Basset F, Corrin B, Spencer H et al (1978) Pulmonary histiocytosis X. Amer Rev Dis 118:811-820

17. James DG, Jones Williams W (1984) Sarcoidosis of the lymph nodes: In: D W Molander (ed) Diseases of the lymphatic system. Springer-Verlag, New York, pp 140-156

18. Jones Williams W, Jones DL, Whittaker JL (1980) Isolated sarcoid like granulomas in Hodgkin's disease. In: Jones Williams W, Davies BH (eds) Sarcoidosis, Cardiff, Alpha and Omega Press, pp 758-763

19. James DG, Jones Williams W (1985) Sarcoidosis and Other Granulomatous Disorders. W B Saunders, Philadelphia, Series No 24, Major Problems in Internal Medicine, pp 45

20. Fagan EA, Moore-Gilson JC, Turner-Warwick M (1983) Multiorgan granulomas and mitochondrial antibodies. N Eng J Med 308:572-575

21. Wallaert B, Bonniere P, Prin L et al (1986) Primary Biliary Cirrhosis: Subclinical inflammatory alveolitis in patients with normal chest roentgenograms. Chest 90:842-848

22. Jones Williams W, Williams WR, Kelland D et al (In Press) Beryllium Skin Disease In: (eds) Proc XI World Congress on Sarcoidosis and Other Granulomatous Disorders (Milan 1987), Elsevier, Amsterdam, pp

23. McClure J (1983) Malakoplakia. J Pathol 140:275-330

24. Mikhail JR, Mitchell DN, Dyson JL et al (1972) Sarcoidosis with genital involvement. Amer Rev Resp Dis 106:465-468

25. Lee G, Shepherd N (1983) Necrotising granulomata in prostatic resection specimens: a sequel to previous operations. J Clin Pathol 36:1067-1070

26. Banik S, Bishop PW, Omerod LP et al (1986) Sarcoidosis of the breast. J Clin Path 39:440-448

27. Going JJ, Anderson TJ, Wilkinson S et al (1987) Granulomatous lobular mastitis. J Clin Path 40:535-540

28. Khang-Loon H (1979) Sarcoidosis of the uterus. Hum Path 10:219-222

© 1988 Elsevier Science Publishers B.V. (Biomedical Division)
Sarcoidosis and other granulomatous disorders
C. Grassi, G. Rizzato, E. Pozzi, editors

A STUDY INTO THE EFFECTS OF DIRECT AND INDIRECT ANTIGENIC
CHALLENGE ON BRONCHOALVEOLAR LAVAGE FLUID FINDINGS IN PIGEON
BREEDERS DISEASE.

S.P. REYNOLDS, E.D. JONES, K.P. JONES, J.H. EDWARDS & B.H. DAVIES.
Asthma & Allergy Unit, Sully Hospital, Penarth, South Glamorgan CF6 2YA.

INTRODUCTION

Pigeon breeders disease characteristically affects the distal airways of the lung;

interstitial and alveolar inflammation, sometimes associated with granuloma formation
being the main pathological finding. Immunological changes occuring in the distal
airspaces following exposure to pigeon antigens can be characterised by analysis of
bronchoalveolar lavage fluid (BALF). We have studied the early cellular and humoral
responses occuring in the human lung following specific antigenic challenge. We have
also compared cell profiles and levels of immune soluble mediators in the BALF of
pigeon breeders and patients with other interstitial pulmonary disease.

MATERIALS AND METHODS

Patient Groups: 25 pigeon breeders (mean age 49 yrs); 14 had clinical, radiological
and physiological abnormalities compatible with the acute phase of pigeon breeders
lung, 4 were diagnosed as having chronic disease and a further 7 were asymptomatic
with at least 5 years exposure. All patients were precipitin positive other than 2 of
the asymptomatic group. In order to compare lavage findings 3 other groups were
studied:- (a) 16 patients with biopsy proven sarcoidosis (3 female, 13 male, mean age
35 yrs). 10 were considered to have high and 6 low intensity alveolitis; (b) 19 patients
with biopsy proven iodiopathic pulmonary fibrosis (4 female, 15 male, mean age 54
yrs). 7 were smokers; (c) 5 men, mean age 40 years, all of whom were referred with
non-specific respiratory symptoms and normal chest x-rays. The study was approved
by the District Ethical Committee.

Bronchcolar Lavage: Segmental bronchoalveolar lavage was carried out according to
standard protocol. Initial and subsequent lavages were carried out on different sub-
segments of the right middle lobe.

Bronchial Challenge: 15 pigeon breeders were considered to by symptomatic on the
basis of a positive response to challenge testing with 1:100 nebulised purified pigeon
serum, i.e., 2 or more of the following changes being documented between 4-24 hours:
(1) constitutional upsets similar to that following loft exposure; (2) a temperature
> 38°C; (3) an increase of > 30% in the peripheral neutrophil count, and (4) a reduction
in FVC and/or FEV1 of > 15%.

Twelve patients agreed to undergo further bronchoscopy 4-6 hours after direct antigenic
challenge. Ten were symptomatic pigeon breeders, 8 of whom were challenged with
nebulised pigeon serum and 2 with saline. Two patients were drawn from the asymptomatic group and given nebulised pigeon serum or nebulised saline. All 25 pigeon breeders
had undergone indirect challenge with antigens in their own lofts within 24 hours of
the study beginning.

Cellular Analysis: BALF was centrifuged at 800g for 5 minutes and the supernatant removed and stored at -70C. The cell pellet was resuspended in phosphate buffered saline, pH 7.4. A different cell count was performed using the Jenner/Giemsa stain. Lymphocyte subsets were estimated using monoclonal antibodies and fluorescence microscopy. T-cell subsets were determined using the OKT series of monoclonal antibodies (Ortho-Diagnostic Ltd.). Ia receptors were visualised using an HLA-DR antibody (Becton-Dickinson Ltd.).

RESULTS

The cellular profile of the BALF in various patient groups is shown in Table 1. Mean values of lymphocyte numbers and lymphocytes expressed as a percentage of other cells are significantly higher in the sarcoidosis and pigeon breeder groups compared to normals ($p = 0.0001$). Total lymphocytes and % lymphocytes in the pulmonary fibrotic group in comparison to normals gave p values of 0.005. On further analysis of the pigeon breeder group both the lymphocyte numbers and the % lymphocytes are higher ($p < 0.005$, $p < 0.05$) for those who suffered an acute attack compared with asymptomatic patients. Five of the asymptomatics with positive precipitins had subclinical alveolitis ($> 28\%$ T-cells recovered from BALF). Distribution of the T-lymphocytes between their subsets showed no statistical significance between any two patient groups or subgroups. Total cell numbers recovered in BALF were not statistically different. Symptomatic pigeon breeders demonstrated significant difference in the levels of total gammaglobulin, anti-pigeon serum IgG and anti-pigeon dropping IgG in BALF compared to asymptomatics ($p < 0.01$, $p < 0.01$ and $p < 0.001$, Figure 1).

Table 1 BALF FINDINGS

DISEASE GROUP (n)	TOTAL CELL x10⁶	TOTAL LYMPHOCYTES x10⁶	% LYMPHOCYTES	% OKT3	4/8 RATIO
PBL acute attack 1/52 (9)	8.23 ± 4.82	6.08 ± 4.10	70.6 ± 4.10	65.4 ± 8.2	1.23 ± 0.36
PBL acute attack 6/52 →52/52 (5)	9.81 ± 4.94	6.12 ± 2.40	68.3 ± 19.0	59.6 ± 8.7	1.86 ± 0.29
PBL chronic (4)	10.21 ± 8.00	7.23 ± 4.84	79.5 ± 5.2	58.4 ± 3.5	1.23 ± 0.29
PB asymptomatic (7)	5.73 ± 2.21	2.43 ± 1.65	43.4 ± 22.7	56.4 ± 3.3	1.84 ± 1.09
High intensity sarcoidosis (10)	8.95 ± 5.47	6.14 ± 4.05	72.5 ± 12.8	65.8 ± 9.5	3.16 ± 2.62
Low intensity sarcoidosis (6)	4.08 ± 1.22	1.32 ± 0.39	33.1 ± 7.7	61.4 ± 4.7	1.17 ± 0.31
Idiopathic pulmonary fibrosis (19)	8.00 ± 5.11	1.48 ± 1.25	24.4 ± 20.2	59.4 ± 6.2	0.58 ± 1.12
Normals (5)	6.20 ± 3.9	0.35 ± 0.33	7.3 ± 3.9	58.5 ± 4.2	1.14 ± 0.30

Cellular profile of bronchoalveolar lavage fluid of the various patient groups. Results are expressed as mean ± S.D.

Values for interleukin-1 (IL-1), interleukin-2 (IL-2) and fibronectin, assessed by the ELISA technique in the pigeon breeder groups failed to show any significant difference on analysis with the student t-test (Figs. 2-4). Following direct antigenic challenge there was a significant increase in the total lymphocytes, T-lymphocytes and neutrophils in those patients who were judged to have had a positive challenge test (p=0.005, 0.005 and 0.01) (Fig. 5-6). Levels of IL-1, IL-2, fibronectin and specific anti-pigeon serum IgG all tended to fall after positive antigenic challenge although their values did not attain statistical significance. (p > 0.1).

DISCUSSION

Previous authors of cellular profile in BALF have reported a predominance of OKT8 labelled cells and a consequential decrease in 4/8 ratios in patients with hypersensitivity pneumonitis[1]. The reverse of this was reported in sarcoidosis[2]. Our work shows that interstitial diseases cannot be distinguished on the basis of 4/8 ratios alone. There was no significant difference between the levels of soluble immune mediators in any group or correlation with progression of the disease. Previous studies of spontaneous release of IL-1 and IL-2 by unstimulated effector cells demonstrated acute synthesis by these cells[3,4]. These studies were on cells cultured outside the lung and as such were not subject to the constraints of immune regulatory factors present in BALF[5]. We were unable to demonstrate increased levels of fibronectin in the lavage fluid of patients with interstitial lung disease compared to normals, as other authors have documented[6]. We would suggest cell studies outside the milieu of the lung are prone to false interpretation and more in vivo studies of immune effector function are necessary before hasty conclusions are reached. Our data shows an increase in lymphocytes and neutrophils 4-6 hours after antigenic challenge in positive responders. The increase in T-lymphocytes was unlikely to have arisen simply due to a repeat lavage as this was not seen in the 4 patients who did not respond to challenge. Fournier et al[7] suggested a neutrophil alveolitis occurring 24 hours after antigenic challenge. However, if cellular events were so clear cut, we would have expected a large proportion of the 25 pigeon breeders initially lavaged to have had a neutrophil alveolitis as they had undergone indirect challenge in their lofts within 24 hours of admission to hospital. We have some evidence to suggest that T-cells recovered in the second lavage in symptomatic pigeon breeders were more activated as a greater percentage expressed the Ia antigen (13.9±2.0 before and 20.73±1.96 after). There was no significant difference in 4/8 ratios (1.54±0.55 before and 2.0±1.14 after positive challenge and 1.72±0.83 and 1.63±0.25 following a negative challenge). The trend towards the fall in IL-1 and IL-2 in symptomatic pigeon breeders in the second lavage is unlikely to be explained by an increased diffusion of urea into the alveolar spaces as has been reported[8], or the failure to produce IL-1 within 4-6 hours. We are currently planning to measure intracellular IL-1 production in these patients to gain a more accurate assessment of the early immune response.

It would be tempting to postulate that the fall in antibody levels observed in those patients who had a positive response to specific challenge was due to complex deposition in tissues or on macrophage receptor sites, but at present no firm conclusion can be drawn because of the small number of patients involved in the negative response group.

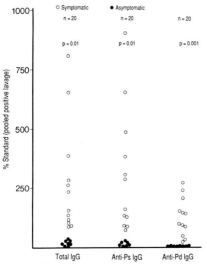

Fig.1. Total IgG / specific anti-Ps / Pd - IgG in symptomatic and asymptomatic pigeon breeders.

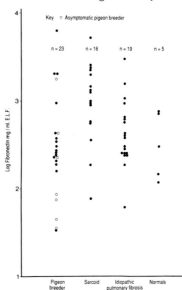

Fig.2.   Log Fibronectin mg/ml. E.L.F. in interstitial pulmonary disease.

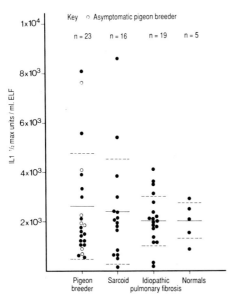

Fig. 3. Interleukin 1 ½ max units / ml. E.L.F. in interstitial lung disease.

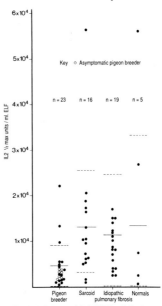

Fig. 4. Interleukin 2 ½ max units / ml. E.L.F. in interstitial lung disease.

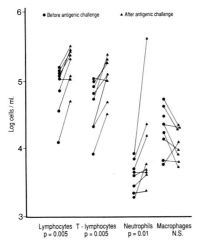

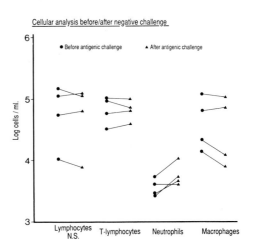

Fig.5. Cellular analysis before / after positive challenge.

Fig.6. Cellular analysis before / after negative challenge.

REFERENCES

1. Costabel U. Bross K.J. Marxen J. Matthys H. T-lymphocytosis in Bronchoalveolar Lavage Fluid of Hypersensitivity Pneumonitis. Changes in Profile of T-cell Subsets During the Course of Disease. Chest 1984:85, No.4:514-518.

2. Hunninghake G.W. Crystal R.G. Pulmonary Sarcoidosis. A disorder mediated by excess helper T-lymphocyte activity at sites of disease activity. N.Eng.J.Med. 1981 305:429-434.

3. Hunninghake G.W. Release of Interleukin-1 by Alveolar Macrophages of Patients with Active Pulmonary Sarcoidosis. Am Rev Respir Dis 1934;129:569-572.

4. Pinkston Paula. Bitterman P.B. Crystal R.G. Spontaneous Release of Interleukin-2 by Lung T-Lymphocytes in Active Pulmonary Sarcoidosis. N.Eng.J.Med. 1983;308: 794-799.

5. Jones K.P. Davies B.H. Inhibition of T-cell Function by Bronchoalveolar Lavage Fluid. Proceedings British Thoracic Society 1985 (Winter Meeting) Thorax 1986; 41:231.

6. Rennard S.I. Hunninghake G.W. Bitamen et al P.B. Production of Fibronectin by the Human Alveolar Macrophage: Mechanism for the Recruitment of Fibroblasts to Sites of Tissue Injury in Interstitial Lung Disease. Proc Nat Acad Sci 1931; 78:7147-7151.

7. Fournier E. Tonnel A.B. Gosset P.H. Wallaert B. Ameison J.C. Voisin C. Early Neutrophil Alveolitis after Antigen Inhalation in Hypersensitivity Pneumonitis. Chest 1986:83, No.4:563-566.

8. Marcy T.W. Merrill W.W. Rankin J.A. Reynolds H.Y. Limitations of Using Urea to Quantify Epithelial Lining Fluid Recovered by Bronchoalveolar Lavage. Am Rev Respir Dis 1987;135:1276-1280.

© 1988 Elsevier Science Publishers B.V (Biomedical Division)
Sarcoidosis and other granulomatous disorders
C. Grassi, G. Rizzato, E. Pozzi, editors

ENVIRONMENTAL AND IMMUNOLOGIC STUDIES ON THE CAUSATIVE AGENT OF SUMMER-TYPE HYPERSENSITIVITY PNEUMONITIS

MASAYUKI ANDO, KAZUKO YOSHIDA, TETSUNORI SAKATA, KYOSEI SODA, MINEHARU SUGIMOTO, MORITAKA SUGA, HIRONORI NAKASHIMA, SHUKURO ARAKI

The First Department of Internal Medicine, Kumamoto University Medical School, 1-1-1 Honjo, Kumamoto 860 (Japan)

INTRODUCTION

Summer-type hypersensitivity pneumonitis (HP) is the most prevalent type of HP in Japan. It is characterized by symptoms that appear during the summer season, provocation of symptoms when at home, familial occurrence, and other manifestations similar to other type of HP. Since 1984, we have reported that *Trichosporon cutaneum* is a likely causative agent of this disease.[1-3] The purpose of the present study was to elucidate the complete features of home environmental fungi, especially yeasts, in the summer-type HP. Moreover, we assayed anti-*T. cutaneum* antibody activities in serum and bronchoalveolar lavage fluids (BALF) samples, and performed the inhalation challenge test with this antigen in many cases. Our results indicate that *T. cutaneum* is a *major* causative agent of summer-type HP.

MATERIALS AND METHODS

Environmental mycological study

Environmental mycological studies were carried out in 26 patients' homes and in 195 control homes. In 13 patients' homes, indoor sampling was performed by open plate culture, house dust culture, and swab culture; but in the other 13 patients' homes, sampling was only by house dust culture.

Immunologic studies

Anti-*T. cutaneum* antibody activities. Anti-*T. cutaneum* antibody activities in serum and BALF samples were assayed by the precipitating antibody method, indirect immunofluorescent antibody (IFA) method, and enzyme-linked immunosorbent assay (ELISA) method.

Inhalation challenge test. The inhalation challenge test was performed on the 13 patients and the 2 asymptomatic family members. Six ml of culture-filtrate antigen of *T. cutaneum* (2.5mg/ml) were inhalated through an ultrasonic nebulizer. During the next 24 h, symptoms and signs were recorded and measurements were made of body temperature, leukocytes, Po_2, vital capacity and diffusing capacity.

RESULTS

Environmental mycologic study

The incidence of fungi in patients' homes was compared with that in control homes. A total of 3,476 strains of fungi were isolated from 26 patients' homes, 424 of which were yeasts. In the 195 control homes, 9,371 strains of fungi were isolated, 926 of which were yeasts. In the data of open plate cultures, the amounts of total fungi and yeasts were not significantly different between the two, and $T.$ $cutaneum$ was the only genus found to be significantly higher in the living rooms of patients' homes than in those of control homes ($P < 0.005$) (Table 1). These findings were also true of the assessment of house dust cultures of patients compared with controls ($P < 0.01$). The swab culture method revealed that genera $Trichosporon$, $Cryptococcus$, and $Candida$ were isolated from patients' homes with significantly higher incidence. The colonizing places

Table 1. Incidence of fungi in patients' homes and control homes

Genera	Yeasts						Total fungi
	Imperfect				$Bas+Asc$	$Total$	
	$T.$	$C.$	$Ca.$	$Others$			
	by open plate culture in living room						
Patients (n=13)	0.54 (3)	0.19 (2)	0.17 (4)	0 (0)	0.31 (4)	1.21 (9)	14.3 [a] (13) [b]
	**						
Controls (n=83)	0.00 (1)	0.04 (4)	0.30 (24)	0.37 (29)	0.30 (31)	1.01 (62)	10.95 (83)
	by house dust culture						
Patients (n=26)	0.42 (11)	0.62 (13)	2.15 (22)	1.03 (19)	0.23 (5)	4.45 (26)	8.27 (26)
	**						
Controls (n=20)	0 (0)	0.25 (4)	1.00 (11)	0.50 (10)	0 (0)	1.75 (16)	4.10 (20)
	by swab culture						
Patients (n=13)	0.09 (10)	0.07 (7)	0.58 (13)	0.25 (9)	0.11 (5)	1.10 (13)	3.15 (13)
	**	*	**				
Controls (n=20)	0 (0)	0.01 (1)	0.17 (2)	0.04 (3)	0.07 (1)	0.29 (14)	0.68 (20)

$T.$=$Trichosporon$, $C.$=$Cryptococcus$, $Ca.$=$Candida$, $Others$=Rhodotorula+Oospori-
dium+imperfect yeasts of other species. $Bas+Asc$=basidiosporogenous yeasts +
ascosporogenous yeasts. a)=Number of strains of the same genus per exposed culture plate. b)=Number of homes from which a genus was isolated. n=Number of
homes. P values (patients homes vs control homes) *$P < 0.01$, **$P < 0.005$.

683

of *T. cutaneum* revealed by the swab culture method were old damp wood (4 homes), floor mats (2 homes), bed clothes (2 homes), and budgeriger droppings (2 homes). Among the 424 strains of yeasts isolated from 26 patients' homes, 175 strains which showed the maximum IFA titers were selected out of strains of the same species in each home. Of these 175 strains, 33 were reactive to the patients' sera at 1:128 or higher in IFA titers: 15 were *T. cutaneum* isolated from 15 patients' homes, and the other 18 were each a different species from a different home except for 2 strains of *Candida parapsilosis*.

Immunologic studies

Anti-*T. cutaneum* antibody activities. Anti-*T. cutaneum* antibody activities were found in almost all serum samples from 68 patients with summer-type HP, but not in those of patients with other pulmonary diseases (except for 1 sarcoidosis patient) or in normal subjects (Table 2). The specific IgG, IgA, and secretory-IgA antibody activities to *T. cutaneum* were also found in all BALF samples from 9 patients with summer-type HP, but not in those of 9 sarcoidosis patients or in 6 normal subjects as assessed by the ELISA method.

Inhalation challenge test. The inhalation challenge test with culture-filtrate antigen of *T. cutaneum* was performed in 13 patients of 10 homes. Nine were positive, 2 were probable, and 2 were negative. The 2 asymptomatic family members were also negative.

Table 2. Anti-*T. cutaneum* antibody activities in serum samples from patients with summer-type HP, asymptomatic family members, and other pulmonary diseases

		Precipitat-ing antibody	IFA titers	ELISA	
				IgG	IgA
Summer-type hypersensitivity pneumonitis	(n=68)	89%	99%	100%	80%
Asymptomatic family members	(n=30)	13	63	84	18
Other pulmonary diseases	(n=100)	0	1*	ND	ND
Normal subjects	(n=100)	0	0	0	0

n=Number of samples tested. Each value represents the percentage of positive sera. ND=Not done. *Sarcoidosis.

DISCUSSION

This study demonstrates that extensive distribution of *T. cutaneum* occurs in home environments of summer-type HP but not in those of normal controls, that

684

the isolated *T. cutaneum* showed high reactivity to the patients' sera as assessed
by IFA titers, that anti–*T. cutaneum* antibody activities were found in almost
all patients' serum and BALF samples, and that many of the patients responded
to the inhalation challenge with the antigen of *T. cutaneum*. Furthermore, this
study reveals the colonizing places of *T. cutaneum* in patients' homes. These
results clearly show that *T. cutaneum* is a *major* causative agent of summer–type
HP. In 1978, Miyakawa et al. reported that all the sera from 41 patients tested
had higher IFA titers against *Cryptococcus neoformans* and proposed that *C.
neoformans* and certain antigen–related fungi could be a causative agent of this
disease.[4] No *C. neoformans*, however, was isolated from patients' homes or
from control homes. In fact, we have demonstrated that anti–*C. neoformans*
antibody activities are highly serologically cross–reactive to *T. cutaneum*.[1]
Thus, *C. neoformans* is *not* a major causative agent of this disease.

Undoubtedly, the climate in western Japan (i.e., muggy summer following the
rainy season) and the living conditions (old wooden houses) influence the occurrence of this unique disease. *T. cutaneum* is distributed worldwide and grows
on old damp wood, floor mats, and bird droppings. Therefore, HP induced by
T. cutaneum may be present in other countries with similar climate and living
conditions.

CONCLUSION

Environmental and immunologic studies revealed that *T. cutaneum* is a *major*
causative agent of summer–type HP in Japan, and that the ELISA method is
very sensitive and useful in the detection of anti–*T. cutaneum* antibody activities in serum and BALF samples.

ACKNOWLEDGEMENTS

We thank Dr. Shimazu K and Tosaka M (Kumamoto University Medical School)
for their assistance in identifying fungi.

REFERENCES

1. Shimazu K, Ando M, Sakata T, Yoshida K, Araki S (1984) Am Rev Respir
Dis 130:407
2. Soda K, Ando M, Shimazu K, Sakata T, Yoshida K, Araki S (1986) Am Rev
Respir Dis 133:83
3. Ando M, Yoshida K, Soda K, Araki S (1986) Am Rev Respir Dis 134:177
4. Miyakawa T, Ochi T, Takahashi H (1978) Clin Allergy 8:501

© 1988 Elsevier Science Publishers B.V. (Biomedical Division)
Sarcoidosis and other granulomatous disorders
C. Grassi, G. Rizzato, E. Pozzi, editors

ABNORMALITIES OF LIPID COMPOSITION OF BRONCHOALVEOLAR LAVAGE (BAL) IN RESPIRATORY DISEASES INDUCED BY DUST INHALATION (RDID)

A. TELES-DE-ARAÚJO, J. M. REIS-FERREIRA, M. FREITAS-E-COSTA AND J. BENVENISTE*

Clínica de Doenças Pulmonares - Faculdade de Medicina de Lisboa - Centro CnL3 Instituto Nacional de Investigação Científica and * I N S E R M - U 200 Av. Prof. Egas Moniz, 1699 Lisboa Codex - PORTUGAL
* 32, rue des Carnets, 92140 Clamart - FRANCE

INTRODUCTION

Respiratory Diseases Induced by Dust Inhalation (RDID) may display several clinical settings. The most frequent syndromes are Occupational Asthma, Alveolitis and Progressive Interstitial Fibrosis[1]. Nevertheless, common pathogenic steps have been described[2].

Surfactant synthesis and secretion may be disturbed in RDID, and this is probably linked to activation of Alveolar Macrophages and involvement of type II Pneumocytes[3].

Phosphatidylcholine (PC), the main component of pulmonary surfactant, may generate ether-linked lipids with a polar headgroup, one of which is 1-0-alkyl 2-acyl glycero-phosphocholine (AAPC). Through the action of Phospholipase A_2, this lipid may switch into 1-0-alkyl 2-lyso glycerophosphocholine, most commonly refered as lyso-paf-acether, the precursor of a powerful proinflammatory mediator, paf-acether[4].

In the present study we analysed the contents in paf-acether and its precursors - lyso-paf-acether, AAPC and PC - of BAL of several groups of RDID, according to syndromes and clinical activity.

PATIENTS AND METHODS

Patients

The patients under study were 24 RDID with lung or bronchial biopsy showing inflammation associated to inclusions of specific dust material. **Alveolitis** was present alone in 12 patients (Group A) and airways involvement with or without alveolitis in other 12 patients (Group B).

Etiology. According to the causative dust, 13 patients had organic dust diseases (6 in group A and 7 in group B) and 11 mineral dust diseases (6 in group A and 5 in group B).

Subgroups. The clinical stage of patients in group A was classified according to clinical, X-ray and lung function worsening and to alveolitis degree (L$\emptyset \geqslant 20\%$)

686

in active forms (both criteria) and less active forms (one or none criteria);
some active forms were on immunosupressive corticotherapy (1 mg/kg/d), and
constituted another subgroup. There was 5 patients classified as active (subgroup A_1), 3 as active on corticotherapy (subgroup A_2) and 4 as less active
(subgroup A_3).

Group B was divided in 5 patients with associated alveolitis ($\geqslant$15% lymphocytes
and/or $\geqslant$5% neutrophils) and 7 without alveolitis, respectively, subgroups B_1
and B_2.

TABLE I

PATIENT CHARACTERISTICS

subgroups, mean $\pm$ standard deviation

charact.	Age	Sex	Smoke	Lymph Ø	Neutroph Ø	EosinophØ
A_1-n=5	51.75±9	3M;2F	3NS;2S	34.8±11.8	1.2±1.6	3.7±7.4
A_2-n=3	33±13.5	1M;2F	2NS;1S	53.7±12	1.2±1.6	1.3±.6
A_3-n=4	52±7.4	1M;3F	3NS;1S	24±7.1	2±1.8	1.75±2.2
B_1-n=5	52.6±6.6	4M;1F	4NS;1S	21.6±5.7	1.6±3.0	1±.7
B_2-n=7	43.6±7.1	6M;1F	3NS;4S	7.9±5.5	.7±.95	.3±.5

M=males; F=females; NS=non smokers; S=smokers (15cig/d); Lymph=% lymphocytes
in BAL; Neutroph Ø=% neutrophils in BAL; Eosinoph Ø=% eosinophils in BAL

Methods

BAL was performed in all patients with 200 ml serum saline 37°C, in 50 ml
syringe aliquots, discarding the first aliquot. Cells were separated by centri-
phugation at 500 G, and supernatant assayed.

PC was titrated by the modified Bartlett phosphore method[5], after separation
of lipids according to Bligh and Dyer[6], and selection of the PC effluent on HPLC.

The etherlipids were assayed by washed rabbit platelet aggregability, by the
method of Benveniste[7].

RESULTS

The results are expressed in tabulated form, by groups and subgroups. Phospho-
lipids are shown in picomoles per mililiter (pmol/mL) overall. Cocients pretend
to be an abstract rate of the activeness of the respective methabolic step. The
statistical comparison used the Student t-test.

TABLE II

GROUP A - RESULTS

subgroup	n	lyso-paf	AAPC	PC	lyso/AAPC	AAPC/PC
A_1	5	81.6±20.8	1073±636	12500±6895	.12±.11	98.5±68.4
stat		p<.01	NS	NS	NS	NS
A_2	3	8.5±8.3	591±416	18300±5351	.02±.02	30.4±13.2
stat		NS	NS	p<.05	NS	NS
A_3	4	13.7±11.1	329.3±221.7	7825±4489	.05±.04	54.9±45.6
st.A_1vA_3		p<.001	.1>p>.05	NS	NS	NS

stat=Student t-test significance intercalated between subgroups compared, except comparison between subgroups A_1 and A_3, in the bottom of the table

TABLE III

GROUP B - RESULTS

subgroup	n	lyso-paf	AAPC	PC	lyso/AAPC	AAPC/PC
B_1	5	9.2±5.4	708±453	23840±15716	.02±.02	35.4±24
stat		NS	p<.02	p<.01	.1>p>.05	NS
B_2	7	11.3±8.1	161.3±133	1983±1383	.17±.16	126.4±115

DISCUSSION

The subgroups of patients are somewhat comparable as general characteristics. Age, sex and smoking habits are not strikingly different; however, smokers are more frequent in group B_2.

Alveolitis was usually lymphocytary and only twice eosinophilic (one asbestosis and one pigeon' breeder) and neutrophilic in another case (asbestosis).

The analysis of BAL composition in phospholipid classes under study displays significant differences between the precedently described groups of patients.

In group A, phosphatidylcholine (PC) is increased in clinically active cases, although statistical significance is reached only between less active and corticoid treated subgroups; this may be due to the well-known stimulant effect of corticoids on surfactant production.

The most interesting variations are found in lyso-paf-acether rates, whose variations cannot be justified only on greater pool of its precursors.

In clinically active forms it is very significantly increased as compared to less active and corticoid treated groups.

Group B, in which airways disorders predomine, yields PC significant increase in the subgroup with interstitial involvement (B_2), suggesting an increased production of surfactant in these patients.

The reported increase of AAPC in this subgroup may depend on the greater PC pool. Lyso-paf-acether does not differ between both subgroups, but is strikingly increased if compared to normals, previously reported by us[3] (lyso-paf-acether: 1.76+ +1.47, n=5 p<.02 - AAPC: 114.4+73.9, n=5 p>.05). This finding is interesting, owing to actual concepts on bronchoconstricting action of lyso-paf-acether.

Our results are even more interesting because lyso-paf-acether to AAPC ratio are greater (borderline significance) in occupational asthma (B_2) subgroup.

The suggested role for lyso-paf-acether is a proinflammatory mediator and neutrophil chemotactic factor. Its decrease with corticotherapy correlates well to clinical improvement.

We were not able to retrieve paf-acether in BAL supernatants overall, and this is probably due to the fast inactivation of this powerful mediator by acetyl-hydrolase[8], into lyso-paf-acether; besides, all the patients under study were free from bronchospasm at the moment of BAL.

In conclusion, the activation of paf-acether pathway in our patients seems clear; at least lyso-paf-acether is probably involved in the pathogenesis of RDID, and its rates correlate with anatomoclinical form of disease, as long as its degree of clinical activity.

REFERENCES

1. Pimentel JC (1973) Am Rev Respir Dis 108:1303
2. Freitas-e-Costa M, Teles-de-Araújo A (1983) Federazioni Medici 36:859-870
3. Teles-de-Araújo A, Arnoux B, Landes A, Freitas-e-Costa M, Benveniste J (1984) Proc 5th Eur Cong Intern Acad Chest Phys, IV/4 (abstract)
4. Snyder F (1985) Medic Res Rev 5:107-140
5. Barlett (1959) J Biol Chem 234:466
6. Bligh , Dyer (1959) Can J Biochem Physiol 37:911
7. Benveniste J, Chignard M, Le-Couedic, Vargaftig BB (1982) Thromb Res 25:375-85
8. Ninio E, Mencia-Huerta JM, Heymans F, Benveniste J (1982) Biochem Biophys Acta 710:23-31

Sarcoidosis and other granulomatous disorders
C. Grassi, G. Rizzato, E. Pozzi, editors

BERYLLIUM SKIN DISEASE

W JONES WILLIAMS[1], WR WILLIAMS[1], D KELLAND[2], PJA HOLT[3]
1-Pathology Department, University of Wales College of Medicine, Llandough Hospital, Cardiff, 2-Department of Metallurgy, University of Cambridge, 3-University Hospital of Wales, Cardiff (UK)

We report on skin lesions in 26 beryllium (Be) workers resulting from cuts and abrasions sustained at work. The series includes 4 previously published UK cases. Our experience with a patient who developed Be lung disease four years following skin disease[1], stimulated us to record and continue to investigate the nature and fate of skin injuries in Be workers.

14 cases satisfy the established criteria for diagnosis[2] and are classified as cases of chronic beryllium disease (CBD).

Six patients had both skin and lung disease and worked with Be metal, alloys and ceramics. Ulcerated nodules were found in four and nodular scars in two. All the skin biopsies showed granulomas and with one exception, conspicuous necrosis. One also has granulomas in the lung. Laser Microprobe Mass Spectrometry (LAMMS)[3] analysis revealed Be within the granulomas in all three examined. The Beryllium Lymphocyte Transformation (BeLT) test[4] using peripheral blood lymphocytes was positive in three of four tested and also with lavage lymphocytes in one. The Kveim test was negative in four tested and all were Mantoux negative. In all but one, lung involvement was present at the initial examination. One patient died from cor pulmonale 10 years after the onset but all the others are alive up to 4 years (2) and between 20 and 30 years (3).

Eight patients had skin lesions only, 5 machinists, 2 ceramic and one flourescent lamp worker (the only one with skin ulceration). All the nodular scars showed granulomas containing Be. Be was also detected in a flattened scar with granulomas and in one of three without granulomas. The BeLT test was positive in three of five. The Kveim test was negative in all four tested. One had a local recurrence at six months, with Be positive granulomas requiring re-excision. None have developed any other local recurrance or lung involvement after intervals of up to six years.

An additional 12 cases, 10 metal machinists and 2 ceramic workers, are classified as "suspect" as the biopsies showed non specific inflammation without granulomas though Be was detected in two scars. All seven tested were BeLT negative. Follow up for 2 years (10), 5 years (1) and 16 years (1) has shown no local recurrance or lung involvement.

690

DISCUSSION

Comparison of our two groups of patients shows that ulcerated skin nodules are more commonly associated with (4 of 6) than without lung involvement (1 of 8). All the nodular scars showed granulomas and two of five flat scars.

We have confirmed our earlier observation that sensitisation is a feature of CBD as the BeLT test was positive in 6 of 9 patients and negative in all the 'suspect' group.

With one exception[2] a careful follow up of patients with isolated skin lesions, to date, have shown no evidence of lung involvement.

Our finding of Be in flattened scars with and without granulomas raises a difficult practical problem. Despite all precautions, machinists inevitably cut their fingers. It is accepted practice in the UK and elsewhere that any such injury be immediately washed with saline, tested for Be and if found, it is washed until free. Though it is impractical to excise all otherwise unremarkable scars in beryllium workers, any which show signs of nodularity and obviously ulceration, must be excised and all kept under surveillance.

We conclude that the diagnosis of beryllium skin disease rests on the finding of Be containing granulomas and supported by evidence of 'in vitro' sensitisation. We advise that patients should avoid further exposure.

ACKNOWLEDGEMENTS

Mr Kelland acknowledges the SERC for financial support and Professor D Hall for research facilities. We are grateful to the many clinicians for case records.

REFERENCES

1.   Jones Williams W, Kilpatrick GS (1974) Cutaneous and pulmonary manifestations of chronic beryllium disease. In: Proc VI Internat Conf Sarcoidosis. Iwai K, Hosoda Y (eds) Univ Tokyo Press pp 141-145

2.   Jones Williams W (1977) Beryllium disease - pathology and diagnosis. J Occup Med 27:93-96

3.   Jones Williams W, Kelland D (1986) New aid for diagnosing chronic beryllium disease: Laser Ion Mass Analysis. J Clin Path 39:900-901

4.   Jones Williams W, Williams WR (1983) Value of beryllium transformation tests in chronic beryllium disease and in potentially exposed workers. Thorax 38:41-44

LIGHT AND ELECTRON MICROSCOPY OF EXPERIMENTAL CUTANEOUS
GRANULOMAS IN MICE TREATED WITH CYCLOSPORINE

C. PINCELLI, A. FUJIOKA, H. SUYA, K. FUKUYAMA and W.L. EPSTEIN,

Department of Dermatology, University of California,
San Francisco, CA. USA

INTRODUCTION

Skin granulomas can develop in mice treated with high doses of
Cyclosporine (Cs) which effectively reduced T-cell function in
lymph nodes and spleen, as determined by mitogenic responses, IL2
activity and IL-2 receptor expression (1). This study reports the
cell components and cell organization of skin granulomas in Cs
treated mice by light and electron microscopy.

MATERIALS AND METHODS

The experimental skin granuloma model of Nishimura et al (2) was
used. BALB/c euthymic mice were injected with Cs (150 mg/Kg/day)
5 times/wk for 5 wks, starting 2 wks before granuloma grafting.
Control mice without Cs treatment received granuloma grafts. Skin
was excised at 3 wks after grafting and prepared for light microscopy.
Granulomas which developed around the eggs were scored and the
percentage calculated for both treated and control mice. Skin
specimens also were fixed in 3% glutaraldehyde, postfixed in 2%
osmium tetroxide, embedded in plastic and cut at 1 um and 60 nm.
The thin sections were stained with uranyl acetate and lead citrate
and examined by a Siemens Elmiskope 1A.

RESULTS AND DISCUSSION

Cs injection resulted in blood levels of 489 ng/ml which was shown
to be sufficient for suppression of T-cell function at the time of
grafting (1). As seen in Table 1, granuloma takes, increased
(p 0.01) in Cs-treated mice compared to untreated mice. Morpho-

692

TABLE 1

PERCENT OF GRANULOMA TAKES

Animals	Eggs Total number	Granulomas Number	%
Cs-treated	519	335	63.2 ± 3.1
Untreated controls	526	204	38.2 ± 4.5

logically, granulomas consisted of similar cells in both groups
(Fig.1 A,B). Cs treatment did not alter accumulation of mononuclear
cells into the skin as reported by others (3). Also, reduced T-cell
function in recipient mice failed to block granuloma initiation,
supporting the view that granulomatous tissue remodeling can be
initiated independent from T-cell function (4). However, these
findings seem to be different from those in BCG granulomas in guinea

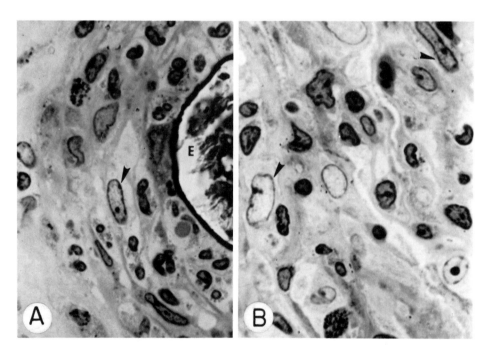

Fig.1. Toluidine blue staining of plastic embedded sections of skin
granulomas from Cs-treated (A) and control (B) mice. Note several
layers of organized cells, mainly macrophages and epithelioid cells
(▼) with scattered mast cells in both groups. Edge of an egg (E).

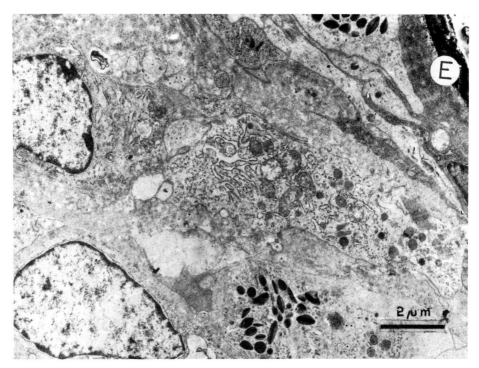

Fig. 2 The edge of an egg (E) surrounded by activated macrophages
and eosinophils with mature appearing granules (x 9.000).

pigs (2) because epithelioid cells with large ovoid nuclei were

readily recognized in the lesions. Ultrastructural observations

confirmed the cell types present in the granulomas (Fig.2). The

cells were tightly packed and cell borders invaginated. Activated

macrophages showed endoplasmic reticulum, with few lysozomal

bodies (Fig.3 A,B). This is thought to be part of the process of

epithelioid cell differentiation. Epithelioid cells may associate

with cell mediated immunity (5). Suya et al (1) detected recovery

in IL-2 activity and mitogen response of regional lymph nodes and

spleen cells in mice after granuloma grafts, despite continued Cs

therapy. Since Cs-insensitive T-cell subsets seem to exist (6),

epithelioid cells may stimulate this T-cell subset. We conclude

that granuloma initiation occurs in the absence of classic T-cell

694

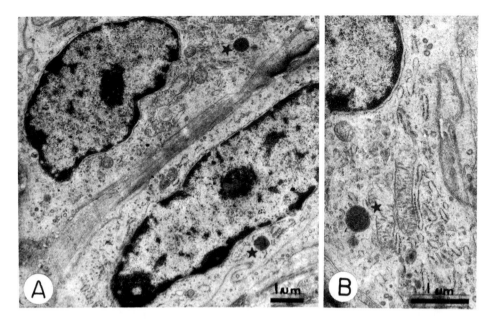

Fig. 3 A,B (A) Two cells revealing characteristics of activated macrophages (x 9.000). (B) Higher power (x 15.000) of a dense body (★) and well developed rough endoplasmic reticulum indicates capacity for phagocytosis and secretory activity, respectively.

function and that the developing granulomas may influence host T-cell function which then help to form organized granulomas.

ACKNOWLEDGMENT

This study was supported by a NIH grant AM.

REFERENCES

1. Suya H., Fujioka A., Pincelli C., Epstein W.L.,(1987) J.Invest. Dermatol.,(submitted).

2. Nishimura M., Higuchi M., Fukuyama K., Epstein W.L.(1985) Arch. Dermatol. Res.,278:61-67.

3. Gupta S.K., Curtis J., Turk J.L.(1985),Cell. Immunol.,93:189-198

4. Epstein W.L., Okamoto M., Suya H., Fukuyama K.(1986/1987) Immunol. Letters,14:59-63.

5. Turk J.L.(1980), J.Invest. Dermatol.,74:301-306.

6. Klausg. G.G.B., Kunkl A.,(1983) Transplantation,36:80-84.

© 1988 Elsevier Science Publishers B.V. (Biomedical Division)
Sarcoidosis and other granulomatous disorders
C. Grassi, G. Rizzato, E. Pozzi, editors

ASSOCIATION OF PULMONARY TUBERCULOSIS AND CROHN'S DISEASE

G.M. MASSAGLIA, A.ARDIZZI, S.BARBERIS, F.GALIETTI, G.E.GIORGIS,
C.MIRAVALLE, P.C.GIAMESIO.
V° DIV.OSP.S.LUIGI GONZAGA ORBASSANO (TORINO) PRIM. DOTT.U.FERRARO

INTRODUCTION

Since the identification of Crohn's disease several pathogenetic
hypothesis have been suggested. Some which included infection
factors:bacterial and viral agents. The pathogenetic possibility
of mycobacteria has been also underlined because of a Crohn like
disease (granulomatous ileitis of ruminants) is due to mycobacterium paratubercolosis. In 1978 Burnham and Lennard obtained a positive culture for M.Kansasii after incubation period of eight months
in one patient with Crohn's disease. Such finding was not confirmed
by others researches. In 1981 White was able to show micolic acid
and acid fast material in cultures of limpho nodes in a percentual
> 50% of patients with Crohn's disease. In 1984 Chiodini repeatedly
obtained, after 3-18 months, the growth of previous unclassified
mycobacteria from bioptic material which inoculated in goats yelded
granulomatous ileitis' patterns. In a following search Thayer found
by ELISA, the presence of antibodies versus a mycobacterial antigen
higher in patients with Crohn's disease than in patients with ulcerative colitis. We decided to contribute to the study of this subject on the clinical background according to Warren's previous reports (I986).

MATERIAL AND METHODS

Data are presented on 7 cases (5 males, 2 females, aged 37-52, mean
age 45.14) with combined Crohn's disease and pulmonary tubercolosis
obseved in 1981-1985. The tubercolosis was nodular in 5 cases, mili
ary in 1 and caused by specific pleuritis in 1. In all cases the
clinical onset of Crohn's disease preceded the TB by 8 months to 2
years. In 3 casea Koch bacilli were not found in direct and cultural
examination of intestinal bioptic material. Before TB was identified
treatment with sulfasalazine gave satisfactory clinical and endo-

scopic results in 2 subjects, poor in 3 and nil in 2. After diagno+
sis of TB, RAMP/INH/EMB was added to treatment in 4 cases and RAMP/
INH/SM/MZA in 3. One patient died a few weeks after admission by
peritonitis complicating Crohn's disease. In the remaining cases
the TB was clinically and radiologically stabilised in 6-8 months.
It is noteworthy that the improvement in the TB was matched by clinical,endoscopic and histological improvement of Crohn's disease in
4 cases in whom there has been no relapses in either the specific
form or the Crohn's disease in an 8-34 month follow up.

CONCLUSION

Our findings may confirm the hypothesis that some cases of Crohn's
disease are microbacterial in haetiology.

REFERENCES

1) BURNHAM WR: Mycobacteria as a possible cause of inflammatory
            bowel disease Lancet 2:693-696,1978

2) CHIODINI RJ: Possible role of mycobacteria in inflammatory bowel
              disease. An unclassified Mycobacterium species iso-
              lated from patients with Crohn's disease.Digestive
              and Sciences 1984,29,1073

3) PATTERSON DSP: Chronic mycobacterial enteritis in ruminants on a
              model of Crohn's disease Proc. R. Soc. Med.,
              65:998-1001,1972

4) THAYER WR : Possible role of mycobacteria in inflammatory bowel
              disease.Mycobacterial antibodies in Crohn's disease;
              Digestive disease and Sciences 1984,29,1080

5) WARREN JB :Remission of Crohn's disease with TB chemotherapy
              New England J.Med. 16,182,1986

6) WHITE SA: Investigation into the density of acid fast organisms
              located from Crohn's disease. The Hague Niihoff Publi-
              shers,1981, pp. 278-282

© 1988 Elsevier Science Publishers B.V. (Biomedical Division)
Sarcoidosis and other granulomatous disorders
C. Grassi, G. Rizzato, E. Pozzi, editors

THE INFLUENCE OF ANABOLIC STEROIDS DURING THE COURSE OF TREATMENT
FOR TUBERCULOSIS.

G.D. RENZI, P.M. RENZI, S. SEKELY, V. LOPEZ MAJANO, P.J. FEUSTEL
AND R.E. DUTTON.
Notre-Dame and St. Luc Hospitals, Montréal, Canada. A.G. Holley
State Hospital, Florida, Cook County Hospital, Chicago and Rensse-
laer Polytechnic Institute, Troy New York, U.S.A.

INTRODUCTION

Definition of problem: Active tuberculosis (TB) affects lung
parenchyma and airways to variable degrees depending on the extent
and severity of the disease. Many TB patients suffer from malnutrition and alcoolism and these conditions will lead to weight loss
with cachexia. Malnutrition may contribute to the decline in respiratory function & respiratory muscle strength and endurance (1, 2,).

Background: Androgens are active in the regulation of muscle
development in relation to their anticatabolic activity in preventing muscle atrophy and to their anabolic activity in stimulating
growth. They also have a tissue building action and can regulate
certain conditions charactarized by protein wastage and negative
nitrogen balance leading to weight loss. (3, 4,).

Object: The object of this study was to determine if anabolic
steroids correct the nutritional components as well as improve
pulmonary function and respiratory muscle force in active TB.

METHODS

We evaluated two groups of male tuberculosis patients on admission and after 4 to 6 months of anti-Tb treatment (cf table 1).
Initial and final evaluation included serum albumin, chest Xray,
spirometry with measurement of forced vital capacity (FVC) & forced
expiratory volume in 1 second (FEV$_1$). Respiratory muscle strength
was obtained using an anaeroid manometer calibrated in cmH$_2$O. We
measured maximal inspiratory mouth pressure (PI MAX) maximal expiratory mouth pressure (PE MAX) and the addition of both (P TOT MAX).

Group AS (23 male subjects) received dianabol 5 mg/die in addition to the anti-Tb treatment. Group NAS (18 male patients) served
as controls during their anti-Tb treatment. Both groups were statistically comparable except for a slightly more decreased observed
FVC in the AS group, but the % predicted FVC were not different.

TABLE 1. Anthropometric Characteristics and Initial Data in 23 male Tb patients receiving anti-Tb treatment and anabolic steroids (AS) compared to 18 male Tb patients with only anti-Tb treatment (NAS).

	AS (MEAN + SEM)		NAS (MEAN + SEM)		SIGNIFICANCE (a)
Age (years)	46.8	2.2	42	2.8	NS
Weight (lbs)	118.0	4.1	121	3.6	NS
Serum albumin (g/dl)	2.7	0.12	2.9	0.15	NS
FVC (Obs. 1)	2.75	0.16	3.2	0.15	$p < .05$
FVC (% of predicted)	64	3.6	70	3.9	NS
FEV_1/FVC (%)	68.9	2.5	70.9	2.3	NS
PI MAX (cmH_2O)	41.3	2.3	48.7	3.4	NS
PE MAX (cmH_2O)	57.7	2.9	62.7	3.5	NS
P TOT MAX (cmH_2O)	99	5.1	111	6.3	NS

(a) Significance was determined using Student's t test.

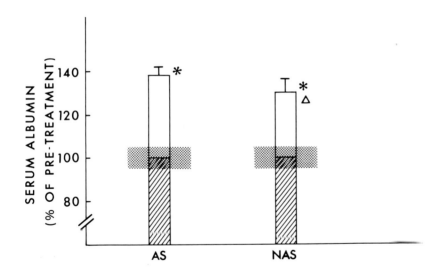

Fig. 1. Serum albumin before (⧄) and after (▭) tuberculosis treatment with anabolic steroids (AS) or without anabolic steroids (NAS). ▨ = 1 standard error of mean (SEM) pre treatment. * = p <0.05 before vs after Tb treatment. △: p= not significant AS vs NAS post treatment.

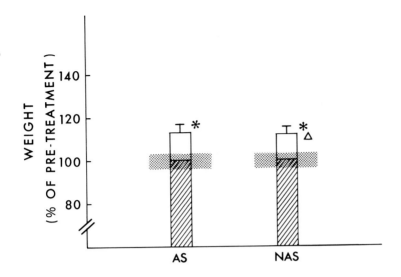

Fig. 2. Weight before (▨) and after (☐) Tb treatment with (AS) or without (NAS). ▨ equals 1 SEM pre treatment. * = p<0.05 before vs after Tb treatment. △: p = not significant AS vs NAS post treatment.

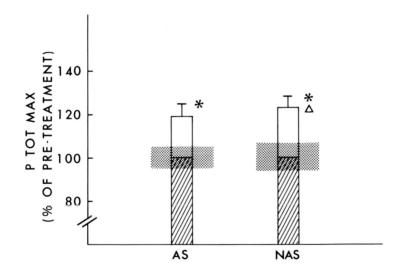

Fig. 3. P TOT MAX (PI MAX = PE MAX) before (▨) and after (☐) Tb treatment with (AS) or without (NAS). ▨ equals 1 SEM pre treatment. * = p<0.05 before vs after Tb treatment. △: p not significant AS vs NAS post treatment.

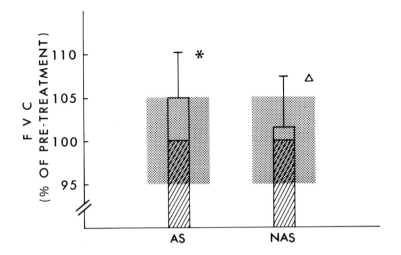

Fig. 4.   FVC before (/////) and after (⬜) Tb treatment with
(AS) or without (NAS). ▨▨ equals 1 SEM pre treatment.
* = p <0.05 before vs after Tb treatment. △ : p not significant
AS vs NAS post treatment.

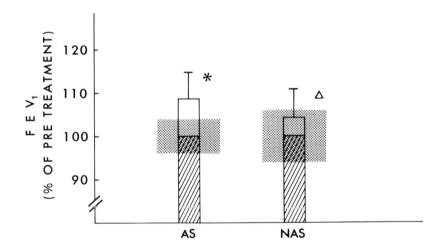

Fig. 5. FEV_1 before (/////) and after (⬜) Tb treatment with
(AS) or without (NAS). ▨▨ Equals 1 SEM pre treatment.
* = p <0.05 before vs after Tb treatment. △ : p not significant
AS vs NAS post treatment.

CONCLUSIONS

1. Serum albumin improves significantly after anti-tuberculous treatment and returns to the lower limits of normal.
2. Weight and respiratory muscle force also improve significantly with anti-Tb treatment but do not return to normal values.
3. Anabolic steroids do not have a positive additive effect on serum albumin, weight and respiratory muscle strength.
4. FVC and FEV_1 increase significantly compared to the control TB group, when anabolic steroids are added to the anti-tuberculous treatment.

REFERENCES

1. Arora NS, Rochester DF (1982) Respiratory muscle strength and maximal voluntary ventilation in undernourished patients. In: Am Rev Respir Dis 126:5-8
2. Renzi G, Renzi P, Feustel P, Dutton R (1985) The influence of weight on exercise limitation in COLD. In: Am Rev Respir Dis 131:A353
3. Hickson R, Davis J (1981) Partial prevention of Glucocorticoid induced muscle atrophy by endurance training. In: Am J Physiol 241:E226-232
4. Evans W, Ivy J (1982) Effects of testosterone proprionate on hindlimb immobilized rats. In: J Appl Physiol 52:1643-1647

© 1988 Elsevier Science Publishers B.V. (Biomedical Division)
Sarcoidosis and other granulomatous disorders
C. Grassi, G. Rizzato, E. Pozzi, editors

STUDIES ON ANTIGENS AND CELLULAR COMPONENTS IN BRONCHOALVEOLAR LAVAGE FLUID
WITH HYPERSENSITIVITY PNEUMONITIS

HITOSHI GEMMA, ATSUHIKO SATO, KINGO CHIDA, MASATOSHI IWATA, IZUMI SHICHI

The Second Department of Internal Medicine, Hamamatsu University School of
Medicine, 3600 Handa-cho, Hamamatsu, 431-31 (Japan)

INTRODUCTION

Hypersensitivity pneumonitis (HP) is an interstitial lung disease which
occurs after exposure to a variety of environmental antigens. Recent studies
have revealed that neutrophil chemotactic factor is potent in bronchoalveolar
lavage fluid (BALF) in patients with HP acute phase[1], and neutrophil increments
in BALF after inhalation challenge[2]. The purpose of this study is to examine
the time course of cellular components in BALF with HP.

MATERIALS AND METHODS

Subjects

21 patients with HP(20 cases biopsy proven, 1 case clinically diagnosed, 11
men and 10 women, mean age 51 years, range from 26 to 70).

Double immunodiffusion and counter immunoelectrophoresis

Sera from 20 patients were tested for precipitins to 18 kinds of antigens.

Bronchoalveolar lavage

BAL was performed at least one time in 15 patients after avoiding further
exposure to antigens.

Environmental challenge test

Four patients were exposed to the presumptive causative environments for 5
hours through 2 days. In all of the 4 patients, the environmental challenge
tests were positive. BAL was performed in the 4 patients within 24 hours after
challenge test.

RESULTS

In 18 out of studied 20 cases, one serum specific precipitins or more were
detected. Results of the positive cases were as follows : i) A. fumigatus, 8
cases ii) Tr. cataneum, 4 cases iii) Budgerigar droppings, 3 cases iv) Pegeon
droppings, 2 cases v) Paddy-bird droppings, 1 case vi) S. granarius, 1 case vii)
other fungi, 7 cases. Five out of 7 cases of group vii also presented anti-A.
fumigatus precipitins.

The BALF lymphocytes % ranged from 21.6 to 89.2 (mean 51.3±21.2) and showed
decrease tendencies after avoiding exposure(Fig.1-A). The mean value of
neutrophil % in BALF was 3.0±5.0. More interesting, in one case which BAL was
performed on the next day of his admission, the neutrophils accounted for 20 %

(Fig.1-B). The OKT4/OKT8 ratios of BALF lymphocytes ranged from 0.05 to 7.03, and there was no relationship between the ratios and the time after admission (Fig.1-C).

In all of the 4 cases challenged by the causative environments, BALF neutrophils were above 20 % (mean 39.7 %)(Fig.2).
In the repeated BAL in 3 out of these 4 cases after 4 days through 20 days, the neutrophil increments were not shown.

DISCUSSION

In the precipitin survey of these 20 cases, 8 cases showed anti-A. fumigatus antibody. Moreover, inhalation challenge of A. fumigatus was positive in one case. These results suggest that A. fumigatus may be one of the potent causative antigens in HP.

Our study demonstrated early and transient BALF neutrophil increments. These data support the concept that the earliest lesion in HP is neutrophil alveolitis[2].

Furthermore, a variety of lymphocytes OKT4/OKT8 ratios were presented, and there was no relationship between the ratios and the time after avoiding exposure. From these results, it seems that the local lymphocytic responses in HP varied according to each exposure pattern, quality and quantity of antigens.

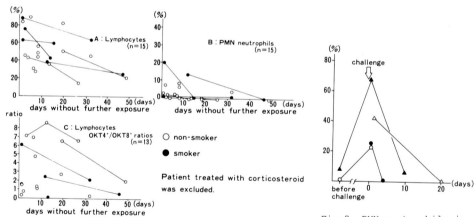

Fig.1 BALF findigs after avoiding exposure.

Fig.2 PMN neutrophils in BALF before and after environmental challenge.

References
1. Yoshizawa,Y. Ohdama,S. Tanoue,M. et al : Analysis of bronchoalveolar lavage cells and fluids in patients with hypersensitivity pneumonitis : possible role of chemotactic factors in the pathogenesis of disease. Int. Arch. Allergy Appl. Immunol. 80 : 376, 1986
2. Fournier,E. Tonnel,A.B. Wallaert,B. et al : Early neutrophil alveolitis after antigen inhalation in hypersensitivity pneumonitis. Chest 88 : 563, 1985

CYTOTOXIC MECHANISMS IN THE LUNG OF PATIENTS WITH HYPERSENSITIVITY PNEUMONITIS.

TRENTIN L[*], ZAMBELLO R, FESTI G, BIZZOTTO R, LUCA M, AGOSTINI C.

Departments of Clinical Medicine, Clinical Immunology, Pneumology and Occupational Medicine, Padua University, Italy.

INTRODUCTION

Cell immunoregulation seems to play an important role in the pathogenesis of hypersensitivity pneumonitis (HP). It has been demonstrated that the alveolitis in these patients is supported by the expansion of CD2+/CD3+/CD8+ cells (1-3). In addition, recent observations pointed out the presence in HP lung of increased numbers of cells bearing cytotoxic related markers which might represent a defensive mechanism to foreign antigens (3).

To better define the nature of cytotoxic mechanisms present in the lung of HP patients, in this study we evaluated the activity of lymphocytes recovered from the bronchoalveolar lavage fluid (BAL) in resting conditions and after in vitro boosting with interleukin-2 (IL-2) against NK-sensitive targets, NK-resistant targets and antigen (Micropolyspora faeni) sensitized autologous monocytes.

MATERIALS AND METHODS

Patients Five symptomatic HP patients were studied. The diagnosis was based on criteria usually reported (4). All patients were non smokers and were studied for at least 1 month after the last acute episode. They had never received therapy. Cytotoxic in vitro assay BAL cells were obtained as previously described (3,5). Effector cells were tested in resting conditions and after in vitro activation for 72 hrs with recombinant interleukin-2 (IL-2, 100 U/ml), for the generation of lymphokine activated killer (LAK) cells, against different targets: NK-sensitive (K-562), NK-resistant (Daudi) and autologous monocytes previously sensitized for 7 days with specific antigen (Micropolyspora faeni, 125μgr/ml/0.5 x 10^6 cells). Cytotoxic tests were assessed and the percent of specific lysis was calculated as previously reported (3).

RESULTS AND DISCUSSION

As shown in Figure 1, at resting conditions, cells obtained from BAL of our HP patients displayed cytotoxic in vitro activity against NK-sensitive targets and were also able to kill the NK-resistant targets. When BAL cells were tested against specific sensitized autologous monocytes, we did not find any lytic activity. Moreover, when BAL cells were activated in vitro with IL-2, an increase of cytotoxic function was demonstrated not only against K-562 targets but also versus Daudi targets.

Milan prize winner for authors under 35 years.

706

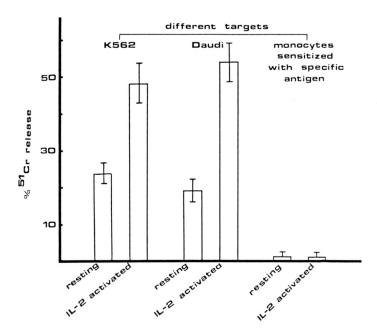

Figure 1. Cytotoxic activity of HP BAL lymphocytes at resting conditions,after in in vitro boosting with IL-2 against different targets. E/T=80/1. Mean ± SE.

These findings substantiate the idea that,other than NK cells (1,3),additional cytotoxic mechanisms are involved in HP lung, such as non-MHC-restricted cyto- toxic T lymphocytes, including LAK cells. The involvement of LAK cells in the lung of these patients is supported by the demonstration of an increased lytic function against NK-resistant targets after in vitro boosting with IL-2. The demonstration of a lytic activity, at resting conditions, versus Daudi targets suggests the hypothesis that BAL lymphocytes had been previously   activated in vivo by lymphokines.

The involvement of different types of cytotoxic cells in the lung of HP patients may help to understand the mechanisms by which the host reacts against the stimulus provided by inhaled antigens.

REFERENCES

1. Leatherman MD, Michael AF, Schwartz BA, Hoidal JR (1984)Ann Intern Med 100:390
2. Costabel U, Bross KJ, Marxen J, Matthys H (1984) Chest 85:514
3. Semenzato G, Agostini C, Zambello R, Trentin L, Chilosi M, Pizzolo G, Marcer G, Cipriani A (1986) J Immunol 137:1164
4. Fink JN (1984) J Allergy Clin Immunol 74:1
5. Semenzato G, Chilosi M, Ossi E, Trentin L, Pizzolo G, Cipriani A, Agostini C, Zambello R, Marcer G, Gasparotto G (1985) Am Rev Respir Dis 132:400

© 1988 Elsevier Science Publishers B.V. (Biomedical Division)
Sarcoidosis and other granulomatous disorders
C. Grassi, G. Rizzato, E. Pozzi, editors

RESPIRATORY DISTRESS FROM MULTIPLE STENOSIS OF THE TRACHEAL AND OF THE BRONCHIAL TREE DURING SYSTEMIC VASCULITIS.

FRANCOIS FORTIN (1), FREDERIC BART (1), JEAN MARC DEGREEF (1), BERNARD GOSSELIN (2), JEAN JACQUES LAFITTE (1)

(1) Département de Pneumologie (2) Laboratoire d'Anatomie et de Cytologie Pathologique, Hôpital A. Calmette, Lille (FRANCE).

Wegener's granulomatosis is characterized by a necrotizing granulomatous vasculitis of the upper and the lower airways together with glomerulonephritis. Subglottic tracheal stenosis are commun, stenosis of the lower respiratory tract are unfrequent and often difficult to manage (1).

CASE REPORT

A 38 yr old male patient was first admitted in 1978 because of loss of weight, facial nerve palsy, purpuric skin lesions, elevated blood pressure and multinevritis. Laboratory investigations showed inflammatory syndrome, normal renal function and no Hbs antigen. Multiple aneurysms were found on renal and coelio-mesenteric arteriography. Renal and skin biopsies yielded vascular lesions compatible with a polyarteritis nodosa. A treatment associating Prednisone (1 mg/kg/day) and Cyclophosphamide (1 mg/kg/day) was initiated; Evolution was favorable. In September 1985 the patient referred because of fever, dyspnea and rhinosinusitis. Chest roentgenogram revealed pulmonary infiltrates and cavitations of the left lower lobe. Fiberoptic bronchoscopy showed a subglottic stenosis and a milder one on the right upper bronchus. Bronchial biopsy yielded gigantocellular granulomatosis without caseum necrosis. Prednisone and Cyclophosphamide were not disrupted. 4 months later dyspnea increased with hemoptysis; chest roentgenogram was unchanged, fiberoptic bronchoscopic examination and inhalation bronchography showed an increase of the subglottic stenosis and the occurence of other stenosis on the right and left main bronchi (figure 1).

Cotrimoxazole (40 mg/kg/day) caused a reduction of the cavitation but was ineffective on the stenosis. Transient improvement was obtained after repeated bronchoscopic dilatation of the subglottic stenosis. An irreversible respiratory distress secondary to the narrowing of the main bronchi occured.

708

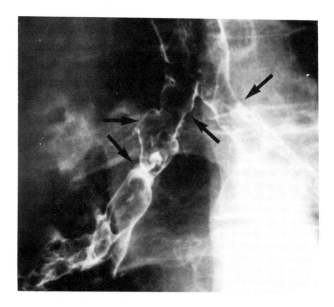

Fig 1 : Inhalation bronchography : stenosis of the two main bronchi, the upper lobe bronchus and the intermediate bronchus.

DISCUSSION

This case illustrates the severity and difficulty of management of multiple stenosis of the lower respiratory tract no responsive to cytotoxic therapy in Wegener's granulomatosis. Subglottic stenosis are accessible to bronchoscopic dilatation and isolated bronchial stenosis to sleeve ressection. Multiple stenosis are still therapic challenge and were not improved by Cotrimoxazole in our case (2). This problem is becoming more frequent because of the improved survival of patients on cytotoxic therapy.

REFERENCES

1) Flye MW, Mundinger GH, Fauci AS (1979). Diagnostic and therapeutic aspects of the surgical approach to Wegener's granulomatosis. J Thorac Cardiovasc Surg 77 : 331 - 337

2) De Remee R, Mc Donald TJ, Weiland LH (1985). Wegener's Granulomatosis on Treatment with anti microbial agents. Mayo Clin Proc 60 : 27 - 32

© 1988 Elsevier Science Publishers B.V. (Biomedical Division)
Sarcoidosis and other granulomatous disorders
C. Grassi, G. Rizzato, E. Pozzi, editors

PNEUMOCONIOSIS CAUSED BY HARD METALS. A CASE SERIES.

G.M. MASSAGLIA°,G. AVOLIO°°,S.BARBERIS°,M. CACCIABUE°°,F. GALIETTI°
G.E. GIORGIS°,C.MIRAVALLE°
° V° DIV.OSP.S. LUIGI GONZAGA ORBASSANO (TORINO) PRIM. DOTT. U.
FERRARO °°Inail Sede Provinciale di Torino

INTRODUCTION
As lung disease caused by hard metals has aroused growing interest
due to the increasing use of these substances (cobalt and metallic
carbides) in various technologies, we decided to give our contribute to the study of such a pathology showing our data.

MATERIAL AND METHOD
The 8 patients studied (6 males and 2 females) were aged 40-64 (mean
57.25). Exposure to inhalation of the pahogen came from employment
in the production of hard metals (sintetitation) in 1 case and in
their processing or use (milling,turning,grinding) in 7.Three
patients reported dyspnoic attacks at work. At diagnonsis the radiological picture showed disseminated roundish (micronodular or nodular) patches of opacity in 5 cases, irregular in 3. In functional
terms 3 cases presented ventilatory restriction, 2 obstruction and
3 both. A cobalt patch test was performed on 5 and was positive
(delayed response) in2. At diagnosis 4 patients were subjected to
fiberoptic bronchoscopy with BAL and 3 to tranbronchial biopsy
as well. The test showed a modest increase in total cell count
(mean $2.98 \pm 0.63 \times 10^5$ cell) with an increase in neutrophilis
(mean 8.2%) and lymphocytes (mean 10.4%). Study of lymphocytes subpopulations showed increased T_{11} (mean 81.34%) and a decreased
T_4/T_8 ratio (mean 1.38%) due to an increase in T_8. Biopsy revealed
immune-type interstitial granulomatosis, reaching an advanced
fibrosing stage in 1 case.

CONCLUSION

The data of our study confirm the points of view of international
literature. It seems very interesting to us that the findings
acquired by BAL are similar to the pneumoconiosis (because of increasing neuttrphilis) and, on the other hand, to the extrinsic
allergic alveolitis (because of increasing lymphocytes and reduction of T_4/T_8 Ratio for increasing T_8). In our casistic, according
to others studies, a further element of analogy with extrinsic allergic alveolitis is the possibility of a regression of the clini-
cal-roentgengraphic pattern following the removal of the patients
from exposure.The cobalt test (performed as this metal is the
greater responsable of this lung disease) is positive index of
sensibilitation rather than of disease.

TABLE 1: TOTAL CELL COUNT (IN 4 PATIENTS WITH BAL)

T.C.C.	N	L	T_{11}	T_4	T_8	T_4/T_8
3.07×10^5	12	6	76	75	59	1.26
2.64 "	6	14	88	70	49	1.42
3.35 "	10	9	69	81	51	1.59
2.87 "	5	13	84	69	54	1.28

REFERENCES

1) DAVISON AG : Interstitial lung disease and asthma in hard
letal workers: bronchoalveolar lavage, ultrastructural and analytical findings and results of
bronchial provocation tests . Thorax 1983,38:119-28

2) SIEGESMUND KA: Identification of metals in lung from a patient
with interstitial pneumonia. Arch. Environ .
HEALTH 28 (1974) 345-349

3) KITAMURA : Effects of cemented tungsten carbide dust on rat
lungs following intratracheal injection of salme
suspension Acta Pathol. Jap. 1980; 30:241-53

4) SJOGREN I : Hard metal lung disease: importance of cobalt in
coolants Thorax 1980;35:653-59

5) HARTUNG M : On the question of the pathogenetic importance of
cobalt for hard metal fibrosis of the lung Int.
Arch. Occup. Environ Health 1982; 50:53-7

6) HILLERDAL G : On cobalt in tissues from hard metal workers
Int. Arch. Occup.Environ Health 1983; 53:89-90

7) KONIETZKO H : Lungenfibrosen bei der Bearbeitung von Hartmetal-
len Dtsch. Med. Wschr. 105 (1980)120-123

8) HARTUNG M : Aktuelle aspekte zur anerkennung einer Hartmetall-
fibrose der lunge als berufdkrankheitIn: Bericht
über die 21 Jahrestagung der Deutschen Gesellschaft
für arbeitsmedizin e.V. Berlin, 13-16 Mai 1981,A.W.
Gentner Verlag, im Druck

© 1988 Elsevier Science Publishers B.V. (Biomedical Division)
Sarcoidosis and other granulomatous disorders
C. Grassi, G. Rizzato, E. Pozzi, editors

CHARACTERISTICS OF THE LYMPHOCYTARY ALVEOLITIS OF SARCOIDOSIS AND MINERAL DUST INHALATION INDUCED PULMONARY GRANULOMATOSIS

A. Teles de Araújo, Ana Cristina Mendes, Jorge Tomás Monteiro, M. Freitas e Costa
- Clínica Doenças Pulmonares - FML and CnL3 INIC - 1699 LISBOA CODEX

INTRODUCTION

The infiltration of the alveolar structures by mononucleated cells - alveolitis - is one of the most common demonstrations of Pulmonary Sarcoidosis (3,4).

In our experience in numerous patients with Mineral Dust Inhalation Induced Pulmonary Granulomatosis (MIPG) it is also possible to evidence the existence of a lymphocytary alveolitis, either through pulmonary biopsy, or through broncho -alveolar lavage (1,2).

The OBJECTIVE of this paper is to study by broncho-alveolar lavage some of the characteristics of the lymphocytary populations of these two types of alveolitis, searching to receive deductions for the pathogenesis of these diseases.

MATERIAL AND METHODS

Seven normal volunteers (average age: 40.5 $\pm$ 10.2), 12 patients with Sarcoidosis histologically demonstrated (average age: 42.5 $\pm$ 14.7) and 22 patients with MIPG histologically demonstrated (average age: 42.6 $\pm$ 11.7) were studied. In the latter group 5 had silicosis, 6 siderosis and 11 had diseases caused by other mineral dusts.

All of them were submitted to a broncho-alveolar lavage with a fiberscope wedged in a medium lobe subsegment and instillations of three to four 50 ml fractions of saline heated to 37°C followed by a gentle aspiration with a syringe, 2 or 3 seconds afterwards.

The cellular counting was carried out and the preparation of cytocentrifuge slides dyed with May-Grunwald-Giemsa for differential cellular counting.

The lymphocytary subpopulations were studied by indirect imunofluorescence after the demarcation of a suspension of 1 x 10^6 cel./ml with monoclonal antibodies OKT_3, OKT_4 and OKT_8.

The statistical study was carried out by Student's t test.

RESULTS

In table I becames evident a significative increase in the number of broncho- -alveolar lavage cells, lymphocytes and T-lymphocytes in both groups of patients.

Moreover a significative increase in T_4 + cells, in Sarcoidosis, and in T_8 + + cells, in MIPG, must be stressed.

TABLE I

NUMBER OF CELLS/ML X 10^4

	TOTAL	MA	LY	PMN	T3	T4	T8	T4/T8
CONTROLS N= 7	16.7±3.8	14.3±2.1	1.3±0.3	0.22±0.5	1.0±0.5	0.8±0.1	0.5±0.2	1.7±0.2
SARCOIDOSIS N= 12	32.5±16.2	18.6±11.7	12.8±10.2	0.90±1.0	10.8±9.0	8.6±7.2	2.2±1.9	3.9±1.1
M.I.P.G. N= 22	33.4±35.9	18.4±10.9	13.7±29.7	1.0±1.6	10.0±20.9	3.2±4.5	6.8±16.5	0.7±0.3

In table II demonstrates that there is not any difference in the characteristics of the T-lymphocytary alveolitis among the subgroups of MIPG considered.

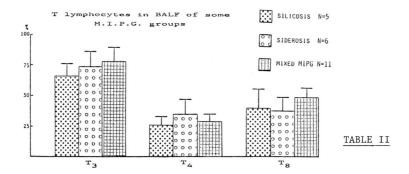

TABLE II

DISCUSSIONS AND CONCLUSIONS

The cellularity study of the broncho-alveolar lavage fluid in these two groups of patients demonstrates an increase of cellularity in both, predominantly caused by a rise of the T-lymphocytes. Thus the existence of an alveolitis lymphocytary T, either in one group or the other, is confirmed.

This alveolitis suggests an activation of the imunological mechanisms. The values discovered are more constant in the Sarcoidosis than in the MIPG, in which the activity of the illness is extremely variable, expressing itself through the intensity of the alveolitis (3).

In the Sarcoidosis the lymphocytary subpopulations shows a predominance of T helpers in the broncho-alveolar lavage and this fact seems to be in the center of the pathogenic mechanisms of the illness, conditioning the histological and clinical manifestations (3,4).

In the MIPG there is an increase in the T_4 + and in the T_8 +, although with predominance of the latter. These facts suggest an attempt to moderate the local imunological procedure, caused, directly or indirectly, by the inhaled particle. The absence of differences between the considered subgroups points in the direction of those modifications translating a similar response in the organism, whatever the aggressive particle.

The existence of the two different types of alveolitis, in the Sarcoidosis and in the MIPG, indicates the existence of different pathogenical pathways in these two situations.

REFERENCES

1. Araújo, A.T.; Alfarroba, E.; Freitas e Costa, M.: "The Role of Monoclonal Antibodies in the Study of Chronic Inflamatory Respiratory Diseases Induced by Dust Inhalation" - Eur. J. Resp. Dis. 1986; 69 (Suppl.146): 201-210.

2. Freitas e Costa, M.; Araújo, A.T.: "Le Fibrosi Polmonari" - Federazioni Medica 1983; 36 = 859-870.

3. Reynolds, H.Y.; Chrétien, J.: "Respiratory Tract Fluids: Analysis of Content and Contemporary Use in Understanding Lung Diseases" - Year Book Med. Publ. Inc. Chicago, 1984.

4. Semenzato, G.: "Immunology of Sarcoidosis" - State of the Art. Proceedings of the IV European Conference on Sarcoidosis and other Granulomatous Disorders: Ed. A. Blasi, D. Olivieri, A. Pezza - Sorrento 1983: 21-36.

Sarcoidosis and other granulomatous disorders
C. Grassi, G. Rizzato, E. Pozzi, editors

PULMONARY INJURY FROM SILICA DUST EVALUATED WITH BRONCHO-ALVEOLAR LAVAGE (BAL)

MIRCO LUSUARDI, ELISA L.SPADA, ARMANDO CAPELLI, ALBERTO BRAGHIROLI, SERGIO ZACCARIA, CLAUDIO F.DONNER

Division of Pulmonary Diseases, "Clinica del Lavoro" Foundation, Institute of Care and Research, Medical Center of Rehabilitation VERUNO (Novara) - Italy

INTRODUCTION

Pulmonary alveoli are the main site of damage caused by silica dust inhalation. BAL adequately samples alveolar lining fluid, so permitting an accurate knowledge of cytologic and biochemical modifications occurring in different pathological conditions affecting the lower respiratory tract. The aim of our study was to assess if BAL can provide cytologic and biochemical data characteristic of pulmonary injury caused by silica dust inhalation.

SUBJECTS AND METHODS

16 patients affected by silicosis (8 nonsmokers, 59 ± 10yr, and 8 smokers, 57 ± 12 yr) and 29 healthy control subjects (13 nonsmokers, 32 ± 15yr and 16 smokers, 39 ± 9yr) were submitted to BAL. Cytologic analysis consisted of total cellularity and single cell fraction determination with the Burker chamber and the May-Grunwald-Giemsa technique respectively. Biochemical analysis consisted of total protein and main protein fraction dosage with the Lowry and the radial immunodiffusion methods respectively. Silicon content of cells was determined by energy dispersive X-ray microanalysis. All the data are expressed as mean $\pm$ standard deviation.

RESULTS

Total cells do not show significant variations between silicotic and the respective control groups (185 ± 56 x 10^3/ml vs 326 ± 335 x 10^3/ml for nonsmoker, 495 ± 226 x 10^3/ml vs 429 ± 192 x 10^3/ml for smokers). So it is for macrophages: 162 ± 53 vs 302 ± 339 x 10^3/ml for nonsmokers and 453 ± 204 vs 372 ± 187 x 10^3/ml for smokers. The most interesting cytologic data are represented by a significant lymphocyte increase in nonsmoker silicotics (33.4 ± 22.2 x 10^3/ml) in comparison with the respective controls (16.2 ± 7.7 x 10^3/ml, $p<0.02$). Smoker controls (27 ± 29 x 10^3/ml) and smoker silicotics (34.5 ± 18.1 x 10^3/ml) do not show significant variations in lymphocyte count. Neutrophils are significantly increased both in nonsmoker silicotics (13.3 ± 17.7 x 10^3/ml vs 1.7 ± 1.6 x 10^3/ml, $p<0.025$) and in smoker silicotics (15.2 ± 17.6 x 10^3/ml vs 3.7 ± 4.1 x

10^3/ml, p< 0.02). On the contrary, eosinophils do not differ appreciably between the compared groups: 0.6+0.6 vs 0.5+0.3 x 10^3/ml for nonsmoker controls and silicotics, 1.14+0.93 vs 1.5+1.7 x 10^3/ml for smoker controls and silicotics respectively.

Biochemical analysis show a slight but significant total protein increase in silicotics (16.0+4.6mg%ml, nonsmokers; 17.1+3.1mg%ml, smokers) compared to controls (10.5+2.8 and 12.4+3.4mg%ml respectively, both p< 0.01). No differences are found in main protein components (albumin, IgG, IgA, α1-antitrypsin, -table 1-) with the ex-ception for IgG which are significantly higher in smoker silicotics (IgG/Albumin=0.46+ 0.19) in comparison to nonsmoker silicotics (0.24+0.16, p< 0.025), who have, in their turn, higher IgG levels than nonsmoker controls (0.12+0.09, p< 0.05).

Cellular silicon content, expressed as silicon/sulphur (Si/S) ratio, shows a highly significant increase between silicotics and the respective controls (Si/S=1.53+0.7 vs 0.6+0.1, p< 0.001 for nonsmokers, Si/S=1.34+0.7 vs 0.6+0.2, p< 0.001 for smokers).

CONCLUSIONS

1) In nonsmoker silicotics BAL reveals a slight intensity lymphocytic increase; 2) both in smoker and nonsmoker silicotics an apparently marked neutrophilic alveolitis is found, but it is quite difficult to establish the component, which is surely important , due to the concomitant chronic airway flogosis; 3) silicosis is associated with an absolute IgG increase, particularly enhanced if tabagism cohexists; 4) charac-teristic alveolar modifications, useful for the diagnosis of silicosis, do not seem there-fore to exist, with the exception of the mineralogic/elemental analysis on cells, which may help in the case of doubtful exposure case history.

TABLE I

Main protein fractions in BAL fluids from nonsmoker and smoker silicotics compared with nonsmoker and smoker healthy controls respectively. Mean $\pm$ standard deviation (in brackets). For statistical comparison (t-test) see text.

	NONSMOKER CONTROLS	NONSMOKER SILICOTICS	SMOKER CONTROLS	SMOKER SILICOTICS
Albumin mg%ml	2.9(0.96)	4.0(2.1)	3.9(2.3)	6.3(5.2)
IgG/Albumin	0.12(0.09)	0.24(0.16)	0.35(0.31)	0.46(0.19)
IgA/Albumin	0.03(0.01)	0.03(0.01)	0.13(0.1)	0.038(0.015)
alAT*/Albumin	0.019(0.01)	0.016(0.017)	0.024(0.01)	0.028(0.021)

* alpha-1-antitrypsin

© 1988 Elsevier Science Publishers B.V. (Biomedical Division)
Sarcoidosis and other granulomatous disorders
C. Grassi, G. Rizzato, E. Pozzi, editors

ANTIGEN-SPECIFIC T CELLS IN A MOUSE MODEL OF BERYLLIUM DISEASE

LEE NEWMAN *

Pulmonary Division and Occupational Medicine Program, National Jewish Center for Immunology and Respiratory Medicine, 1400 Jackson Street, Denver, CO. 80206 USA.

INTRODUCTION

Pulmonary changes in chronic beryllium disease include varying degrees of granuloma formation, mononuclear cell interstitial infiltrates, and fibrosis. Both human and animal studies have implicated cell-mediated immunity in the pathogenesis of beryllium disease (1-3). In most animal models, inhalation of beryllium salts is used to induce disease. However, in a few reports, beryllium disease-like pulmonary infiltrates have been observed after intradermal injection of beryllium salts in the absence of any inhaled beryllium (4). Experiments described here were designed to test the hypothesis that cell-mediated immunity to beryllium is sufficient to induce chronic beryllium disease in mice.

MATERIALS AND METHODS

Eight- to twelve-week old $B6D2F_1$ mice were exposed to beryllium sulfate ($10\mu g$ $BeSO_4$) in complete or incomplete Freund's adjuvant or without vehicle by serial subcutaneous injections. Controls received incomplete or complete Freund's adjuvant alone. Development of disease was determined by lung histologic examination. Development of beryllium-specific cell-mediated immunity was assessed by two methods: 1) delayed-type hypersensitivity response and 2) spleen lymphocyte blastogenic response to $BeSO_4$ in vitro.

Delayed-type hypersensitivity was determined by measurement of mouse foot pad thickness 24 hours, 48 hours and 7 days after pad injection with 0.1 $\mu g/25$ μl $BeSO_4$ in PBS. Lymphocyte blastogenesis was performed in standard culture conditions using 2.5×10^5 splenocytes per well of 96-well plates. Cells were maintained in RPMI 1640 with 2% fetal calf serum for 3, 5 and 7 days. Quadraplicate wells were exposed to Con A, Lipopolysaccharide, or $BeSO_4$ at 1×10^{-3} to 1×10^{-8} M concentrations. Blastogenic response was determined on a well-type gamma scintillation counter, measuring cellular incorporation of [125]Iodouracildeoxyriboside, 20-24 hours after pulsing.

In experiments designed to transfer beryllium-specific immunity, splenocytes from beryllium-exposed mice were passed over nylon wool columns to enrich for T cells. T cells were injected intravenously at two concentrations (1×10^6 cells, 1×10^7 cells) with or without $BeSO_4$ (1×10^{-3} M). Animals received a

---

Milan prize winner for authors under 35 years.

single booster IV injection of $BeSO_4$ (1×10^{-4} M) two weeks after initial T cell transfer. Lung histology and beryllium-specific cell-mediated immunity were studied at serial time points.

RESULTS

Histologic sections of the lungs of $BeSO_4$-injected mice showed focal aggregates of mononuclear cells diffusely throughout the lung as early as three months after the series of subcutaneous injections. Freund control animals' lungs were normal. $BeSO_4$-injected mice showed marked delayed-type hypersensitivity response, (19.6% change in foot pad thickness, S.E. 1.3) compared to control mice (11.9%, S.E. 0.8). Lymphocytes from $BeSO_4$-injected mice showed significantly greater blastogenic response to $BeSO_4$ (8 fold stimulation) than did control mouse lymphocytes (2.5 fold stimulation). Beryllium-naive mice injected with T lymphocytes from beryllium-immunized animals showed increased delayed-type hypersensitivity (16.4%, S.E. 0.5) compared to controls (7.5%, S.E. 0.9) and enhanced lymphocyte blastogenic responses to $BeSO_4$ (6.1 fold stimulation) at four weeks after T cell transfer.

DISCUSSION

These data suggest that 1) pathologic alterations consistent with beryllium disease develop in lungs of mice with demonstrable cell-mediated immunity to beryllium, and 2) since these mice received no inhaled beryllium, this response is independent of local pulmonary toxic or foreign body effects. 3) Beryllium-specific T cells from these mice can transfer immunity to normal animals.

REFERENCES

1. Deodhar SD, Barna B, Van Ordstrand HS (1973) Chest 63:309
2. Barna BP, Chiang T, Pillarisetti SG, Deodhar SD (1981) Clin Immunol Immunopathol 20:402.
3. Votta JJ, Barton RW, Gionfriddo MA et al. (1987) Sarcoidosis 4:71.
4. Eskenasy A (1979) Revroum Morphol Embryol Physiol 25:257.

HISTOLOGY OF GRANULOMATOUS INFLAMMATION IN NUDE RATS LUNGS INDUCED
BY COMPLETE FREUND'S ADJUVANT (CFA).

J. CHANG, J. JAGIRDAR, T. FARAGGIANA, F. PARONETTO.
Veterans Administration Medical Center, Bronx N.Y. and The Mount
Sinai School of Medicine, New York N.Y. U.S.A.

INTRODUCTION

The presence of lymphocytes in the schistosome eggs induced
chronic granulomatous inflammation suggests that a thymus dependent
immune mechanism is involved in the pathogenesis of the disease.
Muramyl dipeptide can induce well organized epithelioid granulomas
in lymph nodes of athymic rat without functional T lymphocytes [1].
However, streptococcal cell wall-induced rat hepatic granulomas and
fibrosis are T-cell dependent processes [2]. We previously reported that CFA induced organized epithelioid granuloma and fibrosis in
rat lung with abundant lymphocytes in the lungs and in the bronchoalveolar lavage (BAL) samples [3]. The purpose of this study is to
evaluate whether CFA-induced granuloma and fibrosis in rats is a T-
cell dependent process.

MATERIAL AND METHODS

Pulmonary granulomas were induced in six week old male athymic
NCR rats (rnu/rnu) and heterozygous littermate controls (rnu/+)
(Frederick Cancer Research Institute, NIH,Bethesda MD) by a single
i.v. injection (1 mg/kg) of CFA (Cappel Lab., Westchester, PA). At
4 days and 1,2,4,6,16 weeks later, groups of 3 to 4 animals were
subjected to BAL and in situ lung fixation with 10% formalin. Lung
sections were stained with hematoxylin-eosin and trichrome. The
total leukocytes count and percent of lymphocytes in each BAL
sample were determined by categorizing 400 leukocytes on Wright-
Giemsa stained smears.

RESULTS

Histology sections of lungs revealed a macrophage aggregation at
4 to 7 days. Well organized epithelioid granulomas associated with
fibrotic ring and scarce lymphocytes (Fig. 1A) were seen at 2 to 6
weeks. At 16 weeks granulomas were loosely organized and associated with numerous lymphocytes at the periphery (Fig. 1B). Lymphocyte count as percent of total leukocytes in BAL samples correlated

with number of lymphocytes in histological sections (0 - 0.5% at 4 days to 2 weeks, 5% at 6 weeks and 16% at 16 weeks). Granulomas in heterozygous littermate were larger, more numerous and with prominent lymphocyte cuffing. Fibrosis was minimal in early stages.

SUMMARY AND CONCLUSION

1. CFA injection in nude rats without functional T lymphocytes induced distinct pulmonary granulomas and early fibrosis.

2. Lymphocytes in BAL and in the lungs were rare in the acute stage (1-4 weeks). The number increased at 16 weeks suggesting that B lymphocytes may play a role in the resolution of granulomas and fibrosis.

3. CFA-induced granulomas in heterozygous littermate rat lung were larger, more numerous and associated with lymphocyte cuffing. Fibrosis was less prominent in the acute stage. This result suggest that T-cells modulate the granulomatous process by augmenting granulomatous formation and inhibiting fibrosis.

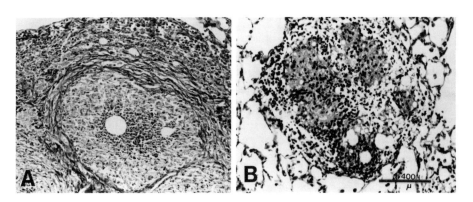

Fig. 1. Appearance of the lung granuloma of nude rats at 2 weeks (A) and 16 weeks (B) after injection of CFA.

ACKNOWLEDGEMENT
Study was supported by the Veterans Administration.

REFERENCES
1. Tanaka A et al (1982) Am J Pathol 106:165
2. Wahl SM et al (1986) J Exp Med 163:884
3. Chang JC et al (1986) Am J Pathol 125:16

© 1988 Elsevier Science Publishers B.V. (Biomedical Division)
Sarcoidosis and other granulomatous disorders
C. Grassi, G. Rizzato, E. Pozzi, editors

OTHER GRANULOMATOUS DISEASES - HOW CAN THEY HELP WITH UNDERSTANDING
SARCOIDOSIS? OUTLOOK

HERBERT Y. REYNOLDS, M.D.

Pulmonary Section, Department of Internal Medicine, Yale University School
of Medicine, 333 Cedar Street, P.O. Box 3333, New Haven, CT. 06510 (USA).

Development of granuloma in tissue is a fundamental response of host
defense and implies heightened cellular immunity (1). Many diseases
feature granuloma formation in various organs especially the respiratory
tract. Although sarcoidosis is the principal focus of this Congress, the
"other" related granulomatous diseases are of relevance in unraveling the
persisting mysteries of sarcoidosis - its enigmatic cause, what drives the
exaggerated T helper cell activity, what stimulates macrophages or why the
disease may ameliorate and spontaneously regress. Without knowing the
etiology of sarcoidosis, all the current lung research giving details about
macrophage and T-lymphocyte interaction leading to the oligoclonal
expansion of T helper cells, activation of latent killer lymphocytes and
stimulation of immunoglobulin producing cells seem as descriptive
epiphenomena and not unique immunologic responses of sarcoidosis, for they
may occur in other sites and with other diseases. However, clues about
immunoregulation in sarcoidosis might be obtained from respiratory
disorders which have a known etiology and elicit a somewhat similar
clinical picture. As yet many of these granulomatous diseases still defy a
clear pathogenesis, particular the systemic vasculitidies. Thus, this
summary will emphasize hypersensitivity pneumonitis (HP) and its possible
parallels with sarcoidosis.

Diseases caused by repeated inhalation of organic dust may produce
distinctive clinical syndromes (2,3) and elicit in the lungs various
histologic responses depending upon the duration or chronicity of exposure.
Early on (and in youthful subjects) an asymptomatic phase of illness may
occur although immunologic changes of lymphocytic alveolitis (4-6) and
specific antibodies are present. With repeat antigen exposure by the

sensitized host, which may be manifested by chills, fever, coughing, <u>etc.</u>, a transient influx of polymorphonuclear neutrophils (PMN) occurs (as sampled by bronchoalveolar lavage of airway challenged subjects, 7-10). With chronic disease resulting from repeated or cumulative exposure to antigen, an interstitial pneumonitis develops which is clinically indistinguishable from other forms of diffuse interstitial pulmonary fibrosis and at this stage is often difficult to diagnose as a hypersensitivity disease. Analysis of BAL fluid and cells (11) reveals the hallmarks of CHP with an impressive recovery of lymphocytes, principally T-cells which in chronic phases will include more T suppressor cells than the T helper variety (12-15), creating a low ratio of T_H/T_S lymphocytes. Also present are foamy alveolar macrophages with large vacuoles and elevated levels of immunoglobulins especially IgG and IgM which may contain specific antibody activity (11,16,17). In lung biopsy material granuloma are usually present in intraalveolar walls and fibrosis can be found (18).

This brief review of HP is intended to point to several practical derivatives that are useful clinically and in research which make this group of diseases satisfying to study. Examples follow. By knowing the etiology, either epidemiologically or through serum and BAL fluid antibody reactivity found from a panel of putative antigens, a rational approach to many facets of the disease can be devised. The diagnosis or symptom complex can be verified with antigen aerosol exposure of the patient (admittedly done with care under close medical surveillance) and the important element of treatment - avoidance - can be reinforced. These airway challenge tests have been instructive in documenting the acute influx of PMN's into the alveolar spaces, giving credence to the idea that a Type 3 or Arthus-like reaction might occur in the sensitized lung through an antigen-antibody reaction (1), thus elucidating immunopathogenic mechanisms. As the in vivo challenge testing of sensitized humans cannot be done in a widespread fashion, in vitro stimulation of blood or airway lymphocytes with specific antigen or measurement of antibodies can provide practical ways to diagnose patients and creative means for exploring cellular interactions for research purposes. Finally, animal models can be constructed to allow research manipulations that cannot be done in humans.

Because avoidance therapy is usually effective, except in advanced CHP, and the clinical syndrome may be mild, it can be difficult, unfortunately, to garner volunteer subjects for research, unless one can target a specific group of motivated volunteers (pigeon handlers) or work with affected patients whose occupational interests are at stake (dairy and grain handlers). Although the enconomic impact of hypersensitivity diseases in aggregate may be even greater than that from sarcoidosis and other rare forms of granulomatous disease, the widespread availability of affected subjects with HP does not seem as plentiful as for sarcoidosis. Again, the lack of an established etiology for sarcoidosis and the possibility that 10-15% of patients will have progressive lung disease or critical other organ involvement serve as the impetus for physicians to refer sarcoidosis patients for tertiary care (and research); such a necessity does not exist for most HP patients.

Thus, after lamenting the fact that it may not be as easy to obtain large numbers of subjects with HP as sarcoidosis, what lessons from HP disease might be relevant to focus on in order to learn (and speed research) more about sarcoidosis. A key difference is the antigen. Without knowing the inciting cause of sarcoidosis, one is investigating the descriptive features of the host's reaction, admittedly now in great detail and at a molecular and genetic level - as lucidly and excitingly presented by Dr. Ronald G. Crystal in his current lecture (19) and at prior meetings of this Congress in 1981 and 1984. The thrusts of research have proceeded simultaneously in two directions from the clinical phase in which sarcoid alveolar spaces are affected with a lymphocytic T-helper cell-activted macrophage-immunoglobulin rich collection of cellular and humoral immune ingredients. In one direction the stimulated T_H cell is producing excessive interleukin 2, presumably from the CD4 DR positive subset (20) which can be documented by activation of the IL-2 gene (21). This lymphokine causes an increased turnover of Il-2 receptors on other T helper cells (with shedding of IL-2 receptors that can be measured in blood - 22) which leads to clonal proliferation of T-cells. Moreover, it can activate other immunocytes such as natural killer cells and B-lymphocytes. T cells also produce gamma interferon spontaneously (23). What the stimulus is that drives this T-lymphocyte response is unclear. Certainly it is not from a lack of T suppressor cell regulation or appropriate function, as reported by Saltini et al at this Congress (24). Yet this cellular reaction (autonomy?) does seem to diminish in intensity once the cells are removed from the immediate milieu of the lung and propagated in vitro, suggesting that a local environmental factor(s) is needed or the full complexity of the mixture of cells found in the alveolar space is required. The question posed: is this a special or unique kind of cellular proliferation and reaction for sarcoidosis, or is it a steriotyped reaction of the host once the cellular stimulus (activated T-cells) is initiated and, therefore, predictable?

Alternatively, the answer to etiology is being sought by working retrograde in the direction of the macrophage-lymphocyte interaction or proximally to the alveolar macrophage itself which is the principal scavenger phagocyte on the alveolar surface and the cell most likely to first encounter an aerosolized antigen arriving in the alveoli. The intricacies of macrophage activation, the ability to present antigen on its surface to adjacent lymphocytes (25), the microstructure of the T-cell antigen receptor (and its possible genetic restriction to part of the variable region of the beta-chain in certain subsets of sarcoid patients - as presented by Dr. Crystal (19) - are all relevant to the processing of an antigen and its subsequent initiation of an immunoproliferative response.

Of relevance at this point was the evidence presented by Dr. Maarsseveen and colleagues from Amsterdam (26) about the composition of lymphocytes found adherent to macrophages lavaged from the sarcoid lung. The observation of so-called spontaneous macrophage-lymphocyte rosettes forming in the airway (or ? in lavage fluid) of sarcoidosis patients was presented by Yeager and colleagues (27,28) and was one of the first cellular studies done on BAL cells in this disease. The observation of Maarsseveen et al, based on phenotypic staining of the lymphocytes, that both T helper and T suppressor lymphocytes were attached was intriguing in thinking about possible antigen processing by T-cells. Moreover, with corticosteroid treatment, the relative proportion of T suppressor lymphocytes increased in the ring of rosetting cells.

Now HP can reenter the discussion and may help with understanding sarcoidosis at this stage. The form in which antigen reachs the alveolar surface may be significant. Aside from its size, particulate shape, solubility and the great variety of organic substances that can sensitize the lung, concomitant substances mixed with the antigen which adhere to or accompany its aerosol journey may give an added effect (3). Consider that the fecal dropping of birds contain albumin (the putative antigen in pigeon handlers disease), fungal and bacterial agents, enzymes and perhaps degraded proteins, etc., all of which dry and are dispersed for inhalation. Ubiquitous bacteria, such as Pseudomonas sp. containing endotoxin, can be found on plants and moldy vegetation, in water and cotton brac, etc. Thus, lipopolysaccharide can contaminate almost everything and could be part of any aerosol generated. Added to the extensive list of organic antigens causing HP is Trichosporon cutaneum (29,30). As reported by Dr. Ando and colleagues (31), this fungus can be cultured from houses in the summer and is the cause of a summer-type hypersensitivity pneumonitis. The causative antigen is a spore between 3-10 microns in diameter. Thus, aerosol antigens that putatively cause HP are potentially accompanied by other substances which may act as an accessory stimulant or adjuvant (3), or the antigen is one that may elicit cellular immunity as well as stimulate specific antibodies. Moreover, it is possible that vegetable particulates may persist within the alveoli or in macrophages because they are not degraded readily, thus prolonging their potential for continued antigen stimulation.

Alternatively, haptens which conjugate with a protein are potent antigenic stimulants. Interesting research with beryllium salts suggests this. This metal which is known to produce a chronic granulomatous disease virtually indistinguishable from sarcoidosis was thought to be well controlled with current industrial standards for air safety, but in fact it seems to be recurring or certainly is being recognized again as a cause of lung disease (32). Saltini and colleagues (33) have extended the above cited immunological studies of human lung lymphocytes (32) in an interesting way. Four patients with beryllium lung disease were lavaged. Their lung lymphocyte analysis indicated the presence of activated (DR positive) T-helper (CD_4) cells in increased numbers. Using blood monocytes exposed to $BeSO_4$ as antigen presenting cells, the lung lymphocytes were stimulated; CD_4 cells proliferated and the clones were expanded (requirements for HLA-DR restriction and IL-2 receptor dependency were demonstrated, also). In brief, this work indicated that beryllium sensitized lung T-lymphocytes could be driven to proliferate and oligoclonally to expand in a way similar to sarcoidosis T helper cells. This addressed two points in the sarcoidosis bi-directional scheme just mentioned - 1) an antigen in this case a hapten within a mononuclear phagocyte could set in motion a cellular sequence; and, 2) once initiated (with previously sensitized lymphocytes) a T cell response occurred which was similar to the spontaneous response of sarcoid lung T-helper cells.

In summary, what we have suggested is that a special kind of antigen and adjuvant or a hapten are needed to induce the combined cell-mediated and humoral response characteristic of HP. As a reminder, animal models developed for HP disease have required the use of an adjuvant for cellular changes in the lungs to persist and granuloma to develop (reviewed in Ref. 3). The identity of this additional stimulant or hapten might explain why the immunologic process blossoms in some people to cause lymphocytic alevolitis and disease but not in others exposed only to the antigen or microbial agent. Also, while the search for the causative antigen or agent of sarcoidosis continues, some attention should be given to searching for a concomitant adjuvant - like substance.

In chronic stages of HP (or for subjects not recently exposed to their antigen), a lymphocytic alveolitis exists which has cellular features that are different from acute sarcoid alevolitis, yet some similarities have been discovered and presented at this Congress. As is well described, the characteristically high percentage of lymphocytes among the BAL cells are

T-cells (11) and the relative proportions of T Helper and T Suppressor cells favor a slight majority of the latter (12-15) giving a reduced ratio of T_H/T_S in contrast to the ratio in normals of about 1.5-1.8 and the high ratio usually found with active pulmonary sarcoidosis. In CHP the percentage of lymphocytes in BAL can be quite elevated (60% range) and often is higher than found in many active cases of pulmonary sarcoidosis (30-40% range). The intricate details about lymphocyte production of mediators in sarcoid (IL-2, IL-2 receptor shedding and interferon gamma) or their effects to activate natural killer cells or stimulate B-cells (in conjunction with other interleukin forms) have not been reported for HP. However, Dr. Trentin and colleagues from Padua (15,34) found spontaneous cytotoxic activity in BAL cells from HP patients against sensitive ^{51}Cr labelled target cells; also additional activity could be induced with specific antigen (Micropolyspora faeni), a lectin or IL-2 (to produce lymphokine activated killer cells). Finding this spontaneous NK activity would lead one to the prediction that T Helper (? DR positive) lymphocytes might be releasing IL-2 into the alveolar lining secretions to simulate these killer cells and, therefore, IL-2 should be detected and quantitated in BAL fluid. In fact, IL-2 could not be measured. In another attempt to find IL-2 and other cellular mediators and cell changes in HP patients, before and after airway challenge of pigeon breeders with pigeon serum, Reynolds and associates from Cardiff (10) could not detect IL-2 either. On balance, it would seem that IL-2 production in the lung of HP subjects is occurring with its excpected impact on other lymphocytes such as NK cells (worthwhile to emphasize the considerable Ig production of IgG, A and M also in this context). In the normal lung NK cells seem to be dormant unlesss stimulated with IL-2 or culture medium (35). Possibly the IL-2 in the HP lung is quantitatively utilized and no reasonable excess can be measured. Also, suspressor cells could modulate this T Helper cell activity as well. Although this mediator's activity is complex and undue speculation may be creeping into this report, the point being suggested is that further research on these cellular interactions in HP needs to be done.

Another observation was made about continued antigen exposure or avoidance in HP patients and their lung T-cell profiles that is relevant to CD_4/CD_8 interactions. Dr. Masciarelli and colleagues from Padua (36) monitored BAL lymphocytes in 16 patients, 8 of whom continued to be exposed at work to etiological antigens and 8 who were not, at 6 month intervals for 24 months. With continued exposure phenotypically CD_8 cells continued to increase; whereas, in the absence of antigen exposure these cells began to decline after six months and the CD_4/CD_8 ratio normalized. However, the BAL lymphocytosis persisted in both groups as did HNK-1 identified cells (killer lymphocytes). Thus, a difference between CHP (and recurrent antigen stimulation) and sarcoidosis is evident, for in the former disease a putative T suppressor cell response seems part of the lung's host defense (possibly an attempt to dampen down immunologic activity); whereas, in sarcoid, the T helper clone increases. Again the role of IL-2 and other lymphokine meadiators in CHP needs further exploration. On the other hand, objective function of suppressor cells needs to be assessed, as done by Saltini et al (24) in sarcoidosis to ascertain in vitro performance of these lung cells. By the same token, perhaps sarcoid T suppressor lymphocytes should be superactive as in CHP, if a persistent antigen really is a cause of sarcoidosis?

At this point another human disease, acquired immunodeficiency syndrome, could be relevant to discuss. At this Congress, it was informally queried around if any of the clinicians had observed AIDS to develop in a person with sarcoidosis? The concensus was that the association was infrequent, if it has occurred (several antidotal cases were mentioned). To pursue a purely immunological lung response, comparison and contrast between sarcoidosis and HP with AIDS is interesting. Many of the respiratory infections that plague the AIDS patient are caused by viruses and microbial agents which are obligate intracellular organisms that can reside in mononuclear phagocytes such as macrophages. Invariably, the host must generate cellular immunity for these phagocytes to adequately contain these organisms. In AIDS, viruses plus organisms such as mycobacteria (M. tuberculosis, M. avium-intracellulare), various fungi (<u>Cryptococcus neoformans</u> and <u>Toxoplasmosis</u> <u>gondii</u>) and perhaps <u>Pneumocystis carinii</u> (PCP) all fall into this category. AIDS by definition denotes an existing deficiency in immunity and the principal defect is the depletion of T-helper/inducer lymphocytes by HIV infection. Although B-lymphocytes and monocytes or macrophages can be infected, this is a secondary phenomenon. AIDS patients can form a granulomatous reponse but it is not optimal; perhaps a more effective response coupled with better CMI would enable the patient to resist these infections - hence the AIDS patient needs some of the sarcoid stimulus and machinery. Perhaps the immune response in the AIDS lungs is "frustrated" in that a more effective granulomatous reaction, and hence cell mediated immunity, reaction cannot be mounted. Noteworthy in the AIDS lung, sampled by BAL in patients with PCP infection (37-40); are the lymphocyte profiles.

Results in lung lavage stand in contrast to the usual lymphocyte pattern in blood and other tissue of AIDS patients, for peripheral blood lymphocyte counts are decreased and a paucity of T-helper lymphocytes are characteristic in blood and in nodal tissue. As these cells are infected with HIV and destroyed, blood lymphocyte counts, while low, show a relative increase in T-suppressor/cytotoxic lymphocytes giving a low T helper/T suppressor ratio.

Summarizing the lung lavage studies and giving emphasis to lymphocyte findings, results from these three studies (37-40) are remarkably similar, suggesting that the pattern of cells recovered and analyzed from AIDS patients with lung infection and from normals is reproducible. In contrast to blood counts that reflected lymphopenia, the alveolar spaces and peripheral airways sampled by BAL had increased numbers of lymphocytes. Although T_4 or Leu3 staining lymphocytes (CD_4), phenotypically identifying T helper cells, might be low in blood, some were present in the lung. Actually, based on absolute lymphocyte counts, T helper cells in AIDS lavage fluid approximated the number of these cells usually found in the alveoli of normals. Whether these T helper (CD_4) cells were latently infected with HIV was not known. Uniformly, the proportion of T_8 or Leu_2 staining cells (CD_8) which identify T suppressor cells was increased,

usually to a marked degree. Alveolar macrophages were recovered in
proportionally smaller numbers, reflecting the greater pecentage of
lymphocytes (ranging from 19.4 to 26.1% of BAL cells in AIDS versus 5.2 to
10.2% in normals). Polymorphonuclear neutrophils (PMN) were increased
(2.1.-18.8% in AIDS) implying that PMN chemotaxis into the alveoli was
occurring.

Only two of these studies examined BAL fluid for immunoglobulins and
antibodies (37,39). All major classes of immunoglobulins were increased in
BAL specimens compared with controls; IgG and IgA were elevated in
respective sera. Perhaps accounting for this local effect in the lung was
an impressive increase in immunoglobulin-releasing cells in lavage fluid
and also in blood. Disordered immunoregulation has been stressed almost
from the onset of the disease and abnormal function of immunoglobulin
synthesis and inapprorpiate or uncontrolled antibody responses have been
noted (41). To summarize the AIDS patients lung is probably deficient in
effective T Helper cells, although some are present, and a relative
increase in T suppressor cells exists. Based on blood studies, it is
probable that NK cytotoxic cell function is impaired also (42).
Immunoglobulin synthesis is excessive, but whether antigen specific
antibody is being generated is questionable. It is evident that the
multiple defects in the impaired AIDS lung represent a mixture of the
immunologic problems that are features of sarcoidosis and HP diseases.
Thus, further dissection of the cellular interactions in AIDS could provide
insight into regualtory mechanisms that might be exaggerated in the
principal diseses under scrutiny at this Congress.

Critique.

For pulmonary sarcoidosis, the description of intraalveolar immunologic
responses, based upon phenotypic identification of T-cell subsets and
macrophages and the manipulation of these BAL recovered cells with
appropriate mediators and reagents, has been spectacular in the past 8
years. These cellular studies have now been extended to the level of gene
expression for regulation of T-helper cell activation and clonal expansion.
Important information about activity of the T-helper's cells antigen

receptor and its molecular characterization has been provided that may help predict what form the putative "antigen" that causes sarcoidosis may have. This may elucidate the critical alveolar macrophage antigen presentation step to receptive T cells which sets in motion the lymphocytic alveolitis that can culminate in the granulomatous response. Of additional importance, as the activated macrophage becomes the focus of intraalveolar events that can inexplicably in some sarcoidosis patients lead to lung fibrosis, is the secretion by alveolar macrophages of various profibrotic polypeptide mediators, such as fibronectin, platelet derived growth factor and macrophage derived growth factor (with insulin like activity) which affect fibroblasts. PMN and their toxic oxygen radicals and lysozomal enzymes also have a role in stimulating this fibrotic reaction. Thus, as well summarized by Dr. Crystal, whose research team has been at the forefront in investigating the immunopathogenesis of sarcoidosis, much is known about macrophage-lymphocyte interaction and what drives, subsequently, the rather autonomous T helper cell response. However, there is a tendency to equate intraalveolar events, using viable cells that can be retrieved from the lung with BAL, with what develops in the interstitial tissue or alveolar and vessel walls where granuloma tend to form, yet little is still known about the micropassage of cells through alveolar walls (even if irritated and inflammed) or the diffusion of mediators beyond the alveolar epithelial surface that might affect other cells at a distance. Permeability studies have disclosed increased clearance across the epithelial surface into the blood in the granulomatous lung (43) this occurs into the interstitium as well. However, it still seems probable that the tremendous cellular reactivity which develops in draining lung nodes of the hilar and mediastinum, causing the prominent adenopathy seen in recent or an early stage of clinical disease, is the site for important activation of lymphocytes or provides a critical intersection with systemic immune cells. Further attention to these processes are needed to fully understand the parenchymal granulomatous response. Animal models may be required for this. Finally, the immense cellular reactivity in the lymph nodes raises questions about initial antigen processing and lymphocyte

stimulation.   Does this require an adjuvant concomitantly with an antigen?
Could this occur or be fostered on the more promixal airway mucosal surface
(as endobronchial grnaulomatous changes are frequent and abnormalities are
not found solely at the alveolar level)?   Is macrophage- T helper
lymphocyte cellular drainage to a lymph node a requisite for optimal
interaction or can it occur, as pictured by spontaneous macrophage-
lymphocyte rosettes found in BAL fluid, on the alveolar surface?   All of
these imponderable ideas may be research ammunition for more work to be
reported at another Congress.

So with these thoughts about sarcoidosis, how do the "other
granulomatous diseases" associate?   Are these diseases such different
entities in their own right that they deserve separate clinical attention
or have unique forms of immunopathogenesis that have little in common with
sarcoidosis?   The granulomatous reactivity may be the histiologic thread
that holds these divergent diseases together as a group, yet different
immunologic pathways may lead eventually to the same tissue reaction.
Thus, should investigators push to look for similarities between HP and
beryllium diseases and sarcoidosis or probe separately for the individual
uniqueness of each?   Some of both approaches are needed for insight might
come from either direction.   In this Review, I have tended to look for
similarities between cell regulation in sarcoidosis and the other diseases,
including AIDS, and this might be a "forced" assumption in retrospect, yet
similar tools of research are being used and many investigators are
studying both sarcoidosis and HP or related diseases.   Perhaps the
respiratory tract's different reaction to organic dust antigens that
elicits more of a T suppressor cell response than an unbridled Thelper
driven reaction in sarcoidosis will prove instructive in understanding
immune cell regulation.   It is commendable that the International Committee
on Sarcoidosis in organizing these World Congresses has had the wisdom to
see the value of studying the "other granulomatous disorders" as a helpful
pathway for solving the mysteries of sarcoidosis and that future meetings
will preserve this avenue.

REFERENCES

1. Reynolds HY (1986) Pathogenic Mechanisms in Immunologic Lung Disease. Hosp. Practice 21:91-108

2. Reynolds HY (1982) Hypersensitivity pneumonitis. In: Clinics in Chest Medicine. W.B. Saunders, Philadelphia, PA., Vol. 3 pp 503-519

3. Reynolds HY (1986) Concepts of Pathogenesis and Lung Reactivity in Hypersensitivity Pneumonitis (Louis E. Siltzbach Lecture) 10th International Conference on Sarcoidosis and Other Granulomatous Disorders. Ann NY Acad Sci 465:287-303

4. Solal-Celigny, P, Laviolette M, Hebert J, Cormier Y (1982) Immune Reactions in the Lungs of Asymptomatic Dairy Farmers Am Rev Respir Dis 126:964-967

5. Cormier Y, Belanger J, Beaudoin J, Laviolette M, Beaudoin R, Hebert J (1984) Abnormal Bronchoalveolar Lavage in Asymptomatic Dairy Farmers - Study of Lymphocytes. Am Rev Respir Dis 130:1046-1049

6. Cormier Y, Belanger J, Laviolette, M (1986) Persistent Bronchoalveolar Lymphocytosis in Asymptomatic Farmers Am Rev Respir Dis 133:843-847

7. Voisin C, Tonnel AB, Lahoute C, Robin H, Lebas J, and Aerts, C (1981) Bird Fancier's Lung: Studies of Bronchoalveolar Lavage and Correlations with Inhalation Provocation Tests Lung 159:11-12

8. Fournier EC, Santorro, F, Aerts C, Lahoute C and Voisin, C (1981) Study of Bronchoalveolar Lavage Before and After the Inhalation Challenge Test in Bird Fancier's Disease: Deduction about Immunological Mechanisms Involved. In: Sarcoidosis and Other Granulomatous Disorders. J. Chretien, J. Marsac and J.C. Saltiel, Eds. Pergamon Press, Paris, pp. 578-583

9. Fournier E, Tonnel AB, Gosset P, Wallaert B, Ameisen JC, Voisin, C (1985) Early Neutrophil Alveolitis After Inhalation Challenge in Hypersensitivity Pneumonitis Chest 88:563-566

10. Reynolds SP, Jones, KP, Trotman, DM, Davies, BH The Effect of Indirect and Direct Antigenic Challenge on Bronchoalveolar Lavage Fluid in Symptomatic and Asymptomatic Pigeon Breeders. Abstract, XI the World Congress on Sarcoidosis and Other Granulomatous Disorders, Milan Italy, page 29, Sept 8, 1987.

732

11. Reynolds HY, Fulmer JD, Kazmierowski JA, Roberts WC, Frank MM and Crystal RG (1977) Analysis of Cellular and Protein Components of Bronchoalveolar Lavage Fluid from Patients with Idiopathic Pulmonary Fibrosis and Hypersensitivity Pneumonitis J Clin Invest 59:165-175

12. Moritz ED, Smiejan JM, Keogh BA. and Crystal RG (1982) Nonfibrotic Pigeon Breeders Syndrome: A Disorder Characterized by a Chronic Suppressor T cell Alveolitis Clin Res 30:453A

13. Leatherman JW, Michael AF, Schwartz BA, and Hoidal JR (1984) Lung T Cells in Hypersensitivity Pneumonitis Ann Intern Med 100:390-392

14. Costabel U, Bross KJ, Ruhle KH, Lohr, GW, and Matthys H Ia-like Antigens on T-cells and Their Subpopulations in Pulmonary Sarcoidosis and in Hypersensitivity Pneumonitis - Analysis of Bronchoalveolar and Blood Lymphocytes Am Rev Respir Dis 131:337-342

15. Semenzato G, Agostini C, Zambello R, Trentin L, Chilosi M, Pizzolo G, Marcer G, Cipriani, A (1986) Lung T-cells in Hypersensitivity Pneumonitis: Phenotypic and Functional Analyses J Immunol 137:1164-1172

16. Calvanico NJ, Ambegaonkar SP, Schulueter DP and Fink JN (1980) Immunoglobulin Levels in Bronchoalveolar Lavage Fluid from Pigeon Breeders. J Lab Clin Med. 9:129-140

17. Patterson R, Wang JLF, Fink JN, Calvanico N and Roberts, M (1979) IgA and IgG Antibody Activities of Serum and Bronchoalveolar Fluid from Symptomatic Pigeon Breeders Am Rev Respir Dis 120:113-118

18. Reyes, CN, Wenzel FJ and Lawton, BR (1982) The Pulmonary Pathology of Farmer's Lung Disease Chest 81:142-146

19. Crystal, RG Sarcoidosis in 1987: From Immune Response Genes to the Bedside. XIth World Congress on Sarcoidosis and other Granulomatous Disorders, Milan, Italy, September 7, 1987.

20. Saltini C, Spuzem JR, Lee, JJ, Pinkston P, Crystal RG (1986) Spontaneous release of Interleukin-2 by lung T-lymphocytes in active pulmonary sarcoidosis is primarily from the Leu3 positive DR positive T cell subset J Clin Invest 77:1962-1970

21. Muller-Quernheim J, Saltini C, Sondermeyer P, Crystal RG (1986) Compartmentalized Activation of the Interleukin 2 Gene by Lung T Lymphocytes in Active Pulmonary Sarcoidosis J Immunol 137:3475-3483

22. Lawrence EC, Berger MB, Brousseau KP, Rodriguez TM, Siegel, SJ, Kurman CC, Nelson DL (1987) Elevated Serum Levels of Soluble Interleukin-2 Receptors in Active Pulmonary Sarcoidosis: Relative Specificty and Association with Hypercalcemia Sarcoidosis 4:87-93

23. Robinson BWS, McLemore, TL, Crystal, RG (1985) Gamma Interferon is Spontaneously Released by Alveolar Macrophages and Lung T-lymphocytes in Patients with Pulmonary Sarcoidosis J Clin Invest 75:1488-1495

24. Saltini C, Spurzen JR, Kirby M, Crystal RG, The Unbalanced Activation of the Helper T-cell Population in the Sarcoid Lung is not Due to a Generalized Suppressor T-cell Defect. Abstract. XI World Congress on Sarcoidosis and Other Granulomatous Disorders, Milan, Italy p. 2, Sept. 7, 1987.

25. Venet A, Hance AJ, Saltini C, Robinson BWS, Crystal RG (1985) Enhanced Alveolar Macrophage - Mediated Antigen-induced T-lymphocyte Proliferation in Sarcoidosis. J Clin Invest 75:293 -

26. Maarsseveen, TV, Mullink H, Stam J, deGroot J, deHaan M Interactions between T Helper/Suppressor Lymphocytes and Macrophages in Sarcoidosis, Abstract. XI World Congress of Sarcoidosis and Other Granulomatous Disorders, Milan, Italy, p. 3, Sept. 7, 1987.

27. Yeager HM, William MC, Beckman JF, Bayly TC, Beaman BL, Hawley RJ (1976) Sarcoidosis: Analysis of Cells Obtained by Bronchial Lavage. Am Rev Respir Dis 113:96-100

28. Reynolds, HY (1978) The Importance of Lymphocytes in Pulmonary Health and Disease Lung 155:225-242

29. Shimazu K, Ando M, Sakata T, Yoshida K and Araki S (1984) Hypersensitivity Pneumonitis Induced by Trichosporon cutaneum. Am Rev Respir Dis 130:407-411

30. Ando M, Yoshida K, Soda K, and Araki S (1986) Specific Bronchoalveolar Lavage IgA Antibody in Patients with Summer-type Hypersensitivity Pneumonitis Induced by Trichosporon cutaneum. Am Rev Respir Dis 134:177-179

31. Ando M, Yoshida K, Sakata T, Soda K, Sugimoto M, Suga M, Nakashima H, Araki, S Environmental and Immunologic Studies on the Causative Agent of Summer-type Hypersensitivity Pneumonitis in Japan. Abstract. XI World Congress of Sarcoidosis and other Granulomatous Disorders, Milan, Italy, p. 29, Sept. 8, 1987.

734

32. Cullen MR, Kominsky JR, Rossman MD, Cherniack MG, Rankin JA, Balmes JR, Kern JA, Daniele RP, Palmer L, Naegel GP, McManus K, Cruz R, (1987) Chronic Beryllium Disease in a Precious Metal Refinery: Clinical Epidemiologic and Immunologic Evidence for Continuing Risk from Exposure to Low Level Beryllium Fume Am Rev Respir Dis 135:201-208

33. Saltini C, Pinkston P, Kirby M, Crystal RG Beryllium Induced Specific Lung Helper (CD_4+) T-cell Activation and the Maintenance of the Alveolitis of Berylliosis. Abstract. XI World Congress on Sarcoidosis and other Granulomatous Disorders, Milan, Italy, p. 31, September 8, 1987.

34. Trentin L, Zambello R, Festi G, Bizzotto R, Luca, M, Agostini C Different Types of Cytotoxic Mechanisms are Involved in the Lung of Patients with Hypersensitivity Pneumonitis. Abstract. XI World Congress on Sarcoidosis and Other Granulomatous Disorders, Milan, Italy, p. 32, September 8, 1987.

35. Robinson BWS, Pinkston P, Crystal RG (1984) Natural Killer Cells are Present in the Normal Human Lung but are Functionally Impotent J Clin Invest 74:942-950

36. Masciarelli M, Trentin L, Mercer G, Gemignani C, Cipriani A, DiVittorio G, Gasparotto G, Semenzato G Persistent Lymphocytic Alveolitis in Patients with Hypersensitivity Pneumonitis: Longitudinal evaluation with monoclonal antibodies. Abstract. XI World Congress on Sarcoidosis and other Granulomatous Disorders, Milan, Italy p. 40, September 8, 1987.

37. Rankin JA, Walzer PD, Dwyer JM, et al: (1983) Immunologic Alterations in Bronchoalveolar Lavage Fluid in the Acquired Immunodeficiency syndrome. Am Rev Respir Dis 128:189-194

38. Venet A, Clavel F, Israel-Biet D, et al (1985) Lung in Acquired Immune Deficiency Syndrome: Infectious and Immunological Status Assessed by Bronchoalveolar Lavage Bull Eur Physiopathol Respir 21:535-543

39. Young KR, Rankin JA, Naegel GP, Paul ES, Reynolds, HY (1985) Bronchoalveolar Lavage Cells and Proteins in Patients with the Acquired Immunodeficiency Syndrome - An Immunologic Analysis Ann Intern Med 103:522-533

40. Wallace JM, Barbers RG, Oishi J, Prince H (1984) Cellular and T-lymphocyte Subpopulation Profiles in Bronchoalveolar Lavage Fluid from Patients with Acquired Immunodeficiency Syndrome and Pneumonitis Am Rev Respir Dis 130:786-790

41. Seligmann M, Pinching AJ, Rosen FS, et al (1987) Immunology of
    Human Immunodeficiency Virus Infection and the Acquired
    Immunodeficiency Syndrome - An Update. Ann Intern Med 107:234-242

42. Bonavida B, Katz J, Gottlieb M (1986) Mechanism of Defective NK
    Cell Activity in Patients with Acquired Immunodeficiency Syndrome
    (AIDS) and AIDS-Related Complex J Immunol 137:1157-1163

43. Mordelet-Dambrine M, Stanislas-Leguern G, Henzel D, Barritaulti L,
    Chretien J, Huchon J Respiratory Clearance of 99mTc-DTPA and
    Granuloma Surface Area in Rat Lung Granulomatous Induced by
    Complete Freund's Adjuvant. Abstract. XI World Congress on
    Sarcoidosis and Other Granulomatous Disorders, Milan, italy, p. 21,
    September 18, 1987

ROUND TABLE:
DIFFUSE PANBRONCHIOLITIS

INTRODUCTION

GIANFRANCO RIZZATO

Sarcoidosis Clinic, Niguarda Hospital, Milan, Italy

When I visited in November 86 the Kyoto Chest Institute, I was surprised to see a number of patients with the diagnosis of diffuse panbronchiolitis. The disease was first described in Japan in 1969 and in the seventies a Japanese survey collected over a thousand cases of probable diffuse panbronchiolitis and 82 histologically confirmed cases. In many cases the chest X ray outlines a diffusely disseminated fine nodular shadows, so that the disease has to be distinguished also from Sarcoidosis stage III. I have asked to myself why this disease has neven been described outside Japan; have we always missed the diagnosis, or is this a disease affecting only Japanese people? On my return to Italy I discussed the problem with the other two members of the Local Organizing Committee. Clearly Diffuse Panbronchiolitus is not a granulomatous disorder; in spite of this, we invited Professor Izumi to organize a Round Table on this disease and asked him to invite from outside Japan two distinguished personalities in the field of pneumology in order to discuss and comment on the problems of diffuse panbronchiolitis. The final aim is to present the existence of this disease to the Western World and to try to understand the reason why this disease is so common in Japan and so unknown outside Japan.

PATHOLOGY OF DIFFUSE PANBRONCHIOLITIS FROM THE VIEW POINT OF DIFFERENTIAL
DIAGNOSIS

MASANORI KITAICHI
Chest Disease Research Institute, Kyoto University, Kyoto, Japan

INTRODUCTION

Diffuse panbronchiolitis(DPB) has been proposed basically as a pathologically
defined disease entity with chronic inflammation predominantly located in the
region of respiratory bronchioles(RBs) (1). Clinical features are a many year
duration of cough, sputa and dyspnea and an obstructive pulmonary dysfunction
with arterial hypoxemia. A chest x-p reveals bilateral small nodular shadows
and hyperinflation of lungs. Very few cases have been reported among non-
Japanese populations and there have been discussions about the identification
and diagnosis of the disorder. The author has made a pathological study of
inflammatory airways disorders(IAD) including DPB.

MATERIALS AND METHODS

92 thoracotomy and 44 autopsy cases of IAD were studied pathologically
(Table 1). All specimens were stained with hematoxylin and eosin. Selected
specimens were also stained using other methods. Special attention was paid
to lesions in areas of RBs.

TABLE 1.
CASES OF INFLAMMATORY AIRWAYS DISORDERS

Disorders	Thoracotomy	Autopsy	Total
DPB	5 (5)*	10 (10)*	15 (15)*
CB		6 (1)	6 (1)
BE	23 (20)	11 (11)	34 (31)
CF		13 (0)	13 (0)
Mycoplasma	7 (2)		7 (2)
HP	15 (11)		15 (11)
BOOP	27 (21)		27 (21)
Cryp OB	3 (2)	4 (0)	7 (2)
SAD	10 (0)		10 (0)
FB	2 (0)		2 (0)
Total	92 (61)	44 (22)	136 (83)

* Numbers in parentheses show numbers of cases among Japanese.

TABLE 2.

A SUMMARY OF HISTOPATHOLOGIC FEATURES OF IAD

	Bronchus	Membranous bronchiole	Respiratory bronchiole	Alveolar duct	Alveolus
DPB	Chronic mural inflammation / Dilation in late stage		Mural and luminal inflammation with foamy histiocytes in the wall		Interstitial accumulation of foamy cells
CB	Increase of glands and goblet cells	Increase of goblet cells with mucin stasis / Mural bronchiolitis	Mucin stasis		
BE	Dilation with inflammation and hypervascularization in the wall / Denudation of epithelial layer		Interstitial accumulation of foamy cells, rare.		
CF	Eosinophilic mucin stasis / Dilation with mural hypervascularization and luminal acute inflammatory exudates / Denudation of epithelial layer		Mural inflammation, mild		
Myco-plasma		Reparative epithelial metaplasia / Mural bronchiolitis / Organizing exudates in air spaces			
HP			Organizing exudates in air spaces / Cellular interstitial infiltrates and sarcoid-like granulomas		
BOOP		Organizing exudates in air spaces		Cellular interstitial infiltrates	
Cryp OB	Mild mural inflammation	Granulation tissue formation in the lamina propria of the wall			
SAD		Mucular hypertrophy, chronic inflammation and subepithelial fibrosis in the wall; stenotic or dilated			
FB	Germinal centers and lymphoid follicles in and around the wall				

RESULTS (Table 2)

Unit lesions of panbronchiolitis(PB)

In the pathological spectrum of IAD known to the author, the most distinctive feature of DPB was found to be an accumulation of foamy histiocytes with lymphoid cells in the wall of RBs and adjacent alveolar ducts(ADs) and alveoli. This feature was named by the author as a unit lesion of PB and could be classified into three degrees (well, moderately and poorly developed) (Fig.).

Diffuse panbronchiolitis(DPB)

Five cases of thoracotomy(M/F: 3/2, age: 19-66 years with a mean of 35.2) and 10 autopsy cases (M/F: 5/5, age: 41-75 years with a mean of 58.5) were studied. All cases showed unit lesions of PB in lung tissues with dilation of membranous bronchioles(MBs) in many cases. A few autopsy cases showed centrilobular fibrotic changes and, in basal segments, centrilobular emphysematous changes. Though one autopsy case showed an incidental primary pancreatic carcinoma, in all autopsy cases extrapulmonary organs were free from long-standing primary lesions such as seen in cystic fibrosis(CF).

Chronic bronchitis(CB)

CB is basically diagnosed from clinical symptoms: expectoration of sputa for more than three months per year for more than two successive years. Pathologic features have been described as increased Reid index or volume of glands, increased goblet cells in bronchiolar epithelium and mucin stasis in bronchiolar air spaces(2, 3). Six autopsy cases (M/F: 2/4, age: 59-88 years with a mean of 68.5) showed similar pulmonary lesions as described in references 2 and 3 without unit lesions of PB in and around the wall of RBs.

Bronchiectasis(BE)

BE is defined in this study as a long-standing pulmonary disorder excluding CF showing dilation of bronchi which was attributable to clinical symptoms or required therapy. 11 autopsy cases (M/F: 7/4, age: 30-79 years with a mean of 59.9) did not show unit lesions of PB. However, among 23 surgical cases (M/F: 8/15, age: 8-66 years with a mean of 39.0), five cases (22%) showed interstitial accumulation of foamy cells in the wall of RBs.

Cystic fibrosis(CF)

CF is an inherited disease, although very rare among Japanese, and often causes pulmonary complications in post-neonatal age (4). 13 autopsy cases (M/F: 4/9, age: 0.4-29 years with a mean of 13.9) were studied. Pulmonary lesions showed marked dilation of bronchi and MBs with eosinophilic mucin stasis in their lumens. Areas of RBs did not show interstitial accumulation of foamy histiocytes.

Mycoplasma pneumonia

Seven biopsy cases (M/F: 3/4, age: 13-65 years with a mean of 36.9) that

proved bacteriologically or serologically to have mycoplasma infection showed
a broad spectrum of inflammatory pulmonary lesions including organized exudates
filling terminal and respiratory bronchioles. A more distinct finding was
reparative epithelial metaplasia of bronchioles (5, 6).

Hypersensitivity pneumonitis(HP)

HP is caused by allergic reactions to inhaled organic substances and shows
bronchioloalveolitis with scattered small granulomas in an aute stage (6, 7).
A majority of 15 biopsy cases (M/F: 2/13, age: 13-68 years with a mean of 42.1)
showed predominantly centrilobular lesions but none showed unit lesions of PB.

Bronchiolitis obliterans organizing pneumonia(BOOP)

BOOP is a type of interstitial pneumonia and shows organizing exudates mainly
in RBs and ADs as well as in MBs (6, 8). Six biopsy cases in U.S.A. (M/F: 1/5,
age: 41-72 years with a mean of 54.5) and 21 biopsy cases in Japan (M/F: 12/9,
age: 40-69 years with a mean of 57.4) were studied. Accumulation of foamy
cells was seen in some alveolar spaces but was not noted in the wall of
bronchioles.

Cryptogenic obliterative bronchiolitis(Cryp OB)

Three biopsy cases (3 females, age: 39, 42 and 51 years) were studied along
with four autopsy cases from a previous study (9). This disorder was labeled
cryp OB in adults (10). The most marked pulmonary lesion was granulation
tissue formation in the lamina propria of MBs with infiltration of plasma cells.
RBs showed much less marked lesions without unit lesions of PB although one
case among them showed accumulation of foamy cells in the subepithelial layer
of several MBs.

Small airways disease (SAD)

SAD is a term introduced by Hogg et al. to encompass pathologic changes
observed in the peripheral conducting airways from patients with COPD. These
lesions included inflammation, fibrosis, smooth muscle hypertrophy, pigment
deposition involving airways and goblet cell metaplasia (11). But no report
showed unit lesions of PB (2, 3).

SAD is also used in North America as a generic term for a disease showing
features of bronchiolitis without any known entities. 10 cases of SAD in this
sense (M/F: 3/7, age: 8-62 years with a mean of 45) were reviewed. They showed
muscular hypertrophy, chronic inflammation and subepithelial fibrosis in the
wall of MBs and RBs which were stenotic or dilated.

Follicular bronchitis/bronchiolitis(FB)

FB has been proposed as a label for pulmonary disorder without COPD or BE
showing formations of germinal centers around airways. FB is reported to be
associated with autoimmune, immunodeficiency or hypersensitivity disorders
(12). Two biopsy cases (2 females, age: 4 and 5 years) were reviewed. They

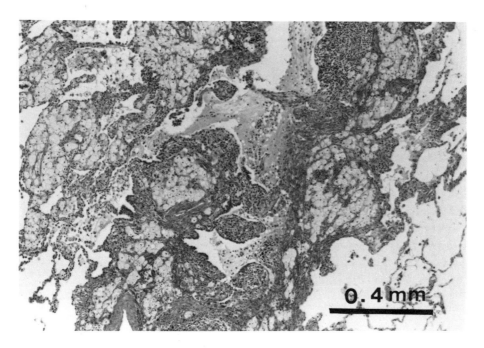

Fig.: A case of diffuse panbronchiolitis showing a well-developed unit lesion of PB.

showed germinal centers or lymphoid follicles in the wall of MBs and RBs while alveolar areas were free from marked lesions. RBs did not show unit lesions of PB.

DISCUSSION

   To consider unit lesions of PB, DPB was separated histopathologically from CB, CF, mycoplasma pneumonia, HP, BOOP, cryp OB, SAD and FB as well as autopsy cases of BE. Although five (22%) out of 23 surgical cases of BE showed accumulation of foamy cells in the wall of RBs, these cells had a tendency to spread out extensively in the interstitium of peripheral lung tissues and BE was localized in these cases. Unit lesions of PB in cases of DPB have been recently classified into three types by serial section analysis (13).

   Among 112 cases of BE reported by CE Gudbjerg, six cases showed involvements in the entire right and left lungs, and of these, four cases (3.6%) showed cylindrical type of BE although unit lesions of PB were not noted (14). The bilateral multiple cylindrical type of BE remains the major problem in the identification and diagnosis of DPB.

746

ACKNOWLEDGEMENTS

This report is a preliminary version of a study which was done with Dr. T.V.
Colby in 1986, which was made possible through the collaboration of many in-
vestigators in Japan, the U.S.A., Canada, West Germany and the United Kingdom.
Among them the author is especially grateful to Drs. F. Kitatani (Sakai),
S. Yamamoto (Sakai), T. Iwata (Tenri), K. Saito (Akita), S. Miyagi (Okinawa),
S. Jinno (Okinawa), A. Churg (Vancouver), B. Corrin (London), W. Jones Williams
(Cardiff), and A. Gibbs (Cardiff).

REFERENCES

1. Homma H, Yamanaka A, Tanimoto S, et al. (1983) Chest 83:63
2. Reid MA (1954) Lancet 1:275
3. Thurlbeck WM (1976) Chronic Airflow Obstruction in Lung Disease, WB
    Saunders, Philadelphia, pp 1-456
4. Harris CJ, Nadler HL (1983) IN: Lloyd-Still JD(ed) Textbook of Cystic
    Fibrosis, John Wright, Boston, pp 1-7.
5. Rollins S, Colby TV, Clayton F (1986) Arch Pathol Lab Med 110:34
6. Flint A, Colby TV (1987) Surgical Pathology of Diffuse Infiltrative Lung
    Disease, Grune & Stratton, Orlando, pp 1-234
7. Kitaichi M (1986) Clin Dermatol 4:108
8. Epler GR, Colby TV et al. (1985) New Eng J Med 312:152
9. Geddes DM, Corrin B et al. (1977) Quart J Med 46:427
10. Turton CW, Williams G, Green M (1981) Thorax 36:805
11. Niewoehner DE (1986) Sem Resp Med 8:140
12. Yousem SA, Colby TV, Carrington CB (1985) Hum Pathol 16:700
13. Maeda M, Saiki S, Yamanaka A (1987) Acta Pathol Jpn 37:693
14. Gudbjerg CE (1954) Acta Radiologica 43:209

RADIOLOGIC FINDINGS OF PATIENTS WITH DIFFUSE PANBRONCHIOLITIS (DPB)

KOICHI NISHIMURA and HARUMI ITOH[*]
Chest Disease Research Institute and Department of Radiology and Nuclear
Medecine[*],
Kyoto University, Sakyoku, Kyoto, 606, Japan

INTRODUCTION

As described by Kitaichi in the previous paper, the most characteristic
histologic feature of DPB is inflammatory foci localized in and around the wall
of the respiratory bronchioles(RBs) and their neighboring structures. These
foci are macroscopic nodular lesions and strictly located near the center of
the secondary pulmonary lobule (centriacinar, cetrilobular). This paper will
describe the macroscopic features of the secondary pulmonary lobule in both
healthy and DPB individuals. Radiologic features of 41 patients with DPB in

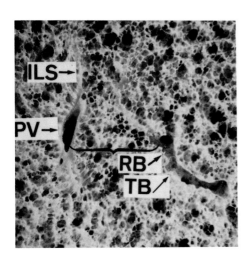
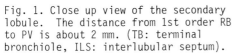
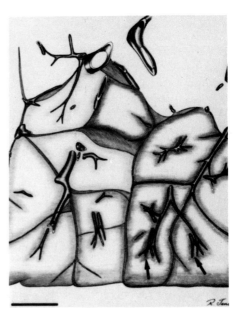

Fig. 1. Close up view of the secondary
lobule. The distance from 1st order RB
to PV is about 2 mm. (TB: terminal
bronchiole, ILS: interlubular septum).

Fig. 2. Schematic drawing of secondary
lobules derived from serial sections
of inflated lung specimens. The
arrows indicate centriacinar regions.
Bar is 5 mm.

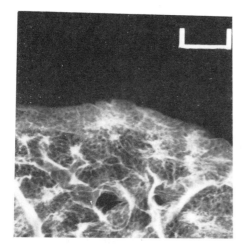

Fig. 3. Radiograph of lung slice specimen of patient with DPB, a 66-year-old
Japanese female with two years duration
of SOB and productive cough who underwent LL lobectomy due to adenocarcinoma.
The nodular shadows are seen at the end
of dilated bronchiolar branchings. Bar
is 5 mm.

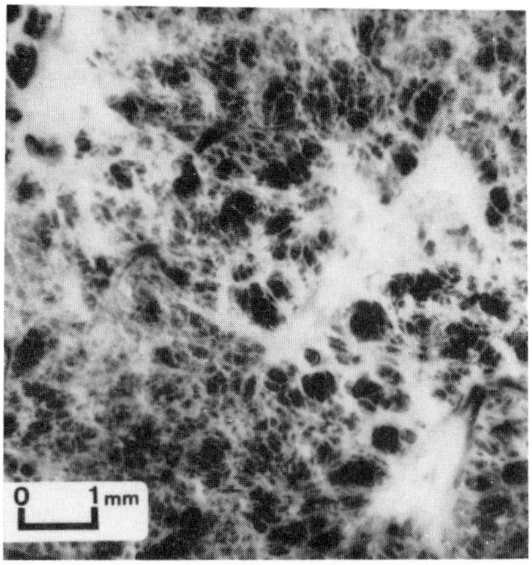

Fig. 4. Stereomicrophotograph of sliced
lung specimen of the same patient as
Fig. 3. Yellowish nodules are seen.
Her preoperative CT is shown in
Fig. 11.

our institute will then be related based on pathologic studies of 3 patients
with DPB.

SECONDARY PULMONARY LOBULE IN NORMAL AND DISEASED CONDITION
Normal structure of secondary lobule (Fig. 1 and 2.)

The secondary lobule is about 1cm wide including 3 to 5 pulmonary acini. The
bronchiole within the lobule divides into the same number of TB every 1 or
2 mm (mm pattern). Each lobule is bordered by ILS, pleura, PV, and extralobular
bronchi and PA. The distance from the first order RB to the border of the
lobule is constant (2-3 mm).

Centriacinar nodules in DPB (Fig. 3 and 4.)

We conducted a radiologic pathologic correlative study on 3 cases of DPB.
The nodular lesions of DPB are distributed at the extreme end of the bronchiolar
branchings. Since the lesions are small in diameter, they do not reach the

lobular margins. In other words, the air space near the lobular margin is spared from the disease assuring a small distance between the nodules and the pleura or PV. This distance is seen with high resolution CT as shown in this paper.

RADIOLOGIC FINDINGS OF DPB
Chest radiographic appearances (Fig. 5 and 6.)

The most characteristic feature is hyperinflation and diffuse nodular shadows with unclear borders, predominantly in lower lung fields. Hyperinflation is reflective of increased total lung capacity(TLC). For the examples, we measured TLC in 17 cases of DPB by use of body plethysmograph, so that TLC was 134.1 ± 28.2% pred.: 6.47 ± 1.17ℓ. Tram lines or peribronchial thickening are often seen, and thin tubular shadows are also detected and related to nodular shadows. The former findings are suggestive of proximal bronchial wall

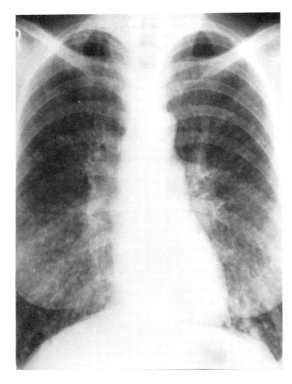
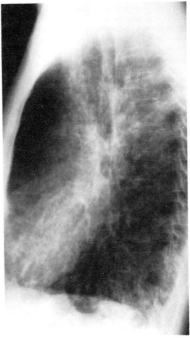

Fig. 5. Posteroanterior chest radio-graph of a 37-year-old Japanese female with SOB and productive cough of 10 years duration. Diffuse nodular shadows and hyperinflation are seen.

Fig. 6. Lateral radiograph of the same DPB patient as Fig. 5.

thickening and the latter findings are suggestive of peripheral airway wall thickening. In case of DPB patients who expectorate excess sputa, sputa itself may modify bronchial wall shadows. After chronic airway infection is intensely treated with antibiotics, diffuse nodular shadows seem to decrease in size and number but hyperinflation is not improved. The characterestic distribution of nodular lesions within secondary lobules can not be seen in chest radiographs but is detectable in X-ray CT.

Bronchographic findings (Fig. 7.)

 Patients with DPB may show mild to moderate cylindrical dilation of airways on their bronchographs, but its degree is usually not so severe as that of typical cases of bronchiectasis. In advanced cases, bronchioloectasis may be detected by their bronchographs (Fig. 7). But often the contrast media passes into the inner lung fields instead of subpleural regions because of the zonal difference in disease intensity.

X-ray CT findings (by use of high resolution CT) (Fig. 8. - 11.)

 X-ray CT was performed in 37 cases of DPB. The major CT findings (Fig. 9, 10, and 11, in comparison with healthy CT in Fig. 8) are as follows: 1) diffuse small nodular shadows located in the centrilobular regions, 2) dilation

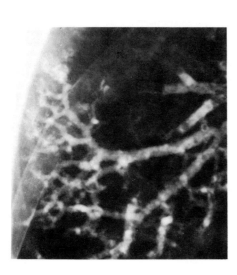

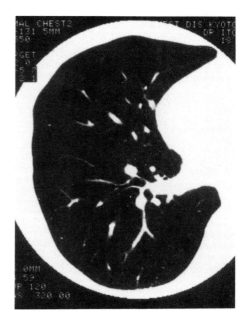

Fig. 7. Bronchographic finding of 65-year-old Japanese female with DPB. Note the peripheral airways are dilated.

Fig. 8. Normal CT, PA and PV shadows are clearly separated.

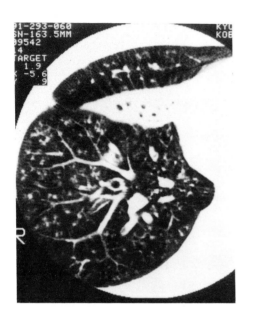 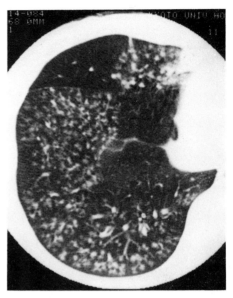

Fig. 9. CT of a 25-year-old Japanese male with DPB. The nodular shadows are separated from PV shadows and pleura on this CT image.

Fig. 10. CT of a 20-year-old Japanese male with productive cough of five years duration. He was diagnosed by open lung biopsy Disseminated nodular shadows are seen clearly on CT.

of small bronchi and bronchioles, 3) thickening of bronchial wall shadows, 4) stratified differences in lung density. Because small nodular shadows on CT of cases of DPB are always 1) separated from the pleura and PV shadows (the edge of secondary lobules) as a constant distance (2 to 3 mm), 2) continuous with PA shadows, and 3) located in the center of areas enclosed by PV shadows, they are distributed in centrilobular regions.

Positron emission tomography(PET) (Fig. 12.)

Ventilation imaging technique using PET and nitrogen 13 provides peripheral air trapping in DPB cases (Fig. 12.) Zonal, subpleural air trapping seems to be reflective of the difference in disease severity between inner and outer lung fields. Such a finding is compatible with stratified differences in lung density on CT and the tendency of contrast media to pass into inner lung fields on bronchographs.

752

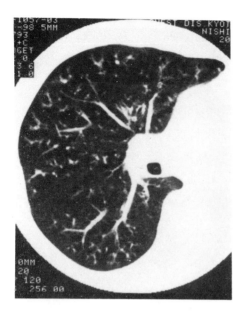

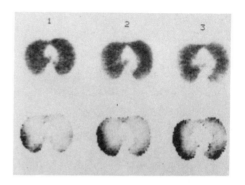

Fig. 11. CT of patient with DPB in
Fig. 3 and 4. Dilation of peripheral
airways as well as small nodular
shadows are seen.

Fig. 12. PET of patient of DPB.
Severe air trapping is visuable in
the outer layer of the lung. His
FEV_1 was 0.62ℓ and FEV_1/FVC was
53.0%.

SUMMARY

The most characteristic radiological findings of DPB are multiple nodular
shadows seen in chest radiograph. Our radiologic-pathologic correlation
showed these lesions to be centriacinar in location. This specific location
is well seen with high resolution X-ray CT. Positron emission tomography
using N-13 showed air trapping is more marked in the outer zone of the lung.

REFERENCES

1. Murata K, et al. Ventilation imaging with positron emission tomography
    and nitrogen 13. Radiology 158: 303-307, 1986.

2. Murata K, et al. Centrilobular lesions of the lung: Demonstration by high
    resolution CT and pathologic correlation. Radiology 161: 641-645, 1986.

3. Itoh H, et al. Recent progress of chest imaging. In: Hayaishi O and
    Torizuka K ed. Biomedical imaging. Academic Press Inc. New York. 1986,
    p. 249-271.

4. Nishimura K, et al. A comparative study of computed tomography and
    pulmonary pathology in diffuse panbronchiolitis. Japanese Journal of
    Chest Diseases 46: 481-486, 1987. (Japanese)

© 1988 Elsevier Science Publishers B.V. (Biomedical Division)
Sarcoidosis and other granulomatous disorders
C. Grassi, G. Rizzato, E. Pozzi, editors

A NATION-WIDE SURVEY OF DIFFUSE PANBRONCHIOLITIS IN JAPAN AND THE HIGH INCIDENCE
OF DIFFUSE PANBRONCHIOLITIS SEEN IN JAPANESE RESPIRATORY CLINICS

TAKATERU IZUMI
Chest Disease Research Institute, Kyoto University, Sakyo-ku, Kyoto 606 (Japan)

INTRODUCTION

A nation-wide survey of diffuse panbronchiolitis (DPB) was conducted in Japan
during a 3-year period from 1980 to 1982 under the sponsorship of the Ministry
of Health and Welfare. In this report, an outline of this survey is presented.
Also, the number of patients with airway obstructive diseases and the disease
type encountered at the Chest Disease Research Institute, Kyoto University,
are described, and the high incidence and consequent significance of DPB in
respiratory clinics in Japan is emphasized.

I. NATION-WIDE SURVEY OF DIFFUSE PANBRONCHIOLITIS IN JAPAN

For this survey, diagnostic criteria of DPB shown in Table 1 were employed.
The country was divided into 17 regions, and regional managers were appointed
to carry out the survey in their regions. In December, 1980, the secretariat
of the Survey sent a questionaire to 1,259 medical institutions with respiratory departments throughout the country asking them whether they have
encountered patients with DPB. In response to this questionaire, 1,237 cases
from 302 institutions were reported to the regional managers. 1) The individual
card, 2) chest X-rays, and 3) pathological slides, if a biopsy or autopsy was
performed, of each DPB case were requested from those institutions. Case

TABLE 1.
DIAGNOSTIC CRITERIA OF DPB USED IN THE NATION-WIDE SURVEY

Clinical DPB 1. Symptoms: chronic cough, sputum, and dyspnea on exertion
              2. Physical signs: rales and rhonchi
              3. Chest X-ray findings: diffusely disseminated fine nodular
                                        shadows with hyperinflation of the lungs
              4. Lung function studies: (at least three of the four
                                         abnormalities listed)
                  (a) FEV_1 under 70%
                  (b) VC under 80% of the predicted value
                  (c) RV over 150% of the predicted value or RV/TLC over 45%
Pathological DPB Histological diagnosis with respiratory bronchiolitis/
                  peribronchiolitis

conferences were held 5 times between July, 1981, and September, 1982, and each case reported was examined to determine whether or not it fulfilled the diagnostic criteria. Through this survey, 319 cases of clinical DPB and 82 cases of pathological DPB were confirmed. Pathological DPB was noted in 48 (15%) of the clinical DPB cases.

Clinical features of the patients obtained in the nation-wide survey of DPB are shown in Table 2.

TABLE 2.
CLINICAL FEATURES IN PATIENTS OBTAINED FROM NATION-WIDE SURVEY OF DPB IN JAPAN

	Clinical DPB	Pathological DPB
1. No. of patients (M, F)	319 (187, 132)	82 (54, 28)
2. Exposure history to noxious gases or dust	21.2% (307*)	20.7% (82)
3. Smoking history	31.3% (313)	35.4% (82)
4. Paranasal sinusitis		
Family history (+)	20.2% (247)	11.0% (82)
Past history	84.8% (301)	80.5% (82)
Operation history	54.8% (261)	43.9% (82)
5. Age of onset		
Cough and sputum	39.5** years (310) (Mode: 20-50)	40.3 years (76) (Mode: 20-50)
Dyspnea	46.8 years (296) (Mode: 30-60)	46.7 years (76) (Mode: 40-50)
6. Initial symptoms		
Cough and sputum	65.8%	69.5%
Dyspnea	1.7% } (295)	2.4% } (72)
Cough, sputum and dyspnea	32.5%	28.0%
7. Chest X-ray findings		
Diffuse nodular shadow	100%	81.3% (80)
Overinflation	100%	88.0% (80)
8. Pulmonary function tests		
%VC	61.0% (135)	65.8% (74)
FEV_1%	55.1% (137)	56.6% (74)
RV/TLC	50.0% (74)	46.5% (52)
DLCO (ml/min/torr)	22.5 (34)	17.6% (27)
PaO_2 (torr)	61.3 (143)	60.7 (60)
$PaCO_2$ (torr)	41.8 (142)	41.8 (60)

	Clinical DPB	Pathological DPB
9. Laboratory findings		
Tuberculin test (+)	34.9% (166)	44.4% (27)
ESR (mm/hr)	46 (279)	36 (57)
CRP (+)	80.0% (272)	65.0% (55)
RA (+)	41.0% (222)	43.0% (37)
Leucocyte count (/mm³)	9,600 (283)	8,700 (58)
Neutrophil	67.4% (257)	65.5% (54)
Lymphocyte	25.6% (268)	27.3% (54)
Eosinophil	1.9% (264)	2.4% (54)
Total protein (g/dl)	7.5 (218)	7.2 (54)
γ-globulin (%)	20.2% (240)	17.6% (49)
Cold hemmaglutinin (> x64)	89% (115)	95.7% (23)
Sputum (ml/day)	73 (230)	56 (50)
H. influenzae	74.4% (184)	77.1% (35)
Pneumococcus	28.7% (94)	61.5% (13)
K. pneumoniae	37.1% (97)	64.7% (17)
Pseudomonas	54.6% (141)	100.0% (12)
10. Prognosis Survival after the appearance of dyspnea		
5 years	80.0% } (306)	74.1% } (77)
10 years	53.9%	42.2%

* No. of examined

** Average

The major findings in the clinical DPB cases were the same as those of the pathological DPB cases, and the following features were especially noted.

1. Smoking history: The percentage of smokers was low, 31.3%, and even the smokers had low Brinkman index values.

2. Chronic paranasal sinusitus: 84.8% of the patients had chronic paranasal sinusitis, which was therefore an important characteristic of diffuse panbronchiolitis.

3. Onset: Cough and sputum were first often noted from the 2nd to 5th decade (average 39.5 years old) and dyspnea from the 3rd to 6th decade (average 46.8 years old). Dyspnea rarely (1.7%) developed prior to cough and sputum, but occurred 7-8 years (average) after the appearance of cough and sputum in 65.8% of the patients. All these symptoms occurred within 1 year in 32.5% of the patients.

4. Serum cold agglutinin titer and RA test: 88.7% of the patients exhibited x64 or higher cold agglutinin titers, but none showed elevation in the anti-mycoplasma antibody titers. These findings were not observed in patients with pulmonary emphysema and bronchial asthma. Joint symptoms were completely absent and RA was positive in 41% of the patients.

5. Sputum: The amount of sputum was about 50 ml/day in early stages, but increased to more than 100 ml/day with the advancement of the disease. Predominant bacteria changed from *Hemophilus influenzae* to *Pseudomonas aeruginosa*.

6. Prognosis: The disease becomes chronic and progresses as patients suffer repeated infections. The 5 year survival of patients from the onset of dyspnea on exertion was 80.0%, and the 10 year survival was 53.9%. Infection by *Pseudomonas* greatly affects prognosis.

Further investigation is in progress as to whether patients with clinical DPB without pathological materials had pathological DPB or not.

II. PATIENTS WITH AIRWAY OBSTRUCTIVE DISEASES AT THE CHEST DISEASE RESEARCH
     INSTITUTE, KYOTO UNIVERSITY

One hundred and five patients were diagnosed as having airway obstructive diseases except asthma from June, 1982 to July, 1987, at the Chest Disease Research Institute, Kyoto University, complaining of cough, sputum, and dyspnea and were found to have FEV_1/FVC of 70% or lower. Table 3 shows the diagnoses made in these 105 patients.

A diagnosis of pulmonary emphysema (PE) was made on the basis of $FEV_1/FVC < 50\%$ and/or alveolar destruction pictures by selective alveolo-bronchography. Patients with DPB were those in the clinically diagnosed group described above.

TABLE 3.
PATIENTS WITH AIRWAY OBSTRUCTIVE DISEASES (JUNE, 1982 - JULY, 1987)

Diseases	No. (M, F)	Age of onset	Smoking history (+)	Paranasal sinusitus (+)
Pulmonary emphysema	53 (50, 3)	53.2 ± 14.0*	100.0 %	25.5 %
Diffuse panbronchiolitis	47 (25, 22)	36.0 ± 16.2	28.9 %	95.4 %
Chronic bronchitis ?	5 (4, 1)	39.8 ± 13.8	60.0 %	60.0 %

* Mean ± SD

A diagnosis of chronic bronchitis was made in patients who were considered to have neither PE nor DPB, but this diagnosis is not certain.

We would like to emphasize that the number of patients with DPB is comparable to that of patients with PE. This observation was made also in other regions of Japan, and PE caused by smoking and DPB probably due to an inherent factor of increased susceptibility to infection are considered to be the main airway obstructive diseases besides asthma. In the light of these findings, the very strong interest in DPB among Japanese doctors appears to be reasonable.

SUMMARY

A nation-wide survey demonstrated that DPB is not a rare disease in Japan. Moreover, according to our experience in Kyoto, the incidence of DPB was comparable to that of pulmonary emphysema. DPB, therefore, is a disease of great significance in respiratory clinics in Japan.

The term diffuse panbroncholitis is used only in Japan, but whether there is DPB in other areas of the world is a very important problem.

DIFFUSE PAN BRONCHIOLITIS

MARGARET TURNER-WARWICK
The Cardiothoracic Institute, Brompton Hospital, Fulham Road, London SW3 6HP

INTRODUCTION

The symposium has, in a series of elegant presentations from Japan, reviewed the clinical, pathological and radiological characteristics of the respiratory disorder described as diffuse Pan bronchiolitis (DPB).

The contributors clearly recognised the difficulties of attempting to separate definitively DPB from many other variants of airflow limitation. However when all the features were put together, there is a convincing case that this condition can be distinguished from others. Now that the condition has been so clearly defined, further studies can be undertaken to identify its cause(s).

THE DISTINCTION FROM OTHER WELL RECOGNISED TYPES OF BRONCHIOLITIS

Not only does DPB differ from many other types of airway obstructive diseases as described in the preceding papers, but it is also very different from other groups of patients with proven predominant injury to the smaller airways. Some of the striking differences are summarised on table 1.

BRONCHIOLITIS

Selective clinical features contrasting Diffuse Panbronchiolitis (DPB) from other types

Cause/cofactors	X-ray shadows	Airway Obstruction	Sputum	Pathology/Course
INFANTS				
Viral	++	?	-	Acute often recovering
ADULTS				
Post viral	+ or -	++	-	Obliterative - stable
Chemicals e.g. NO_2	-	++	-	Obliterative - stable
Post - Transplant	-	++	-	Obliterative - stable
Rheumatoid Arthritis	-	++	-	Obliterative - stable
BOOP	++	-	-	Organizing pneumonia steroid responsive
DPB	+ Nodular	++	++ and crackles	Slowly progressive (Foamy macrophages)

The outstanding contrasting features of DPB are the widespread nodular shadows on the chest radiograph (and strikingly confirmed on the CT scans), the long history of sputum production becoming increasingly productive and infective over the years and the prominent coarse and fine crackles on auscultation. The remarkable pathological feature of foamy macrophages densely packed in the alveoli surrounding the respiratory bronchioles is characteristic.

An epidemiological clue of great potential importance is the extremely high prevalence of persisting sinusitis which occurred as we were told in over 85% of these largely non smoking patients.

THE URGENT QUESTIONS

Why is it that this disease reported now in some 319 Japanese patients has not apparently been observed in other countries? The syndrome is so well characterised that it seems improbable that lack of recognition alone counts for the exceptional focus of cases in Japan.

Does the peribronchiolar distribution of foamy macrophages provide a clue? Can electron microscopy of these cells give more information about the nature of the damaging agent?

Finally is it possible that these patients are receiving some special form of inhaled medication, perhaps used over prolonged periods, for their sinusitis? The foamy macrophages are not dissimilar to those seen in some patients habituated to oily nose drops. Their peribronchiolar distribution strongly suggests an inhalation bronchiolii injury. Is it possible that a Japanese remedy accounts for the limitation of DPB in that country? This is but speculation. However it has the advantage of being testable and could lead to eradication of this disabling and progressive disease.

© 1988 Elsevier Science Publishers B.V. (Biomedical Division)
Sarcoidosis and other granulomatous disorders
C. Grassi, G. Rizzato, E. Pozzi, editors

DIFFUSE PANBRONCHIOLITIS – HOW TO PLACE IT INTO THE FRAMEWORK OF CHRONIC BRONCHIOLITIS IN ADULTS?

By J. MEIER - SYDOW

Division of Pneumology, Dept. of Internal Medicine
J.W. Goethe-University Frankfurt/Main
Theodor Stern-Kai 7, D-6000 Frankfurt/Main/FRG

The Round Table Conference on Diffuse Panbronchiolitis can be summarized in three steps:

1) To grasp the striking elements of the condition presented in the proceeding contributions
2) To assess whether the condition in question is a well defined nosological entity
3) To place this condition into the framework of chronic bronchiolitis in adults

Ad 1): The striking elements of Diffuse Panbronchiolitis

1) Diffuse multifocal inflammmatory lesions in both lungs, often associated with atelectasis (middle lobe respectively lingula)
2) Histological pathology: "Unit lesion" (M. Kitaichi, this conference), consisting of:
   a) Foamy histiocytosis (and lymphocytes) in the walls of the respiratory bronchioles and the alveolar ducts
   b) No obliterative polypoid narrowing of the airways
3) Considerable, often excessive sputum production
4) Concomitant sinusitis
5) Severe airflow obstruction with corresponding hyperinflation of the lung
6) Several serological phenomena like elevated cold agglutinine titer and positive rheumatoid factor
7) Relatively poor prognosis
8) Cases described only in Japan
9) No obvious relation to smoking habits.

762

Ad 2) <u>Is Diffuse Panbronchiolitis a nosological entity?</u>
On the base of the details presented by the proceeding
speakers I think we are justified to call Diffuse Panbronchiolitis a nosological entity. The morphologist
(M. Kitaichi, this confe-rence) has stressed the differential diagnosis to bronchial asthma, pulmonary emphysema,
chronic bronchitis, and bronchiectasis. One must of course
be aware of the fact that in this assessment the etiology
and the pathogenesis nor the treatment have been taken in
consideration.

Ad 3: <u>How can we place Diffuse Panbronchiolitis into the</u>
<u>framework of chronic bronchiolitis in adults?</u>
At first two remarks:
a) The condition seems to be unspecific or even cryptogenic as the patient´s history and morphology do not
   give us any idea of the etiology. Chronic bronchiolitis of extrinsic origin, e.g. sequel of gas
   poisening has to be excluded in our considerations.
b) Local factors - the condition has been described only
   in Japan - have not been elucidated.

Despite our limited knowledge we tried to separate seven
entities of chronic unspecific bronchiolitis in adults (4),
Diffuse Panbronchiolitis being included (table 1).

Further investigations are necessary in order to bring
more insight into the interesting field of chronic bronchiolitis in general and Diffuse Panbronchiolitis in particular
with its relation to alveolitis, bronchitis and emphysema
(4).

1. Small airways disease: Hogg et al. 1968 (2)
   Chronic obstructive bronchiolitis:
      Fletcher and Pride 1984 (1)
2. Diffuse Panbronchiolitis: Homma et al. 1983
3. Cryptogenic obliterative bronchiolitis:
      Turton et al. 1981
4. Progressive airway obliteration ...
      (rheumatoid disease): Geddes et al. 1977
5. Bronchiolitische pulmonale Fibrose:
      Kartagener et al. 1964
   Interstitial pneumonia with obliterative bronchio-
      litis (BIP): Liebow 1968
6. Interstitial lung disease, rapidly progressive
      to bronchiolitis/bronchitis with emphysema:
      Colp et al. 1967
      Meier-Sydow, et al. 1977
      Sopko et al. 1979
      McCarthy et al. 1980
7. Secondary bronchiolar/bronchial damage in diffuse
      fibrotic conditions: McClement et al. 1953 (3)

Table 1 - Chronic bronchiolitis in adults

References

1) Fletcher, C.M., N.B. Pride: Definitions of emphysema,
      chronic bronchitis, asthma, and airflow obstruction:
      25 years on from the Ciba symposium.
      Thorax 1984, 39, 81-85
2) Hogg, J.C., P.T. Macklem, W.M.Thurlbeck: Site and
      nature of airway obstruction in chronic obstructive
      lung disease. New Engl.J.Med. 1968, 278, 1355-1366
3) McClement, J.H., A.D. Renzetti, A.Himmelstein,
      A.Cournand: Cardiopulmonary function in the
      pulmonary form of Boeck´s sarcoid and its modification
      by cortisone therapy. Am.Rev.Tuberc. 1953, 67,
      154-172
4) Meier-Sydow,J., M.Schneider, M.Rust: Chronic bronchio-
      litis in adults. Eur.J.Respir.Dis. 1986, 69
      (Suppl. 146), 337-344 (with further references)

INDEX OF AUTHORS

Agostini, C., 109, 187, 255, 263, 705
Ainslie, G.M., 105
Albera, C., 259, 441
Alberts, C., 321, 373, 545
Alexandre, C., 499
Alguetti, A., 185
Ando, M., 509, 681
Andrews Jr, J.L., 291
Angi, M.R., 493
Angomachalelis, N., 503
Aoki, K., 307
Aprile, C., 563
Arakawa, K., 147
Araki, S., 509, 681
Ardizzi, A., 695
Armstrong, E.M., 313
Asai, M., 147
Auzeby, A., 575
Ávila, R., 657
Avolio, G., 709
Ayalon, D., 185
Azzolini, L., 641

Bacchella, L., 563
Badrinas, F., 317, 545
Balbi, B., 441
Bambery, P., 311
Barberis, S., 695, 709
Bardessono, F., 259
Barritault, L., 367
Bart, F., 455, 707
Barth, J., 155, 183, 371
Bartone, B., 259
Basset, F., 235
Baughman, R.P., 593
Baur, R., 429
Begiomini, E., 375
Behera, D., 311
Bellia, V., 191
Benveniste, J., 685
Beretta, L., 505
Berger, M.B., 407
Berton, G., 263
Bertorelli, G., 557
Bianco, S., 135, 369, 567
Biot, N., 595
Bizzotto, R., 705
Blaschke, E., 271
Blasi, A., 273

Bonanno, A., 191
Bonniere, P., 35
Bonsignore, G., 191
Bourguet, P., 227
Bouros, D., 453
Braghiroli, A., 713
Breebaart, A.C., 321
Brousseau, K.P., 407
Brown, L.K., 7, 351

Cacciabue, M., 709
Calle, A., 247
Campbell, T.C., 291
Capelli, A., 713
Capelli, O., 641
Capelli, P., 255, 493
Capuana, G., 571
Cardoso, L.E., 247
Care, S.B., 123
Carriero, G., 567
Casorati, G., 187
Cassatella, M.A., 263
Castrignano, L., 383, 645
Castriotta, R., 517
Chang, J., 717
Chappard, D., 499
Charrin, C., 457
Chase, C.C., 591
Check, I., 581
Chida, K., 703
Chilaris, N., 369
Chilosi, M., 255
Chretien, J., 367, 449, 525
Chretien, M.F., 433
Christ, R., 325
Cintorino, M., 135
Cipriani, A., 109, 255, 263, 451, 493, 545
Collodoro, A., 135, 369, 567
Conrad, A.K., 213
Cooper Jr, J.A.D., 123
Coral, A.P., 587
Cordier, J.-F., 247
Cortot, A., 35
Costabel, U., 429
Coviello, G., 567
Cozon, G., 457

Davies, B.H., 675
Degreef, J.M., 707

De Groot, J., 101
De Haan, M., 101
Delaval, P., 227, 545
Delerive, C., 455
Deodhar, S.D., 311
DeRemee, R.A., 51, 201
De Rose, V., 563
Desrues, B., 227
Di Vittorio, G., 451
Djuric, B., 323, 325
Donner, C.F., 713
Dragonetti, C., 641
Dubois, M., 157
Dubois, R.M., 105
Dugas, M., 35
Durante, F., 645
Dutta, S.K., 651
Dutton, R.E., 697

Edel, J., 411
Edwards, J.H., 675
Efraim, S.B., 185
Eishi, Y., 143
Eklund, A., 271
Ellison Jr, P.S., 513
Elo, J.J., 515
Emonot, A., 499
Entzian, P., 183, 371
Epstein, W.L., 691

Fantini, F., 485
Faraggiana, T., 717
Fasolini, G., 383
Fayolle, M.P., 595
Ferrara, A., 369
Festi, G., 451, 705
Feustel, P.J., 697
Fireman, E., 185
Fité, E., 317
Fitzgerald, M.X., 89, 315, 585
Fleming, H.A., 19
Foley, N.M., 587
Fonlupt, P., 157
Fontana, A., 641
Forattini, F., 493
Formichi, B., 375
Fornai, E., 375
Fortin, F., 707
Foster, C.S., 177
Freitas e Costa, M., 329, 685, 711
Frija, J., 449
Froldi, M., 557
Fröseth, B., 297
Fujioka, A., 691
Fukuda, K., 355
Fukuyama, K., 691
Fyhrquist, F., 203

Galietti, F., 695, 709
Garbisa, S., 109

Garovoy, M.R., 291
Gasparini, S., 441
Gattinara, M., 485
Gemma, H., 703
Gerloni, V., 485
Germain, D., 457
Ghio, P., 259, 441
Giagnoni, E., 505
Giamesio, P.C., 695
Giobbi, A., 649
Giorgis, G.E., 695, 709
Giuntini, C., 375
Glasius, E., 321
Gormand, F., 157, 457
Gosselin, B., 707
Gottlieb, J.E., 599, 605
Gougoulakis, S., 319
Gourgoulianis, K., 319
Gozzelino, F., 259
Graham, D.Y., 161
Granata, M., 545
Gray, J.W., 601
Grayston, J.T., 297
Greif, J., 185
Grimaud, J.-A., 247
Grönhagen-Riska, C., 203, 297
Guaglianone, M.O., 641
Gupta, A., 311
Gupta, S.K., 377, 397, 643, 651

Hackney Jr, R.L., 313
Hällgren, R., 271
Hance, A.J., 235
Hanngren, Å., 271
Harf, R., 595
Hatakeyama, S., 143
Hayashi, S., 165
Heidorn, K., 155
Henzel, D., 367
Hernbrand, R., 271
Herzog, H., 385
Hiraga, Y., 307, 489, 579
Hirsch, A., 449
Holland, V.A., 407
Holt, P.J.A., 689
Holter, J.F., 139
Hoppe-Seyler, S., 371
Horton Jr, E.S., 445
Hosoda, Y., 279, 307, 309, 579
Hourzamanis, A., 503
Huchon, G., 367

Ikeda, T., 447
Ina, Y., 147
Israel, H., 151, 599, 601, 605
Itoh, H., 747
Iwai, K., 309
Iwata, M., 703
Izumi, T., 129, 193, 307, 423, 545, 579, 753

Jagirdar, J., 717
James, D.G., 1, 587
Jansen, H.M., 373
Jindal, S.K., 311
Joensuu, H., 515
Johns, C.J., 417
Johnson, J.L. 97
Johnson, N.McI., 587
Jones, E.D., 675
Jones, K.P., 675
Jones Williams, W., 661, 689
Jordanoglou, J., 453
Joubert, J.R., 591

Kalter, D.C., 161
Kamikawaji, N., 165
Karma, A., 511
Kataria, Y.P., 139
Kaur, U., 311
Kelland, D., 689
Khomenko, A.G. 325
Kidd, M., 581
Kijlstra, A., 321
Kitaichi, M., 423, 741
Klatt, E., 421
Klech, H., 115, 461
Kleinhenz, M.E., 97, 169
Klemi, P.J., 515
Knapp, W., 115
Kobayashi, F., 489
Koga, T., 589
Kohrogi, H., 509
Koivisto, V., 203
Kotoh, H., 447
Kraft, D., 115
Kreipe, H., 155, 183
Kunkel, S.L., 267
Kurman, C.E., 407

Lacronique, J., 575
Lafitte, J.J., 707
Langer, B.G., 541
Laval-Jeantet, M., 449
Lawrence, E.C., 407
Leggieri, E., 557
Lestani, M., 255
L'Huillier, J.P., 227
Licata, G., 571
Lieberman, J., 221
Loglisci, T., 645
Lopez-Majano, V., 519, 521, 541,
  603, 697
Lower, E.E., 593
Luca, M., 109, 705
Luger, Th., 115
Luisetti, M., 563
Lusuardi, M., 713

Maffre, J.Ph., 433
Malik, S.K., 311

Mallette, L.E., 407
Mañá, J., 317
Marcuse, H.R., 373
Markesich, D.C., 161
Marsac, J., 575
Martignoni, G., 649
Martinot, J.B., 35
Masciarelli, M., 109, 187
Massaglia, G.M., 695, 709
Massart, V., 455
Matsuba, K., 165, 589
Matsui, Y., 143, 309
Matthys, H., 429
Mayer, M., 325
Meier-Sydow, J., 761
Melissinos, C., 453
Mella, C., 631
Mendes, A.C., 711
Merendino, A., 191
Merrill, W.W., 123
Merritt, J.C., 513
Miadonna, A., 557
Michalopoulos, A., 653
Mikami, R., 489
Miller, A., 351
Mirabella, A., 191
Miradoli, E., 649
Miravalle, C., 695, 709
Mishra, B.B., 151
Mitra, K., 651
Mochizuki, I., 489
Montagna, L., 255
Monteiro, J.T., 711
Montemurro, L., 631, 645
Mordelet-Dambrine, M., 367
Morel, P., 449
Morera, J., 317
Morishita, M., 147
Mounier, D., 499
Mullink, H., 101
Murelli, M., 485
Muthuswamy, P., 519, 521, 603

Naegel, G.P., 123
Nagai, S., 129, 423
Nakashima, H., 509, 681
Negro, A., 109, 485
Nelson, D.L., 407
Neuchrist, C., 115
Newman, L., 715
Nishimura, K., 747
Nishimura, M., 589
Noda, M., 147, 579
Nozza, M., 383

O'Connor, C., 89, 585
Odaka, M., 307
Odlum, C., 89, 585
Ogata, K., 165
Oksanen, V., 381

Olivieri, D., 557
Oshima, S., 129, 423
Oury, M., 433

Pacheco, H., 157
Pacheco, Y., 157, 457
Panayeas, S., 653
Papadopoulos, S., 653
Papapaschali, A., 653
Park, H.K., 139
Paronetto, F., 717
Parrinello, G., 571
Parwaresch, M.R., 155, 183
Patrick, H., 151, 599, 601, 605
Pencole, C., 227
Peona, V., 563
Perari, M.G., 135, 567
Perez, R., 581
Perrella, A., 369
Perrin-Fayolle, M., 157, 457, 545
Pescetti, G., 259
Pescetti, L., 259
Pesci, A., 557
Petermann, W., 155, 183, 371
Peyrol, S., 247
Phan, S.H., 267
Phillips, S.M., 151
Pieroni, M.G., 369
Pietra, R., 411
Pilipski, M., 351
Pincelli, C., 691
Pizzolo, G., 255
Pohl, W., 115
Polk Jr, O.D., 313
Poulter, L.W., 105, 173
Povazan, D.J., 323
Pozzi, E., 563
Prandi, E., 641
Prediletto, R., 375

Radzun, H.J., 155, 183
Ranginwala, M., 603
Refini, M., 369
Reis-Ferreira, J.M., 685
Renzi, G., 361, 519, 697
Renzi, P.M., 361, 697
Reynolds, H.Y., 123, 719
Reynolds, S.P., 675
Rhee, R., 541
Riccobono, L., 191
Riska, H., 203, 297
Rizzato, G., 325, 411, 545, 631, 739
Rocklin, R.E., 291
Rockoff, S.D., 437
Rohatgi, P., 545
Rohrbach, M.S., 213
Rohtagi, P., 437
Rømer, F.K., 327
Roos, C.M., 373

Rossi, G.A., 441
Rossouw, D.J., 591
Rothova, A., 321
Rottoli, L., 135, 369, 567
Rottoli, P., 135, 369, 567
Roy, M., 651
Rudolph, P., 155
Rühle, K.H., 429
Ruiz-Manzano, J., 317
Ryujin, Y., 489

Sabbioni, E., 411
Sachero, A., 505
Sado, S., 147
Saikku, P., 297
Sakata, T., 681
Sanguinetti, C.M., 441
Sansi, P., 521
Santolicandro, A., 375
Sastre, A., 221
Sato, A., 579, 703
Scaglione, R., 571
Scagliotti, G., 259
Scharkoff, T., 303
Scheiner, O., 115
Schenk, E., 115
Schieppati, A., 383
Schonfeld, S.A., 417
Schweiger, O., 325
Sciascia, T., 485
Scott, P.P., 417
Scotti, F., 319
Secen, N., 325
Sehgal, S., 311
Sekely, S., 697
Sekiguchi, M., 489
Selroos, O., 637
Semenzato, G., 73, 109, 255, 263, 493
Shapiro, H., 517
Sharkoff, T., 545
Sharma, O.P., 341, 421
Sharma, S.K., 377
Shepley, K.J., 601
Sherlock, S., 59
Shichi, I., 703
Shigematsu, N., 165, 447, 589
Shima, K., 355, 579
Shimada, Y., 489
Siafakas, N., 653
Sibille, Y., 35, 123
Sider, L., 445
Sisti, S., 631
Siviero, F., 187
Soda, K., 681
Soler, P., 235, 575
Sorg, C., 115
Spada, E.L., 713
Spatafora, M., 191
Specks, U., 213

Spencer, R., 517
Spigos, D.G., 541
Spiteri, M., 173
Stam, J., 101
Stanislas-Leguern, G., 367, 449
Staton, G., 581
Stefis, A., 319
Steiner, R.M., 599, 605
Strohofer, S., 593
Sturman, A., 369
Suga, M., 681
Sugimoto, M., 509, 681
Sulavik, S.B., 517
Suya, H., 691

Tachibana, T., 307, 309, 579
Takada, K., 147
Takemura, T., 143
Takenaka, S., 355
Takeuchi, M., 129
Takiya, C., 247
Tamura, S., 489
Tedeschi, A., 557
Teirstein, A.S., 7, 351
Teles-de-Araújo, A., 685, 711
Teramoto, K., 355
The EMMEANS Cooperative Study
 Group, 595
Tommasini, A., 187, 451
Topilsky, M., 185
Tosi, G., 631
Touitou, Y., 575
Trainor, W.D., 603
Traore, B.M., 575
Trentin, L., 187, 255, 263, 705
Tsakraklides, V., 319
Tsiroyiannis, C., 653
Tuchais, E., 433
Tung, K., 587
Turner-Warwick, M., 621, 759

Valverde, J., 317

Van Breda, A., 89, 585
Van Maarsseveen, T., 101
Vassallo, F., 441
Velluti, G., 641
Vergnon, J.M., 499
Veslemes, M., 453
Viberti, L., 259
Vidal, R., 317
Viegi, G., 375
Vindigni, C., 135
Voisin, C., 35
Von Willebrand, E., 203
Vuk-Pavlovic, Z., 213

Wagner, D.J., 429
Wallace Jr, R.J., 407
Wallaert, B., 35
Ward, K., 89, 315, 585
Watanabe, K., 129, 447
Weed, D., 517
Williams, W.R., 689

Yagawa, K., 165
Yamaguchi, M., 307
Yamamoto, M., 147, 579
Yoshida, K., 681
Yoshimura, H.H., 161
Young Jr, R.C., 313

Zaccaria, S., 713
Zafran, N., 323
Zahariadis, M., 453
Zaiss, A., 429
Zakria, F., 221
Zambello, R., 109, 187, 255, 263,
 705
Zanni, D., 631
Zanussi, C., 557
Zarifis, D., 453
Zwijnenburg, Z., 373

SUBJECT INDEX

ACE 89,201,203,227,467,513,527, 595,599,601,603,605
ACE in CSF 381
ACE in tears 513
ACE inducing factor 213
ACE inhibitors 221,653
acellular sarcoid granuloma 24
activity 525
aerosols 643
AIDS 64,726
airway obstruction 341,351,371,3
aluminium 665
alveolitis 35,101,129,238 545,587, 711
anabolic steroids and TB 697
angiotensin I 129
angiotensin II 129
anti OK T3-Ab 129
antigen presenting capacity 147
arthritis 485
autopsy 285,309,421

BAL 36,73,89,101,105,109,115, 123,129,135,173,271,369,371, 423,429,473,509,533,545,557, 567,579,581,585,587,595,675, 685,703,713
BAL in elderly 441
beryllium disease 664,689,715
biochemical markers 516
biopsy 515,591
blood pressure 653
bone mineral content 631
bone quantitative histomorphometry 499
bronchial hyperreactivity 351,355, 369,389
bronchoscopic abnormalities 453

budesonide 637
bullae 352

calcitonin 631
cancer and sarcoidosis 327
captopril 221,653
cardiac failure 27
cardiac sarcoidosis 313,503
cell wall defective acid fast bacteria 161
cerebrospinal fluid 381
chemiluminescence 36,156
chemotaxins 123
chest X ray,atypical 437
Chlamidia 297
chromosomal analysis 457
chronic active hepatitis 59
chronic respiratory failure 313
chronic tonsillitis 165
circulating immune complexes
clearance of 99Tc-DTPA 367,389
climate 287
clinical activity 105
clinical aspects 5,397
clinical presentation 398
collagen alterations 531
computed tomography 445,449
cor pulmonale 421
criteria of activity 4
Crohn 695
cutaneous granulomata 139
cyclophosphamide 55
cyclosporin 67,691

death 19,313,421
deflazacort 641,657
diagnosis 280,451
diffusing capacity 347,385

echocardiography 503
elderly 441
embolotherapy 419
enalapril 221
environmental factors 286
epidemiology 3,279,303,329
erythema nodosum 585
experimental granulomas 691,717
extrapulmonary sarcoidosis 466
extrathoracic granulomatous
   disorders 35
extrinsic allergic alveolitis 719

familial sarcoidosis 291,398
fibroblasts 89,271
fibronectin 89,259,271,589
fibrosis 273
fibrotic changes 242
follow up 323,545,567
functional impairment 5,341,385

Gallium 470,517,519,521,532,545,
   571,579, 581,609
giant cells 155
glucocorticosteroids and ACE 207
   – and breathing pattern 361
granuloma formation 76,143, 235
granuloma index 154
granuloma load 603
granulomas 151,661,691
granulomatosis, mineral induced
   711

hard metal workers disease 411,
   709
heart block 11
heart disease 19,421
hemoptysis 417
hepatocellular disease 59
histiocytosis X 666
histoplasmosis 662
HLA typing 291
hospitalizations 645
hyaluronan 271
hydrogen peroxide 593

hydroxiproline 251
hypercalcaemia 499
hypercalciuria 499
hypersensitivity pneumonitis 703,
   705

idiopathic pulmonary fibrosis 455
Ig levels in the epithelial lining
   fluid 191
IL-1 89,98,123,155,
   255
IL-1 B 89
IL-2 73,97,407
immune complexes 165
immunohistochemical analysis of
   granulomas 255
immunology 1,73
in vitro granulomas 151
incidence rate 280
incidence in GDR 303
India 311
indomethacin 267
infections 662
injection with autologus BAL cell
   preparations 139
Italy, the role of a sarcoidosis
   clinic 645

Japan prevalence 307

Kveim-like activity 139
Kveim-Siltzbach test 2,7

laminin 589
leukotriene B4 123
lipids in BAL 685
liver failure 59
liver involvement 59
liver-lung interface 59
Lofgren syndrome neutrophil
   alveolitis 433
Lofgren syndrome spring cluster
   317
lung epithelial permeability
   471

lung function tests 464,609
lymph-nodes 143
lymph-nodes TB 319
lymphocytes kariotypes 457
lymphocytes subpopulations 36,105
   173,429
lysozime 468,528,595

macrophages 101,105,109,115,123,
   147,173,183,263,593

macrophage chemiluminescence 36
macrophage-lymphocyte aggregates
   101
magnetic resonance 541
markers of activity 227,591
mast cells 135,557
metalloendopeptidase 529
metals 411
microangiopathy 489
monoclonal antibodies 105,109,
   169,183,187
monocytes 109,147,203,589
mononuclear cells 97,129
morbidity 280
mortality 283
mouse model of beryllium disease
   715
Muramyl dipeptide 143,267
mycetomas 417
Mycobacterium tuberculosis 143,162

needle aspiration biopsy 515
neopterin 530,575
neurosarcoidosis 381
neutron activation analysis 411
neutrophil alveolitis in Lofgren 433
neutrophil mobility 123

ocular manifestations 177,321,
   493,509,511,513
oesophageal sclerotherapy 65
open lung biopsy 591
origin of ACE 201

osteoporosis 631
other granulomatous disorders 6

panbronchiolitis 741,747,753,
   759,761
Panda sign 517
pathogenesis of granuloma
   formation 143,193
pathology 1,26,273
PGE$_2$ production 185
phosphatidylethanolamina
   methyltranferase activity 157
phosphocalcium metabolism 499
pigeon breaders 675
prednisolone 101
prednisolone induced osteoporosis
   631
prednisone therapy 191,641,657
prevalence 397
   - in Japan 307
primary biliary cirrhosis 59
procoagulant activity of BAL
   cells 581
procollagen peptide 89
prognosis 579,595,603
pulmonary fibrosis 463
pulmonary function tests 37

race 397,607
radiological staging 377
regulation of ACE synthesis 201
relapse 611
respiratory muscles dysfunction
   347,392
retroperitoneal involvment 383
risk factors 285,421

sarcoid activity 605
sarcoid-like granulomas 235
sarcoid matricial complex 247
sarcoidosis clinic 645
seasonal variations 287
sex 398

silica dust 713
skin biopsy 139,161
skin lesions 161
skin testing 169
smoking 315,423
small airway obstruction 352
socio economic factors 286
Spain 317
staging 377
stenosis of large bronchi 353, 707
steroid aerosols 643
subclinical alveolitis 35
sudden death 19
sulfathiazole 649
summer type hypersensitivity pneumonitis 681
superoxide anion 263
suppressor cell activity 185
synovial sarcoidosis 485
T cell activation 73
T cells 157,715
T cells subsets 89,165,169,557,567
T8+ lymphocyites 101
T4+ lymphocytes 101

T4/T8 ratio 429
T helper/suppressor ratio 101

tonsillitis 447
transbronchial lung biopsy 451
treatment 5,101,621,637,651,657
treatment decisions 605
trimethoprim-sulfamethoxazole 56
tuberculosis 319,695,697
TWAR antibodies 297
type III procollagen peptide 89, 563
type IV collagenase 109

upper airways obstruction 353
uronic acid 251
uveitis 177,321,493,509,511

vascular involvment 240,664
vectorcardiography 505
ventilation perfusion relationship 373,375,390

Wegener 51,707
worldwide study 325